Practical Guides in Radiation Oncology

Series Editors
Nancy Y. Lee
Department of Radiation Oncology
Memorial Sloan-Kettering Car
New York, NY, USA

Jiade J. Lu
Department of Radiation Oncolc
Shanghai Proton and Heavy Ion
Shanghai, China

The series Practical Guides in Radiation Oncology is designed to assist radiation oncology residents and practicing radiation oncologists in the application of current techniques in radiation oncology and day-to-day management in clinical practice, i.e., treatment planning. Individual volumes offer clear guidance on contouring in different cancers and present treatment recommendations, including with regard to advanced options such as intensity-modulated radiation therapy (IMRT) and stereotactic body radiation therapy (SBRT) and proton beam therapy (PBT). Each volume addresses one particular area of practice and is edited by experts with an outstanding international reputation. Readers will find the series to be an ideal source of up-to-date information on when to apply the various available technologies and how to perform safe treatment planning.

More information about this series at http://www.springer.com/series/13580

Nancy Y. Lee • Jonathan E. Leeman
Oren Cahlon • Kevin Sine • Guoliang Jiang
Jiade J. Lu • Stefan Both
Editors

Target Volume Delineation and Treatment Planning for Particle Therapy

A Practical Guide

Springer

Editors
Nancy Y. Lee
Department of Radiation Oncology
Memorial Sloan-Kettering Cancer Center
New York, NY
USA

Oren Cahlon
Department of Radiation Oncology
Memorial Sloan Kettering Cancer Center
New York
USA

Guoliang Jiang
Department of Radiation Oncology
Shanghai Proton and Heavy Ion Center
Shanghai
China

Stefan Both
Department of Radiation Oncology
University Medical Center Groningen
Groningen
The Netherlands

Jonathan E. Leeman
Department of Radiation Oncology
Memorial Sloan Kettering Cancer Center
New York
USA

Kevin Sine
Department of Medical Dosimetry
ProCure Proton Therapy Center
Somerset
New Jersey
USA

Jiade J. Lu
Department of Radiation Oncology
Shanghai Proton and Heavy Ion Center
Shanghai
China

ISSN 2522-5715   ISSN 2522-5723   (electronic)
Practical Guides in Radiation Oncology
ISBN 978-3-319-42477-4   ISBN 978-3-319-42478-1   (eBook)
https://doi.org/10.1007/978-3-319-42478-1

Library of Congress Control Number: 2017962011

© Springer International Publishing Switzerland 2018
This work is subject to copyright. All rights are reserved by the Publisher, whether the whole or part of the material is concerned, specifically the rights of translation, reprinting, reuse of illustrations, recitation, broadcasting, reproduction on microfilms or in any other physical way, and transmission or information storage and retrieval, electronic adaptation, computer software, or by similar or dissimilar methodology now known or hereafter developed.
The use of general descriptive names, registered names, trademarks, service marks, etc. in this publication does not imply, even in the absence of a specific statement, that such names are exempt from the relevant protective laws and regulations and therefore free for general use.
The publisher, the authors and the editors are safe to assume that the advice and information in this book are believed to be true and accurate at the date of publication. Neither the publisher nor the authors or the editors give a warranty, express or implied, with respect to the material contained herein or for any errors or omissions that may have been made. The publisher remains neutral with regard to jurisdictional claims in published maps and institutional affiliations.

Printed on acid-free paper

This Springer imprint is published by Springer Nature
The registered company is Springer International Publishing AG
The registered company address is: Gewerbestrasse 11, 6330 Cham, Switzerland

Acknowledgments

This publication is partially supported by the following grants: (a) Shanghai Hospital Development Center (Joint Breakthrough Project for New Frontier Technologies, Project No. SHDC 12015118); (b) Science and Technology Commission of Shanghai Municipality (Project No. 15411950106).

Contents

1 **Physics Essentials of Particle Therapy** 1
 Dennis Mah, Michael Moyers, Ken Kang-Hsin Wang,
 Eric Diffenderfer, John Cuaron, and Mark Pankuch

2 **Proton Treatment Delivery Techniques** 17
 Xuanfeng Ding, Haibo Lin, Jiajian Shen, Wei Zou,
 Katja Langen, and Hsiao-Ming Lu

3 **Proton Treatment Planning** 45
 Chuan Zeng, Richard A. Amos, Brian Winey, Chris Beltran,
 Ziad Saleh, Zelig Tochner, Hanne Kooy, and Stefan Both

4 **Tumors of the Nasopharynx** 107
 Jeremy Setton, Pamela Fox, Kevin Sine, Nadeem Riaz,
 and Nancy Y. Lee

5 **Oral Cavity Tumors** 117
 Jennifer Ma, Benjamin H. Lok, Kevin Sine, and Nancy Y. Lee

6 **Oropharyngeal Cancer** 131
 Suchit H. Patel, Amy J. Xu, Kevin Sine, Nancy Y. Lee, and
 Pamela Fox

7 **Sinonasal Cancers** 141
 Roi Dagan and Curtis Bryant

8 **Salivary Gland Tumors** 153
 Jonathan E. Leeman, Paul Romesser, James Melotek,
 Oren Cahlon, Kevin Sine, Stefan Both, and Nancy Y. Lee

9 **Thyroid Cancer** 165
 Mauricio Gamez, Aman Anand, and Samir H. Patel

10 **Non-melanoma Skin Cancer
 with Clinical Perineural Invasion** 175
 Curtis Bryant and Roi Dagan

11 **Head and Neck Reirradiation** 187
 Carl DeSelm, Upendra Parvathaneni, and Kevin Sine

12	**Lung Cancer**	197
	Daniel Gomez, Heng Li, Xiaodong Zhang, and Steven Lin	
13	**Esophagus Cancer**	211
	Steven H. Lin, Heng Li, and Daniel Gomez	
14	**Carbon Ion Radiation Therapy for Liver Tumors**	221
	Zheng Wang, Wei-Wei Wang, Kambiz Shahnazi, and Guo-Liang Jiang	
15	**Pancreatic and Stomach Malignancies**	235
	Pamela J. Boimel, Jessica Scholey, Liyong Lin, and Edgar Ben-Josef	
16	**Lower Gastrointestinal Malignancies**	257
	John P. Plastaras, Stefan Both, Haibo Lin, and Maria Hawkins	
17	**Breast Cancer**	271
	Robert Samstein, David DeBlois, Robert W. Mutter, and Oren Cahlon	
18	**Gynecologic malignancies**	289
	Jessica E. Scholey, Pamela J. Boimel, Maura Kirk, and Lilie Lin	
19	**Prostate Cancer**	303
	Neil K. Taunk, Chin-Cheng Chen, Zhiqiang Han, Jerry Davis, Neha Vapiwala, and Henry Tsai	
20	**Adult Intracranial Tumors**	317
	Natalie A. Lockney, Zhiqiang Han, Kevin Sine, Dominic Maes, and Yoshiya Yamada	
21	**Primary Spine Tumors**	329
	Anuradha Thiagarajan and Yoshiya Yamada	
22	**Sarcoma**	347
	Curtiland Deville, Matthew Ladra, Huifang Zhai, Moe Siddiqui, Stefan Both, and Haibo Lin	
23	**Mediastinal Lymphoma**	369
	Bradford S. Hoppe, Stella Flampouri, Christine Hill-Kayser, and John P. Plastaras	
24	**Pediatric Tumors**	381
	Paul B. Romesser, Nelly Ju, Chin-Cheng Chen, Kevin Sine, Oren Cahlon, and Suzanne L. Wolden	

Physics Essentials of Particle Therapy

Dennis Mah, Michael Moyers, Ken Kang-Hsin Wang, Eric Diffenderfer, John Cuaron, and Mark Pankuch

Contents

1.1	History of Light Ion Teletherapy...	2
	1.1.1 Rationale for Light Ion Beam Teletherapy.....................................	2
1.2	Basic Physics	4
	1.2.1 Penumbra	4
	1.2.2 In Patient	5
1.3	Relative Biological Effectiveness (RBE)	6
	1.3.1 Terminology...	8
	1.3.2 Ions Heavier than Protons	9
1.4	Range Uncertainty	11

D. Mah (✉)
ProCure New Jersey, Somerset, NJ, USA
e-mail: dennis.mah@nj.procure.com

M. Moyers
Shanghai Proton and Heavy Ion Center, Shanghai, China
e-mail: Michael.F.Moyers@sphic.org.cn

K. Kang-Hsin Wang
Johns Hopkins Hospital, Baltimore, MD, USA
e-mail: kwang27@jhmi.edu

E. Diffenderfer
University of Pennsylvania, Philadelphia, PA, USA
e-mail: Eric.Diffenderfer@uphs.upenn.edu

J. Cuaron
Memorial Sloan Kettering Cancer Center, New York City, NY, USA
e-mail: cuaronj@mskcc.org

M. Pankuch
Northwestern Medicine, Chicago Proton Center, Warrenville, IL, USA
e-mail: mark.pankuch@nm.org

© Springer International Publishing Switzerland 2018
N. Lee et al. (eds.), *Target Volume Delineation and Treatment Planning for Particle Therapy*, Practical Guides in Radiation Oncology,
https://doi.org/10.1007/978-3-319-42478-1_1

1.5	Beam Generators	12
	1.5.1 Synchrotron	12
	1.5.2 Cyclotron	13
1.6	Future Developments	14
1.7	References	15

1.1 History of Light Ion Teletherapy

1.1.1 Rationale for Light Ion Beam Teletherapy

- There are three reasons for using light ion beams for teletherapy: (1) the low entrance dose and almost zero dose delivered distal to the target results in the ratio of nontarget tissue dose to target dose being smaller than with other radiation beams; (2) with appropriate collimation, the dose gradients at the lateral and distal sides of the targets are higher than with other radiation beams thereby offering higher dose gradients between the target and normal tissues; (3) for ions heavier than helium, the increase in RBE with increasing depth results in the target receiving a higher RBE dose than the tissues on the entrance side.
- Light ions are a subset of heavy charged particles and are defined as ions with atomic numbers less than 20 [1–3]. Although six different ions have been used for human treatments, the majority of patients have been treated with protons, helium ions, and carbon ions. Figure 1.1 shows the approximate number of patients treated with different heavy charged particle beams between 1954, when

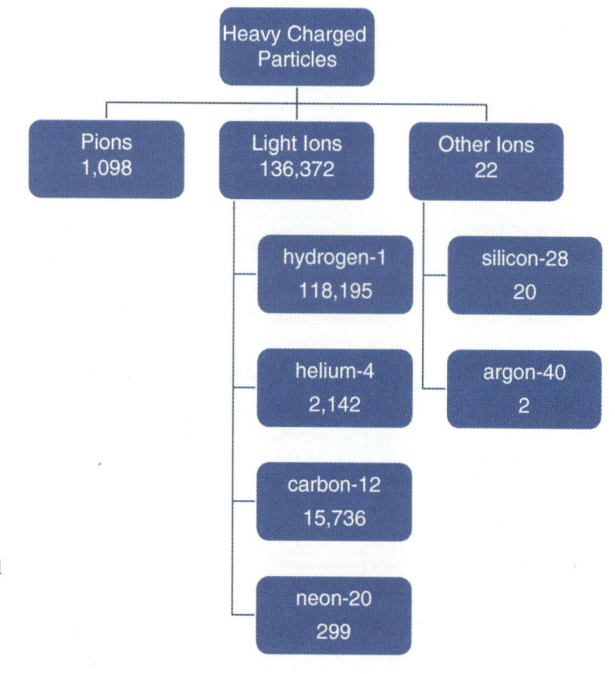

Fig. 1.1 Approximate number of patients treated with different heavy charged particle beams from 1954 to 2015. Figure adapted from Vatnitsky and Moyers [4] and updated with data from Jermann [5] to reflect recent data

treatments commenced, through 2015. Table 1.1 is a list of major milestones since the first patient was treated with a proton beam in 1954.

- As of 2015, there were approximately 50 facilities in the world treating patients with light ion beams. Figure 1.2 plots the number of operating facilities according to continent.

Table 1.1 Major milestones in light ion teletherapy according to year and location

Year	Location	Milestone
1954	Berkeley	First patient treated with protons
1957	Uppsala	First patient treated with uniform scanning with protons
1958	Berkeley	First patient treated with helium ions
1965	Boston	First AVM treated with protons
1975	Boston	First ocular melanoma treated with protons
1977	Berkeley	First patients treated with carbon and neon ions
1979	Chiba	First patients treated with modulated scanning with protons
1989	Tsukuba	First proton patients treated with respiratory beam gating
1990	Loma Linda	First patient treated in hospital with protons
1991	Loma Linda	First use of rotating gantry for proton beams
1996	Loma Linda	First electronic x-ray imaging with computerized analysis for daily alignment of proton beams
1997	Darmstadt	First patients treated with modulated scanning with carbon ions
1998	Loma Linda	100 patients treated with protons in 1 day at a single facility
2005	Loma Linda	173 patients treated with protons in 1 day at a single facility
2012	Heidelberg	First use of rotating gantry for carbon ion beams

Table from Vatnitsky and Moyers [4] and used with permission from Medical Physics Publishing

Number of Light Ion Facilities

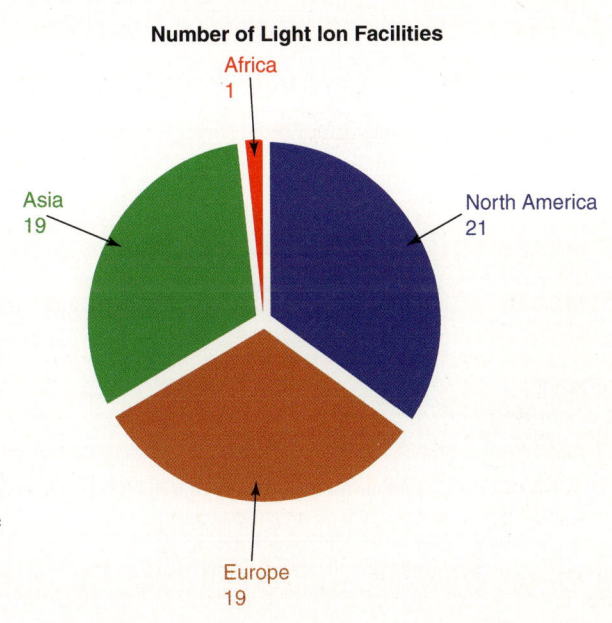

Africa 1
Asia 19
North America 21
Europe 19

Fig. 1.2 Number of light ion facilities operating worldwide as of 2015 according to continent. Data compiled from Jermann [5]

1.2 Basic Physics

- Like electrons, protons interact with material through ionization and Coulomb scattering, but because protons are 1836 times heavier than electrons, they are not deflected much by scattering with electrons. With a much lower probability, protons can interact with the nucleus resulting in lateral deflections and an increasing lateral spreading of the beam at depth [6].
- The maximum energy of protons used to treat patients is typically between 220 and 250 MeV. The velocity of protons having these energies is about 0.6 times the speed of light. As protons slow down, they spend more time passing by molecules thus causing more ionization resulting in a larger dose deposition toward the end of their range. The shape of the most distal region is called the Bragg peak (Fig. 1.3a). To treat finite size targets in depth, beams of multiple energies may be combined to generate a spread out Bragg peak (SOBP). Proton range depends on the beam energy with higher-energy beams being more penetrating. Proton range is typically defined as the depth of the 90% isodose on the distal edge of the Bragg peak (Fig. 1.3b). The modulation width is typically defined as the width of the SOBP between the depth of the proximal 90% dose and the depth of the distal 90% dose.

1.2.1 Penumbra

- Lateral penumbra may be defined as in photon beams, i.e., the distance between the 80 and 20% dose levels. The lateral penumbra width increases with increasing depth. The 90–50% penumbra width is about ~3% of the depth for double

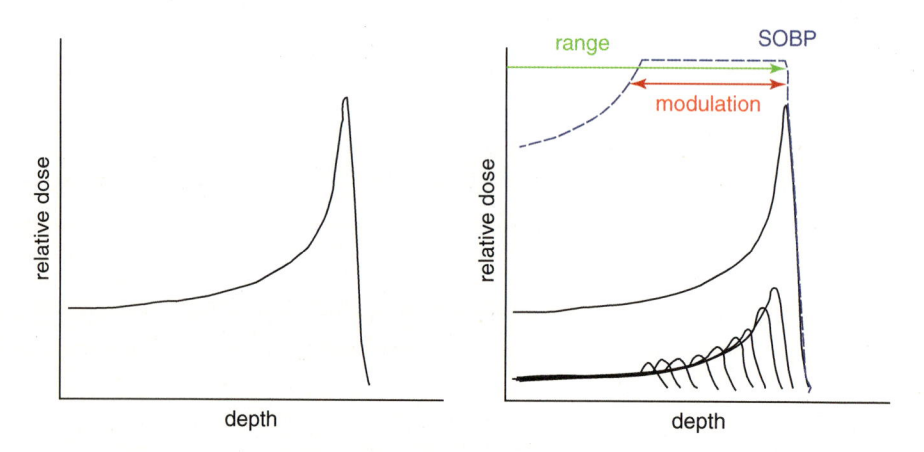

Fig. 1.3 (a) Pristine (monoenergetic) energy proton beam depth dose distribution in water. (b) A weighted average of the depth dose distributions in water from several energy proton beams results in a spread out Bragg peak. The modulation width is characterized by the difference between the depths of the 90% isodose at the proximal and distal ends of the SOBP

80-20 Penumbra vs Depth

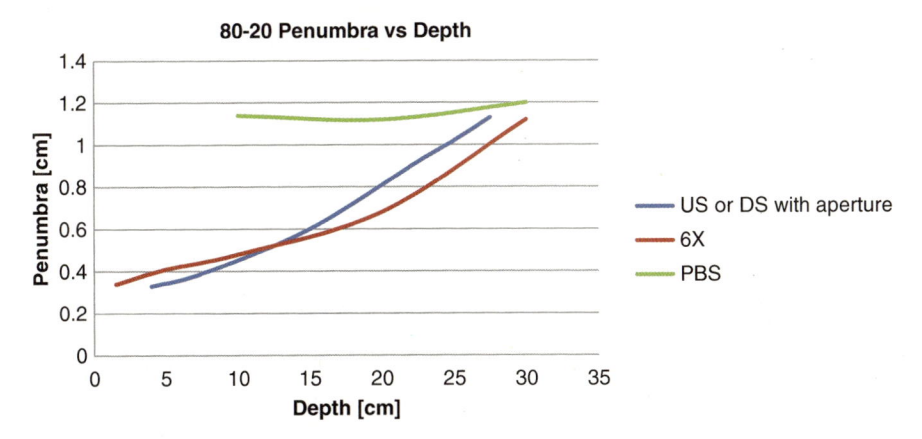

Fig. 1.4 Comparison of lateral penumbra for proton double-scattered beam with aperture, proton pencil beam scanning without collimation, and collimated 6 MV x-rays in water. The 6 MV x-ray data were taken from [8]. The proton data were generated for an IBA universal nozzle using a Raystation treatment planning system. The results are meant to show the trend, and results will vary between centers due to differences in the delivery systems (e.g., nozzle design)

scattering systems [7]. Figure 1.4 compares lateral penumbra for a collimated proton beam, collimated 6 MV x-ray beam, and proton pencil beam scanning without collimation. In general, the penumbra for pencil beam scanning (PBS) is constant with depth. The penumbra for PBS delivered beams can be improved by an aperture [9, 10].
- The distal penumbra results primarily from range straggling (which is ~1.2% of the range) and from beam energy spread (which depends upon the proton source) [11].
- Ions heavier than protons, such as carbon ions, have both sharper lateral and distal penumbra because their larger mass results in less scatter. While in theory, carbon could have a penumbra 1/3 that of protons, scanning with such a small spot would result in unacceptable delivery times. Consequently, spots larger than the minimum possible are used. However, it is the RBE (see below) effects that make these particles heavier than protons more compelling.

1.2.2 In Patient

- Tissue inhomogeneity issues are much worse in protons than photons, but protons also have dose homogeneity advantages over photons and fewer proton fields are often used. Patients have inhomogeneities in terms of composition and density. Scatter increases with atomic number. Changes in density alter the range in a manner that is difficult to fully account for using CT-based planning (see range uncertainty). Interfaces between different materials can lead to in and out scatter resulting in hot or cold spots at the interfaces. These effects are not fully calculated in pencil beam-based treatment planning systems but can be modeled using Monte Carlo [12]. Additionally, not only the range, but also the shape and distal penumbra of the SOBP can be affected by inhomogeneities; in many cases, the slope of the distal penumbra is enlarged by inhomogeneities.

1.3 Relative Biological Effectiveness (RBE)

- In radiation therapy, much of the clinical experience has been gained through photon treatments, which is based on the physics parameter dose, not directly related to the biological end points, such as tumor control probability (TCP) or normal tissue complication probability (NTCP) [13, 14]. Biological endpoints for an identical physical dose can be different for proton and photon therapy, *i.e.*, equal doses of photon and proton therapy do not produce the same clinical or biological outcomes.
- To take advantage of the clinical experience gained from the photon therapy and account for the difference of the biological effect between the two modalities, proton prescriptions are based on a factor (relative biological effectiveness, RBE) times the physical proton dose.
- The RBE for proton therapy (or another particle therapy) can be defined as—given the same biological effect—the ratio of the physical doses between the reference beam, *e.g.*, photon, and the proton beam.

$$\mathrm{RBE} = \frac{\mathrm{Dose}_{\mathrm{reference}}(\mathrm{Biological\ effect})}{\mathrm{Dose}_{\mathrm{proton}}(\mathrm{Biological\ effect})}$$

- From the available in vitro and in vivo data, recent publications [13, 14] have suggested that RBE is a function of:
  - *Dose*: From clonogenic cell survival curve (cell survival fraction *versus* dose, Fig. 1.5), within the low dose region, protons typically show a less pronounced shoulder compared to photons, which implies larger α/β (α is the parameter describing the cell killing per Gy of the initial linear component and β describes the killing per Gy^2 of the quadratic component of the linear-quadratic survival curve). It renders that for a given survival fraction, the ratio between photon and proton dose (RBE) can be different at low dose region than that of the high dose region (Fig. 1.5).
  - *Tissue type:* Recent findings from clonogenic cell survival data [14] has suggested that the RBE increases with decreasing $(\alpha/\beta)_x$ {α_x and β_x are the dose response parameters in the linear-quadratic model in photon therapy}, although large uncertainties existed in these data. This finding suggests that proton treatments can potentially induce larger RBEs for late responding normal tissues than for tumor tissue with high $(\alpha/\beta)_x$ values.
  - *Proton beam properties (linear energy transfer, LET):* Given the energy of clinical proton beams, in general, RBE increases with increasing LET. The LET is

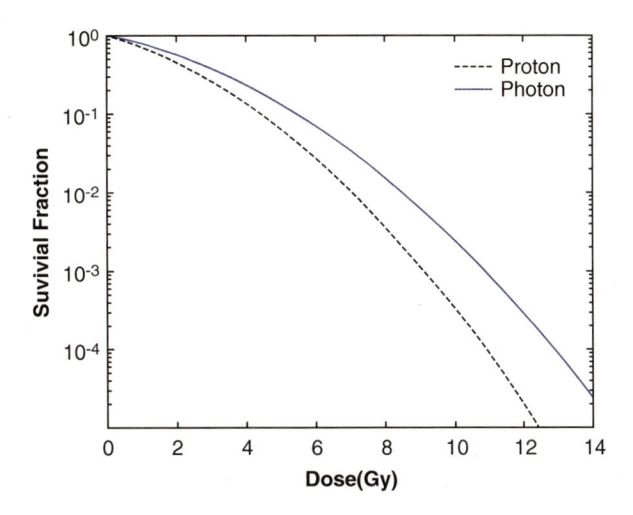

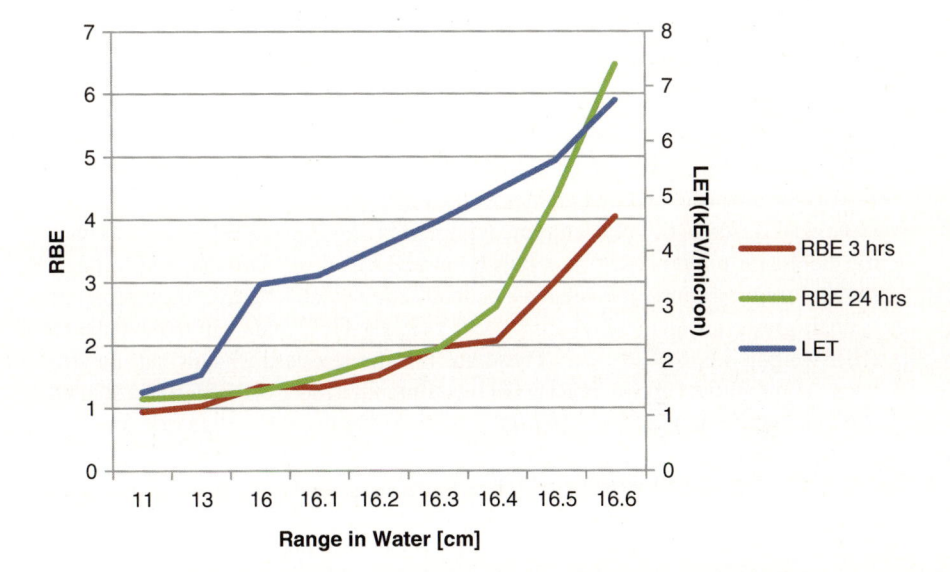

Fig. 1.5 Schematic cell survival curves for photon radiation (*solid*) and proton radiation (*dashed*)

Fig. 1.6 LET and RBE as a function of depth along the distal edge of a proton beam

also a function of depth in a proton beam, which results in an increase of RBE with depth. This effect can be demonstrated using Monte Carlo simulation of LET of a 152 MeV proton beam, plotted alongside RBE values of the same beam using DNA double strand breaks as a biological endpoint (Fig. 1.6) [15].
- The increase of RBE also increases the effective range of the RBE-weighted depth dose, which can result in an effective 1–3 mm shift of the depth of the distal penumbra region. It is also important to keep in mind that the LET values depend on the treatment field, particularly the SOBP modulation width.

- Clinical (generic) RBE value: Although proton RBE depends on the above mentioned factors and considerable uncertainties in RBE values remain, the use of a constant RBE of 1.1, recommended by ICRU 78 report [16], does not seem unreasonable if an average value of is desired cross the proton ranges used clinically. To follow the same convention given in the ICRU report,

$$D_{RBE} = 1.1 \times D,$$

where D is the proton absorbed dose in Gy and D_{RBE} in Gy is the RBE-weighted proton absorbed dose equivalent to the dose of photons that would produce the same clinical outcome as a proton dose D. For example, one prescribes the proton absorbed dose to the target as $D = 63$ Gy, and the RBE-weighted dose can be expressed as $63 \times 1.1 \rightarrow D_{RBE} = 70$ Gy(RBE). In other words, to deliver a photon equivalent dose 70 Gy(RBE) to a target, one would deliver a proton dose of 63 Gy.

1.3.1 Terminology

1. *RBE-weighted dose* is a biologically weighted quantity used to define a dose of protons that would produce an identical biological effect as a dose of photons. Due to the consistent characteristics of the cobalt-60 beam and the undetectable biological differences between typical photon beams and Co-60 beams, all photon fields are referenced to a cobalt-60 equivalent dose. This has led to commonly used terminology such as "cobalt equivalent," "gray equivalent" or "cobalt-gray equivalent" with units such as Gy(E), GyE, and CGE to describe an RBE-weighted absorbed dose. These are not the standard SI unit but are still used. As mentioned above, ICRU [16] recommended to report the RBE-weighted dose in DRBE [in units of Gy(RBE)].

   It is common practice to incorporate the doses in the treatment planning system in RBE-weighted dose so that clinicians can evaluate in terms of equivalent doses rather than physical doses.
   - Clinic considerations: Because proton RBE is a function of dose, tissue type, and LET, the following points potentially affect clinic outcome [13].
     - *Dose effect*: Because RBE depends on dose, the RBE can be potentially reduced, less than 1.1, with increasing dose, especially for hypofractionated cases.
     - *Tissue type*: Tumors with low $(\alpha/\beta)_x$ values, such as prostate tumors, might show a RBE higher than 1.1. In contrast, tumors with very high $(\alpha/\beta)_x$ values could have lower RBE.
     - *The RBE increases with depth* and recent data suggests that RBE values are significantly higher than previously estimated, especially at the distal edge (24). During planning, one should be cautious if aiming a beam toward an organ at risk (OAR) even if it is behind the target, because the combination

of the high-LET/RBE region at the distal falloff region and range uncertainties can potentially result in an undesirable radiobiological dose to the downstream OAR.
- *Delivery modalities*: Investigators recently indicate [17] LET variation appears to be potentially significant in IMPT delivery, such as distal edge tracking (DET)-IMPT where the DET-IMPT plans resulted in considerably increased LET values (increased RBE) in critical structures. In contrast, the 3-D IMPT shows more favorable LET distributions than does DET-IMPT. It is important to be aware of the LET variation for different delivery techniques.
- Considering these uncertainties, it is crucial that physicians, treatment planners, and physicists work together to mitigate, track, and report acute and long-term toxicities and outcomes among patients treated with proton therapy. Clinical data will help to determine whether these uncertainties should guide refinement of treatment planning and delivery, or alternatively, can be safely disregarded.

1.3.2 Ions Heavier than Protons

- Heavier charged particles (such as argon, neon, silicon, and carbon ions) and fast neutrons are considered high-LET radiation. Currently, carbon ions are the most often used high-LET therapy worldwide because of a number of potential advantages over photon and proton therapy in both physical and biological aspects [18, 19];
  - *Dose distribution*: Both the lateral and distal penumbras are narrow. The energy spread and range straggling of the particles are smaller for carbon ions. The dose ratio between the SOBP and entrance plateau is higher than protons. Nuclear fragmentation after the distal end of the Bragg peak can be a potential disadvantage when using carbon. However, this aspect is usually minimal because the dose is low and the fragments are lower-LET particles.
  - *Therapeutic gain*: The LET in a clinical ion beam increases with depth, leading to the increase of RBE. Among the heavier ions, carbon ions have the advantage of the highest peak-to-plateau RBE ratio. At the position of the SOBP, where the target regions are located, high-LET radiation makes ion beams specifically effective for the treatment of some tumor types that are resistant to low-LET radiation. These features open the potential to treat tumors that are deeply located and resistant to proton or photon treatment. Other advantages for carbon ions include reducing the oxygen enhancement ratio (OER), radiosensitivity of the cell cycle dependency, and suppressing the repair of radiation damage.
- The RBE of SOBP carbon beam exhibits substantially greater variation with depth than that of a proton beam, being dependent upon the position within the SOBP, dose, dose per fraction, and tissue type. For the same depth and tissue, the RBE at the center of the SOBP can vary between three and five, and the ratio between target and skin doses may vary by a factor of two [18, 19].

- Treatment planning: Since large RBE variations are seen for carbon ion therapy, unlike proton therapy, a single value is not sufficient to accurately/safely describe the biological effective dose. For treatment planning, RBE values must be estimated as accurately as possible. Two different strategies and modeling approaches were chosen by two leading carbon facilities, the National Institute of Radiological Sciences (NIRS) in Japan and Gesellschaft für Schwerionenforschung (GSI) in Germany, respectively.
    - NIRS employed an experimentally oriented approach [3]. It is based on the measurements of RBE in vitro, which are used to determine the shape of the biological effective depth dose profile. The clinical RBE value is then determined by establishing equivalency between carbon and neutron beams to make use of the experience in neutron therapy. The NIRS group found a carbon beam which possesses a dose averaged LET of 80 keV/μm results in an equivalent biological response to those from the neutron beams. The clinical RBE was defined as 3, the same as that used in neutron therapy at the point where the dose averaged LET value is 80 keV/μm. Figure 1.7 shows the physical dose distribution required in the SOBP to yield a constant biological response (dose) across the SOBP. To further obtain the clinical/prescribed dose, the biological dose at every depth is multiplied by the ratio of the biological and clinical RBEs at the neutron equivalent position.

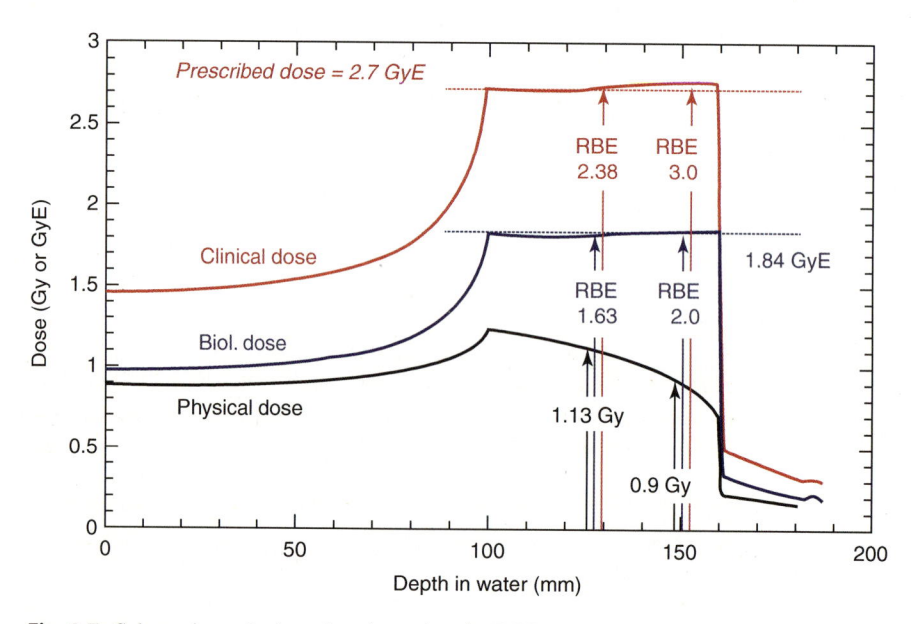

Fig. 1.7 Schematic method used to determine the RBE at the SOBP for the clinical situation (Reproducing the Figure with permission by the IAEA from International Atomic Energy Agency, MIZOE J. et al. "Clinical RBE determination scheme at NIRS-HIMAC," Relative Biological Effectiveness in Ion Beam Therapy, Technical Reports Series No. 461, IAEA, Vienna 135–152 [18])

- The GSI strategy is based on biophysical modeling [18]. The goal is to develop a model, which should be able to predict the response of the charged particle radiation from the known response of the biological object to photon radiation. This links the treatment planning for carbon therapy to the clinical experience with photon radiation. An example of such a model, the local effect model (LEM), has been implemented in treatment planning for carbon ion irradiation. The clinical results obtained at GSI are consistent with the predicted RBE values in that there is no significant clinical complication observed.

1.4 Range Uncertainty

The stopping power of an ion beam describes the energy loss of ions passing through matter per unit path length and determines the range of the ions and the ultimate depth of the Bragg peak. The stopping power is dependent on the energy of the ion beam and the atomic composition of the material. Uncertainty in the calculation of the stopping power then translates directly into uncertainty in the range and depth of the distal edge of the Bragg peak and in the dose distribution that is displayed by the treatment planning system.

All ion treatment planning is currently done using 3-D computed tomography (CT) images. The volumetric image consists of a 3-D voxel array of CT Hounsfield numbers (HU) that correspond to the attenuation coefficients of the material. To calculate the ion dose distribution, the HU must be converted to stopping power.

There are uncertainties in the HU to stopping power conversion that translate into significant uncertainties in the ion range and have a marked effect on the target margins that are used for treatment planning. Additionally, there are sources of uncertainty in HU resulting which are a function of patient size, CT scanner, scanning protocol, and reconstruction algorithm. In the HU to stopping power conversion, these uncertainties are combined with degeneracy in the mapping of HU to stopping power in the HU. Care must be taken in calibrating the CT scanner and HU to stopping power conversion to minimize the impact that this uncertainty has on target margins [20].

To ensure target coverage, despite these uncertainties, margins are added to the target during planning. The size of the margin is determined by the overall range uncertainty, which is typically proportional to 2.5–3.5% of the ion range with an additional 1.0–3.0 mm to account for range uncertainty that is not dependent on the dose calculation (e.g., setup error, measurement uncertainty, etc.) [21]. This margin is added to the distal and proximal extent of the target during treatment planning. Thus, the margin in the beam direction may be different from the lateral setup margin. The formula for calculating range uncertainty is as follows:

$$\text{Range Uncertainty}(\text{mm}) = \left(\text{Range}(\text{mm}) \times \text{Uncertainty}(\%)\right) + \text{Margin}(\text{mm}).$$

Figure 1.8 shows some common choices of uncertainty parameters and the significant effect that it has on the necessary target margins.

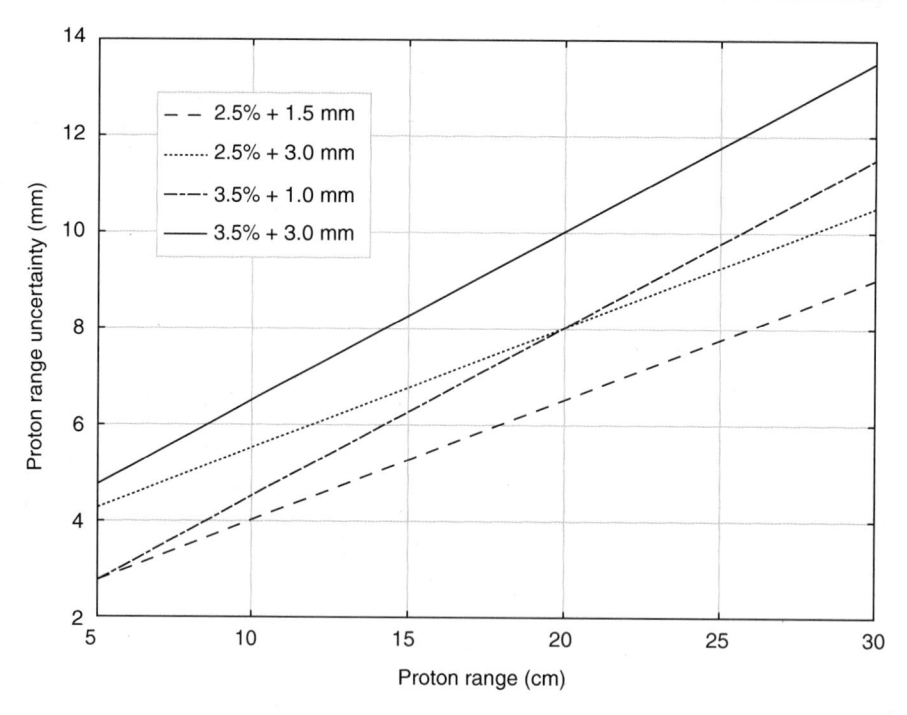

Fig. 1.8 Proton range uncertainty in millimeters plotted as a function of proton range in centimeters for various common choices of uncertainty parameters. The range uncertainty is calculated at the distal and proximal edges of the target and added to the target volume during planning (adapted from [21])

1.5 Beam Generators

- Clinically useable proton kinetic energies vary from ~70 to 250 MeV corresponding to 4 to 37 cm range in water. There are two types of accelerator systems used for proton therapy, a synchrotron and a cyclotron. In 2016, for ions heavier than protons, all accelerators were synchrotrons.

1.5.1 Synchrotron

- Figure 1.9 shows a photograph of a synchrotron.
- The synchrotron accelerates protons in a ring with a fixed radius orbit by boosting the proton's energy in each revolution in a fixed orbit.
- Low-energy particles are injected into the ring and are accelerated in an RF cavity placed within the ring. The generation of higher kinetic energy protons requires additional revolutions through the RF acceleration cavity. During each rotation the magnetic field that keep the protons constrained within the ring must be synchronously increased to maintain a stable proton orbit.

1 Physics Essentials of Particle Therapy

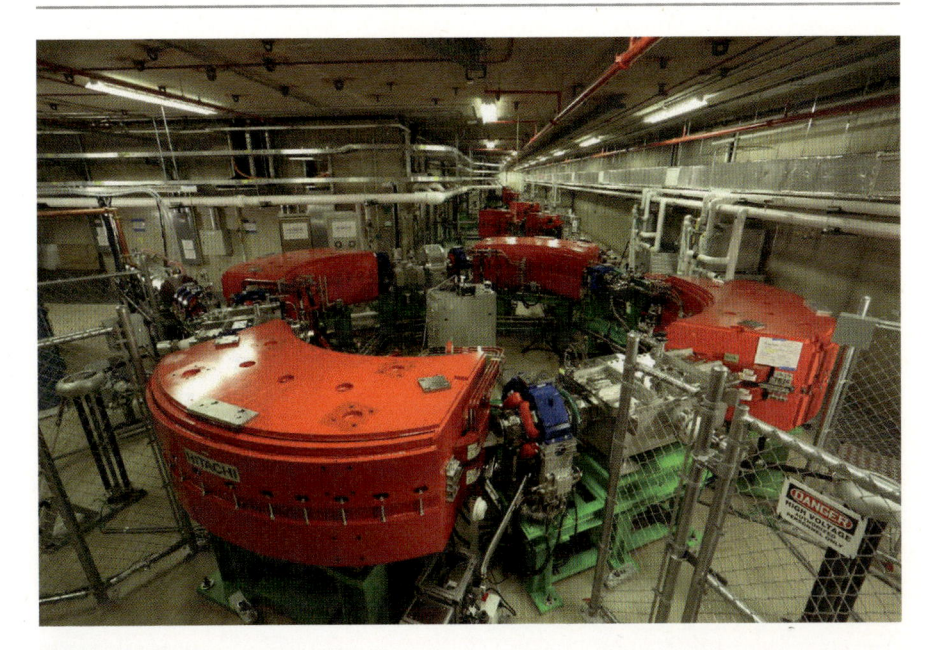

Fig. 1.9 Synchrotron at Mayo Clinic, Arizona. Photograph courtesy of Martin Bues

Once the protons are at the energy needed for treatment, they are "spilled" into the beam line and directed to the treatment room by a series of focusing and bending magnets. Synchrotrons produce beams in a pulsed beam structure requiring a period to "fill" for acceleration, then "spill" into the treatment rooms. This process typically takes 2–5 s per energy layer.

1.5.2 Cyclotron

Figure 1.10 shows a photograph of a cyclotron. A cyclotron accelerates protons within a fixed magnetic field. Low-energy protons are injected into the center of disk-shaped accelerating cavity. Particles gain kinetic energy by passing through RF accelerating cavities within the disk. The constant magnetic field binds the protons to a circular path within the disk, but, with each rotation, the protons that pass through the accelerating cavities gain energy and spiral radially outward incrementally increasing the energy. At the outer most orbit, the protons are "peeled" off and directed down the beam line for clinical use. All protons leaving the cyclotron are at the maximum clinically available energy. Since energies lower than the maximum are most commonly used, the proton beam is directed through low atomic number materials of variable thicknesses which interact with the protons to lower their energy to the required clinical energy. The cyclotron delivers a nearly continuous output of protons once the range and beam line magnets are set. Table 1.2 summarizes the differences between the two delivery systems.

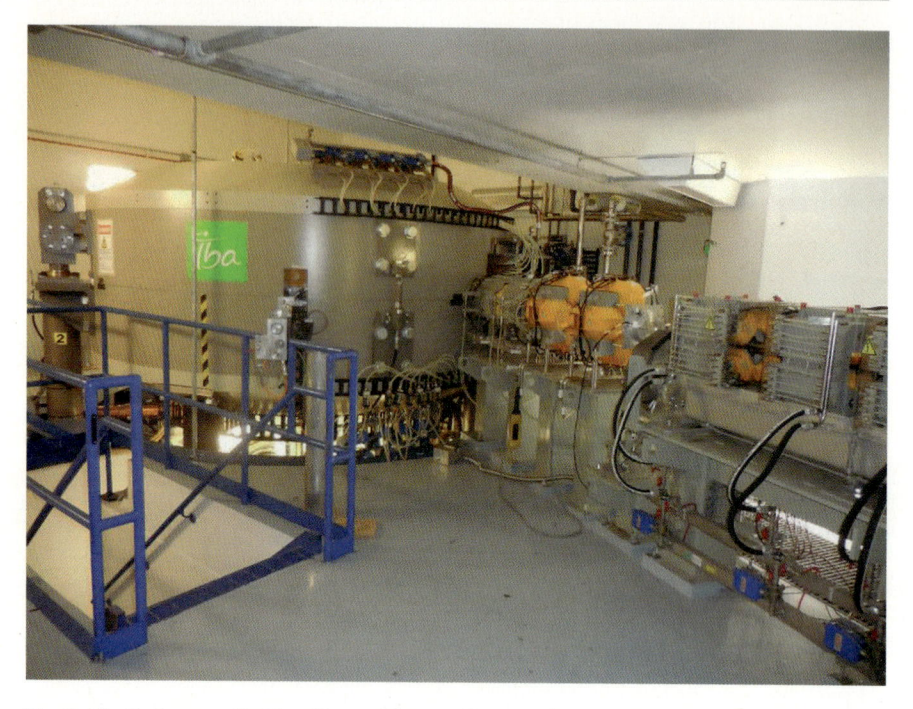

Fig. 1.10 Cyclotron at ProCure Proton Therapy Center, NJ. Photograph courtesy of Dennis Mah

1.6 Future Developments

Light ion teletherapy is growing rapidly globally. Future developments are difficult to predict, but some developments include:

- Superconducting bending magnets and cyclotrons lead to more compact systems, but more complicated systems may have challenges with maintenance and downtime [22, 23].
- Range uncertainty is being addressed by a variety of different approaches including:
  - Proton CT—A proton beam is used like an x-ray to create a proton transmission CT image; the CT number to stopping power uncertainty is thus reduced. For some existing systems, this technique might be limited to thinner body sections because the maximum energy may not penetrate thick portions of the body. In addition, the energy/range relationship is dependent upon precise models of the proton trajectory [24].
  - Real-time diode dosimetry—A diode system is implanted into a body cavity, and the range is varied allowing the diode system to determine the range at which the protons can just be detected [25].
  - Prompt gamma imaging—Excited nuclei decay to the ground state emitting gamma rays up to 7 MeV. Knife edge slits collimate the gamma rays to within 2 mm. Initial results appear to be promising [26].

Table 1.2 Comparison of accelerator characteristics

	Magnetic field	Beam structure	Output energy
Synchrotron	Dynamic	Pulsed	Variable
Cyclotron	Constant	Continuous	Constant

- Dual energy CT—Different energy CT scans are used to minimize uncertainties in CT numbers and provide additional information to convert CT numbers to stopping powers. The technique has not yet been proven to be sufficient over the range of compositions found in human body [27].
- PET imaging—Ions can generate short-lived positron-emitting isotopes which in turn produce annihilation photons which are detected by PET scanners. Biological and temporal wash out limit the utility [28].
- MRI—For craniospinal irradiation, the fatty replacement of vertebral bone is visible on MRI thereby illustrating where the beam stops [29]
- Interplay effects between the scanning beam and the internal motion of the patient may lead to hot and cold spots not represented in the plan. A variety of approaches are being actively studied including repainting, breath hold, abdominal compression, and robust optimization [30].
- Relative biological effectiveness—New calculation models are being studied to include the combined effects of LET and fractionation while simultaneously reducing calculation times [31]
  - Further characterization of the clinical and biological effects of the enhanced RBE at the distal edge:
    - possible exploitation of end of range effects
    - Development of "biological dose painting" [32]

References

1. Blakely EA, Tobias CA, Ludewigt BA, Chu WT, Some physical and biological properties of light ions. In: Chu W, editor. Proceedings of the Fifth PTCOG Meeting & International Workshop on Biomedical Accelerators. Lawrence Berkeley Laboratories Report LBL-22962; 1986.
2. Chu WT, Ludewigt BA, Renner TR. Instrumentation for treatment of cancer using proton and light-ion beams. Lawrence Berkeley Laboratories Report LBL-33403, UC406; 1993.
3. Wambersie A, Deluca PM, Andreo P, Hendry JH. Light or heavy ions: a debate of terminology. Radiother Oncol. 2004;73(S2):iiii.
4. Vatnitsky SM, Moyers MF. Radiation therapy with light ions. In: van Dyk J, editor. The modern technology of radiation oncology v.3: A compendium for medical physicists and radiation oncologists. Wisconsin: Medical Physics Publishing; 2013. p. 183–222. ISBN: 978-1-930524-57-6.
5. Jermann M. Particle therapy statistics in 2014. Int J of Particle Therapy. 2015;2(1):50–4.
6. Goitein M. Radiation oncology: A Physicist's-eye. New York: Springer-Verlag; 2008.
7. Moyers MF, Stanislav V. Practical implementation of light ion beam treatments. Madison, WI: Medical Physics Publishing; 2012.
8. Metcalfe P, Kron T, Hoban P. The physics of radiotherapy X-rays from linear accelerators. Madison, WI: Medical Physics Publishing; 2007.
9. Dowdell SJ, Clasie B, Depauw N, Metcalfe P, Rosenfeld AB, Kooy HM, Flanz JB, Paganetti H. Monte Carlo study of the potential reduction in out-of-field dose using a patient-specific aperture in pencil beam scanning proton therapy. Phys Med Biol. 2012;57:2829–42.

10. Moteabbed M, Yock TI, Depauw N, Madden TM, Kooy HM, Paganetti H. Impact of spot size and beam-shaping devices on the treatment plan quality for pencil beam scanning proton therapy. Int J Radiat Oncol Biol Phys. 2016;95:190–8.
11. Paganetti H, editor. Proton therapy physics. Boca Raton, FL: CRC Press; 2011.
12. Paganetti H, Jiang H, Parodi K, Slopsema R, Engelsman M. Clinical implementation of full Monte Carlo dose calculation in proton beam therapy. Phys Med Biol. 2008;53:4825–53.
13. Paganetti H. Relating proton treatments to photon treatments via the relative biological effectiveness-should we revise current clinical practice? Int J Radiat Oncol Biol Phys. 2015;91:892–4.
14. Paganetti H. Relative biological effectiveness (RBE) values for proton beam therapy. Variations as a function of biological endpoint, dose, and linear energy transfer. Phys Med Biol. 2014;59:R419–72.
15. Cuaron JJ, Chang C, Lovelock M, et al. Exponential increase in relative biological effectiveness along distal edge of a proton Bragg peak as measured by deoxyribonucleic acid double-strand breaks. Int J Radiat Oncol Biol Phys. 2016;95:62–9.
16. ICRU. Prescribing, recording, and reporting proton-beam therapy. J ICRU. 2007;78:7.
17. Grassberger C, Trofimov A, Lomax A, et al. Variations in linear energy transfer within clinical proton therapy fields and the potential for biological treatment planning. Int J Radiat Oncol Biol Phys. 2011;80:1559–66.
18. Relative biological effectiveness in ion beam therapy. IAEA Technical Reports Series. 2008;461:1–165.
19. De Laney TF, Kooy HM. Proton and charged particle radiotherapy. Philadelphia: Lippincott Williams & Wilkins; 2008.
20. Ainsley CG, Yeager CM. Practical considerations in the calibration of CT scanners for proton therapy. J Appl Clin Med Phys. 2014;15(3):4721.
21. Paganetti H. Range uncertainties in proton therapy and the role of Monte Carlo simulations. Phys Med Biol. 2012;57(11):R99–117.
22. Blosser HG. Compact superconducting synchrocyclotron systems for proton therapy. Nucl Inst Methods Phys Res Sec B. 1989;40–41:1326–30.
23. Robin DS, Arbelaez D, Caspi S, Sun C, Sessler A, Wan W, Yoon M. Superconducting toroidal combined-function magnet for a compact ion beam cancer therapy gantry. Nucl Instrum Methods Phys Res A. 2011;659(1):484–93.
24. Schneider U, Pedroni E. Proton radiography as a tool for quality control in proton therapy. Med Phys. 1995;22:353–63.
25. Tang S, Both S, Bentefour EH, Paly JJ, Tochner Z, Efstathiou J, Lu HM. Improvement of prostate treatment by anterior proton fields. Int J Radiat Oncol Biol Phys. 2012;83:408–18.
26. Richter C, Pausch G, Barczyk S, Priegnitz M, Keitz I, Thiele J, Smeets J, et al. First clinical application of a prompt gamma based in vivo proton range verification system. Radiother Oncol. 2016; 118:232–7.
27. Yang M, Virshup G, Clayton J, Zhu XR, Mohan R, Dong L. Does kV-MV dual-energy computed tomography have an advantage in determining proton stopping power ratios in patients? Phys Med Biol. 2011;56:4499–515.
28. Knopf A, Parodi K, Bortfeld T, Shih HA, Paganetti H. Systematic analysis of biological and physical limitations of proton beam range verification with offline PET/CT scans. Phys Med Biol. 2009;54:4477–95.
29. Krejcarek SC, Grant PE, Henson JW, Tarbell NJ, Yock TI. Physiologic and radiographic evidence of the distal edge of the proton beam in craniospinal irradiation. Int J Radiat Oncol Biol Phys. 2007;68:646–9.
30. Rietzel E, Bert C. Respiratory motion management in particle therapy. Med Phys. 2010;37:449–60.
31. Wedenberg M, Lind BK, Hårdemark B. A model for the relative biological effectiveness of protons: the tissue specific parameter α/β of photons is a predictor of the sensitivity to LET changes. Acta Oncol. 2013;52:580–8.
32. Ling CC, Humm J, Larson S, Amols H, Fuks Z, Leibel S, Koutcher JA. Towards multidimensional radiotherapy (MD-CRT): biological imaging and biological conformality. Int J Radiat Oncol Biol Phys. 2000;47:551–60.

Proton Treatment Delivery Techniques

2

Xuanfeng Ding, Haibo Lin, Jiajian Shen, Wei Zou, Katja Langen, and Hsiao-Ming Lu

Contents

2.1	Introduction of Proton Treatment Delivery System	18
2.2	Treatment Delivery Techniques of Proton Therapy	20
	2.2.1 Passive-Scattering	20
	2.2.2 Pencil Beam Scanning	24
2.3	Imaging for Proton Beam Therapy	25
2.4	Intra-fractional Motion Management for Proton Therapy	28
2.5	Proton Beam Therapy Systems and Specifications	30
2.6	Quality Assurance (QA)	33
	2.6.1 System QA	33
	2.6.2 Patient-Specific QA (PSQA)	37
2.7	Future Developments	42
References		43

X. Ding
Beaumont Health, Royal Oak, MI, USA

H. Lin • W. Zou
University of Pennsylvania, Philadelphia, PA, USA

J. Shen
Mayo Clinic, Phoenix, AZ, USA

K. Langen
University of Maryland, Baltimore, MD, USA

H.-M. Lu (✉)
Massachusetts General Hospital, Boston, MA, USA
e-mail: HMLU@mgh.harvard.edu

© Springer International Publishing Switzerland 2018
N. Lee et al. (eds.), *Target Volume Delineation and Treatment Planning for Particle Therapy*, Practical Guides in Radiation Oncology,
https://doi.org/10.1007/978-3-319-42478-1_2

2.1 Introduction of Proton Treatment Delivery System

Proton therapy systems include three major components, the accelerator which raises the energy of the proton to a sufficient level, the energy selection and beam transportation system which modifies the proton energy, if necessary, and transports them from the accelerator to the treatment delivery system, and the treatment delivery system which modifies the proton beam characteristics for specific treatment needs. Currently, three types of accelerator, synchrotron, cyclotron, and synchrocyclotron, are commercially available, as discussed in the previous chapter. Protons generated from a cyclotron have a fixed energy, and energy reduction and selection systems are required, as shown in Fig. 2.1a. A synchrotron, on the other hand, can produce protons at any desired energy level. A synchrocyclotron is a special type of cyclotron that is typically used for a compact proton system. The beam transportation system (Fig. 2.1b), consisting of a sequence of dipole (bending and steering) magnets and quadrupole (focusing) magnets, delivers the proton beam from accelerator to treatment room through its vacuum beam pipeline. The beam switching from one treatment room to another is achieved by controlling the dipole deflector units along the beam transportation system.

The treatment delivery system is one of the main components of a proton therapy facility. It consists of several major subsystems: gantry, nozzle, snout, and patient positioning system in a treatment room. Proton beams are transported into a treatment room containing either fixed-beam lines or an isocentric gantry, as shown in Fig. 2.2.

A fixed-beam treatment room can have either one horizontal beamline (Fig. 2.2a) or the combination of a horizontal beamline and an angled beamline (e.g., 30° and

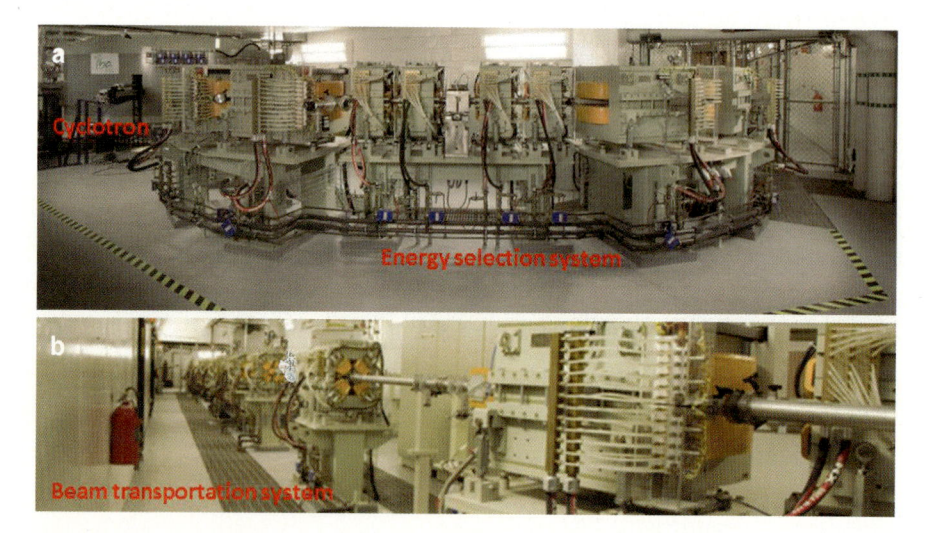

Fig. 2.1 Cyclotron and energy selection system (**a**) and a section of the beam transportation system (**b**) for a proton therapy facility (Courtesy of IBA, SA). Vacuum tube with multiple steering or bending magnets guide and focus the narrow proton beam to treatment rooms

90° for IBA inclined-beam gantry in Fig. 2.2c). The motivation of this design is to reduce the treatment room size and the overall cost. In the current stage, most fixed-beam and incline gantry rooms have been used for bilateral prostate cancer treatment as well as some cranial tumor with non-coplanar beam angles, e.g., vertex direction.

A gantry room provides either full 360° rotation (Fig. 2.2b) or limited rotations 0–220° (Fig. 2.2d) for the treatment. These gantry configurations are able to treat most of complicated cases which require different beam angles, e.g., the head and neck, lung, abdomen, etc. The standard full gantry is typically about 10 m in diameter with a total weight of up to 200 tons. A room with floor-to-ceiling height of about 20 m is required to accommodate such a structure and its base. Some compact gantries were designed with much smaller size and lighter weight around 100 tons.

The nozzle is the final element of the beam delivery system, which not only delivers the beam to the patient but also monitors the beam quality, alignment, and the dose delivery during treatment. There are two main types of nozzles: the nozzle that houses scattering components for passive-scattering (PS) delivery and the nozzle that houses components for pencil beam scanning (PBS) delivery.

- The PS nozzle contains first scatterers, range modulators, second scatterers, dose and field monitor chambers, patient-specific beam-shaping apertures, or other collimation components and compensators, as shown in Fig. 2.3a.

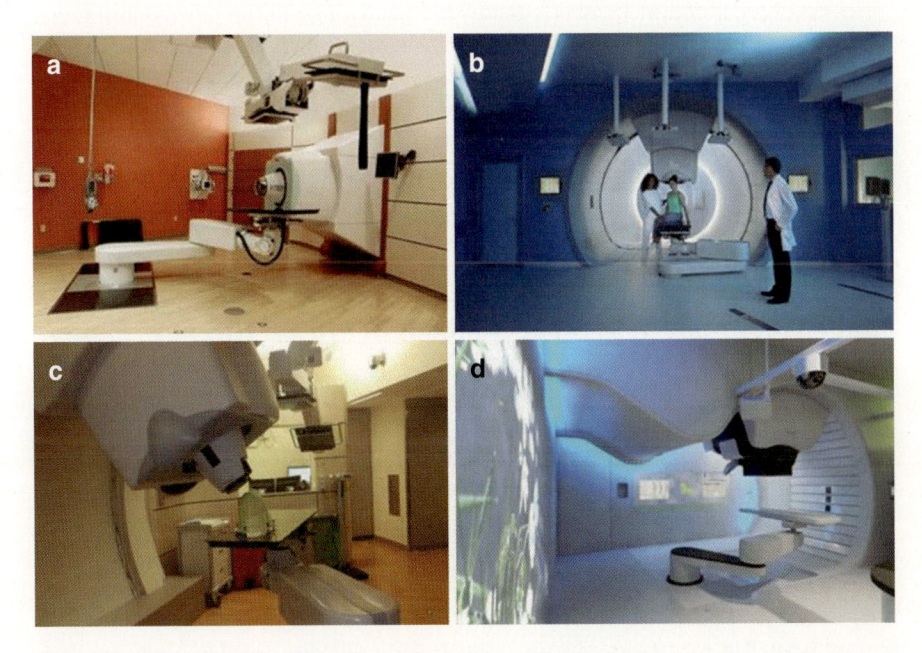

Fig. 2.2 Treatment rooms with different flexibilities of beam angles: (**a**) horizontal fixed-beam room, (**b**) 360° full gantry room, (**c**) inclined fixed-beam room (beam at 90° and 30° only), and (**d**) compact gantry (beam from 0° to 220°) (Courtesy of IBA, SA)

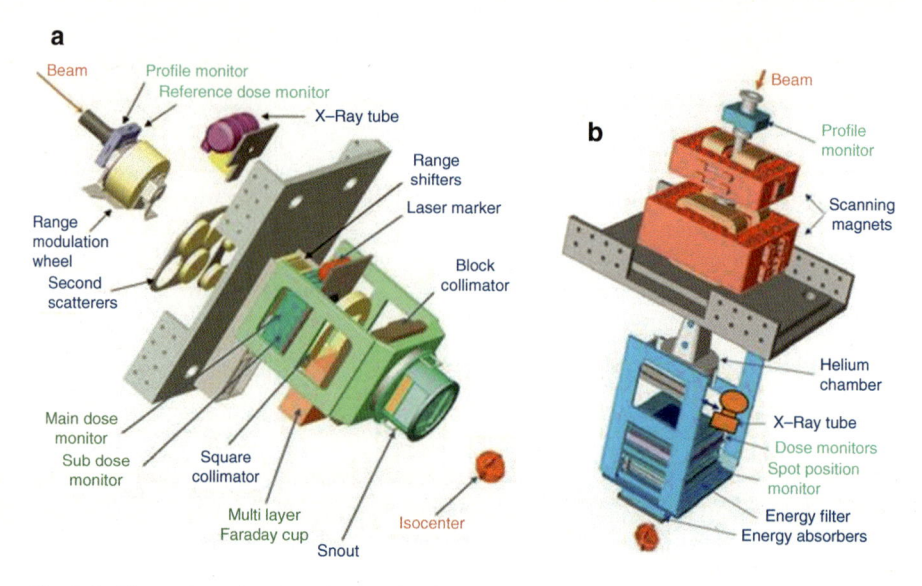

Fig. 2.3 Three-dimensional rendering of (**a**) the passive-scattering nozzle and (**b**) the scanning beam nozzle of the M.D. Anderson proton system (Hitachi Inc.) [1]

- The PBS nozzle contains the beam profile monitor, scanning magnets, dose and spot position monitor chambers, energy filter and range shifter (energy absorber), and possibly vacuum or Helium chambers on the beam path as well (Fig. 2.3b).

In addition to nozzles dedicated either for PS or PBS treatment delivery, some vendors provide nozzles with both scattering and scanning delivery capabilities, e.g., universal nozzle. However it can take a substantial amount of time to switch between different delivery modalities (e.g., IBA universal nozzle at the University of Pennsylvania).

2.2 Treatment Delivery Techniques of Proton Therapy

2.2.1 Passive-Scattering

Passive scattering is a conventional treatment technique in proton therapy. It utilizes the focused proton beam transported from the accelerator and scatters it through single or double scatterers to obtain a beam with large field size. In the proton beam scattering process, other components in the beam line will further modify the beam, for example, absorbers adjust the beam to the desired energy; modulator wheels or ridge filters modulate the beam to form a spread-out Bragg peak (SOBP) with a dose plateau. The scatterers, absorbers, modulator wheels, or ridge filters are usually installed in the treatment nozzle. At the end of the nozzle before the beam reaches patient, other devices such as apertures or MLC are inserted to the beam

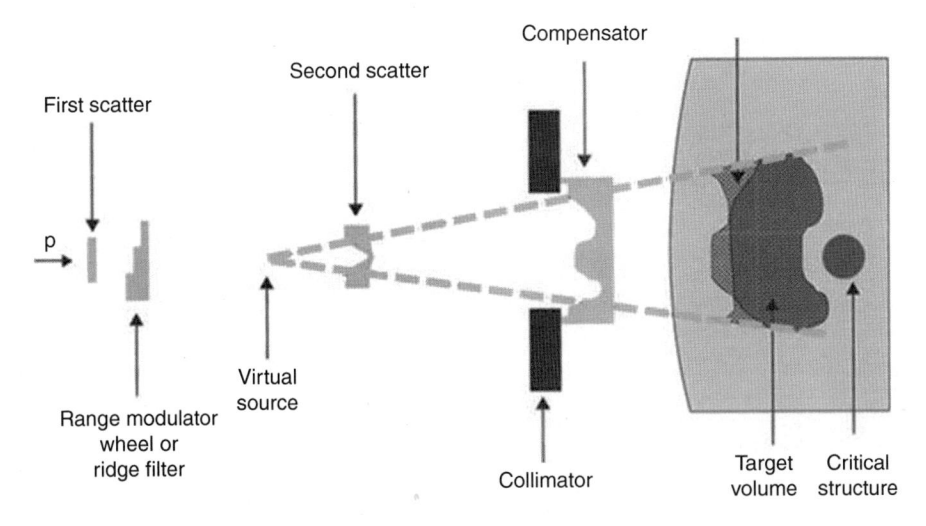

Fig. 2.4 Illustration of passive-scattering delivery technique [2]. Beam monitoring ionization chambers are not shown

line to collimate the beam to the shape of the treatment target. A compensator with varying thickness profile is also used to shape the distal penetration of the beam to the distal shape of the treatment target (Fig. 2.4).

2.2.1.1 Single Scattering
Single-scattering technique utilizes one scatterer in the beam line to scatter the focused proton beam into a large field. The scatterer is usually made from high atomic number foil such as lead. The proton beam passing through the single scatterer is laterally dispersed. The resulting proton field can be of nonuniform Gaussian-shaped intensity across the field. However, the central portion of the beam can be sufficiently uniform for treatment of small targets such as eye lesions. A single-scattering system generally produces sharper lateral beam penumbra than double-scattering systems and is therefore more often used for eye or brain tumor treatments.

2.2.1.2 Double Scattering
In double-scattering system, downstream from a first scatterer foil that scatters the proton beam into a Gaussian-shaped intensity field, a second scatterer is used to flatten the transverse intensity across the field. The second scatter is usually made of high Z material such as lead with a compensating thin layer of low Z material such as polycarbonate. The shape of the high Z material is close to a Gaussian with the thickest portion at the center. The double-scattering system can achieve uniform field intensity at a large field size up to 40 cm in diameter.

In a passive-scattering system, the delivery of a uniform dose across the depth of the target is usually achieved through the construction of SOBP. The SOBP is made of a series of intensity and energy-modulated pristine Bragg peaks. The system

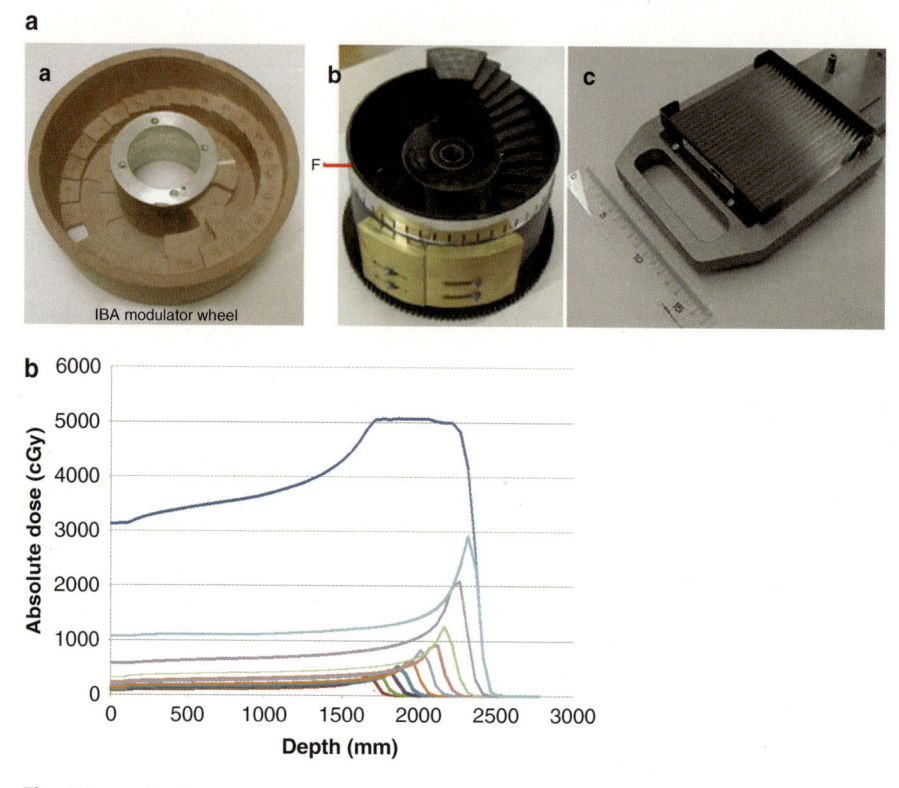

Fig. 2.5 (**a**) Devices for SOBP construction: *a* IBA three-track modulator wheel, *b* Mevion single-track modulator wheel, *c* HIBMC ridge filter [3]. (**b**) Generation of SOBP using passive-scattering technique. *Red line graph* shows the spread-out Bragg peak (SOBP) peak. There are ten lines of pristine Bragg peak which indicates the different proton energies and dose depositions after going through the modulation wheel in order to treat a target uniformly using the SOBP (*dark blue line*). The sum of the individual line equals to the *dark blue line*

achieves this through a range modulator wheel or ridge filter (Fig. 2.5a, b). The modulator wheels are made of a series of steps from low Z material with varying step heights and widths. As the wheel rotates at a constant speed, the proton beam passes the steps in sequence so that the beam energy is reduced to produce the group of Bragg peaks with the required proton energies and intensities for the construction of SOBP. The ridge filter modulates the proton beam through a series of stationary localized ridge-shaped bars. The ridge profile, taking into the account of beam scattering and energy reduction, is designed with the height and the spread to construct the desired SOBP [3].

2.2.1.3 Uniform Scanning

Uniform scanning utilizes a first scatterer to scatter the beam to a slightly larger beam spot, typically several centimeters. The scanning magnets downstream in the beam line have two perpendicular sets of magnets to sweep the proton spot, with a fixed frequency (e.g., 30 Hz) across the transverse plane over a rectangular or circular (so-called wobbling) area that covers the maximum projected dimension of the target volume. Longitudinally, the target volume is covered layer by layer, usually from deep to shallow, by changing the beam energy. In one particular implementation, the energy change is achieved by building a special track on the modulator wheel but with equal length steps and equal thickness difference between subsequent steps (e.g., the outmost track in Fig. 2.5). During treatment, the modulator wheel rotates in a "step and shoot" manner to produce the desired beam energy for each corresponding scanning layer. Thin range shifters may also be used upstream to reduce further the layer spacing down to a millimeter. The beam intensity stays uniform within each layer, but relative intensities between layers are adjusted in order to produce a SOBP depth dose distribution with a dose plateau when measured in water. The second scatterer is not needed, but patient-specific field apertures/MLC and compensators are used as in passive scattering.

In both the passive-scattering and uniform-scanning treatment delivery mode, apertures are custom cut from brass (or cerroband). Brass has a high proton stopping power ratio of 5.6 to water. Some proton beam systems have utilized MLC in place of apertures. MLC can save the effort of block cutting and block mounting; however, it often has a restricted field size. The compensators are milled from a block of PMMA or wax. PMMA compensators are more rigid and transparent but non-recyclable as opposed to wax. The thickness profile of the compensator is patient beam specific and is usually calculated in the patient treatment plan and exported to the milling machine (Fig. 2.6).

Current treatment planning systems (TPS) do not usually support the calculation of beam MU values for passive-scattering treatments. The MUs are determined either from direct measurements with ion chambers in water or water equivalent materials or from analytic models with parameters derived from measured data [4]. A major disadvantage of scattering systems are that the use of compensators only conforms the dose distribution to the distal shape of the target but not the proximal side (see Fig. 2.4). It does not provide the capability to actively spare the organ at risk on the proximal side, although such dose spill can sometimes be mitigated by using multiple beam angles.

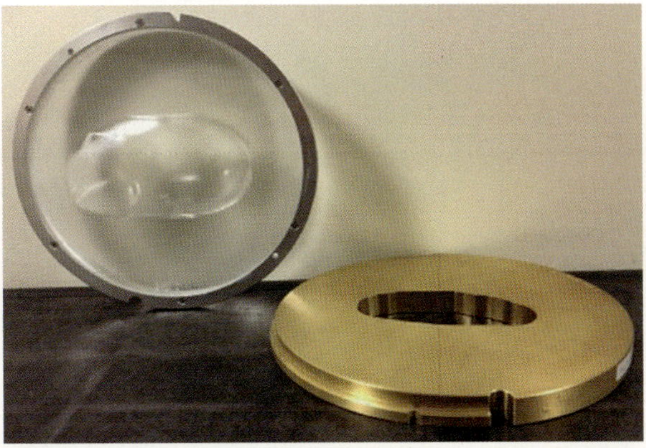

Fig. 2.6 Patient beam-specific brass aperture and PMMA compensator

The use of scatterers in the beam line results in a larger virtual source size and therefore increases the penumbra substantially. In addition, penumbra increases with the depth of penetration. During treatment, the apertures should be brought to as close to the patient as possible to reduce penumbra. The penumbra may also be slightly reduced by having the aperture cut divergently through its thickness, although such improvement is very small for systems with large SAD values (>200 cm).

2.2.2 Pencil Beam Scanning

The pencil beam scanning (PBS) technique was first introduced for patient treatment a couple of decades ago, and the technique has gone through a rapid expansion and development in the last decade. PBS is becoming the new standard technology in proton therapy, and for new centers PBS is often the only treatment modality.

In pencil beam scanning systems, two pairs of orthogonal dipole magnets (scanning magnets) are used to steer protons laterally (Fig. 2.7).

The scanning magnets sequentially direct a small size pencil beam to predetermined positions with desired intensity, i.e., the number of protons. The dose to the entire tumor is the superposition of each individual small size pencil beams. The PBS system is very complex because it requires a very fast and reliable control with adequate risk mitigation measures [5].

Proton pencil beam scanning technology naturally provides intensity-modulated proton therapy (IMPT) technique by varying the location of each pencil beam and the number of protons delivered to it. Its intensity modulation in the lateral direction is similar to IMRT. However, it also provides modulations in depth by varying proton energies, which IMRT cannot provide. As a result, PBS is capable of true 3D dose painting [6]. With the typical pencil beam size of a few mm, PBS can deliver highly conformal dose to any arbitrary shape. The IMPT technique vastly increases the proton applications in radiation therapy.

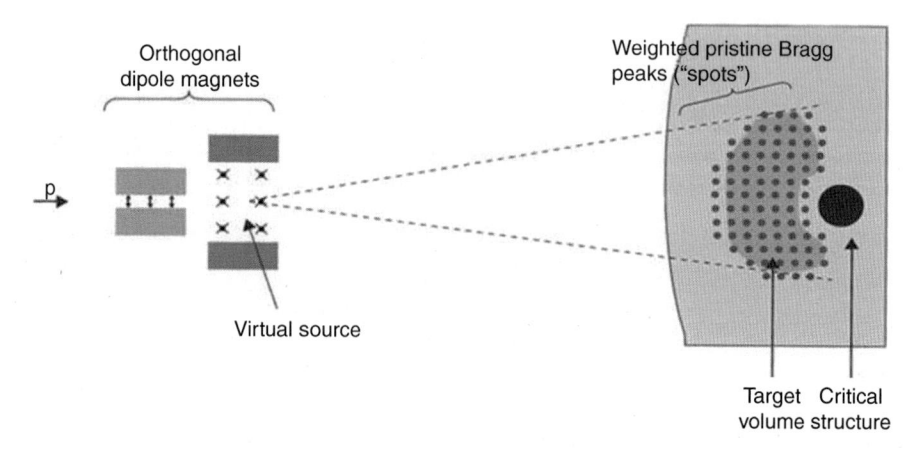

Fig. 2.7 A schematic representation of a scanning proton beam delivery system [2]

The delivery of pencil beam spots can be discrete or continuous. In continuous scanning, the beam is not turned off between spots, while in discrete spot scanning, it is completely turned off. Discrete spot scanning could avoid the transient dose uncertainties when beam moves to the next spot. However, the beam delivery is slowed due to the dead time (~several milliseconds) between spots. Although most of the current proton systems use discrete spot scanning, continuous scanning is being implemented in future systems by some manufactures.

Pencil beam scanning treatments generally do not need apertures and compensators as in passive scattering and uniform scanning. However, apertures may still be used to sharpen lateral beam penumbra, when the pencil beam spot size is too large to produce the desired dose gradient between the target volume and the organs nearby [7].

There are currently two main approaches to PBS treatment: single field optimization (SFO) technique, where each individual field uniformly covers a target, and multi-field optimization (MFO) technique, where each individual field only partially covers a target, but uniform target coverage is provided by the combination of all the fields included in the optimization. SFO and MFO are also regarded as SFUD and IMPT, respectively, in ICRU78. This book chapter uses SFUD and IMPT definition for consistency. The details of these optimization techniques and standards will be discussed in the next chapter.

Compared to passive scattering, pencil beam scanning has the following major advantages:

- Delivers 3D conformal dose to tumor in a single beam: distally, proximally and laterally (refer to treatment planning section).
- Reduces target dose heterogeneity due to presence of severe tissue heterogeneity, for example, in the treatment of head and neck cancers.
- Neutron production in air is significantly reduced due to the absence of beam-modifying hardware in the beam line.
- Eliminates time and resources required for the use of apertures and compensators.

Since each PBS beam is composed of thousands of individual spots, the final accuracy of the dose delivered to patient relies on how accurately each spot is delivered. The typical parameters that affect the dose accuracy are the spot position, spot shape, and the number of protons of each spot. For the scanning beam, it is very important to have a reliable and rapid-response control system that could deliver each spot to the desired position with the correct number of protons. Physicists design various quality assurance (QA) procedures to validate the system performance and patient-specific treatment delivery.

2.3 Imaging for Proton Beam Therapy

A variety of patient-specific imaging techniques are routinely used or still under development for planning, image guidance, or verification of proton treatment, which are summarized in Table 2.1. All the imaging techniques can be simply

Table 2.1 Summary of imaging techniques for proton therapy

Type of imaging	Application	Routine practice	Advantage	Challenges
CT	Anatomic structure delineation; dose and range calculation	Yes	High resolution; high bone-tissue contrast; anatomical imaging; fast acquisition time	Requires proton stopping power calibration; uncertainties due to calibration and CT artifacts translate to the proton beam range uncertainties
Dual-energy CT	Tissue decomposition	No	Increase the accuracy of the proton range calculation	Theoretical improvements in range predictions with DECT data in the order of 0.1–2.1% were observed [9]
MRI	Anatomic structure delineation	Yes	High spatial resolution and soft tissue contrast	Possible geometric distortion; direct use for dose calculation still under investigation
PET (for PET/CT)	Target volume delineation and identification	Yes	High sensitivity	Limited anatomic resolution and need to combine with CT
CT on-rails	Patient positioning; treatment verification	Yes	High resolution; fast acquisition time; allows adaptive planning and treatment	Require extra space in the treatment room; increase patient in-room time; unable to assess intra-fractional motion
Orthogonal kV planar imaging	2D patient positioning	Yes	High image quality especially for bone-tissue contrast	Low soft tissue contrast
CBCT	3D patient positioning; treatment verification	Yes	High spatial resolution of soft tissue	Poor image quality compared to CT, potential value for dose calculation and adaptive therapy under investigation
Optical imaging	Patient surface tracking and positioning	Yes	Fast, high sensitivity and real time acquisition; no radiation dose; large field of view; ideal for superficial target	No visualization of internal anatomy and relies on surrogates rather than target itself; skin needs to be visible and may have clearance issue
PET (treatment activated)	3D verification of treatment delivery	Only at limited institutions	In vivo verification of treatment	Require short time delay between treatment and imaging; reduced signals due to limitations of the imaging protocol (e.g., biological washout et al.)

2 Proton Treatment Delivery Techniques

Table 2.1 (continued)

Type of imaging	Application	Routine practice	Advantage	Challenges
Prompt gamma	Verification of proton ranges	No	In vivo verification of treatment; no biological washout effect	Require bulky equipment for signal collimation and detection. Clinical value remain to be demonstrated
Proton radiography and proton CT	Planning and treatment verification	No	Direct measurement of proton stopping power	Require high proton energy sufficient to penetrate the patient; limited spatial resolution due to multiple coulomb scattering

divided into three groups based on their purposes of applications. The first group including CT, MRI, and PET/CT is mainly used for structure delineation and dose calculation, which is very similar to photon/electron therapy. Since CT data does not provide directly proton stopping power ratio (SPR) required for proton dose calculation, a calibration procedure is required to establish the relationship between CT HU values and proton SPR. However, uncertainties in the HU to SPR calibration exist, and these uncertainties eventually translate to range uncertainties that have to be carefully accounted for during the planning stage [8]. Dual-energy CT improves the SPR production and has the potential to reduce the range uncertainties associated with HU to SPR calibration [9, 10]. However, more studies and evaluations are needed for future implementation in routine clinic. The second group is mainly used for patient alignment, verification of the treatment position before each treatment, and adaptive planning. It includes techniques such as orthogonal kV, CBCT, CT on rails, body surface imaging, etc. The third group includes particle therapy unique imaging techniques such as proton radiography, proton CT [11], treatment-activated PET imaging [12], or prompt gamma [13] imaging, many of which are in the process of being adopted or under development for the purpose of range and dose verification. Since the anatomical and physiological variations have greater impact on the proton dosimetry compared to their impact on the photon dosimetry, imaging may be frequently repeated during the proton treatment course for monitoring and validating the treatment.

Successful proton treatment delivery requires reproducible patient positioning during daily treatment. IGRT is essential for patient positioning and placement of devices used for treatment such as immobilization devices. Immobilization devices in the beam path should be considered consistently through simulation, planning, and treatment in terms of their locations and physical properties.

- Devices intersecting beam paths during treatment should be homogeneous, indexed, and included in the proton dose calculation during the planning stage; devices present during CT simulation, but not during treatment, should be excluded from the body contour for proton dose calculation. Couch overlay should be utilized consistently with what is planned.

- Any HU override for devices and artifacts during the planning stage should be carefully evaluated on a case by case basis. Inappropriate override of HU can lead to significant dose errors.
- Immobilization devices should be indexed to the treatment couch top when they are positioned in the treatment area or whenever possible.
- Partial beam blocking by any devices (couch, bolus et al.) is difficult to reproduce and should be avoided (e.g., large-angle posterior oblique field passing through the couch edge).
- Positions of range shifter and bolus should be minimized and consistent with those in planning. Air gaps between device and patient should be confirmed routinely. Air gaps between the range shifter (or bolus) and the patient should be kept the same to maintain the spot profile. The couch top is generally made of uniform low-density material, but some institutions have purposely used thicker substitutes as range shifters for spot-scanning treatment.

2.4 Intra-fractional Motion Management for Proton Therapy

The management of intra-fractional target motion during proton therapy depends on the specific proton treatment technique.

- Passively scattered proton beams are more akin to 3D photon treatment techniques in the sense that the whole treatment field is delivered simultaneously. A modified ITV concept ensuring that the target is covered during all motion phases may be used to provide sufficient target coverage. The variations in WET due to intra-fractional motion may be accounted for in the compensator design. Kang et al. described the treatment planning strategies for mobile lung tumors treated by passively scattered proton beams. A 4D CT scan is used to derive the internal gross tumor volume (IGTV). For planning purposes the average CT scan is used; however, the IGTV volume density is overwritten with uniform density value of 100HU [14] or established based on the average ICTV HU values for each case.
- The use of pencil beam scanning presents a different challenge in the sense that it is more akin to IMRT because only subsections of the target volume are treated at any given time. The dynamics of the treatment delivery and a moving target can lead to interplay effects that need to be assessed and managed.

For either delivery technique, it is beneficial to restrict the amount of motion during beam delivery. Abdominal compression as well as gating have been successfully employed by some groups during proton therapy treatments [15, 16].

On the other hand, it is unlikely that a target in motion can be managed to a degree that it can be treated as stationary.

- For unmanaged or a given residual motion, it is of interest to assess the dosimetric impact of the target motion. This simulation requires accurate knowledge and synchronization of the proton delivery dynamics and moving patient anatomy. A number of research groups have developed in-house simulators to assess the dosimetric impact of motion [15, 17]. The dosimetric impact depends on the timing of the treatment with respect to the breathing phases. While researchers demonstrated that the dosimetric effect of a single fraction delivery can be concerning, it has also been demonstrated that the dosimetric effect averages out quickly after the delivery of several fractions [17, 18]. However, the effect is treatment site and patient specific.
- The cumulative dosimetric effect of target motion after the completion of a fractionated course of treatment is of interest has been investigated. Using a realistic interplay simulator, Li et al. showed that after the delivery of a regular fractionated treatment, the cumulative dose distribution approaches that of the 4D dose distribution [17]. The latter is obtained by recalculating the nominal plan into each 4DCT phase and accumulating the dose distributions from the individual phases onto the nominal treatment planning CT using deformable image registration. The calculation of the 4D dose does not require an interplay simulator and is relatively easy to implement in commercial treatment planning systems.
- The magnitude of the dosimetric effect will be a function of plan and patient parameters.
  - Grassberger et al. reported that the dosimetric effect of motion is reduced with increasing spot size [18]. While the spot size is typically not variable for a given scanning nozzle, it can be manipulated by the use of external range shifters and by varying the air gap between the range shifter and the patient's skin.
  - Grassberger et al. reported an increase of the motion effect with motion magnitude.
  - Li et al. reported that motion effects may be enhanced if the CTV is small with respect to motion magnitude [17].
  - With respect to dose modulation, Dowell et al. report that the amount of dose modulation for targets that moved less than 20 mm had no significant effect [19].
  - Zeng et al. [20, 21] report that for single-beam PBS treatments of mediastinal lymphomas, the cumulative dosimetric degradation (D98%) was less than 2% and up to 5% for single factions. Actual breathing phases as measured at time of 4DCT were used for this simulation.
- Other groups have investigated modified delivery techniques to make spot-scanning plans more robust against intra-fractional motion.
  - Repaint the target volume, i.e., each spot location is revisited by the scanning beam multiple times which is a widely discussed option. In general two techniques have been developed. In the first technique, termed layered repainting, each energy layer is repainted several times until all MUs are delivered. This is repeated for each subsequent layer. In the second

technique, termed volumetric repainting, the complete target is painted multiple times [22]. A disadvantage of the techniques is that each volumetric repaint requires each energy layer to be revisited. This will increase the treatment time and hampers the use of this technique for systems that have a longer layer switching times. The latter technique is, however, relatively simple to implement by increasing the fractionations by multiples of n. Each repainting technique however has to account for machine delivery limitations such as the minimum MU per spot limit. A spot which is planned to deliver MUs close to the minimum MU cannot be repainted with either method. To manage these machine limitations various refined repainting techniques have been reported.

- In a recent publication Li et al. investigated a spot sequence optimization technique to increase the plan's robustness against motion. The spot map delivery was altered to increase the distance between subsequent spot deliveries [23]. This sparser delivery sequence resulted in more robust plans.
- Motion robust treatment planning techniques have also been developed. Yu et al. reported the use of 4D robustness optimization in conjunction with beam angle optimization [24]. For 4D optimization, plans were robustly optimized on multiple 4D CT phases. In addition beam angles were evaluated for changes in WET with respiration and angles with minimal changes in WET were selected for treatment planning.

To summarize, the dosimetric impact of motion on proton therapy treatments has been studied widely for proton plans. While no single solution has emerged, multiple techniques have been reported to be useful for target motion management during proton therapy.

2.5 Proton Beam Therapy Systems and Specifications

In recent decades, due to the increasing demands for proton beam therapy, many manufacturers have started to join the market. So far, there are many proton system configurations, techniques, and combinations developed to fit the needs of various institutions. In the meanwhile, proton beam therapy technology has continued to evolve rapidly. The goal of this section is to summarize the clinical systems currently available commercially to provide the reader with a brief account of the important machine parameters and characteristics which could have a significant clinical impact on treatment and protocol development. The clinical parameters quoted in Table 2.2 are based on proton centers actively treating patients as of May 2016 (Tables 2.3 and 2.4).

Table 2.2 The summary of proton system specifications in clinical operation

Manufacture	Model	Accelerator type	Clinical beam ranges	Treatment room options	IGRT system	Treatment modality
IBA	ProteusPlus	Cyclotron	32.0 g/cm^2; 4.1 g/cm^2	Fix beam line, inclined gantry, and full gantry	2D orthogonal imaging; CBCT; CT on rail	PBS[a], US[b], DS[b], SS[b]
IBA	ProteusONE	Superconducting synchrocyclotron	32.0 g/cm^2; 4.1 g/cm^2	220° compact single-room gantry	Stereotactic imaging; CBCT	PBS only
VARIAN	ProBeam	Superconducting cyclotron	36.0 g/cm^2; 4.1 g/cm^2	Fix beam line and full gantry	2-D orthogonal imaging; CBCT	PBS only
HITACHI	ProBEAT	Synchrotron	32.4 g/cm^2; 4.0 g/cm^2	Fix beam line, 180° gantry, and full gantry	2-D orthogonal imaging; CT on rail	PBS, US, DS, SS
Mevion	S250	Superconducting synchrocyclotron	32.0 g/cm^2; 5.0 g/cm^2	180° compact single-room gantry	2-D orthogonal imaging; CT on rail (planned)	DS
Sumitomo	P235	Cyclotron	32.0 g/cm^2; 3.8 g/cm^2	Full gantry	2D orthogonal imaging; CBCT (planned)	US, DS, PBS

PBS Pencil Beam Scanning treatment delivery technique; *US* Universal-scanning treatment delivery technique; *SS* Single-scattering treatment delivery technique
DS Double-scattering treatment delivery technique

[a]PBS Pencil Beam Scanning treatment delivery technique
[b]DS Double-scattering treatment delivery technique

Table 2.3 Pencil Beam Scanning clinical parameters (spot scanning)

Parameters	Clinical significance	Most common values
Maximum field size	The maximum lateral dimension of the target that can be treated without using multi-iso fields	From 20×24 cm^2 to 30×40 cm^2
Energy layer switch time (ELST)	A major factor of spot-scanning beam delivery efficiency	Cyclotron <1 s synchrotron 1 ~ 2 s
Spot switch time	A minor factor of spot-scanning beam delivery efficiency	2–10 ms
Spot size (1 sigma in air)	The lateral penumbra of the dose distribution	2.2–4.4 mm at 32 g/cm
Spot symmetry	The quality and consistency of the proton beam for all gantry angles and energies	10%
Spot position accuracy	The quality and consistency of the proton beam position accuracy for all gantry angles and energies	1 mm
Length of time for irradiating a 1 L target to a uniform dose of 2 Gy	Overall estimation of the treatment delivery efficiency of a proton system	30–120 s
Remote air gap tuner	Capable of adjusting air gap between range shifter to patient' skin in order to optimize the spot size for the treatment	Continuous/fixed/discrete position
Room switch time (RST)	The operation efficiency of a multiroom proton therapy center	10–60 s

Table 2.4 Passive-scattering clinical parameters

Parameters	Clinical significance	Most common values
Maximum field size	The maximum lateral dimension of the target that can be treated without using multi-iso fields	15 cm; 25 cm diameter (DS); 30×40 cm (US)
Dose rate	Major factor of passive-scattering beam delivery efficiency	2 Gy/min; 1 Gy/min
Number of modulation wheels and options	Number of combinations of SOBP and beam range	14 modulator wheels, 24 options (Mevion) 3 modulator wheels and 8 options (IBA)
Modulation wheel warm up time before irradiation	A minor factor of passive-scattering beam delivery efficiency	30–60s
Collimation system	Manual or auto configuration of the beam lateral shape	MLC/brass aperture
Room switch time (RST)	The operation efficiency of a multiroom proton therapy center	10–60s

2.6 Quality Assurance (QA)

2.6.1 System QA

A detailed and comprehensive physics QA protocol is needed to ensure system performance and patient safety. Table 2.5 summarizes the major mechanical and dosimetry-related QA items and procedures of most common proton therapy systems. It includes the daily, weekly, monthly, and annual QA items followed by a

Table 2.5 QA tasks and procedures for proton therapy systems

Items	Frequency	Description	Measurement devices
Beam dosimetry parameters for PBS			
Output	Daily; monthly; annually	*Purpose*: verify monitor chambers' integrity and reliability, as well as beam characteristics and fluence consistency *Method*: measure the beam output at the center of modulation (the center of the SOBP) using a broad uniform field. Criteria: 2%	Cylindrical farmer type; parallel plate ionization chamber (PPIC) Fig. 2.8a
Range	Daily; monthly; annually	*Purpose*: verify the stability of the machine for delivering predetermined beam energies *Method*: range of individual spots and a uniform large field. Commonly used phantoms with varying thickness, e.g., a custom-made wedge phantom Criteria: 1 mm	PPIC with scanning water tank; multilayer ionization chamber (MLIC) Fig. 2.8b
Dose flatness and symmetry	Daily; monthly, annually	*Purpose*: verify beam stability and reproducibility of the beam optics at nominal and all gantry angles *Method*: measure 2D dose distributions and compare with commissioning data in TPS Criteria: 1%	Scintillator/CCD camera system; ion chamber array; film
Distal dose falloff	Monthly; annually	*Purpose*: verify the constancy of beam energy spread which could affect the integral depth dose distributions (IDDD) *Method*: measure depth dose distributions Criteria: 1 mm	PPIC with scanning water tank; multilayer ionization chamber (MLIC) (may be combined with range check procedure)
Spot profile	Daily; monthly; annually	*Purpose*: verify spot profile consistency. *Method*: measure individual spot profile Criteria: 10% (1-sigma)	Film, ion chamber array, strip chambers, or scintillator/CCD detecting system. (Fig. 2.8c)

(continued)

Table 2.5 (continued)

Items	Frequency	Description	Measurement devices
Spot position	Daily; monthly; annually	*Purpose*: verify spot position accuracy *Methods*: deliver several sets of spot pattern and verify their positions Criteria: 1 mm	Film, ion chamber array (Fig. 2.8d), strip chambers, or scintillator/CCD detecting system (can be combined with spot profile procedure)
Pencil beam depth dose distribution	Annually	*Purpose*: verify integral dose of the pencil beam at different depths *Method*: measure depth dose using a Bragg peak ion chamber in a water tank equipped with scanning capabilities	Bragg peak ion chamber
Spot angular-spatial distribution and lateral dose profiles	Annually	*Purpose*: verify spot dose lateral profiles and at different depths *Methods*: measure individual spot profile Criteria: 20% (spot symmetry)	Film, small volume ion chambers, scintillator/CCD camera system
Inverse square correction test	Annually	*Purpose*: verify the distance of the point of measurement for broad fields from the "effective source" position *Method*: measure dose with an ionization chamber at different distances relative to isocenter and compare it with the predicted dose using the inverse square correction factor	2D ion chamber array
Monitor chamber linearity, reproducibility, and min/max checks	Annually	*Purpose*: verify linearity, reproducibility, minimum and maximum dose criteria of the monitor chambers for PBS delivery *Method*: measure dose by decreasing/increasing the intensity of spots to the tolerance levels Criteria: 1%	PPIC
	Patient setup verification		
Laser	Daily	*Purpose*: verify the laser-projected position relative to isocenter of the imaging system *Method*: position a phantom with fiducials at isocenter using the imaging system and verify the laser projections on the phantom Criteria: 1 mm	IGRT phantom (Fig. 2.8f)

2 Proton Treatment Delivery Techniques

Table 2.5 (continued)

Items	Frequency	Description	Measurement devices
IGRT system	Daily; monthly	*Purpose*: verify imaging system vs. radiation isocenter, as well as imaging quality *Method*: position IGRT phantom at isocenter using the imaging system and deliver proton beam at center of the field Criteria: 1 mm	IGRT phantom (combined with laser check procedure)
Communication and interface	Daily	*Purpose*: verify the interface between delivery and IGRT system and record and verification system *Method*: load a plan, acquire images, deliver treatment beams, and send records back to record and verification system. Check if all images and delivered dose are recorded	The procedure should be tested in treatment mode during one of daily QA testing items
Safety	Daily	Audiovisual monitor; visual monitor; beam-on indicator; X-ray on indicator; search/clear button; beam pause button; emergency beam stop button, monitor units interlocks; collision interlocks; radiation monitor system (neutron or X-ray); door interlock	N/A
Emergency stop	Monthly	*Purpose*: verify the emergency-stop buttons stop not only the mechanical movements but also the particle and/or the X-ray radiation	N/A
Mechanical systems			
Gantry angle vs. gantry angle indicators	Weekly	*Purpose*: verify the accuracy of the gantry angle as indicated on the gantry angle indicators or digital readout Criteria: 1°	Digital level
Snout extension	Weekly	*Purpose*: verify the mechanical accuracy of the snout positions with respect to the treatment plan Criteria: 1 mm	Meter stick
Collision sensors	Weekly	*Purpose*: check nozzle and imaging component collision sensors functionality	N/A
Couch positional	Weekly	*Purpose*: verify the accuracy of couch position with respect to treatment plan; normally 6° of freedom Criteria: 1 mm	Meter stick and digital level

(continued)

Table 2.5 (continued)

Items	Frequency	Description	Measurement devices
Gantry radiation Isocentricity	Monthly; annually	*Purpose*: verify the radiation isocenter accuracy with respect to the gantry angles *Method*: gantry star shot technique for central beam axis Criteria: 1 mm	Film Fig. 2.8h; XRV-100 Fig. 2.8f
Couch Isocentricity	Monthly; annually	*Purpose*: verify the radiation isocenter accuracy with respect to the couch rotations *Method*: couch star shot technique for central beam axis Criteria: 1 mm	Film
Additional QA items for passive-scattering systems			
SOBP width	Monthly; annually	*Purpose*: verify beam extraction and intensity that synchronized with the rotation of the modulator wheel in order to produce flat SOBPs *Method*: measure depth dose distributions for specified SOBP fields covering all options, that is, the use of the all beam-modifying components for SOBP construction Criteria: 1 mm	PPC with scanning water tank system; multilayer ionization chamber (MLIC) (can be combined with range check procedure)
Multi-leaf collimator	Monthly; annually	*Purpose*: alignments; leaf position; activation; interlock functionality	Survey meters; film
MLC leakage	Monthly; annually	*Purpose*: verify the requirements for the leakage dose from intraleaf, interleaf, leaf-end, leaf banks, and other MLC components *Method*: use the highest proton energy to check the leakage	Film

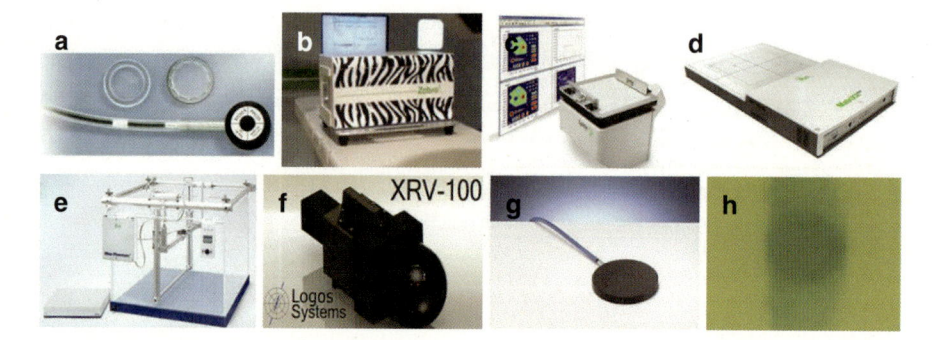

Fig. 2.8 Dosimetry equipments. (**a**) Parallel plate ion chamber: PPC05. (**b**) Multilayer ionization chamber: Zebra (IBA, Belgium). (**c**) Scintillator/CCD camera detector: Lynx (IBA, Belgium). (**d**) 2D ion chamber array: MatriXX (IBA, Belgium). (**e**) Water tank: Blue phantom 2 (IBA, Belgium). (**f**) IGRT phantom for PBS QA: XRV-100 (Logos Systems International, Scotts Valley, CA). (**g**) Bragg Peak Chamber: PTW (Freiburg GmbH). (**h**) Radiochromic films (Ashland, NJ)

brief description of the procedure and measurement devices required. Detailed IGRT QA procedures are not included here, since IGRT systems for proton therapy are in rapid transition, for example, toward volumetric imaging. CBCT for proton treatment has just been implemented at the University of Pennsylvania in 2015, and several centers have started using CT on rails recently. For 2D orthogonal imaging systems, interested readers may consult corresponding sections in AAPM task force report 142 (TG142) on image guidance in external beam therapy.

2.6.2 Patient-Specific QA (PSQA)

Patient-specific quality assurance (PSQA) has been one of the most important programs in radiation therapy workflows to ensure the accuracy of dose delivery for each treatment plan prior to the patient's treatment. Similar to clinical practice in QA procedures for intensity-modulated radiation therapy (IMRT), PSQA for proton therapy includes (1) absolute dose verification and (2) dose distribution verification. One major difference between IMRT and proton therapy is that the latter uses much fewer fields for each treatment fraction. In many cases, a single treatment field is sufficient to produce the satisfactory fractional dose distribution. Even in the case of IMPT multi-field optimizations for pencil beam scanning, the number of fields required is usually two to four, compared to IMRT where most treatments use five or more. As a result, PSQA for proton treatment has been conducted for each field, even in the case of IMPT, rather than for the composite dose from all fields as in the case of IMRT QA. This also results from the lack of reliable and efficient techniques for measuring three-dimensional dose distributions. Such QA measurement techniques, e.g., 3D gel dosimetry, are still not feasible for routine clinical practice due to various limitations. Overall, given the ongoing development of new treatment delivery, planning, and measurement techniques, PSQA for proton beam therapy is in the stage of rapid evolution and no gold standard exists currently for procedures and guidelines. The purpose of this section is therefore limited to providing a general idea about the most common PSQA procedures and dosimetry tools used at different institutions.

2.6.2.1 PSQA for Pencil Beam Scanning

As mentioned above, two types of optimization techniques are used for planning PBS treatment, SFUD, and IMPT. Treatment fields obtained from both techniques have modulated beam energies and intensities and generally do not produce homogeneous dose distributions in a phantom, creating challenges for measurements, although understandably substantially more so for IMPT than SFUD fields.

SFUD QA

SFUD is often used where the target is simple, and no critical organs at risk (OARs) are present along the beam path such as prostate cancer. A very comprehensive SFUD PSQA procedure based on prostate planning has been published by Zhu et al. [25]. The procedure includes three parts, (1) point dose verification, (2) central axis depth dose verification, and (3) relative 2D dose measurements, as listed in Table 2.6.

Table 2.6 An example of PSQA components for SFUD fields

Items	Procedure	Dosimetry device
Point dose verification	*Purpose*: (1) an end-to-end test of data transfer integrity from the TPS to the scanning beam accelerator control system (ACS); (2) verify the beam steering magnets are working properly for different gantry angles; (3) uploading of the required bending magnet field strengths *Methods*: measure point dose in the mid-SOBP position	MatriXX; PPC05; solid water phantom; scanning water tank
Central axis depth dose verification	*Purpose*: verification of spot energy and position and dose calculation by the TPS *Methods*: measure point dose at several depths (Fig. 2.9a)	MatriXX; PPC05; solid water phantom; scanning water tank
Relative 2D dose measurements	*Purpose*: 2D dose measurement at multiple depths allows detection of potentially large errors in spot lateral position as well as TPS dose modeling *Methods*: use 2D ion chamber array detector to measure three depths within the SOBP (proximal, middle, and distal). The γ-index was used for comparison of 2D dose distribution with a requirement of a 3% dose or 3-mm distance to agreement (Fig. 2.9b)	MatriXX; solid water phantom; (Fig. 2.10 is the example of 2D dose distribution comparison of RT and LT prostate fields)

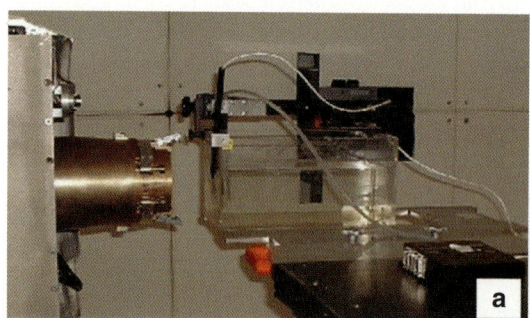

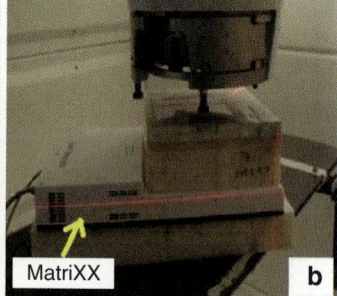

Fig. 2.9 (a) Rectangular water phantoms for depth dose measurements. (b) MatriXX 2D ion chamber array detector with plastic water phantoms

The average time based on this comprehensive PSQA procedure for each patient's plan was approximately 2 h for all three types of measurements and data analysis. For a busy center running 16-h treatment days and thus on average five new plans to start daily, it requires significant QA beam time after treatment and weekends. Therefore, it is highly desirable to simplify the procedure and improve the efficiency of PSQA. In most clinics today, measurements at the exact treatment gantry angle are not always performed due to the complicated workflow which requires a special couch mount device to hold heavy solid water and the MatriXX detector. Lomax et al. reported PSI's QA experiences using orthogonal dose profiles acquired by an ionization chamber array, typically at two different depths in water

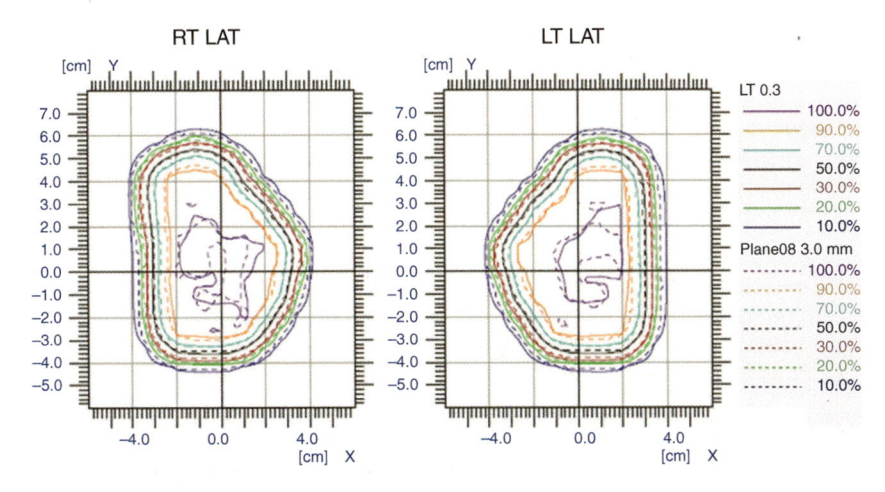

Fig. 2.10 Comparison of the two-dimensional dose distribution for a prostate proton SFUD plan at a depth of 23.4 cm. *Solid lines* indicate measurements obtained using MatriXX detector, and *dashed lines* indicate calculations obtained using the treatment planning system. (**a**) Right lateral field, (**b**) left lateral field

Fig. 2.11 Setup photo of DigiPhant with beam coming from the left (*red arrow*). The detector array automatically stops and acquires data at multiple programmed locations within the water tank during measurements (Permission pending IBA dosimetry)

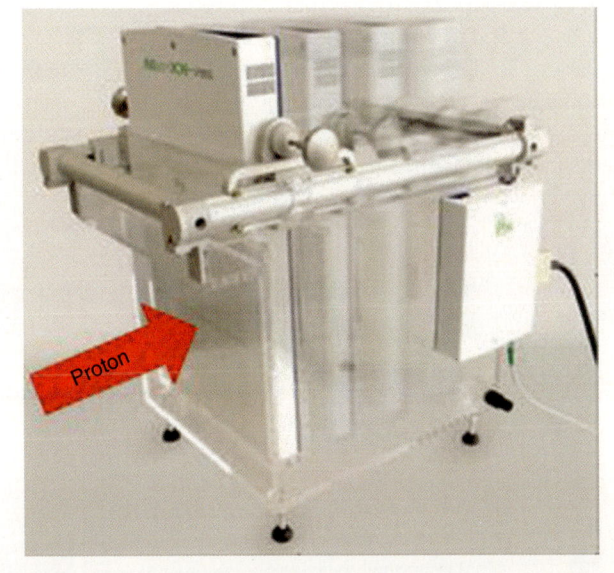

[6]. Lin et al. [26] investigated the feasibility of using a waterproof housing to hold the MatriXX that is scanned in a water phantom (DigiPhant, IBA dosimetry) (Fig. 2.11). This new dosimetry tool could combine point dose, depth dose, and 2D dose distribution in one setup and significantly reduce the time and QA workload. Unfortunately such QA tools are not able to verify the gantry dependent parameters, e.g., current settings of all bending and steering magnets.

To further reduce the PSQA workload, Mackin et al. proposed a second-check dose calculation engine, HPlusQA. The study concluded that it could reduce the need for PSQA measurement by 64%. Zhu et al. [27] suggested incorporating both independent dose calculation and treatment log file analysis to reduce the time required for measurements.

IMPT QA

IMPT is most often used in situations with complex patient anatomy and target, e.g., head and neck, CNS, and thoracic/GI. Compared to SFUD, each field in an IMPT plan is highly modulated in both energy and spot position. Although the principles of PSQA procedures are very similar to SFUD, they require more measurements and more detailed analysis. To the best of our knowledge, there is still no publication on comprehensive PSQA procedures for IMPT yet. In some institutions, IMPT field is normally measured in more different depths compared to SFUD. At MD Anderson, HPlusQA is implemented for IMPT PSQA as well.

Range Shifter Effects on PSQA for PBS

Range shifters (RS) are used often in PBS treatments for shallow targets, e.g., HNC and CNS. Beam modeling of RS is a separated option in some TPS. The QA result might be affected by the air gap and beam modeling. Initial result reported by Mackin et al. [17] suggested that the dose algorithm in certain planning system is accurately modeling the dose from the secondary radiation but not so for the effects on the distal falloff.

2.6.2.2 PSQA for Passive-Scattering

Passive-scattering beam delivery involves more hardware and system configurations compared to spot-scanning beam delivery, such as apertures, compensators, and the beam options with the specific scatterer settings, modulation wheels, etc. For each treatment field, apertures and compensators were manually checked; apertures must match with the treatment plan; compensator thickness tolerance is 0.5 mm (see Fig. 2.12). To make the process more quantitative and comprehensive, Yoon et al. [28]

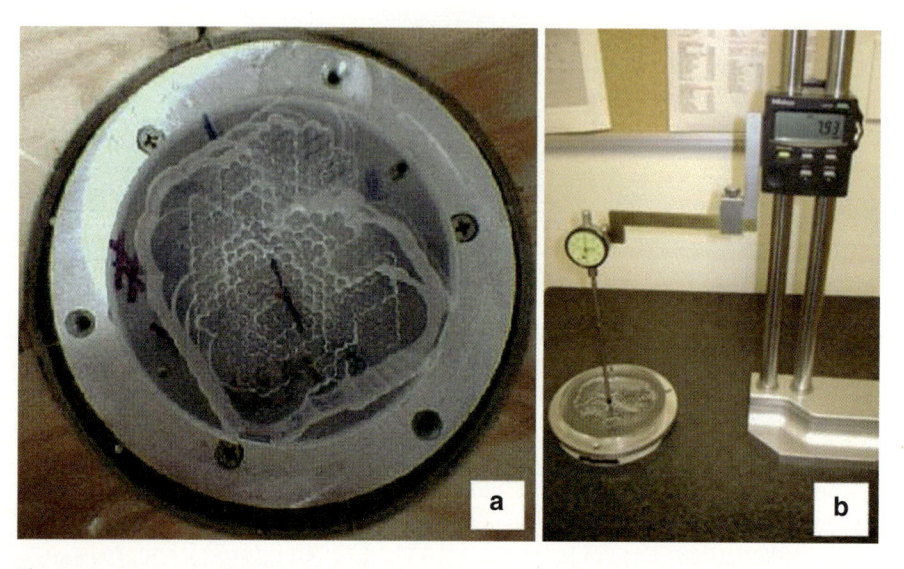

Fig. 2.12 (a) An example of an actual compensator used for proton beam treatment. (b) The device used to verify the thickness manually by measuring the height relative to the surface for a single-sided compensator

2 Proton Treatment Delivery Techniques

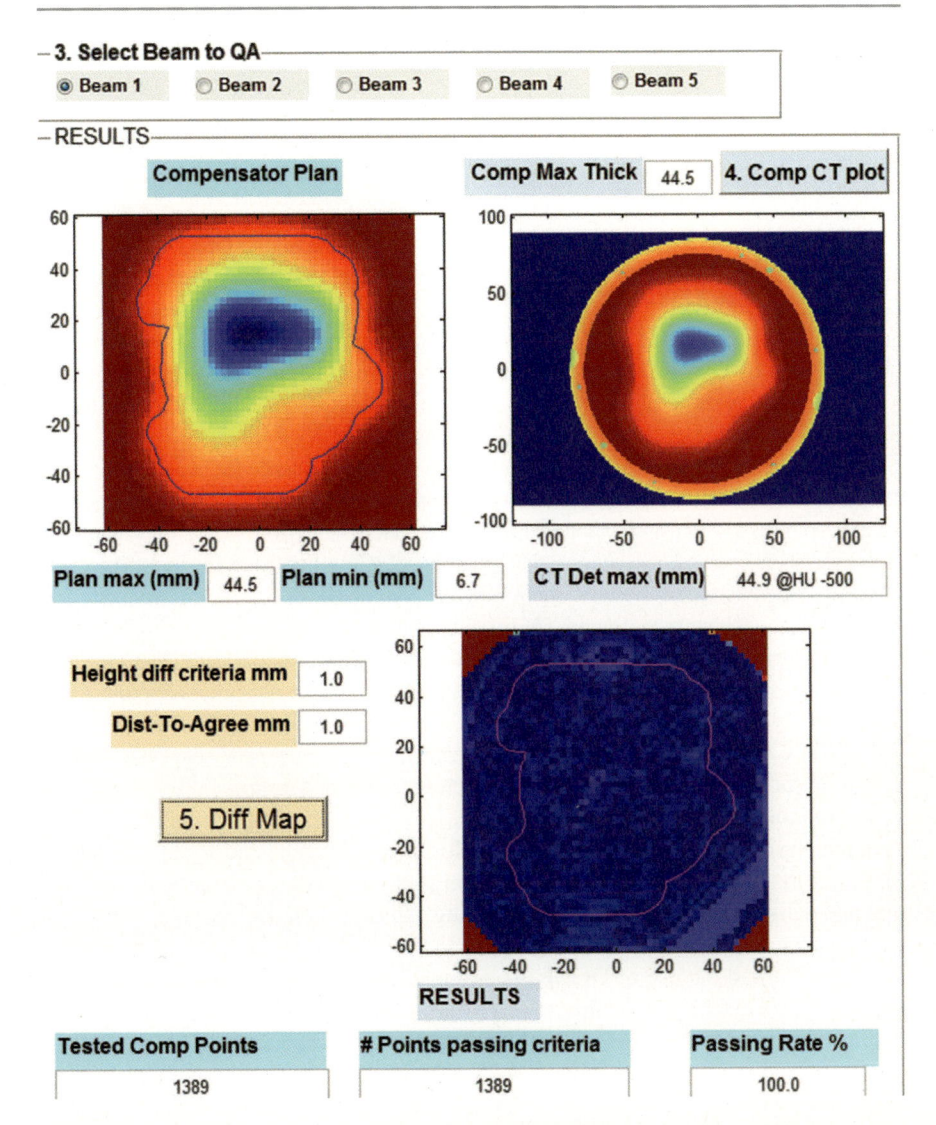

Fig. 2.13 User interface of an in-house developed compensator QA software based on CT image of the compensator at the Robert Wood Johnson Cancer Institute

suggested using CT to assess the quality of the compensator instead of the manual measurement. Figure 2.13 shows the workflow and user interface for the CT-based compensator QA method used at the Robert Wood Johnson Cancer Institute.

As described above, current TPS systems do not generally support the calculation of beam MU values for PS. The MUs are determined from measurements with ion chamber in water or water equivalent materials. Normally absolute dose is checked through measurement in the center of SOBP using a water tank or solid water combining with the PPC or ion chamber array. An analytic model based secondary check system is generally used.

2.7 Future Developments

Proton beam therapy technique has been advancing rapidly within this decade. Considering that PBS treatment technology became commercially available only less than 10 years ago [1], it is remarkable that nearly all new proton centers now are configured with a PBS only technique. However, treating moving targets remains the biggest challenge for PBS technique, owing to the interplay effects, as described above [6, 18, 20, 22–24]. A number of delivery techniques have been proposed to compensate the interplay effects by using, e.g., repainting [29], breath-holding [30], gating [31], and tracking [31]. Some of these techniques have been successfully implemented by certain vendors in some clinics. We are expecting more new techniques as well as more clinical data coming in the next decades to demonstrate the feasibility and value of treating moving tumors with PBS.

Another area with rapid improvement expected is image guidance for treatment, specifically the use of volumetric imaging. Although proton therapy once led the way to image guidance in radiotherapy by using orthogonal X-rays for patient setup from the very beginning, in recent years it fell behind conventional therapy where CBCT is now routinely used. The value of volumetric imaging has been recognized by the community of particle therapy now, and adoption of this technique has started. The first CBCT for proton system was just implemented commercially at the Roberts Proton Therapy Center at the University of Pennsylvania in 2015 which opens a new area of precise patient positioning and dose evaluation to improve treatment accuracy [32]. The use of in-room CT, or CT on rails, is another approach taken by certain vendors. Daily CT-/CBCT-based dose calculation and treatment adaptation should become a routine treatment option to further improve treatment outcomes [32].

Beam range uncertainties in patients have always been a major challenge to utilizing the full potential of the proton beam for target coverage and organ avoidance. Major efforts have been focused on increasing accuracy of the proton range calculation and delivery by using innovative imaging and detection devices such as prompt gamma camera [13], ultrasound detectors [33, 34], PET imaging [35], proton beam imaging [36] and the use of DECT [9]. Some of these new imaging techniques are expected to be clinical available soon. A prompt gamma camera system is currently in clinical testing at the University of Pennsylvania.

The technique of volumetric-modulated arc therapy (VMAT) has been widely used in photon therapy, with significantly shorter treatment time and possibly improved dose distribution when compared to standard intensity-modulated radiation therapy using static fields. It is a natural question if proton arc therapy can also improve dose distributions and robustness given the well-known issues of beam range uncertainty, anatomical variations, distal-end RBE uncertainties, limitations of spot sizes, etc. Exploration in this direction has started recently. Ding et al. proposed a novel spot-scanning proton arc (SPArc) algorithm to generate a robust, delivery-efficient and continuous proton arc plan, showing a promising dosimetric improvement over current IMPT technique especially in the reduction of integral dose and target conformity with comparable delivery time [37]. It is demonstrated for the first time that the concept of proton arc therapy could be clinical valuable and feasible through continuous delivery. Although implementing such treatment technique will need to overcome tough technical challenges, some of which may be more difficult than ever, efforts in this direction are expected to continue.

References

1. Smith A, Gillin M, Bues M, et al. The M. D. Anderson proton therapy system. Med Phys. 2009;36:4068–83.
2. Christopher G. Ainsley, James McDonough. Physics considerations in proton therapy. Radiation medicine rounds: proton therapy. C. Thomas and J. Metz (eds). Demos Medical Publishing LLC; New York: 2010.
3. Akagi T, Higashi A, Tsugami H, et al. Ridge filter design for proton therapy at Hyogo Ion Beam Medical Center. Phys Med Biol. 2003;48:N301–12.
4. Kooy HM, Schaefer M, Rosenthal S, et al. Monitor unit calculations for range-modulated spread-out Bragg peak fields. Phys Med Biol. 2003;48:2797–808.
5. Gillin MT, Sahoo N, Bues M, et al. Commissioning of the discrete spot scanning proton beam delivery system at the University of Texas M.D. Anderson Cancer Center, Proton Therapy Center, Houston. Med Phys. 2010;37:154–63.
6. Lomax AJ. Intensity modulated proton therapy and its sensitivity to treatment uncertainties 2: the potential effects of inter-fraction and inter-field motions. Phys Med Biol. 2008;53:1043–56.
7. Wang D, Dirksen B, Hyer DE, et al. Impact of spot size on plan quality of spot scanning proton radiosurgery for peripheral brain lesions. Med Phys. 2014;41:121705.
8. Ainsley CG, Yeager CM. Practical considerations in the calibration of CT scanners for proton therapy. J Appl Clin Med Phys. 2014;15:4721.
9. Hünemohr N, Paganetti H, Greilich S, et al. Tissue decomposition from dual energy CT data for MC based dose calculation in particle therapy. Med Phys. 2014;41:61714.
10. Xie Y, Yin L, Ainsley C, et al. TU-FG-BRB-01: dual energy CT proton stopping power ratio calibration and validation with animal tissues. Med Phys. 2016;43:3756.
11. Arbor N, Dauvergne D, Dedes G, et al. Monte Carlo comparison of x-ray and proton CT for range calculations of proton therapy beams. Phys Med Biol. 2015;60:7585–99.
12. España S, Paganetti H. The impact of uncertainties in the CT conversion algorithm when predicting proton beam ranges in patients from dose and PET-activity distributions. Phys Med Biol. 2010;55:7557–71.
13. Verburg JM, Riley K, Bortfeld T, et al. Energy- and time-resolved detection of prompt gamma-rays for proton range verification. Phys Med Biol. 2013;58:L37–49.
14. Kang Y, Zhang X, Chang JY, et al. 4D Proton treatment planning strategy for mobile lung tumors. Int J Radiat Oncol Biol Phys. 2007;67:906–14.
15. Richter D, Saito N, Chaudhri N, et al. Four-dimensional patient dose reconstruction for scanned ion beam therapy of moving liver tumors. Int J Radiat Oncol Biol Phys. 2014;89:175–81.
16. Hong TS, DeLaney TF, Mamon HJ, et al. A prospective feasibility study of respiratory-gated proton beam therapy for liver tumors. Pract Radiat Oncol. 2014;4:316–22.
17. Li Y, Kardar L, Li X, et al. On the interplay effects with proton scanning beams in stage III lung cancer. Med Phys. 2014;41:21721.
18. Grassberger C, Dowdell S, Lomax A, et al. Motion interplay as a function of patient parameters and spot size in spot scanning proton therapy for lung cancer. Int J Radiat Oncol Biol. Phys. 2013;86:380–6.
19. Dowdell S, Grassberger C, Paganetti H. Four-dimensional Monte Carlo simulations demonstrating how the extent of intensity-modulation impacts motion effects in proton therapy lung treatments. Med Phys. 2013;40:121713.
20. Zeng C, Plastaras JP, James P, et al. Proton pencil beam scanning for mediastinal lymphoma: treatment planning and robustness assessment. Acta Oncol Stockh Swed. 2016;55(9–10):1132–8.
21. Zeng C, Plastaras JP, Tochner ZA, et al. Proton pencil beam scanning for mediastinal lymphoma: the impact of interplay between target motion and beam scanning. Phys Med Biol. 2015;60:3013–29.
22. Rietzel E, Bert C. Respiratory motion management in particle therapy. Med Phys. 2010;37:449–60.
23. Li H, Zhu XR, Zhang X. Reducing dose uncertainty for spot-scanning proton beam therapy of moving Tumors by optimizing the spot delivery sequence. Int J Radiat Oncol Biol Phys. 2015;93:547–56.

24. Yu J, Zhang X, Liao L, et al. Motion-robust intensity-modulated proton therapy for distal esophageal cancer. Med Phys. 2016;43:1111–8.
25. Zhu XR, Poenisch F, Song X, et al. Patient-specific quality assurance for prostate cancer patients receiving spot scanning proton therapy using single-field uniform dose. Int J Radiat Oncol Biol Phys. 2011;81:552–9.
26. Lin L, Kang M, Solberg TD, et al. Use of a novel two-dimensional ionization chamber array for pencil beam scanning proton therapy beam quality assurance. J Appl Clin Med Phys. 2015;16:5323.
27. Zhu XR, Li Y, Mackin D, et al. Towards effective and efficient patient-specific quality assurance for spot scanning proton therapy. Cancers (Basel). 2015;7:631–47.
28. Yoon M, Kim J-S, Shin D, et al. Computerized tomography-based quality assurance tool for proton range compensators. Med Phys. 2008;35:3511–7.
29. Zenklusen SM, Pedroni E, Meer D. A study on repainting strategies for treating moderately moving targets with proton pencil beam scanning at the new Gantry 2 at PSI. Phys Med Biol. 2010;55:5103–21.
30. Mast ME, Vredeveld EJ, Credoe HM, et al. Whole breast proton irradiation for maximal reduction of heart dose in breast cancer patients. Breast Cancer Res Treat. 2014;148:33–9.
31. Shimizu S, Miyamoto N, Matsuura T, et al. A proton beam therapy system dedicated to spot-scanning increases accuracy with moving tumors by real-time imaging and gating and reduces equipment size. PLoS One. 2014;9:e94971.
32. Veiga C, Janssens G, Teng C-L, et al. First clinical investigation of CBCT and deformable registration for adaptive proton therapy of lung cancer. Int J Radiat Oncol Biol Phys. 2016;95:549–59.
33. Jones KC, Stappen FV, Bawiec CR, et al. Experimental observation of acoustic emissions generated by a pulsed proton beam from a hospital-based clinical cyclotron. Med Phys. 2015;42:7090–7.
34. Patch SK, Covo MK, Jackson A, et al. Thermoacoustic range verification using a clinical ultrasound array provides perfectly co-registered overlay of the Bragg peak onto an ultrasound image. Phys Med Biol. 2016;61:5621.
35. Zhu X, Fakhri GE. Proton therapy verification with PET imaging. Theranostics. 2013;3:731–40.
36. Bentefour EH, Schnuerer R, Lu H-M. Concept of proton radiography using energy resolved dose measurement. Phys Med Biol. 2016;61:N386.
37. Ding X, Li X, Zhang JM, et al. Spot-scanning proton arc (SPArc) therapy—the first robust and delivery-efficient spot-scanning arc therapy. Int J Radiat Oncol Biol Phys. 2016;96(5):1107–16.

Proton Treatment Planning

3

Chuan Zeng, Richard A. Amos, Brian Winey, Chris Beltran, Ziad Saleh, Zelig Tochner, Hanne Kooy, and Stefan Both

Contents

3.1 Differences Between Photon and Proton Treatment Planning 46
   3.1.1 Physics 48
   3.1.2 Geometric Uncertainties, Range Uncertainty, and the PTV Concept 49
   3.1.3 Particularities of the Delivery System Proton Versus Photon 52

C. Zeng
Procure Proton Therapy Center, Sumerset, NJ, USA
e-mail: chuan.zeng@nj.procure.com

R.A. Amos
University College London, London, UK
e-mail: r.amos@ucl.ac.uk

B. Winey • H. Kooy
Department of Radiation Oncology, Massachusetts General Hospital, Boston, MA, USA
e-mail: Winey.Brian@mgh.harvard.edu; HKOOY@mgh.harvard.edu

C. Beltran
Mayo Clinic, Rochester, MI, USA
e-mail: Beltran.Chris@mayo.edu

Z. Saleh
Memorial Sloan-Kettering Cancer Center, New York, NY, USA
e-mail: SalehZ@mskcc.org

S. Both (✉)
Department of Radiation Oncology, University Medical Center Groningen, Groningen, The Netherlands
e-mail: s.both@umcg.nl

Z. Tochner
University of Pennsylvania, Philadelphia, PA, USA
e-mail: Zelig.Tochner@uphs.upenn.edu

© Springer International Publishing Switzerland 2018
N. Lee et al. (eds.), *Target Volume Delineation and Treatment Planning for Particle Therapy*, Practical Guides in Radiation Oncology,
https://doi.org/10.1007/978-3-319-42478-1_3

3.2	Proton-Specific Treatment Simulation and Immobilization Principles	53
	3.2.1 CT Protocol, 4D CT, DIBH, DECT, and Contrast/Non-contrast CT	53
	3.2.2 Materials and Positioning in the Beam	58
	3.2.3 PET/MR Imaging	61
	3.2.4 Image Registration and Fusion	61
3.3	Anatomy Modeling, Overrides, CT, Average CT, and MIP	65
	3.3.1 Artifact Reduction	65
	3.3.2 Delineation and CT Number Override	66
3.4	Anatomy Modeling	67
	3.4.1 4D CT	67
3.5	Beam Design Characteristics	70
	3.5.1 Passive Scattering	70
	3.5.2 Pencil-Beam Scanning	76
3.6	Treatment Plan Design and Site Considerations	83
	3.6.1 Site Considerations	83
	3.6.2 Fraction Management	83
	3.6.3 TPS Algorithm and Features	86
	3.6.4 PBS Optimization Volumes, Concept, and Examples	87
	3.6.5 Patient Field QA	89
3.7	SRS Treatment Planning	90
	3.7.1 Treatment Planning Considerations for Proton SRS	92
	3.7.2 Proton SRS with Scattered Beam	92
	3.7.3 Proton SRS with Scanned Beam	92
	3.7.4 Commissioning and QA Considerations Specific for Proton SRS	93
	3.7.5 Clinical Benefits of Physical Dose Properties of Proton SRS	94
	3.7.6 Benign Lesions	94
	3.7.7 Metastatic Lesions	94
3.8	Image Guided Radiation Therapy (IGRT)	96
	3.8.1 Purpose	96
	3.8.2 In-Room Digital Radiography	96
	3.8.3 Out-of-Room CT	97
	3.8.4 Radiopaque Markers	97
	3.8.5 In-Room CT	97
	3.8.6 CBCT	97
	3.8.7 CT on Rails	98
	3.8.8 Other Auxiliary Methods	98
	3.8.9 Impact of Anatomical Changes and Adaptive Radiotherapy	100
3.9	Emerging Technologies and Future Developments	100
References		101

3.1 Differences Between Photon and Proton Treatment Planning

The differences between planning proton-beam therapy and photon-beam therapy derive from the differences in the physics of protons and photons, namely [1]:

- That protons have a finite and controllable (through choice of energy) penetration in depth with virtually no exit dose (Fig. 3.1).
- That the penetration of protons is strongly affected by the nature (e.g., density) of the tissues through which they pass, while photons are much less affected (density changes generally give rise to only small intensity changes, except for the lung). Therefore, heterogeneities are much more important in proton-beam therapy than in photon-beam therapy (Fig. 3.2).

3 Proton Treatment Planning

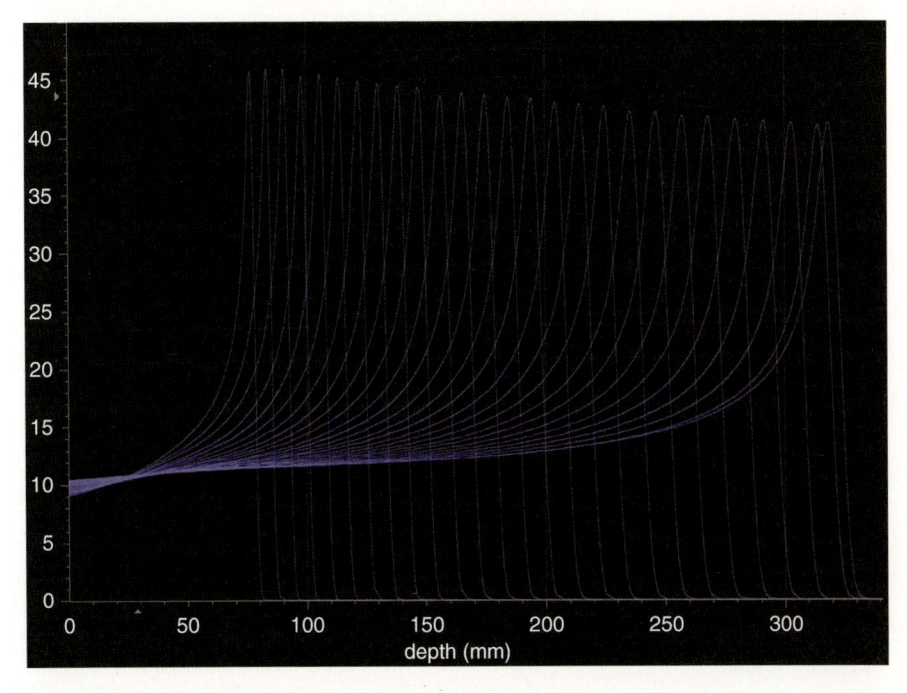

Fig. 3.1 Example integrated depth dose curves (arbitrary unit) corresponding to proton beams with different energies (100–230 MeV). Beams with higher energies penetrate deeper

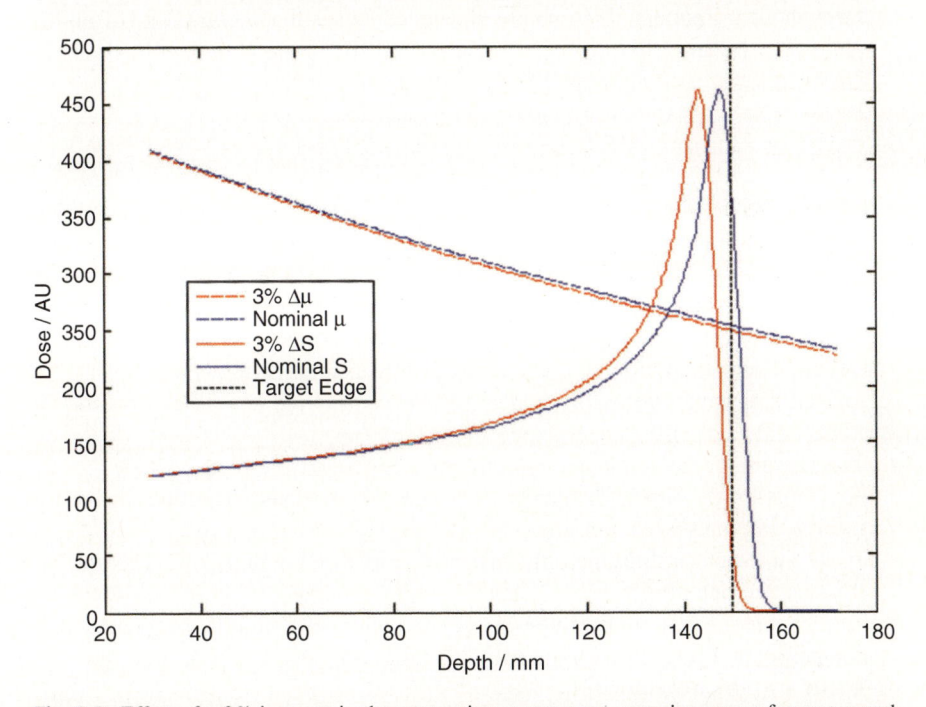

Fig. 3.2 Effect of a 3% increase in the attenuation parameters—stopping power for proton and attenuation coefficient for photon—on the proton and photon field. Note that the proton field shift causes a full underdose at the target edge, while the photon field is minimally affected

- The apparatus for proton-beam delivery is different, and its details affect the dose distributions (Chap. 2).

3.1.1 Physics

3.1.1.1 Rationale for Proton Therapy
Advantage of proton therapy comes from the physical characteristics of the proton beam:

- Finite range and ability to define depth of penetration.
- Intrinsic 3D shaping feature, in depth and laterally, compared to the 2D lateral controls in a single photon beam.
- Inserting a material of certain thickness in a proton beam results in a proportional energy reduction (range $\propto$ energy1.77; [2]) and a known shift downward of the range; proton-beam intensity *does not* change (in contrast to a clinical photon beam where the mean energy is minimally affected while the intensity reduces exponentially as a function of thickness).
- Intrinsically sharp penumbral edge due to near-straight tracks of protons (intrinsically sharper compared to a single photon-beam penumbra at depths below ~ 18 cm in water).
- Proton beams deposit virtually no dose beyond the distal edge of the Bragg peak. Photon beams, in contrast, have no localization ability along the depth and "pass" throughout the patient. This simple difference means that a composite of multiple proton beams will have approximately half the integral dose of a similarly arranged set of photon beams [3].
- Proton dose distributions are biologically equivalent to photon dose distributions except for a constant RBE factor of 1.1 (more detail later in the chapter; Table 3.1).

3.1.1.2 Heterogeneities
Because of the influence of heterogeneities, a map of heterogeneities along the beam path must be made and compensated for (to the extent feasible); finally, the dose distributions must reflect the remaining effects of the heterogeneities. The map of heterogeneities is built up from fine-resolution CT images converted to water-equivalent densities in order to compute three-dimensional dose distributions.

The resulting requirements for planning proton-beam therapy imply the following [1]:

- To ascertain the CT number to water-equivalent density conversion table
- To compensate, either physically or virtually, for heterogeneities, including metallic implants when present
- To be aware of, and mitigate the effect of, possible hot and cold spots due to lateral scattering effects
- To take into account uncertainties associated with possible misalignment of the compensator (Chap. 2) with the patient's tumor, organs, and tissues for passive scattering proton therapy
- To take into account uncertainties in proton-beam penetration. For example, it is common practice to partially or completely avoid using beam directions for

3 Proton Treatment Planning

Table 3.1 Major sources of uncertainty in proton therapy

Source of uncertainty	Comments
Range uncertainty	Proton-beam range varies as a function of proton energy and relative stopping power (RSP) of the absorbing material. A significant source of range uncertainty comes from the conversion of Hounsfield units (HU) in the planning CT to RSP (Fig. 3.4a). This uncertainty is approximately 2% for soft tissue and as high as 5% for lung, fat, and bone. An average value of 3.5% is assumed for clinical practice [4–6]. Much greater uncertainty exists for high-Z materials such as metal hip prostheses (Fig. 3.11) and dental fillings. Traversing these implants should be avoided wherever possible. CT image reconstruction artifacts also increase range uncertainty [7]
Patient setup uncertainty	Proton dose distributions are highly sensitive to patient positioning. Daily image guidance is recommended to ensure accurate alignment with the machine isocenter as well as alignment of patient relative to the patient support system and immobilization equipment traversed by the proton beams [8, 9]
Anatomical variability	Protons are highly sensitive to intrafractional and interfractional variations in anatomy. Variations may be caused, for example, by respiratory motion, weight loss, tumor shrinkage (Fig. 3.14), bladder filling, bowel gas, or changes in sinus filling. Mitigation techniques include 4D CT-based planning for respiratory motion, adaptive replanning for weight loss or tumor shrinkage, and careful beam angle selection to avoid traversing anatomy susceptible to variation wherever possible
Biological uncertainty	The relative biological effectiveness (RBE) is accepted as 1.1 for clinical practice. This is based on a meta-analysis of in vivo and in vitro data obtained in the middle of the SOBP [10]. However, linear energy transfer (LET) increases toward the distal end of the SOBP, with a corresponding increase in RBE [11]. The biological dose is extended distal to the physical range [12]; 2–3 mm is a reasonable approximation for this extension

which there would be a tight margin between the target and a sensitive structure lying distal to it (e.g., the spinal cord)

3.1.2 Geometric Uncertainties, Range Uncertainty, and the PTV Concept

The primary physical and conceptual difference between protons and photons passing through matter is that protons lose energy but not intensity and photons lose intensity but not energy (Sect. 1.1). An uncertainty in tissue density thus has a direct effect on the proton penetration and the position of the Bragg peak. If this Bragg peak was assumed to be at the distal edge of the target, it may "stop short" and the target edge may receive zero dose due to the sharp distal falloff of the Bragg peak. Figure 3.2 illustrates the effect on a proton Bragg peak with respect to the target and the effect on a photon field both for a 3% increase in the relevant physical attenuation parameter.

The difference in consequence is the root cause of the difference in uncertainty mitigation strategies between protons and photons.

As can be seen in Fig. 3.2, the photon field intensity and thus dose is minimally impacted by changes in density. As a consequence, a photon dose distribution has (almost certainly within the range of uncertainties of therapy) a static 3D shape in the patient space unaffected by acceptable uncertainties. This means that if we are able to position the patient with respect to this static 3D shape, we will achieve our intended doses within the patient. This is the sole reason why geometric imaging suffices in photon radiotherapy: we only need to shift the patient to the intended location to align with the 3D dose. Any residual uncertainties are accounted for by PTV margin, to ensure that the CTV within remains covered.

The proton dose distribution is a composite of numerous pristine Bragg peaks whose terminal locations are the main loci of dose. Uncertainty in stopping power translates into a proportional uncertainty in all these loci. This direct correlation between geometric error and dose error (unlike in photon fields) means that an expansion of the CTV into a PTV does not apply directly to protons.

Uncertainties arise from:

1. Uncertainty in local stopping power in the patient
2. Changes in the patient's internal and external anatomy
3. Setup errors
   All causes have the same effect: a potential shift of the Bragg peak location. Stopping power uncertainties arise from (1) the conversion of CT number to stopping power based on a population average conversion curve and (2) the inherent uncertainty in the stopping power itself. Typically, the practical uncertainty in this conversion is assumed to be about 2.5%, which can vary from one institution to another (values up to 3.5% are used in clinical practice). Thus, a 150 mm range proton may have its (worst case) locus between 146.25 mm and 153.75 mm, i.e., an uncertainty range of 7.5 mm, which would be unacceptable.
   Changes in the patient's internal and external anatomy require repeated verification volumetric imaging depending on the treatment site. Over the course of treatment, the anatomy of the patient can change. Weight gain/loss is a typical example where thickness of a patient's subcutaneous fat layer may change significantly during the course of radiotherapy. Changes in the size of a bulky tumor or lymph nodes can affect the delivered dose. Gas in the rectum or bowels can create large perturbations if the proton beam is traversing these areas. The repeated image set should be used to reassess the dose to the patient as apparent geometric fidelity may *not* translate into dosimetric fidelity. This can be practically checked on a biweekly basis.
   Daily imaging, either minimally by means of orthogonal X-rays or maximally by cone beam CT (CBCT) or diagnostic quality CT, is required to ensure that patient setup errors are within tolerances and representative of the assumed errors.
   The known effect of uncertainties yet their unknown magnitude in a given patient requires mitigation at the treatment planning level to ensure that the resultant dose distribution maintains its integrity, qualitatively expressed as robustness against those uncertainties, in the presence of these uncertainties.
   Robustness assessment is a difficult computational and practical problem and depends on the mode of proton field delivery. We identify two practical modes of delivery and their mitigation:

1. SOBP fields composed of a fixed set of pristine Bragg peaks with a fixed modulation and shaped by apertures in the lateral dimensions and by range compensator in depth. To the first order, an uncertainty shifts the field proportional

to the uncertainty. Thus, an expansion of the SOBP field in the proximal and distal directions will ensure proximal and distal coverage. This can be considered as a one-dimensional PTV expansion. An aperture expansion, to first order similarly, will ensure that the target remains covered in the lateral dimensions barring large heterogeneity differences. Note, however, that the first mitigation along depth is because of stopping power uncertainty, while the second is because of setup error. In addition, lateral setup errors are, in practice, corrected by assuming a worst case penetration in the shape of the range compensator (see Fig. 3.3).

2. PBS (pencil-beam scanning) fields composed of individual Bragg peaks. We identify two modes for PBS (nomenclature is not uniform in the radiotherapy community, and we follow the ICRU Report 78 [1]):
   (a) Single-field uniform dose (SFUD) where each field in the set of PBS fields achieves a uniform dose over the entire target. The fields are thus geometrically decoupled and can be considered independently in the uncertainty mitigation. Their individual mitigation is considered adequately handled by the considerations in SOBP fields. The SFUD technique is also called single-field optimization (SFO). The SFO may be used in the case of a simultaneous integrated boost (SIB) or when a single field is optimized together with constraints to OARs which partially overlap with the target.

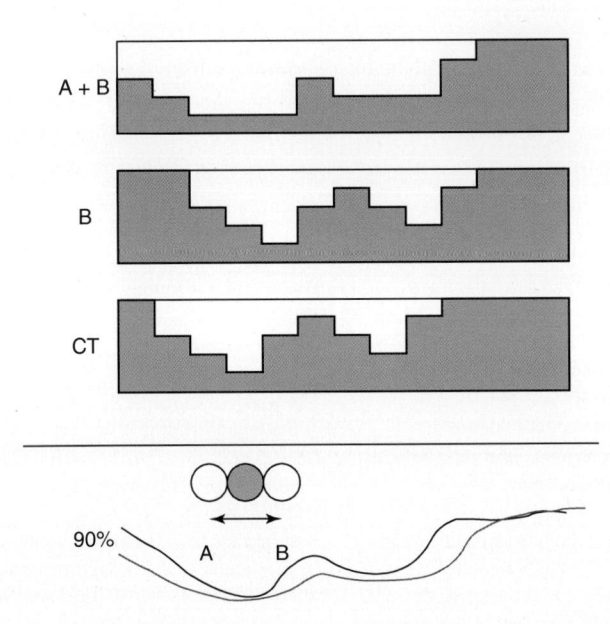

Fig. 3.3 Consider a beam entering from the top of the three range compensators. The range compensator "CT" is derived from the CT in the nominal position and has a profile as indicated and results in the top 90% dose profile. A setup error (e.g., to location B) results in a shifted compensator profile. The worst case range compensator profile (A + B, where A refers to the setup error to opposite direction of B) considers the deepest required penetration anywhere in the field given the range of uncertainties and results, as a consequence, a nominally deeper 90% dose profile

(b) Intensity-modulated proton therapy (IMPT) where each field delivers a heterogeneous dose to the target and only the composite dose from all fields covers the entire target and achieves the desired dose shape. The IMPT fields are strongly coupled and must be considered as a single set in the uncertainty mitigation. The uncertainty mitigation in IMPT may be achieved through robust optimization, which requires an explicit computation of individual uncertainty scenarios to assess that the dose in each scenario remains clinically acceptable. We will return to this topic in Sect. 6.4. The IMPT technique is also referred to as multi-field optimization (MFO) (Table 3.2).

3.1.3 Particularities of the Delivery System Proton Versus Photon

3.1.3.1 Proton Delivery Techniques

In proton-beam therapy, a number of different beam-shaping and delivery techniques can be used, and these techniques strongly affect the selection of beams and their resulting dose distributions [1]. The planning software must therefore be able to simulate all techniques of proton-beam delivery available to the user. For example, it might be required to compute the dose distributions of scatter beams, scanned beams (continuous or discrete), or wobbled beams (a special case of beam scanning, using relatively wide finite pencil beams):

- Protons have a sharp lateral beam penumbra which decreases with increasing beam energy.
- Proton-beam penumbra is widest in the Bragg peak region where the proton energy is least.

Table 3.2 Proton delivery techniques

Passive scattering	Pencil-beam scanning
An SOBP field is of constant modulation, thus in general *cannot* conform to the proximal volume of target	The dose distribution of one field can conform to the volume proximal to the target
The width of SOBP is determined by the widest part of the target in depth	The width of SOBP is determined by the width of the target in depth along each line of spots
Dose distributions are determined laterally by the collimation system	Dose distributions are determined laterally by the placement and weights of the spots on each energy layer
Penumbra will be affected by the air gap between the aperture and patient	Penumbra is largely determined by size of spot perpendicular to the beam direction and distance between range shifter (if any) and patient
Field size is usually limited. The limit may depend on range/modulation due to the different hardware options involved for different range/modulation combinations	

- Penumbra is narrower for protons compared to photons for depths of penetration less than 17–18 cm (This is the result of proton interaction with tissue, which is independent of delivery technique.).

3.2 Proton-Specific Treatment Simulation and Immobilization Principles

CT simulation is mandatory for proton therapy and it provides:

- 3D and/or 4D model of patient for geometric treatment planning
- Reference images for daily treatment guidance
- Material composition information, specifically proton stopping power, for heterogeneity corrections and substrate for dose distribution calculation

The processes of simulation and immobilization are essential when advanced technologies are employed in conjunction with tight treatment margins. In general, the use of tighter margins is employed to protect normal tissues and requires precise knowledge regarding geometric uncertainties (patient setup, motion, etc.) in radiation therapy.

The data on geometric uncertainties established in conventional external beam is of similar value to charged particle radiotherapy. However, the additional challenges of range uncertainty in particle therapy, a dimension in patient positioning not present in photon radiotherapy, raise a new challenge for particle therapy:

- Proton therapy demands repeatable, reliable simulation to successfully leverage the advantages of very selective dose distributions.
- Robust treatment planning can help accommodate a small amount of variation.
- Proton plans are highly susceptible to deterioration due to interference between the proton beam and the immobilization equipment.

The whole process of simulation and immobilization includes patient preparation, patient positioner (typically 6D), patient position verification system, patient immobilization, and patient imaging (preferably 3D).

3.2.1 CT Protocol, 4D CT, DIBH, DECT, and Contrast/Non-contrast CT

CT images are used to map the patient anatomy in terms of proton stopping power ratio properties. The accuracy in estimating the stopping power ratio from CT numbers is critical, and stoichiometric calibration, described below, is typically used to minimize range uncertainties due to CT imaging [13, 14]. This method has the advantage of not being affected by the differences in elemental composition between substitute material used in calibration and actual biological tissues. However, stoichiometric calibration does not eliminate the uncertainty in estimated stopping power ratios; and imaging is not the only source of range uncertainty.

As a consequence, a distal margin of approximately 2.5–3.5% of the range is usually taken into account during planning. This uncertainty can perhaps be reduced using DECT [15], proton radiography [16], etc. In general:

- 3D and 4D CT-based simulations are standard in particle therapy.
- Use only calibrated protocols corresponding to particular kVp, since CT numbers are dependent on kVp.
- Scanner-specific calibration is recommended.
- The planning CT should fully include the immobilized patient.
- Treatment table and all immobilization equipment need to be included in the planning CT.
- The CT field of view must include all materials that are potentially in the beam's path.
- Setup reproducibility is paramount; therefore, indexed immobilization devices should be employed.
- CT artifacts and contrast materials are of concern and should be minimized or corrected as necessary.

3.2.1.1 Stoichiometric Calibration [13]

The error of relative stopping power distribution originates from a number of sources. Firstly, the measurement of CT number of homogeneous material can vary between 1% and 2% and is also dependent on the location of the material in the image, a variation that can reach up to 3%. In addition, the measurement of high CT numbers can vary from scanner to scanner and can strongly influence the calibration. It is also known that scanner-specific parameters such as the scan diameter and the matrix size may affect the measurement of CT number. A final source of error is the approximation of real tissue with tissue substitutes used for the measurement of the relationship of CT number to stopping power. The chemical composition of commonly used tissue substitutes is different to that of real tissue. A possible solution to this problem is a stoichiometric calibration:

1. Acquire CT scan of phantom with tissue equivalent materials with known relative electron density and elemental compositions (Figs. 3.5 and 3.6).
2. Measure CT numbers for each tissue equivalent material.
3. Use measured CT numbers to determine coefficients k^{ph}, k^{coh}, and k^{KN} for stoichiometric equation

$$\mu = (\langle Z^{3.62}\rangle_e k^{ph} + \langle Z^{1.86}\rangle_e k^{coh} + k^{KN})\rho N_A Z/A,$$

where chevrons $\langle\rangle_e$ denote an average weighted by number of electrons (Fig. 3.4).

4. Using coefficients to calculate CT numbers for a full range of "real" tissues using their published elemental compositions and physical densities [17, 18].

5. Calculate the stopping power ratio for each "real" tissue based on elemental composition (Bethe formula).
6. Use calculated SPR versus calculated CT numbers to establish respective calibration for TPS.

The overall accuracy of the range control of proton beams in the human body by using this stoichiometric calibration was estimated to be 1.8% and 1.1% for bone and soft tissue, respectively [14].

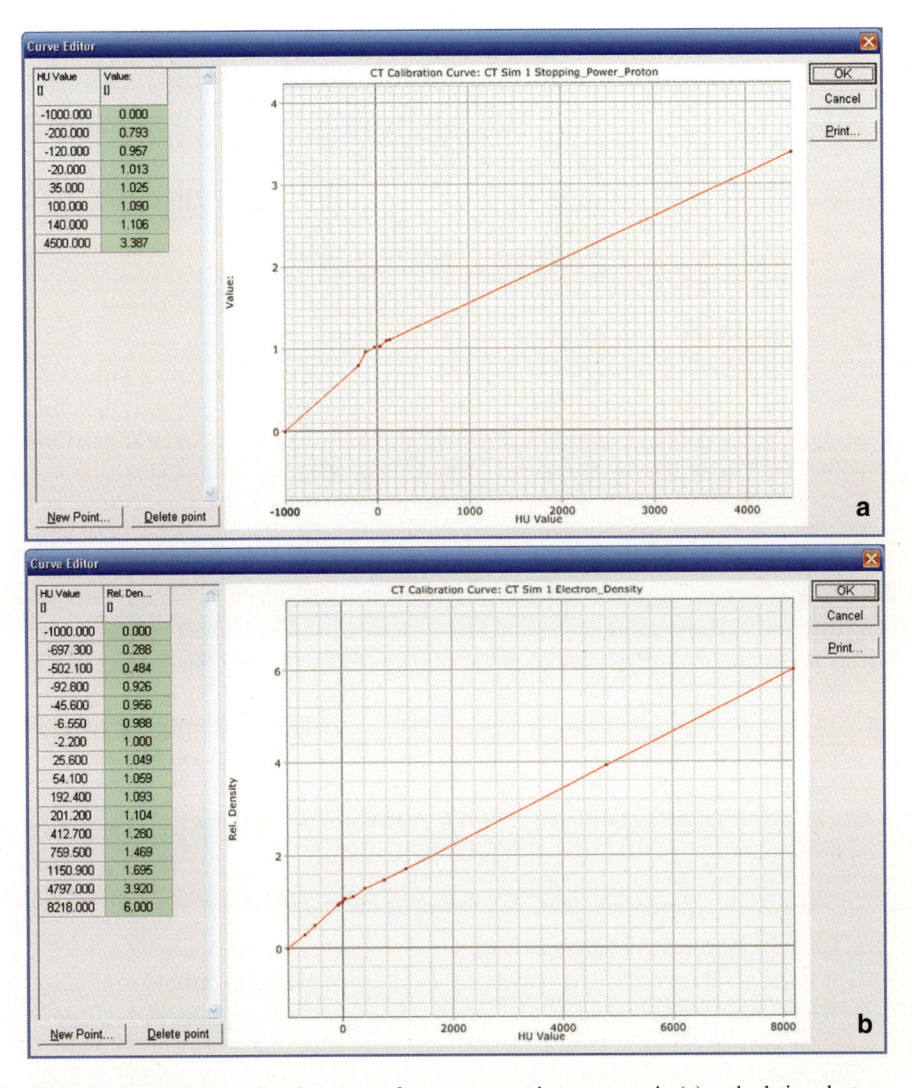

Fig. 3.4 Example CT calibration curves for proton stopping power ratio (**a**) and relative electron density (**b**). Hospital of the University of Pennsylvania (SIEMENS Sensation Open; 120 kVp)

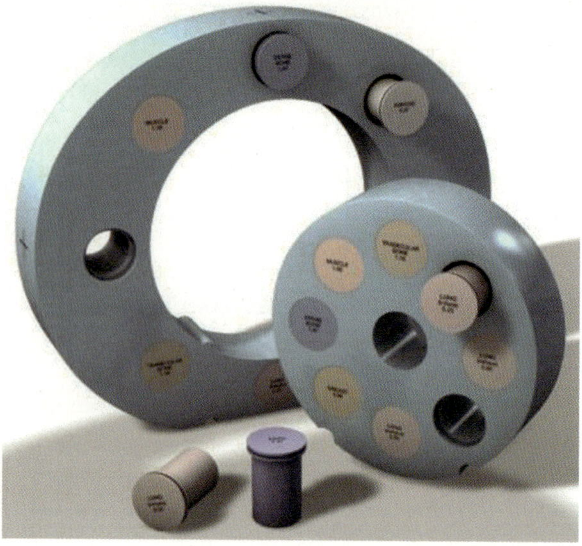

Fig. 3.5 CIRS electron density phantom (Courtesy of Computerized Imaging Reference Systems, Inc.)

3.2.1.2 DECT [15]

Schneider et al. [19] have demonstrated that a single CT number cannot differentiate between a change in density or chemical composition of an imaged material. Dual-energy CT (DECT), however, is able to attribute changes in X-ray attenuation to either density or chemical composition. This is achieved by decomposing two simultaneous single-energy CT (SECT) scans into relative electron density and effective atomic number. The process exploits the energy dependency of kilovoltage X-ray interaction atomic cross sections and the energy-independent parameter. The extra information gained in DECT, compared to SECT, can be used to estimate two material-specific parameters, and these are then used in a direct calculation of the SPR instead of a fitted value as in the stoichiometric method. The use of DECT has been shown to reduce the range uncertainty in PT compared to SECT [20]:

- DECT has the potential to better characterize patient composition and stopping power.
- Reduce SPR uncertainties from 1.1 (SECT) to 0.4% for soft tissue [21] and from 13 to 3% for a silicone-based dosimeter [22].
- Reduce maximum dose calculation error from 8 to 1% [23].

3.2.1.3 CT Contrast Avoidance [24]

- The use of contrast agents is common in CT studies employed in treatment planning.
- Contrast agents accumulate, and their iodine content increases the CT number of soft tissues significantly, creating artifacts and degrading the quality of CT images.
- Whenever a contrast agent is needed for target delineation purposes, the contrast CT has to be acquired after a simulation CT is acquired without contrast.
- Treatment planning calculations must be done on the non-contrast CT scan to avoid significant range errors

3 Proton Treatment Planning

Fig. 3.6 (a) Gammex tissue characterization phantom. (b) Arrangement of tissue substituting rods (Courtesy of Sun Nuclear)

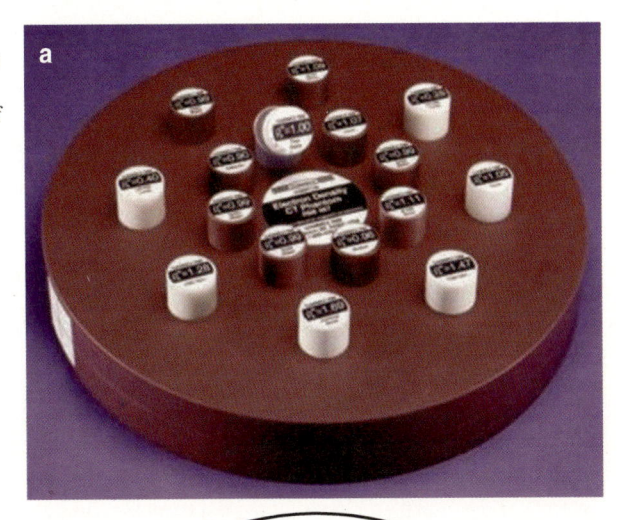

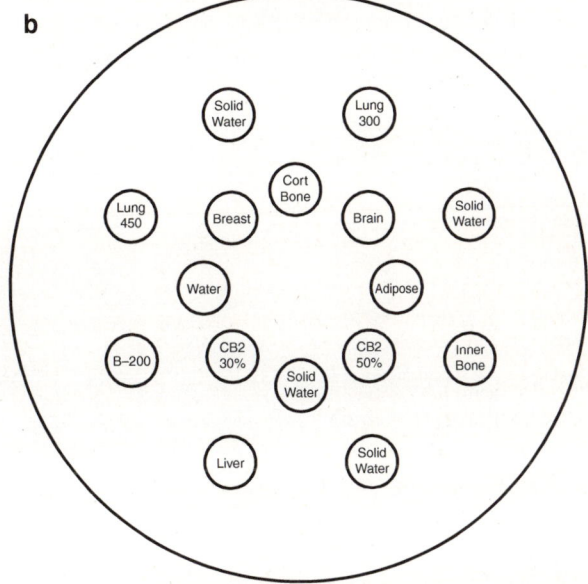

3.2.1.4 4D CT
- Four-dimensional CT is routinely used to acquire target motion amplitude, allowing moving target treatment planning and active motion mitigation strategies for proton beams:
  - Proton centers may have motion thresholds above which PBS or proton therapy in general is not used.
  - Common thresholds for moving targets treated with PBS are established based on the motion mitigation techniques available and planning techniques (selecting beam direction along the largest component of motion,

smaller spot spacing, use of larger spots) and delivery techniques (optimized delivery sequence, layered/volumetric rescanning); a typical value that is commonly used is 1 cm.

3.2.1.5 DIBH [25, 26]

- Deep inspiration breath-hold (DIBH) has been used to reduce the motion of moving targets and is commonly used in the treatment of breast, lung, mediastinal, and gastrointestinal targets.
- DIBH increases lung volume, can displace normal lung and/or heart away from irradiated regions, and may displace the target volume away from the spinal cord in some cases [27].
- DIBH can significantly reduce heart and lung doses in some cases [28].

3.2.2 Materials and Positioning in the Beam

Like for conventional radiotherapy, patient immobilization materials are adjusted to patient-specific geometry for particle therapy (Fig. 3.7).

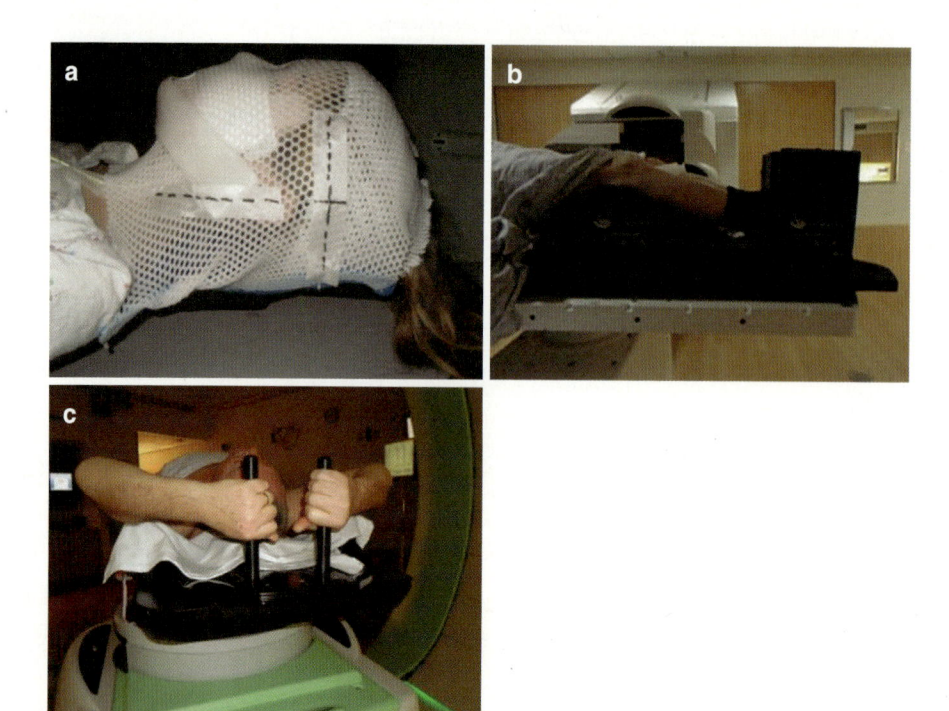

Fig. 3.7 Examples of patient immobilization used at the Hospital of the University of Pennsylvania (**a–d**), (**a**) CNS, (**b**) pelvis, (**c**) thorax, and (**d**) shoulder, and Massachusetts General Hospital (**e, f**), (**e**) cranial SRS and (**f**) cranial SRS

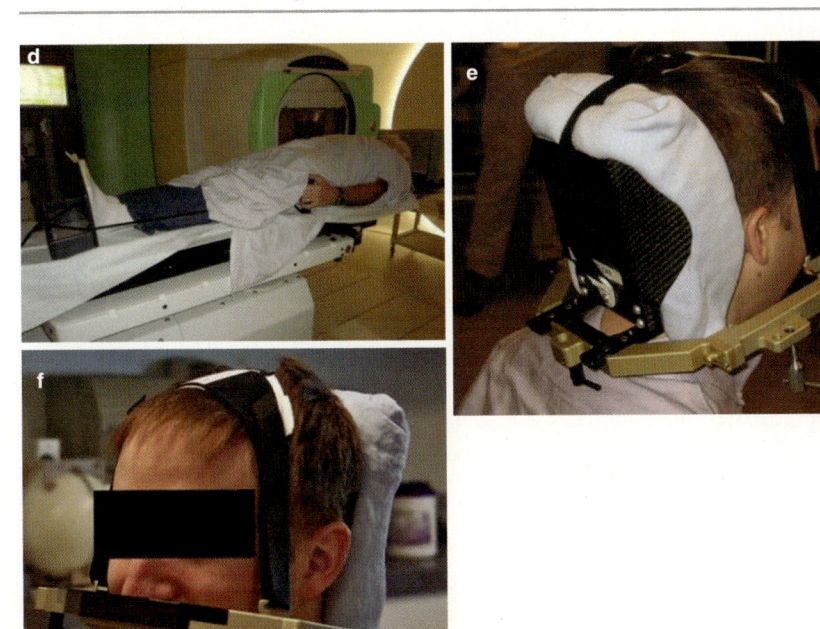

Fig. 3.7 (continued)

For particle therapy, the following additional principles apply [29]:

- Immobilization devices can be used in contact with skin, as there is no buildup effect for heavy charged particle beams.
- Immobilization devices present in the treatment beam should be minimal and indexed as particle beams are highly sensitive to changes in radiologic depth due to the sharp distal falloff of the Bragg peak.
- Immobilization devices should be radiologically thin in order to minimize the lateral penumbra (due to scattering) and thus preserve dose conformality and lateral sparing of OARs.
- For fixed beam or partial gantry, when the patient rotates with the couch, extra immobilization may be needed to reinforce lateral support.
- Patients have to be positioned in the most comfortable treatment position in order to achieve reproducibility.

3.2.2.1 Treatment Couch

While the attenuation of treatment beam by the couch for X-ray treatments is usually negligible, there is a clinically meaningful shift in range of proton beam for proton treatments [30] (Table 3.3).

Table 3.3 Examples of couch tops currently used for proton therapy

Device	Vendor	WET
Hitachi couch extension QFIX proton kVue couch QFIX Standard Couch	Hitachi Ltd., Japan WFR Aquaplast, Avondale, PA WFR Aquaplast, Avondale, PA	1.1 cm 0.55 cm 1 cm

- Determine WET experimentally. This should be done by:
  - Measure proton PDD and range through multiple points in each device.
  - Traditionally with a water-scanning parallel plate chamber:
  - Ensure homogeneity within a given device.
  - Check consistency between devices within a clinic.
  - If measured WET matches calculated value, include full couch top in simulation CT dataset and incorporate couch into calculation. If measured WET does not match calculated value, contour couch top in the treatment plan and override CT numbers to achieve correct.

3.2.2.2 WET
1. Edge effects can be mitigated by:
   - Indexing all immobilization equipment to treatment couch
   - Avoiding treatment beams that traverse couch edges
2. The couch should be designed to be:
   - Free of heterogeneities
   - Base end mounted on robotic positioners with six degrees of freedom
   - Contoured surfaces:
     - Excessive adipose tissue may exhibit widely varying shapes from day to day:
        Posterior neck in H&N treatments [31]
        Pelvis contour in prostate and GYN treatments
     - Variable external contour leads to changes in target depth
     - A customized, contoured couch surface can help present a consistent external contour to the proton beam

3.2.2.3 Range Shifter
- Minimum range for most proton therapy systems is at least ~ 4 g/cm^2 (70 MeV).
- Treatment of superficial lesions requires a range shifter—typically mounted in the head of the machine.
- Range shifters have nonzero scattering power, and so any air gap between range shifter and patient can lead to dramatic increase in spot size [32, 33].
- Place range shifter on or in the couch.

3.2.2.4 Endorectal Balloons
- Reduce interfractional and intrafractional variation of prostate position within the body [34, 35].

3 Proton Treatment Planning

- Reduce rectal toxicity by limiting volume of rectal wall within high-dose treatment volume.
- Generally more widely adapted in proton centers because localization of soft tissue target alone does not guarantee adequate target coverage.
- Typically filled with water to avoid gas pockets and heterogeneities along the path of beams.
- May be used for treatment of GYN cancer [36].

3.2.2.5 Collision Detection
In order to avoid delays in treatment, it is important to determine the possibility of patient collision during the treatment planning stage in proton therapy [37]:

- Alpha Cradle, leg abductors, and beanbag used in the thoracic, pelvic, or extremity regions are much less motion limiting.
- Size of devices may limit the choice of beam direction or close proximity of aperture, compensator, or range shifter to the patient.
- The close proximity of these devices is critical to maintain sharp lateral dose falloff for double scattering and to preserve beam spot size for scanned beam.

Current commercial treatment planning systems do not allow automated patient collision detection.

3.2.3 PET/MR Imaging

Besides CT, positron emission tomography (PET) and/or magnetic resonance (MR) imaging studies may have been performed with primarily diagnostic intent, even before the decision to use radiation therapy has been taken. These images are also vital for the planning of the radiation treatment as they give essential information about the anatomic site and extent of disease and the location of nearby uninvolved normal tissues.

3.2.4 Image Registration and Fusion

- There has been a proliferation of medical images through the increased use of functional PET for tumor segmentation, staging, and assessment of treatment response. In addition, MR images are being utilized for accurate tumor and organ delineation due to superior soft tissue contrast. Moreover, patients are being imaged routinely using weekly CBCT and repeated CT scans to monitor anatomical changes as part of adaptive treatment (Fig. 3.8).
- Rigid registration is used in the clinic on a routine basis to fuse daily kV images with DRR and CBCT with planning CT to ensure accurate patient setup (Fig. 3.8).

In addition, rigid registration is utilized to fuse inter- and intra-modality images by overlaying information from diagnostic PET/CT and MRI scans over the planning CT. The fused images are used to delineate tumors and organs at risk for treatment planning purposes (Fig. 3.9).

- Deformable image registration plays an essential role in radiotherapy process for tracking anatomical changes (Fig. 3.10), contour propagation and internal target volume (ITV) generation on 4D CT, and dose accumulation for the purpose of adaptive RT (Sect. 8.9).

3.2.4.1 Uncertainties in Registration

- Deformable image registration is an ill-posed problem, and different solutions may exist which leads to uncertainties. Uncertainties are encountered near

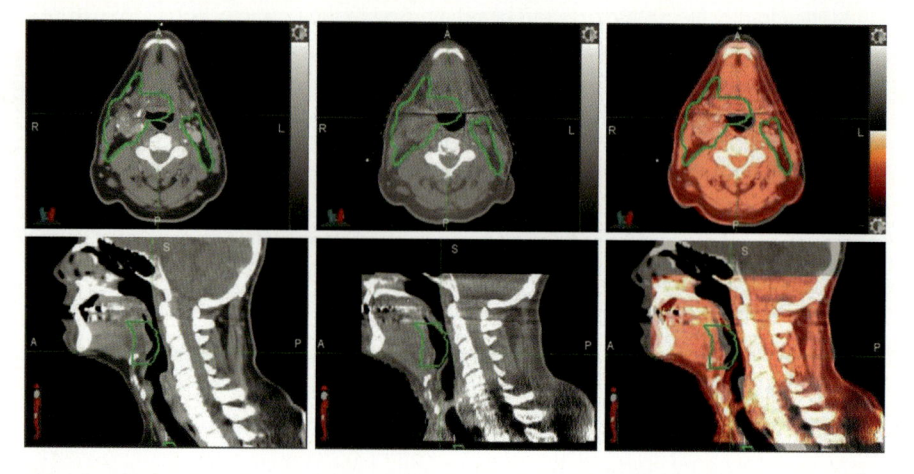

Fig. 3.8 Axial and sagittal views from a planning CT (*left*), CBCT at week 2 (*middle*), and rigidly fused images (*right*) of an example H&N patient. CTV 54 Gy shown in green is overlaid on the CT and CBCT. Notice the tumor shrinkage near the base of tongue which necessitates adaptive planning

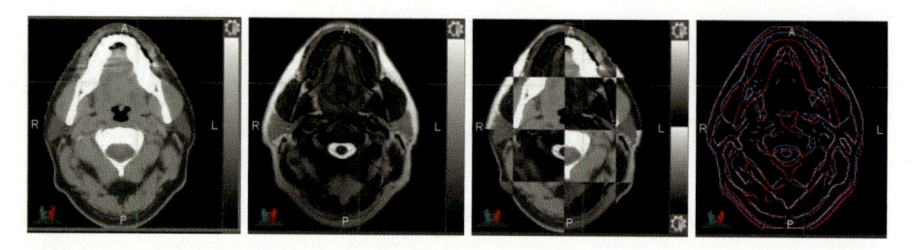

Fig. 3.9 An axial slice of an example H&N patient from a planning CT and follow-up T2-weighted MRI scan. MRI provides better soft tissue contrast compared to CT. Visual inspection of the registration is performed using checkerboard display for image alignment. This process can be facilitated utilizing edges generated from CT and MRI as shown in *blue* and *red*, respectively

3 Proton Treatment Planning

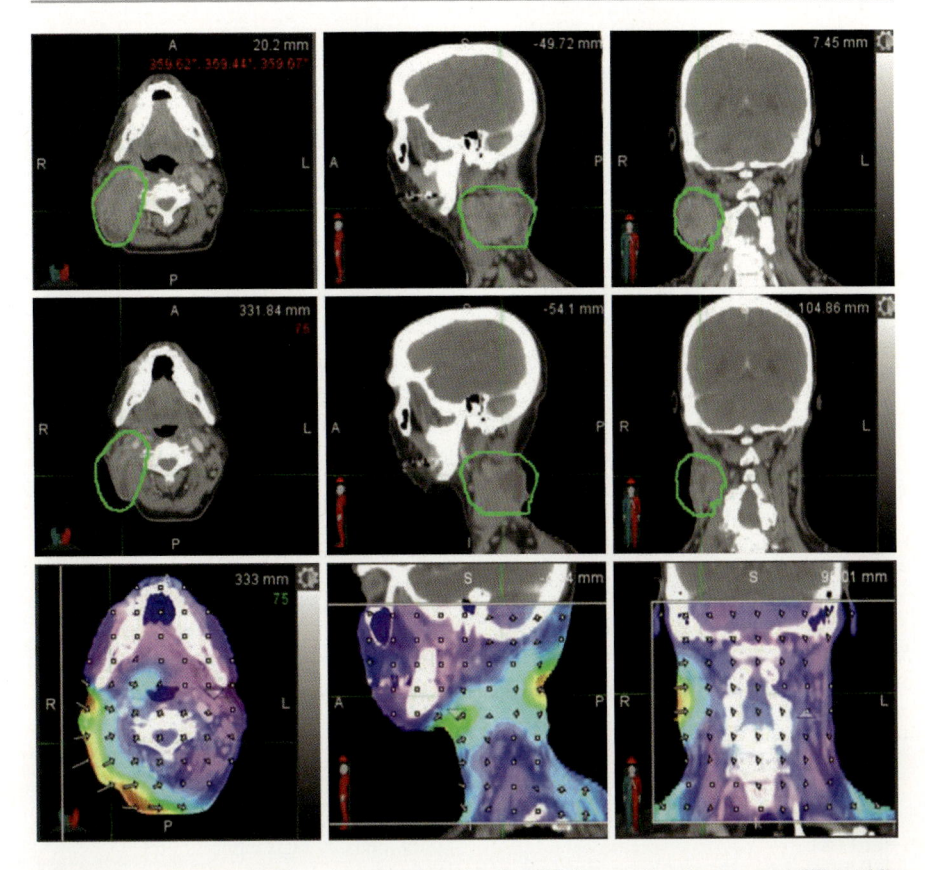

Fig. 3.10 An example H&N patient showing planning CT (*top row*) and a repeated CT (*middle row*). Tumor regression is observed in response to treatment. The deformation grid (*bottom panel*) illustrates regions with large deformation as shown in *red*. Deformation vector fields are also displayed where *large arrows* correspond to large deformations

> misaligned edges (bones, tissue-air interface), inside regions of uniform intensity (liver) and of low contrast (lung). These uncertainties are more relevant in proton therapy as compared to photon therapy and must be incorporated into the uncertainty margins of the target (PTV) during the TP process [38].
> - Uncertainties in deformable image registration have a direct impact on the dose propagation and accumulation. The spatial uncertainty can lead to large dose errors in the regions of high-dose gradients near the tumor [39]. Larger deformations are usually associated with large registration errors. Consult with physics team to assess the range of dose uncertainty.
> - Dice similarity coefficient (DSC; [40]) and Hausdorff distance (HD; [41]) are commonly used metrics to evaluate the quality of the registration based on

physician-drawn contours for segmentation purposes. Several other metrics have been proposed to evaluate the accuracy and underlying uncertainties of the registration such as inverse consistency error (ICE; [42]), transitivity error (TE; [42]), and distance discordance metric (DDM; [43]). However, none of these metrics are considered ground truth, and they need further validation. Several of these metrics rely on the deformation vector field (DVF) of the registration. Guidelines for qualitative and quantitative assessment of deformable registration are emerging but have not been published (AAPM TG 132; [38]). The clinical practices outlined in Table 3.4 are necessary, but not sufficient, to ensure a reasonably accurate registration [38, 44, 45].

- The registration accuracy varies among anatomical sites (H&N, liver, lung, etc.), across image modalities (CT, CBCT, MR), and the choice of registration algorithms (B-spline, Demons, fast free form, etc.). Table 3.5 gives a summary of the absolute registration error reported in literature based on "ground truth" of anatomic landmarks [46–48].
- Overall, the accuracy of deformable registration is on the order of 2–3 voxels. Due to its relevance in proton therapy which is susceptible to range uncertainty, the accuracy of the registration must be investigated for each treatment site for clinical use.

Table 3.4 Guideline for qualitative and quantitative evaluation of deformable image registration

Methodology/metric	Technique	Relevance	Ground truth?
Qualitative			
Color overlay of image difference	Visual	Intensity matching for intra-modality registration	✗
Checkerboard display	Visual	Edge alignment for intra- and inter-modality registration	✗
Quantitative			
Dice similarity coefficient (DSC)	Contour based	DSC ~ 1 corresponds to better volume overlap	✗
Hausdorff distance (HD)	Contour based	Small HD value corresponds to better registration	✗
Average surface distance (ASD)	Contour based	Small ASD value corresponds to better registration	✗
Anatomic landmarks/ implanted markers	Landmark based	True registration error (TRE)	✓
Jacobian determinant of DVF	Voxel-wise	$J < 0$ corresponds to tissue folding (nonphysical)	✗
		$0 < J < 1$ corresponds to shrinkage (tumor regression)	✗
		$J > 1$ corresponds to expansion (tumor progression)	✗
Curl of the DVF	Voxel-wise	Check presence of swirls (nonphysical deformations)	✗
Physical or digital phantom (InSimQA)	Voxel-wise	End-to-end test	✓

3 Proton Treatment Planning

Table 3.5 Range of absolute registration error for different anatomical sites

Modality	Site	Landmarks	Range of mean abs. error	Standard dev.	Max. error
CT/CT [39]	Head and neck	Physical phantom	2.1 mm	2.2 mm	N/A
4D CT [46]	Lung	Bronchial bifurcations	2.0–2.5 mm	2.5 mm	12.0 mm
	Heart and aorta	Calcifications	2.5–5.0 mm	2.5–5.0 mm	6.7 mm
	Liver	Vessel bifurcations	2.5–5.0 mm	2.5 mm	10.0 mm
	Left kidney	Vessel bifurcations	2.5 mm	3.0 mm	3.3 mm
MRI/CT [46]	Liver	Vessel bifurcations	1.1–5.0 mm	2.5 mm	7.0 mm
MRI/MRI [46]	Prostate	Gold seeds	0.4–6.2 mm	0.3–3.4 mm	8.7 mm
CT/CT [47]	Lung	Bronchial branch pts	1.6–4.2 mm1	N/A	15.0 mm
CT/CT [48]	Head and neck	Bone and tissue	2.01–5.16 mm	1.29–2.52 mm	N/A

3.3 Anatomy Modeling, Overrides, CT, Average CT, and MIP

An accurate 3D or 4D model of the patient is established through CT simulation, which is essential for geometric treatment planning. CT images are used to map the patient anatomy to a distribution of proton stopping power ratio.

3.3.1 Artifact Reduction

3.3.1.1 Beam-Hardening Artifacts
- Besides uncertainty of the CT-SPR calibration curve, beam hardening contributes additional uncertainty in SPR values.
- Lower-energy photons have a higher cross section for the photoelectric effect and are absorbed with a higher probability than higher-energy photons. This results in a hardening of the spectrum.
- In all diagnostic scanners, a correction for this effect is applied in the calculation by the scanner software.
- This is only perfect for a standard situation (16 cm cylindrical water phantom) but is incorrect if high-Z materials (e.g., metals) are present.
- Beam hardening makes the calibration curve dependent on patient size [14].

3.3.1.2 Artifact Reduction Algorithms
- Projection completion method [49]
- Iterative artifact reduction methods [50]

3.3.2 Delineation and CT Number Override

- The standard practice to deal with metal CT artifacts is to delineate artifact regions and to reset the CT number of these regions to average soft tissue or bone values measured in similar areas of the body where no artifacts are present [51] (Fig. 3.11).
- The average values may be obtained from artifact-free regions of the same CT dataset.
- High-Z materials which are included in the treatment fields will be contoured and assigned a CT number consistent with the proton stopping power of that material.

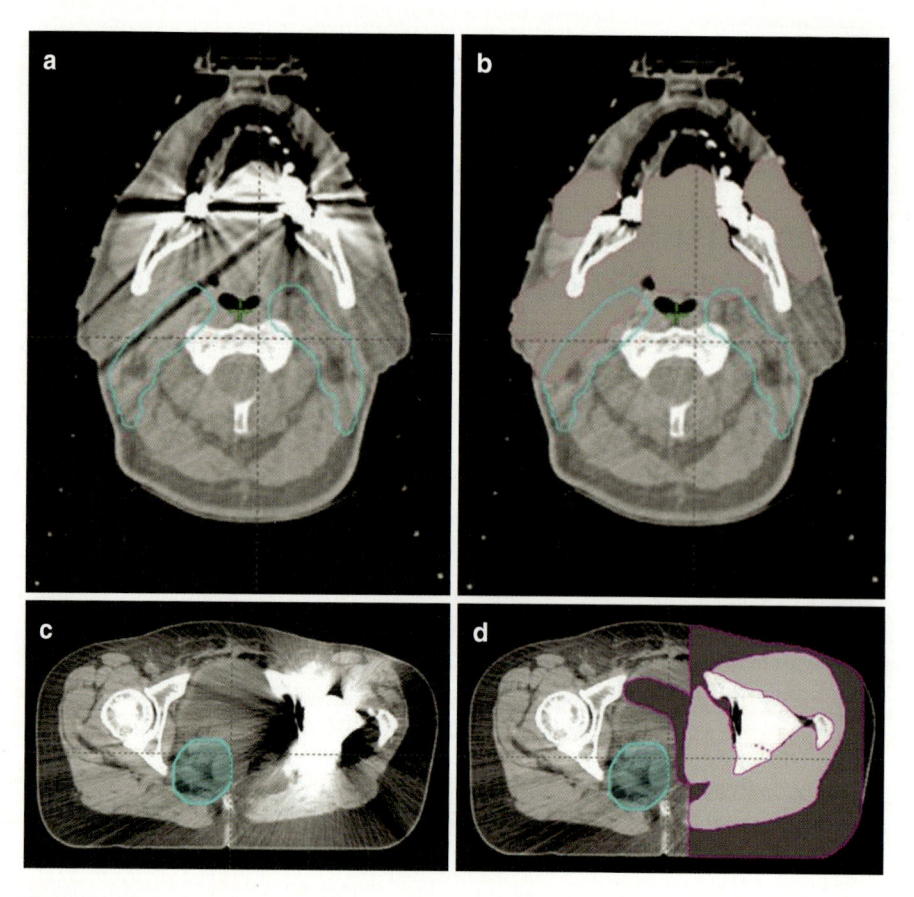

Fig. 3.11 Examples of image artifacts overriding. (**a**) Before overriding, (**b**) after overriding, (**c**) before overriding, (**d**) after overriding

3.4 Anatomy Modeling

1. Barium-doped plastic catheters will be overridden with 0 HU or the CT number of the tissue displaced by the catheter.
2. Metal (small clips and mesh) that does not saturate the CT scanner will not be overridden, although any imaging artifacts resulting from this material will be corrected as described above (sampling similar tissues without artifacts):
   - While this is a time-consuming process, it usually leads to adequate results.
   - Bowel gas is overridden as tissue for dose calculation in order to improve target coverage robustness with respect to daily bowel gas variation.
   - The override could cause the beam to overshoot into neighboring OARs, which can be evaluated by calculating the plan on the same CT without gas overridden (Fig. 3.12).

3.4.1 4D CT [52]

- Average CT—average density values of slices:
  - Better approximation of breathing motion
  - Used for treatment plan dose calculation and display (Fig. 3.13)

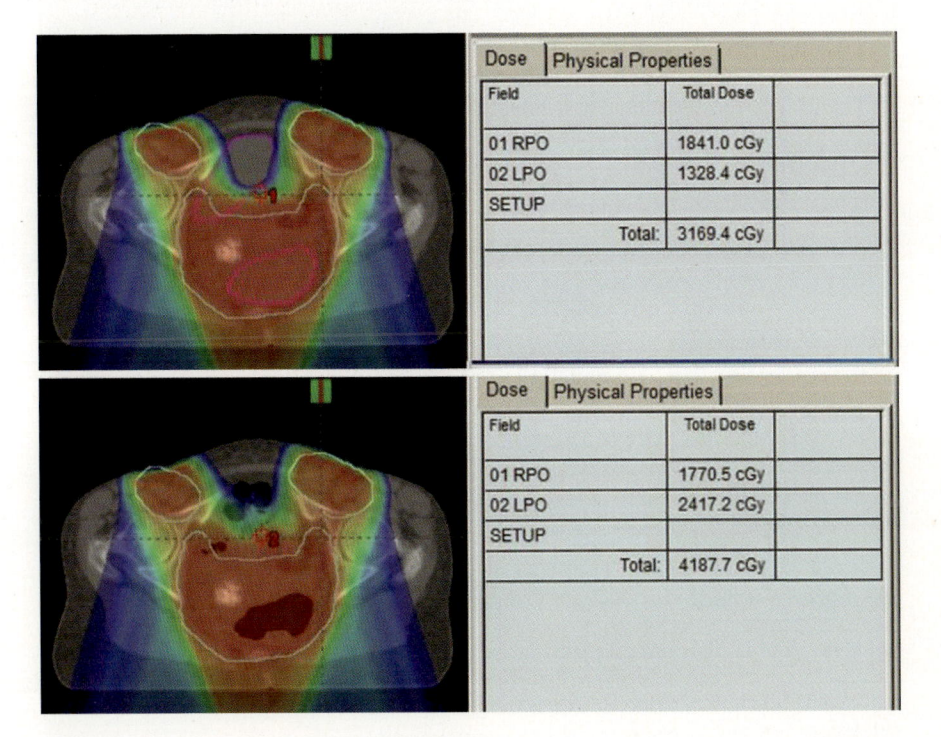

Fig. 3.12 Example of the effect on OAR dose from overshoot. *Top*, dose calculated with bowel gas overridden; *bottom*, dose calculated *without* overridden

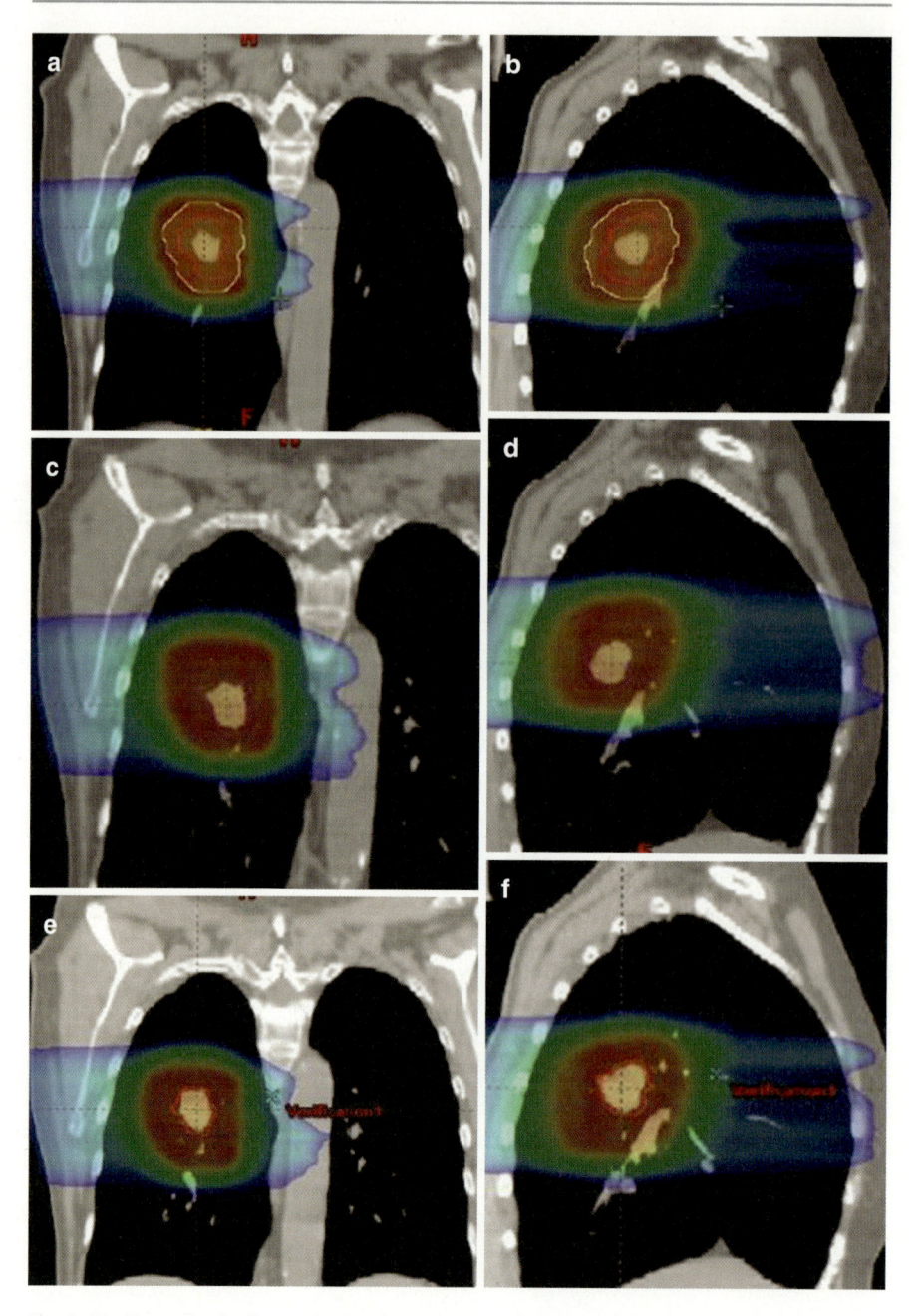

Fig. 3.13 Dose distributions calculated on average CT (**a**, **b**), (**a**) average CT, frontal, and (**b**) average CT, sagittal; end-inhalation CT (**c**, **d**), (**c**) end of inhalation, frontal, and (**d**) end of inhalation, sagittal; and end-exhalation CT (**e**, **f**) with identical beamline, (**e**) end of exhalation, frontal, and (**f**) end of exhalation, sagittal

- May need CT number override of IGTV with a conservative estimation of densities in order to ensure tumor coverage. However, this approach may compromise OAR sparing
- Any single phase:
  - Extreme phases (inhale and exhale) used to evaluate coverage by forward calculation using planned beamline (Figs. 3.13 and 3.14)
- MIP image—maximum intensity projection; maximum density value of slices:
  - Conservative since maximum density is provided
  - Should guarantee dose coverage of distal target
  - Lose coverage in proximal target region
  - Employed for targets located in the lung
- End-expiration phase (e.g., in Fig. 3.13):
  - Provides better stability and reproducibility [53]

4D CT-based planning is described in further detail in Sect. 5.

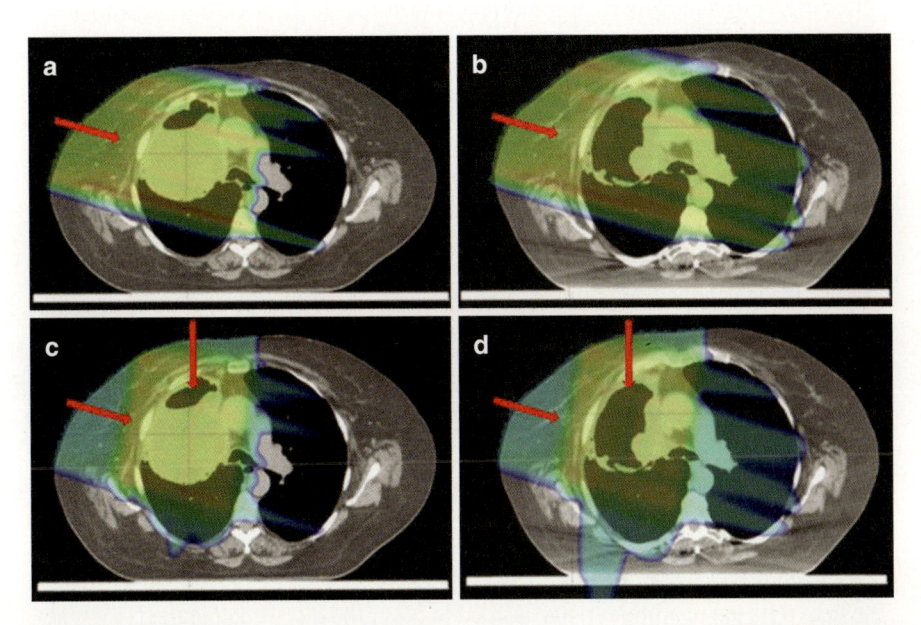

Fig. 3.14 The effect of lung tumor shrinkage on proton dose distribution. The second CT scan was taken at 3 weeks into treatment course. (**a**) shows a single RAO field from the nominal treatment plan; and (**b**) shows the effect of tumor shrinkage on the RAO field. (**c**) shows the complete two-field nominal plan; and (**d**) shows the effect of tumor shrinkage on the two-field plan

3.5 Beam Design Characteristics

3.5.1 Passive Scattering

With passive scattering (PS) beam delivery, the beam is broadened as it passes through the delivery nozzle and spreads uniformly over a large area (Chap. 2). A major difference between proton beams and photon beams is that individual proton beams may be designed to cover the entire target volume with a uniform dose distribution, characterized by the proton range, field size, and modulation width of the spread-out Bragg peak (SOBP). Field shaping is achieved by customizing the field aperture, proton beamline, and range compensator designs to ensure conformal coverage of the CTV with appropriate lateral margins and beam-specific distal and proximal margins to account for proton range uncertainties.

3.5.1.1 Beam Design Characteristics
- Field aperture: Typically manufactured from brass plates; however, some facilities use Cerrobend blocks or multi-leaf collimators (MLC). Designed to conform dose to the CTV in the beam's eye view (BEV), including margin for internal motion of target (IM), margin for setup uncertainty (SM), and a dosimetric margin to account for the physical and geometrical lateral penumbra, typically defined from the field edge (50% isodose level) to the prescription isodose, ($P_{50\%, Rx\%}$).

Aperture lateral margin (LM) (Fig. 3.16b) from the CTV at the isocenteric plane is given by
$$LM = IM + SM + P_{50\%, Rx\%}.$$
The physical dimensions of the aperture will be a function of nozzle position relative to the isocenter.

- Distal and proximal margins: Distal margins (DM) and proximal margins (PM) are defined from the CTV (Fig. 3.15) and are realized by appropriate combination of beam range and SOBP width. Both DM and PM are range dependent, with 3.5% of the range [4–6] plus 1 mm used typically.

Required range (R) is given by
$$R = R_d + DM = 1.035 R_d + 1 \text{ mm},$$
where R_d is the maximum range needed to cover the distal edge of the CTV without margin (Fig. 3.15). R_d is established by initial calculation of the water-equivalent thickness (WET) along the beam path to the most distal point of the CTV.

The required SOBP width is given by
$$SOBP = R_d - R_p + PM + DM = 1.035 R_d - 0.965 R_p + 1.0 \text{ mm},$$
where R_p is the minimum range needed to cover the proximal edge of the CTV without margin (Fig. 3.15).

The beam-specific distal and proximal margins give rise to the concept of the beam-specific PTV (bsPTV) [54], defined by the prescription isodose curve of each individual beam (Fig. 3.16).

3 Proton Treatment Planning   71

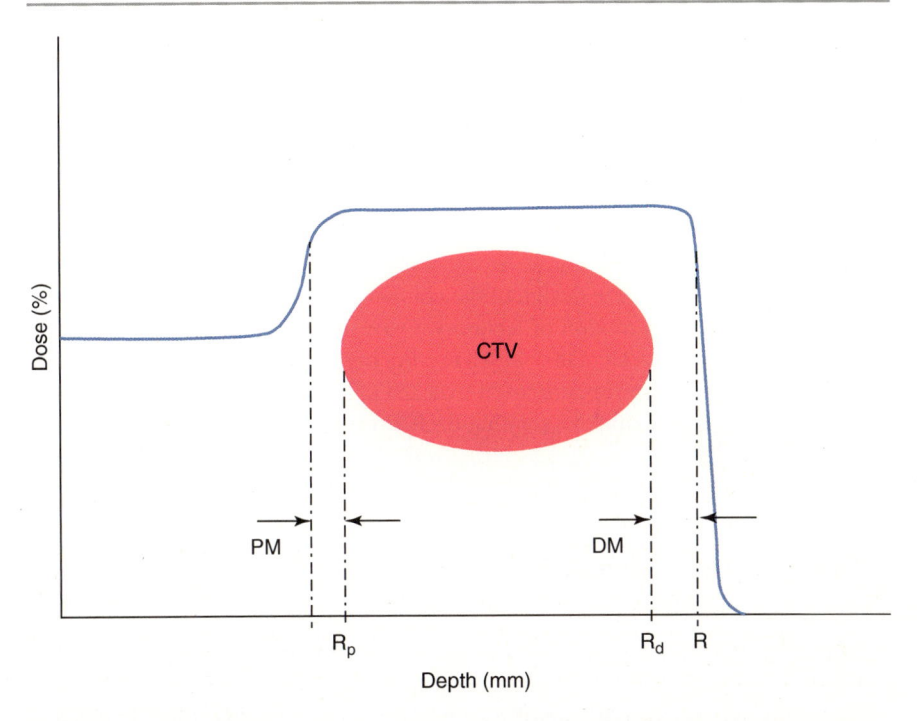

Fig. 3.15 SOBP covering CTV with distal margin, DM, and proximal margin, PM, where R is range, R_d is maximum range needed to cover CTV distal edge, and R_p is minimum range needed to cover proximal edge of CTV

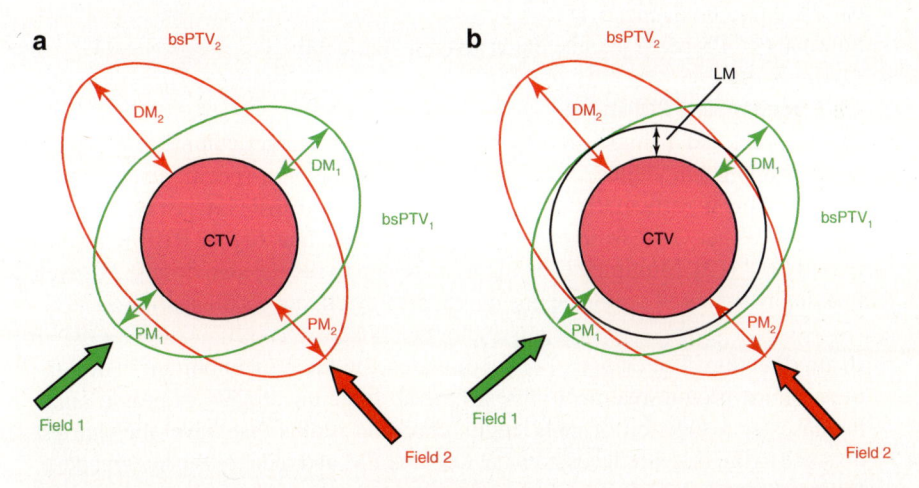

Fig. 3.16 (**a**) Beam-specific distal margins (DM) and proximal margins (PM) giving rise to a beam-specific PTV (bsPTV) for each field. (**b**) Lateral margins (LM) for both fields, similar in concept to the photon PTV

- Range compensator: Typically manufactured from PMMA, although some facilities use wax. Designed to conform the distal end of the beam to the distal edge of the CTV with DM and account for heterogeneities along the beam path, by pulling back the distal end of the beam. This is achieved with the compensator designed to be of varying thicknesses along each ray line across the BEV. It should be noted that the calculated range, R, includes the minimum WET of the compensator.

Smearing is applied to the design of the compensator to account for lateral setup uncertainty and internal motion of anatomy. Once the ideal thickness of the compensator at each point is calculated with a ray-tracing algorithm, circles of a specific smearing radius (SR) are superimposed over the calculation grid, centered at each point. The compensator thickness within each circle is reduced to the minimum at any point within the circle.

The SR is given by

$$SR = \sqrt{(IM + SM)^2 + (0.03R)^2},$$

where the first term accounts for internal motion and setup uncertainty and the second term accounts for proton lateral scatter [4, 55, 56].

Smearing has the effect of making the distal dose less conformal on a static treatment plan but ensures distal coverage with positional uncertainty (Fig. 3.17).

While the range compensator conforms the dose to the distal edge of the target, a major limitation of PS proton beams is the inability to conform the dose to proximal side of the target. This is because the beam is modulated to a fixed SOBP width across the entire field (Fig. 3.18).

Summary of PS beam parameters is given in Table 3.6.

3.5.1.2 Treatment Planning

Despite the fact that a single proton beam can cover the target volume, it is typical to use multiple beam angles to mitigate the effect of proton-specific uncertainties (Table 3.1). This is particularly useful if an organ at risk (OAR) lay just distal to the target to spare that OAR from end-of-range effects such as higher RBE related to increased LET [12]. Multiple beam angles also help to reduce skin dose [57], given that passively scattered proton beams do not display effective skin sparing.

- Beam direction: The choice of beam direction is extremely important in designing a robust proton treatment plan. As the absolute uncertainty in proton range increases as a function of path length, choosing beams that travel the shortest distance to the target reduces both the DM and PM and reduces the integral dose. However, beam directions are often chosen so as to protect OAR that lay distal to the target from end-of-range effects [12]. In such circumstances, a beam direction may be chosen such that its lateral edge, rather than its distal edge, is used to block an OAR. Furthermore, as protons are sensitive to the radiological path

3 Proton Treatment Planning

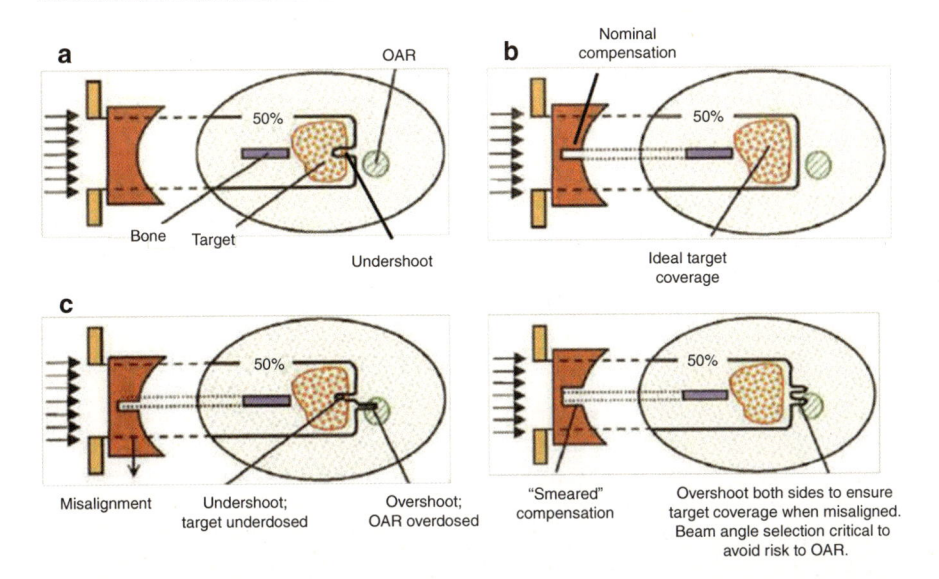

Fig. 3.17 The effect of the range compensator with and without smearing: (**a**) no compensation; (**b**) nominal compensation, without smearing; (**c**) effect of misalignment without smearing; (**d**) compensation with smearing

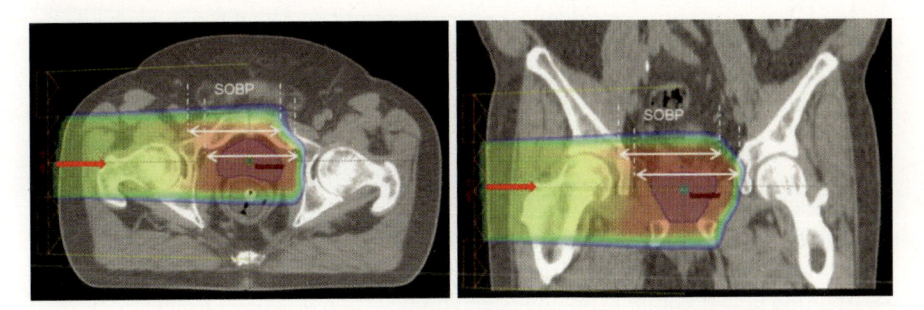

Fig. 3.18 Single right lateral field to the prostate. The distal end of the SOBP conforms to the target shape because of the compensator; however, the proximal side of the SOBP is not conformal because of the fixed SOBP width

along which they travel, choosing beam angles that avoid variations in the anatomy caused by, for example, bladder filling, bowel gas variation, stomach filling, respiratory motion, or other such processes is preferable. If at all possible, directions with abrupt changes in proton stopping power (highly heterogeneous) should be avoided. Directions, for example, that are oblique to the patient surface, or that travel through high-density materials such as titanium rods, or that travel through the edge of patient immobilization devices or the couch edge, are all highly susceptible to range uncertainty and therefore have to be avoided (Table 3.1).

Table 3.6 Formulae for calculating passive scattering beam-specific parameters

Beam-specific parameter	Formulae
Aperture lateral margin from CTV	$IM + SM + P_{50\%, Rx\%}$
Range margins	$1.035R_d + 1.0$ mm
SOBP width	$1.035R_d - 0.965R_p + 1.0$ mm
Smearing radius	$\sqrt{(IM+SM)^2 + (0.03R)^2}$

R range, R_d maximum range needed to cover CTV distal edge, R_p minimum range needed to cover proximal edge of CTV, SM setup uncertainty, IM internal margin, $P_{50\%, Rx\%}$ penumbra width from field edge to prescription isodose

- 4D CT-based planning: Treatment planning of thoracic and abdominal targets with significant respiratory motion is typically based on 4D CT. 4D CT data are acquired and binned into 3D datasets representing different phases of the respiratory cycle. Maximum-intensity projection (MIP) and intensity-weighted average projection (average CT) datasets are generated. The envelope of motion of the GTV—the internal GTV (iGTV)—is contoured either on the MIP (when the target has large contrast in CT, e.g., in the lung) or from the union of GTV contours from all phases. The iGTV contour is copied onto either the average CT or a mid-ventilation dataset on which the nominal plan is calculated. The iGTV is uniformly expanded to be the iCTV to encompass microscopic clinical disease. The CT numbers are overridden according to tumor density throughout the iGTV in order to provide a conservative estimate of radiological path lengths for all positions of the GTV, ensuring distal coverage of the target throughout the respiratory cycle (Fig. 3.19). This results in proton-beam overshoot across much of the field; and so distal OARs need to be considered when choosing beam direction. Planning to the iCTV is done using the margins described above. IM is set to zero in the calculation of LM and SR as the internal motion has been accounted for. Nominal treatment plan may be reviewed on the end-inhalation and end-exhalation phases to verify target coverage in these extremes (Fig. 3.20).
- Abutting fields: For large or elongated volumes, two or more adjacent fields may need to be used from any given beam direction. This typically requires multiple isocenters and dosimetric matching of field penumbrae at depth. The classic example of this is craniospinal irradiation (CSI) with PS proton beams (Fig. 3.21) [58]. Due to the sharp lateral falloff of dose for PS fields shaped with an aperture, numerous sets of match fields are planned with the match line displaced 1 cm or so to reduce uncertainty at match line locations. Each set of fields is only delivered for a proportion of the total number of fractions. This is labor intensive and expensive as new apertures are required for each set of fields. By comparison, pencil-beam scanning (PBS) techniques for CSI can use intensity modulation to improve matching field robustness [59, 60].
- Patch fields: Patch-field planning may be used when a target wraps around an OAR in very close proximity. To avoid directing a beam toward the OAR, a "shoot-through" beam is used to cover part of the target, while a "patch" field,

3 Proton Treatment Planning

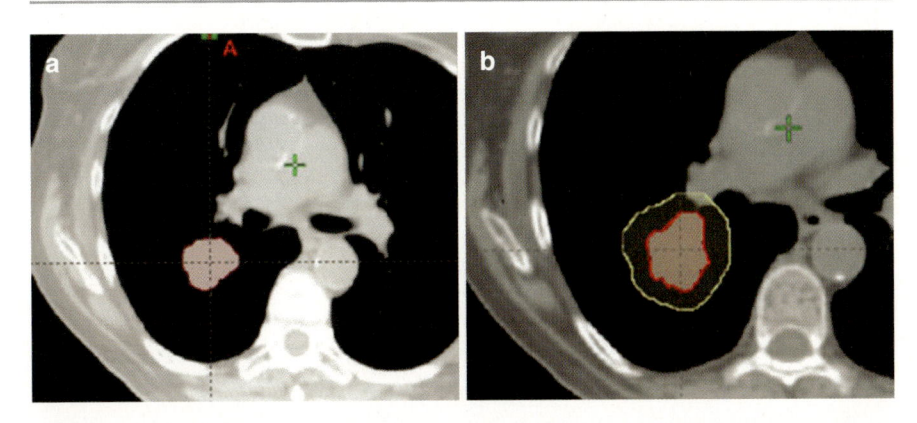

Fig. 3.19 (a) iGTV contour on average CT (or mid-ventilation) dataset with CT numbers overridden to provide a conservative estimate of radiological path lengths throughout the respiratory cycle; (b) uniform expansion to the iCTV

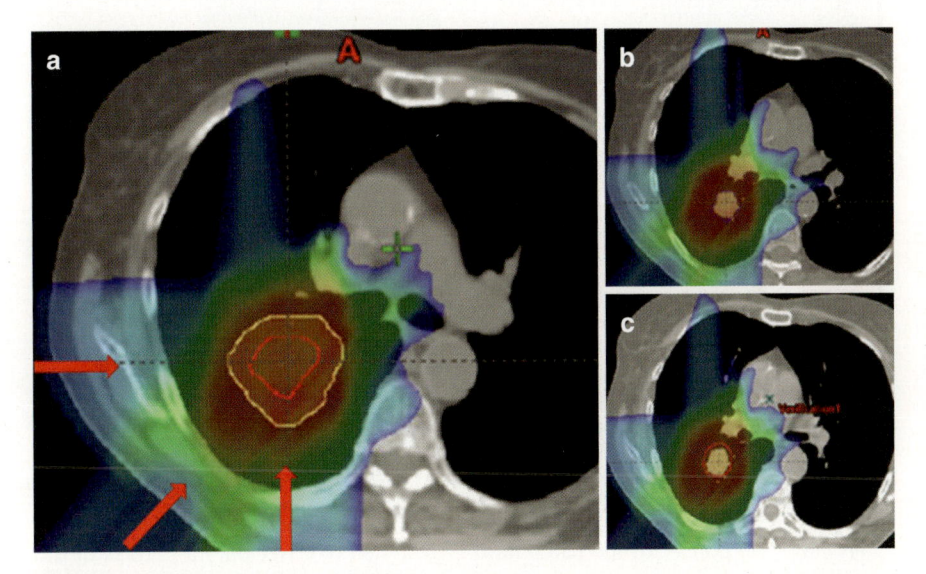

Fig. 3.20 (a) Nominal plan on average CT (or mid-ventilation) dataset, with plan evaluated on (b) end-inspiration phase and (c) end-expiration phase

covering the remaining part of the target, is designed such that its distal edge matches the lateral edge of the "shoot-through" beam [61]. Both beams block the OAR with their lateral edges (Fig. 3.22). The distal penumbra of the "patch" field is typically sharper than the lateral penumbra of the "shoot-through" field. As a consequence, matching the 50% isodose lines of these beams at the patch line produces hot and cold spots. As the patch line is typically within the CTV, the match is planned erring slightly toward being hot rather than cold. To mitigate the overall effect, the beam direction of the "shoot-through" and "patch" are reversed on alternating fractions, thus changing the location of the patch line.

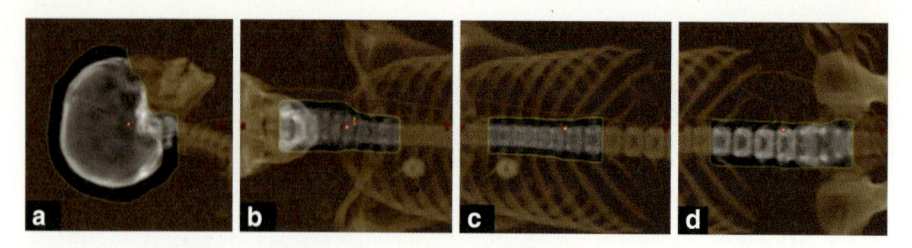

Fig. 3.21 Field-defining apertures for (**a**) cranial, (**b**) upper spine, (**c**) mid-spinal, and (**d**) lower spine fields matched for total craniospinal irradiation (CSI). Four isocenters are used in this example

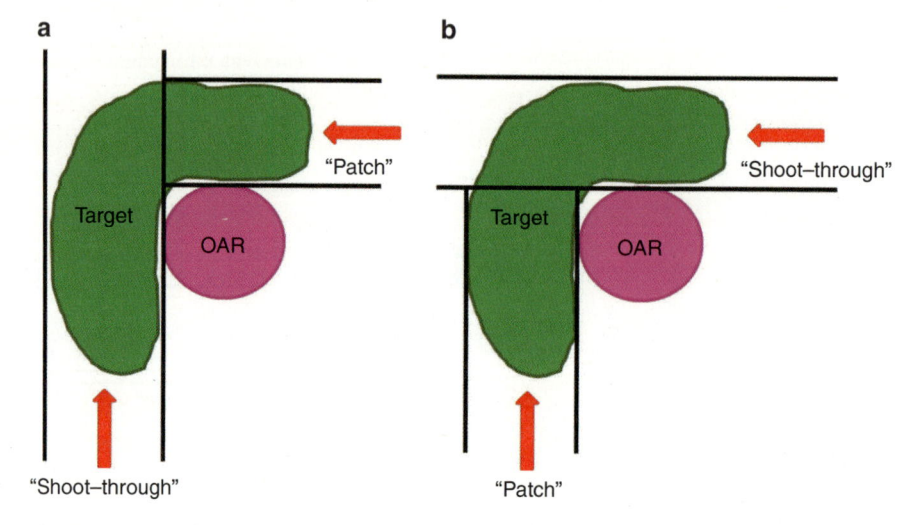

Fig. 3.22 Patch-field setup to cover the target while sparing the OAR. (**a**) shows "shoot-through" and "patch" field directions chosen to avoid range uncertainty risk to the OAR; and (**b**) shows beam arrangement used on alternating days to mitigate dose heterogeneity within the target at the patch line

As each component of the patch field is designed to cover only a portion of the target, they are inherently less robust than other PS field designs. It is therefore recommended that robustness analysis be performed to evaluate the dosimetric consequences of uncertainties.

3.5.2 Pencil-Beam Scanning

3.5.2.1 Proton Pencil-Beam Features

Any radiation beam has two features:

- Geometry: its orientation and placement with respect to the patient and target
- Dosimetry: its ability to deposit dose within the patient

3 Proton Treatment Planning

The geometric approach of a radiation beam correlates with its dosimetric abilities. That is, for example, a single photon beam has little or no dosimetric control along the penetration axis of the field. This limitation is mitigated by adding many other photon fields to achieve conformal abilities. A single proton beam, however, has the ability to achieve full conformality and less or sometimes even no additional fields are needed. Thus:

- Geometric placement of proton fields can be used to greater advantage, compared to photon fields, to achieve normal tissue sparing. That is, proton field placement can completely avoid normal structures if desired.
- Geometric placement of proton fields can enhance the penumbral falloff between target and OAR. Since fewer fields are needed, the field-intrinsic penumbra can be preserved. In contrast, a complex photon field arrangement (such as IMRT) inherently creates a washout of the penumbra as a consequence of the continuous overlap of fields. In practice, IMRT penumbra can only be preserved along a narrow surface parallel to the rotation axis as in rectal wall sparing in prostate treatment (see Fig. 3.23).
- Geometric placement for PBS beams pragmatically aims to achieve the least healthy tissue between the skin and the target and achieves maximal OAR avoidance.

The dosimetric ability of a proton pencil-beam field is defined by numerous spots with the ability to modulate the dose within each spot contained in a three-dimensional sub-volume of the target:

- A spot is a "narrow" single-energy proton pencil beam deflected magnetically to a location (x, y) in the isocentric plane with a penetration proportional to the energy and of a particular intensity defined by the number of protons in the pencil beam. The spot location is typically indicated with the radiological depth of its 90% range, R_{90}.
- The set of all beam spots is, initially, chosen such that the spot locations form a regular grid (rectangular or hexagonal) at a constant energy (range) (see Fig. 3.24):
  - Spots placed at a constant energy are referred to as a spot "layer."
  - The spot grid spacing, typically, is proportional to the spot size σ in air. This overpopulates the spot layer as it excludes the effect of inpatient scatter which increases the spot size to $\sqrt{\sigma^2 + 0.03R^2}$.
  - Multiple layers are stacked across the depth of the target to cover the target. Typical layer spacing is 5–8 mm.
  - Margins in proximal and distal depths are used to allow for range uncertainties and proximal and distal dose equilibrium.
  - Lateral margins (>3σ and see above on the effect of inpatient scatter) are used in each layer to achieve lateral dose equilibrium.
  - For a 100 mm cube, the set of spots could be as many as 10,000 for a small spot (σ ~ 5 mm) given a brute force geometric spot placement algorithm as suggested above.

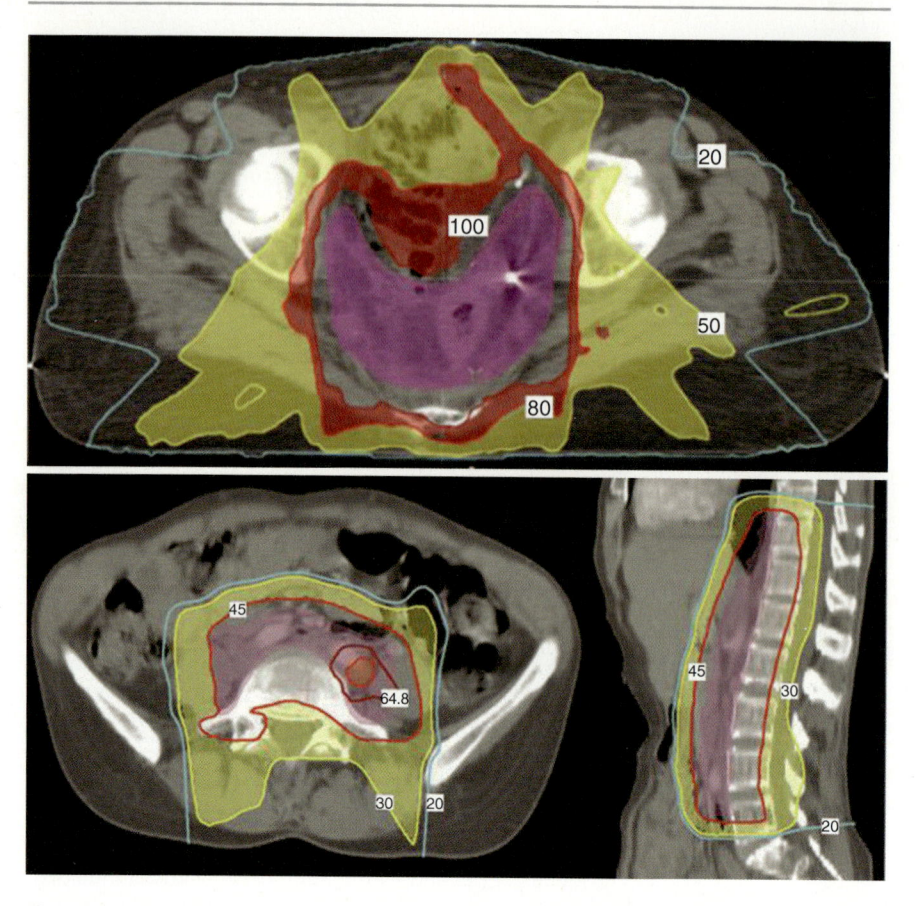

Fig. 3.23 Patient treated for endometrial cancer. The conformality of a single proton field, as in the lower panel, exceeds that of, for example, the IMRT fields shown in the upper panel. The IMRT treatment has an unavoidable dose path throughout the abdomen. Note that the IMRT is in relative dose, while the PBS plan is in absolute dose; 100% equals 45 Gy(RBE) (Image courtesy of Dr. A. Russell and J. A. Adams, Massachusetts General Hospital)

- Spot placement is per beam and ignores (as currently implemented) the spot placement in another beam. The overall consequence of current spot placement algorithms is that there are too many spots in the total set of all beams.

The spot intensities, specified in charge (number of protons) or monitor units, of a set of beams, where a minimum set includes the beams delivered in a treatment fraction, are determined by the optimization algorithm. The spot placement algorithm and spot size affect the spot intensities because:

- The fraction dose to the target volume determines (to the first order) the total number of protons that are required. A rule of thumb is that 1 Gp (giga-protons) is required to deliver 1 cGy(RBE) to 1000 cc. Thus, 2 Gy(RBE) to a liter requires about 200 Gp. Table 3.7 illustrates some consequences of delivery.

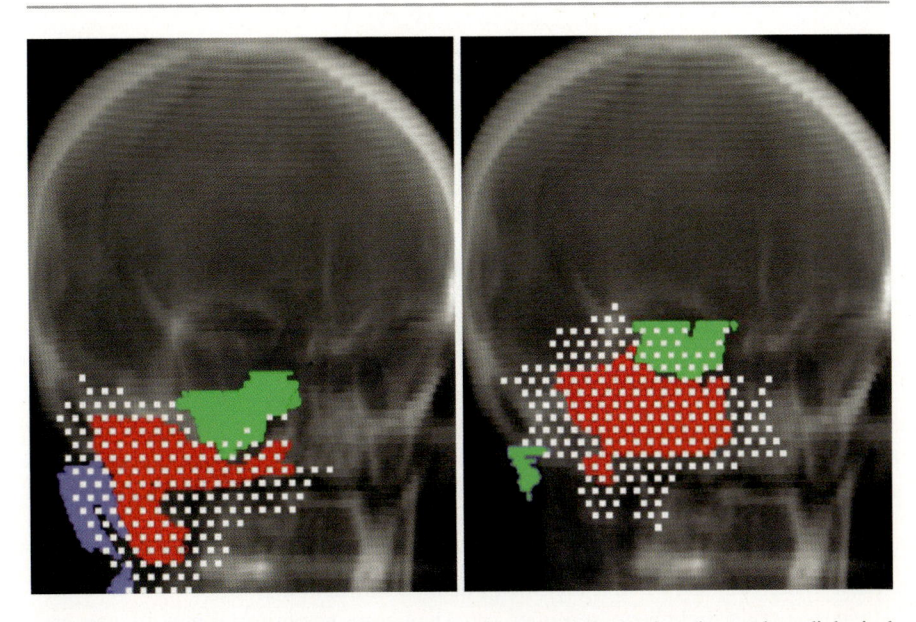

Fig. 3.24 Two spot layers (at different energies). The spot terminal points (i.e., at the radiological depth equal to R_{90}) intersect the patient at different positions as is evident from the volume (target, red; brainstem, green; etc.) intersections. The intersection surface is not a plane (per se) but a surface at constant water-equivalent (in terms of proton stopping power) depth in patient

Table 3.7 Some rule-of-thumb considerations in spot charge and delivery

Desired treatment time	60 s		
Total number of protons	2.00×10^{11}		
Number of layers	15		
Total number of spots	10,000		
Layer switching time/s	2	1	0.005
Spot rate/s	333	222	167
Maximum number of protons per layer	1.40×10^{11}		
Maximum number of protons per spot	2.10×10^{8}		
Maximum current/nA	11	7	6

A desired irradiation of 1 L cube to 2 Gy(RBE) requires 200 Gp (Gp: 10^9 protons). We wish to treat in 60 s. The delivery uses 15 layers with about 10,000 spots (implying a spot size $\sigma \sim 4$ mm). If the layer switching time is 2, 1, or 0.005 s, spots need to be delivered at the rate indicated. Of note, spot rate is primarily limited by the ability to change the magnetic field. The maximum number of protons per layer and spot is approximated by assuming the deepest, distal layer delivers 70% of the total charge. This results in the maximum currents indicated in the bottom row

- A typical charge density across the field is on the order of 1,000,000 protons per mm². Much higher local densities are common. It should be obvious, however, that larger spots will have higher mean charges. Thus, a spot twice as large as another spot will have four times the mean charge. The number of protons is distributed over the spots: the more spots, the lower the mean charge of a spot.

- The accelerator typically has a lower limit on the possible spot intensity. If there are too many spots, there may be many spots that have an intensity below this limit.
- All these effects may affect the plan quality in terms of optimization efficiency and quality and in terms of treatment delivery efficiency.

3.5.2.2 Beam Set and Fractions

Proton fractions can readily alternate different combinations of beams, or fraction beam sets, within a particular treatment phase. For example, of a total of five individual beams in a phase, three sets may be defined as (1, 3, 5), (2, 5), and (4, 5). The set combinations may be chosen to alternate healthy dose areas or even be based on practical considerations such as effects on overall treatment time for a fraction. Such beam rotations are not used in IMRT treatments and, as a consequence, are not well established in general clinical practice.

Each beam set must deliver the desired fraction dose. Thus, beam 5 in the above example really has three different dosimetric representations, one for each set. Beam 5 simply refers to its geometric features but its dosimetric features depend on its fellow members. Each beam is thus defined by its geometry (say 5) and its dosimetric state, i.e., beam 5 in fraction 1 or beam 5 in fraction 2.

The use of different beam sets over a phase requires an optimizer that can consider the membership of a beam within the fraction while considering the objectives of the whole course. In the asteroid system (.decimal, Sanford, FL), the user can define:

- Course constraints, e.g., maximum dose to the brainstem less than 54 Gy(RBE), minimum dose to the CTV is 52 Gy(RBE), and so on.
- Course objectives, e.g., try to minimize the brainstem mean dose, try to maximize the minimum dose to the CTV.
- Fraction constraints, e.g., in the five fractions for this beam set, the maximum dose to the brainstem is 10 Gy(RBE).

Table 3.8 shows a fraction group subdivision for a simultaneous optimization for a chordoma treatment. Figure 3.25 shows the dosimetry for the GTV fraction group, obtained while simultaneously optimizing all fraction groups, and the total dosimetry of all fraction groups.

3.5.2.3 Field Matching and Patching

For SOBP fields in PS (see previous section on PS; Sect. 5.1):

- Matching requires two to three feathers to avoid hot or cold spots possible with the sharp SOBP penumbra.
- Patching requires alternate through/patch combination due to the range uncertainty. In practice, a single through/patch combination should not be used for more than five fractions. For PBS fields:

1. Matching is greatly simplified by specifying an overlap volume left/right of the match line and allowing the optimizer to produce a gradient in the region (see Fig. 3.26).

3 Proton Treatment Planning

Table 3.8 Three fraction groups to CTV, CTV II, and GTV, each with fraction group constraints and beam allocations. The multiple fractions and constraints are optimized as a single problem

Fraction groups		Number of fractions
1 CTV	Type: IMPT Target: CTV + 5 mm Total dose: 26 Gy(RBE) Constraint: CTV + 3 mm minimum 24 Gy(RBE) beams: R35A CTV, L50P CTV	13
2 CTV II	Type: IMPT Target: CTV + 5 mm Total dose: 24 Gy(RBE) Constraint: CTV + 3 mm minimum 22 Gy(RBE) beams: R50P CTV, L25A CTV	12
3 GTV	Type: IMPT Target: GTV Total dose: 28 Gy(RBE) Constraint: GTV minimum mean 28 Gy(RBE) beams: L70P GTVp3, R50P GTVp3	14

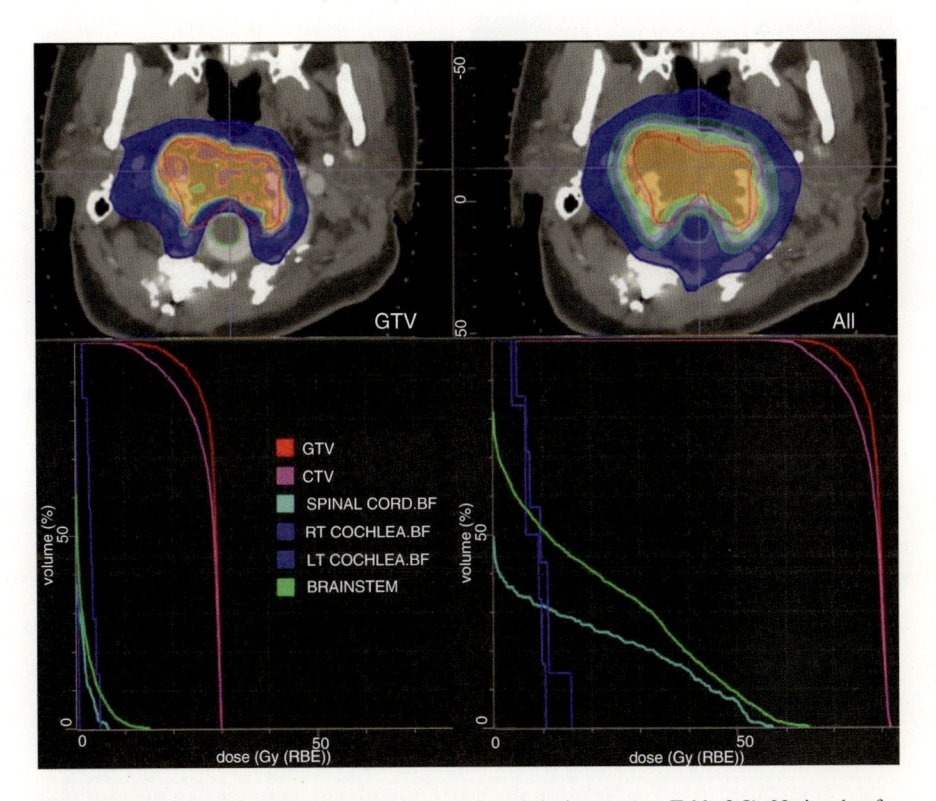

Fig. 3.25 Dosimetry for GTV fraction group and total dosimetry (see Table 3.8). Notice that for the GTV fraction group, the constraint is specified as a minimum mean dose of 28 Gy(RBE)

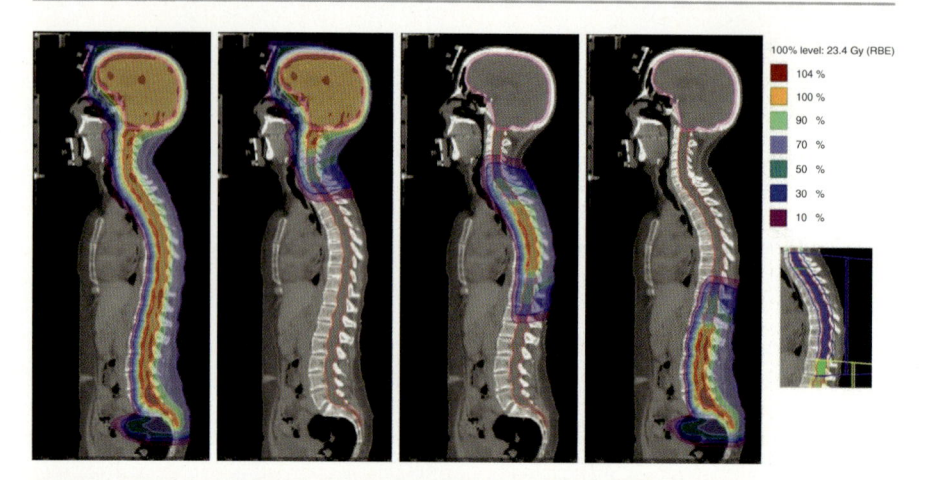

Fig. 3.26 Medulloblastoma patient treated with two cranial fields (to ensure lens sparing) and two posterior fields. Two overlap regions, in the cervical spine and lower thorax, ensure a smooth and long gradient that ensures dose continuation with ±3 mm setup uncertainty. The inset (*right*) shows the overlap region between the thoracic (*blue*) and lumbar fields (*yellow*)

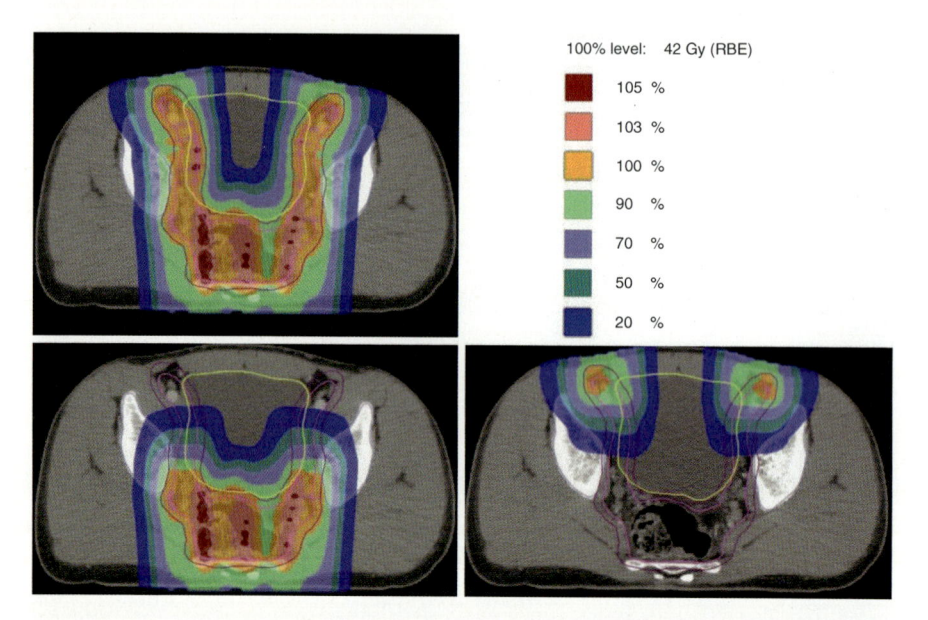

Fig. 3.27 Rectal cancer patient, composite dose top left. Anterior and posterior field patches along the distal edges are allowed to range out over an overlap volume (bottom left/right). Note that the spot size in this example is large which causes the size of the penumbral lateral falloff

2. Patching is obviated as fields are allowed to range out into the each other. This, of course, is subject to robustness considerations (see Fig. 3.27).
   - This does not necessarily imply IMPT fields. SFUD fields can overlap to a lesser extent or otherwise achieve smooth gradients.

3.6 Treatment Plan Design and Site Considerations

3.6.1 Site Considerations

- The effect of treatment site specifics influences the approach and quality of proton fields.
- Range uncertainties and increased LET (ionization density per unit length) at the end of range demand that proton fields cannot range out into a critical structure. Instead, penumbral separation between target and critical structure must be achieved by the lateral edge:
  - Of note, the distal penumbra is typically twice as sharp compared to the lateral penumbra in SOBP fields that use a range compensator. Nevertheless, the distal penumbra should not be used for separation between target and OARs.
  - The distal penumbra in a PBS field is essentially equivalent to the lateral penumbra because the distal penumbra in such a field is comprised of multiple, near arbitrarily positioned, spots.
- Motion effects are particularly troublesome as the motion periodicity requires a consideration of the dose perturbation at every time point:
  - 4D CT can accurately establish the periodicity of the patient's anatomy.
  - In principle, a plan can be designed that simultaneously meets the dosimetric constraints over the whole periodic interval. Such a plan, by definition, increases the dose to the uninvolved tissues.
  - Reduction of the covered time interval compared to the total periodicity interval improves the treatment plan quality at the expense of increased treatment time.
  - For SOBP treatment fields, typically, a site-specific motion mitigation strategy can be established using, for example, ITVs or by using the most likely point in the periodicity.
  - For PBS treatment fields, the frequency of motion may interfere destructively with the spot delivery sequence and cause "interplay" effects that produce hot/cold spots in the target. Such interplay effects can only be evaluated through explicit temporal simulation of the delivery sequence in conjunction with the target motion (e.g., [53, 62, 63]).

Typical beam arrangements for various anatomical sites are summarized in Table 3.9.

3.6.2 Fraction Management

- Even a single proton field may achieve sufficient dose conformality.
- Fractions over the course of treatment may use alternating sets of one or more proton fields to decrease fraction time while maintaining, over the course, the benefit of integral dose reduction with many fields.

Table 3.9 Summary of typical beam arrangements for various anatomical sites for proton therapy plans

Site	Number of fields	Orientation	Comments
Craniospinal	4–5	Left and right posterior oblique fields to the brain, cribriform plate, and upper C-spine, with abutting PA fields to the spine	3–4 sets of these fields are planned to allow junction shifts during treatment course
Brain	2–4	Noncoplanar, multidirectional	Angles depend on tumor location and chosen to reduce integral dose and risk to OARs from end-of-range effects
Ocular melanoma	1	AP	Specialized technique with specific ocular horizontal beamline. Patient treated in seated position. Eye rotated into optimal position for OAR sparing by defining a gazing angle at simulation and indicating this on the delivery nozzle for individual patients
Head and neck, unilateral	2–3	PA/lateral/anterior oblique/posterior oblique	Beam angles chosen to reduce integral dose or traversing heterogeneous tissue wherever possible and to reduce end-of-range effects to OAR
Head and neck, bilateral	2–3	PA/lateral/posterior oblique	Anterior beams traversing the oral cavity and nasal sinuses should be avoided wherever possible. The heterogeneity of these structures, and variation in sinus filling, increase uncertainty. Patch fields (combinations of PA and lateral fields) are often used to spare the brainstem
Breast, partial	2–3	Noncoplanar, multidirectional	Multiple beams to reduce area of skin receiving full dose and to not have all beams ranging out on the same rib

3 Proton Treatment Planning

Table 3.9 (continued)

Site	Number of fields	Orientation	Comments
Breast, whole	1–2	Anterior oblique	En face, avoiding obliquity, to minimize range uncertainties caused by respiratory motion
Mediastinum/chest wall	1–2	AP/anterior oblique	En face, avoiding obliquity, to minimize range uncertainties caused by respiratory motion
Hemithorax	3	PA/posterior oblique/lateral, or AP/anterior oblique/lateral	Beam angles depend on tumor location. Typically, three fields or used to improve plan robustness 4D CT-based treatment planning approach to account for respiratory motion
Upper GI	2–3	PA/posterior oblique	Beam angles to reduce lung/cardiac dose and to avoid traversing anatomy with significant respiratory motion
Lower GI	3	PA/posterior oblique/lateral	Avoid anatomy that varies due to bowel gas changes, stomach filling, and respiratory motion. Multiple beams increase robustness and reduce risk of end-of-range effects on radiosensitive OARs. The use of multiple angles also reduces dose to spinal cord and kidneys from entry plateau of passing beams
Prostate	2	Right and left laterals	Typically, patient treated with a full bladder and water-filled rectal balloon in situ to immobilize the prostate. Some centers utilize a spacer between the prostate and rectum instead of using a rectal balloon to spare the anterior rectal wall

- Multiple fraction groups allow for per fraction optimization of certain constraints (i.e., one fraction may allow dose to the brainstem while another must avoid it).
- The use of multiple fraction groups for a single plan requires effective support in the TPS for optimization and dose accumulation over these multiple fraction groups.

3.6.3 TPS Algorithm and Features

- A dose calculation algorithm must, at a minimum, model all the available geometric and dose-modifying features of the delivery system:
  - The user must ensure proper commissioning and use per validated protocols.
  - Extension beyond both the delivery system or calculation capabilities requires careful specification and validation.
  - Geometry features comprise those that model the position of the patient with respect to the beam axis.
  - Dosimetry features comprise those that model the beam itself, scatter effects in the patient and from external materials, apertures, range compensators, and range shifters.
- Proton dose calculation must use, at a minimum, pencil-beam algorithms (PBA):
  - The use of Monte Carlo has not yet been clinically integrated.
  - PBA, depending on their implementation, decreases in spatial resolution as a function of depth. At best, the spatial sensitivity is about 0.03ρ where ρ is the radiological depth.
  - The use of PBA in lung dose calculations should be accompanied by Monte Carlo validation (either per patient or per site standard) because of range straggling effects in the lung that are not modeled by PBA.
  - PBA should consider secondary proton interactions, where the proton interacts with the nucleus and creates a broad secondary dose effect, especially for field sizes, either confined by apertures or limited by scanning size, less than 100 mm diameter (see Fig. 3.28) [64].

The use of halo corrections often is included implicitly if patient fields are calibrated on a per field basis. The user should analyze the effect and necessity of this correction in their practice.

  - There is, theoretically, no difference in PBA for scattered, uniform scanning, or PBS fields. There may be significant implementation differences.
- Proton dose calculations (i.e., the context in which a PBA is used) must consider the effect of proton uncertainties. These include geometric and dosimetric uncertainties:
  - Geometric uncertainties are in common with those in photon radiotherapy.
  - Geometric uncertainties, however, cannot be readily accommodated by the definition of a PTV because the geometric uncertainty has an effect on the dose distribution itself unlike in photon radiotherapy.

3 Proton Treatment Planning

Fig. 3.28 Depth doses for primary and secondary proton dose depositions in water for an infinite broad field with infinite SAD. Note the specification of the depth dose in absolute dose per Gp. Alternatively, MU can be used as a specification in the treatment planning system. Note the use of the log scale on the ordinate axis

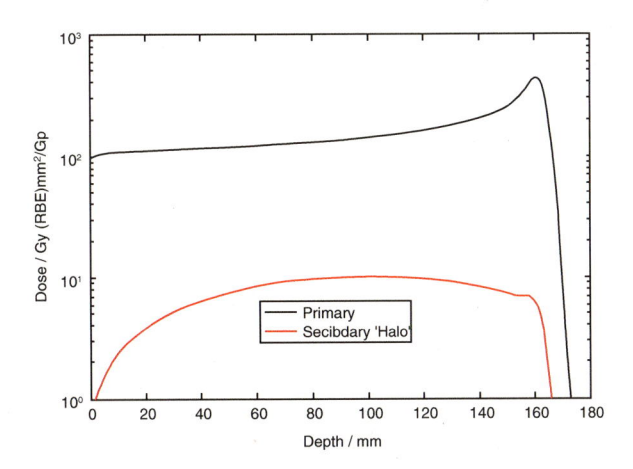

- Range uncertainties (apart from those caused by geometric uncertainties) arise from uncertainty in the patient-specific (relative to water) stopping power, the proton equivalent of "attenuation." This uncertainty, in clinical practice is managed as follows:

For SOBP fields: increase of distal range penetration and decrease in proximal range penetration. Typical correction is $0.035R + 1$ mm.

- For PBS fields: the explicit modeling of variation in the isocenter position and CT values.
- Proton dose calculations currently use water-relative stopping powers (RSP) derived from CT-number-to-RSP conversion.
- The CT-number-to-RSP conversion uses a population average curve whose anchor points are (typically) water, air, and bone. This conversion carries an intrinsic uncertainty in the stopping power which contributes to the uncertainty in range.
- The dose to water calculation may differ from the effective dose to tissue [65].
- The biological equivalent proton dose relative to cobalt-60 is assumed to have an RBE = 1.1 throughout. The RBE = 1.1 is largely an empirical equivalence with minimal experimental confirmation and assumed for similar clinical end points as in photon radiotherapy. Thus, dose equivalences at extreme situations, such as in SBRT, remain subject to scrutiny.

3.6.4 PBS Optimization Volumes, Concept, and Examples

- PBS optimization computes the spot intensities, quantified in number of protons (giga-protons or Gp) or equipment-specific monitor units, such that the total dose from all spots meets the dosimetric criteria of optimization:
  - A spot is a proton pencil beam quantified by energy (range in patient), position in the isocentric plane achieved by magnetic deflection, and intensity.

- A spot is typically "positioned" at a radiological depth equal to its distal range (typically the depth of 90% of peak value).
- An optimization algorithm typically uses a dosimetric transfer function D_{ij} that maps the dose from a unit charge to spot j to all points i. For that function, the dose to a point i is $D_i = \sum_j Q_j D_{ij}$. The use of the D_{ij} function allows the optimizer to rapidly compute the dose anywhere during the manipulation of the spot charge Q:
  - The dose calculation in PBS computes the *Dij* function prior to optimization. The patient dose is subsequently computed when the charges have been optimized.
- PBS optimization uses a spot placement algorithm that must ensure that the total set of spots of all fields can achieve the desired dosimetric result:
  - This primarily implies that the set of spots sufficiently covers the target volume, including lateral and distal extents, that ensures dose equilibrium at the target surface.
- The scale of optimization for protons is an order of magnitude larger than for photon IMRT due to the large number of spots.
- The larger solution space benefits from multi-criteria optimization (MCO) because a single-valued optimization result may, in fact, not be the most optimal in terms of clinical objectives:
  - Pareto optimization is an MCO technique that specifies a set of inviolable constraints (such as target minimum dose greater than 50 Gy(RBE)) and a set of objectives (such as, given the constraints, minimize the maximum dose to the brainstem).
  - Pareto optimization creates a multidimensional (proportional to the number of objectives) surface, the Pareto front, that contains a set of Pareto-optimal treatment plans given the constraints and treatment approach.
  - Each Pareto-optimal treatment plan is optimal given a unique set of objective values. The surface can be interrogated to assess the impact of one trade-off versus another (see Fig. 3.29).
- Current optimization techniques often require "guidance" volumes to achieve some local optimal effect. This is primarily a consequence of the limited ability to quantify the desired constraints.
- Robust optimization produces optimized plans which are insensitive, i.e., guaranteed to maintain the desired dose constraints and objectives, to uncertainties. This applies to both proton and photon optimization:
  - For photon optimization, however, robustness can be achieved through the definition of planning targets and avoidance regions around critical structures.
  - For proton optimization, the optimization must include robustness in its computation of charges.
  - Proton robust-optimized plans are currently most readily visualized through uncertainty bands around the nominal non-robust plan in a DVH (see Fig. 3.30) [66].

3 Proton Treatment Planning

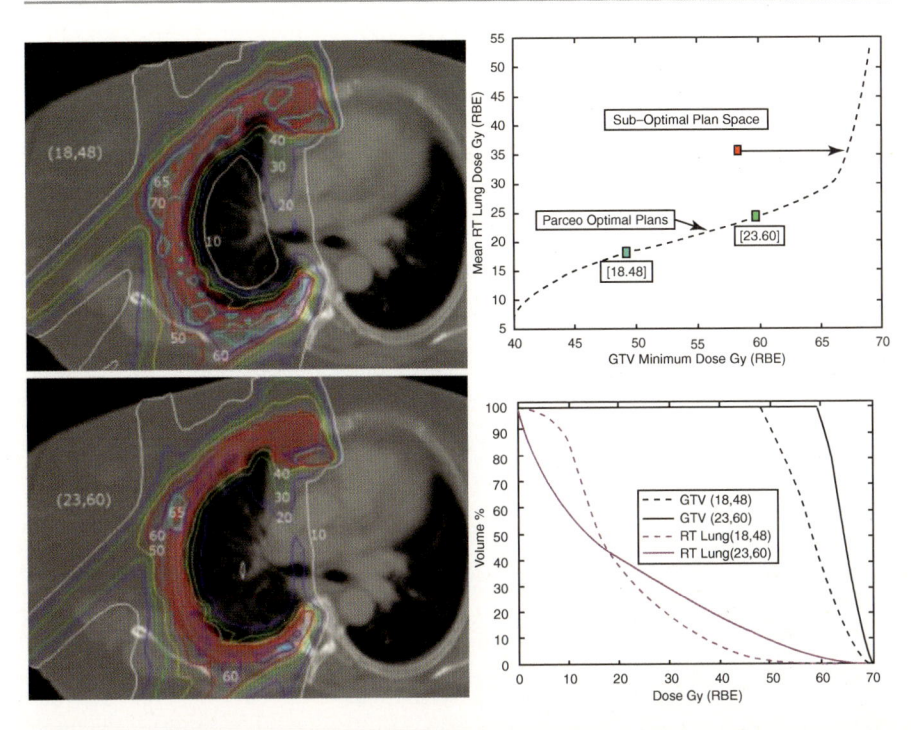

Fig. 3.29 Example trade-off analysis based on Pareto-optimal plans. Optimal mesothelioma GTV dose is in conflict with minimal lung dose. The top graph shows a curve that indicates the plans that balance the optimal trade-off of the achievable values (indicated in parentheses for two example points). The "red" point indicates a suboptimal plan because for its achieved mean lung dose, a still much higher minimum GTV dose is physically achievable. The DVHs in the bottom graph indicate the trade-off between the two plans indicated on the curve. The left figures are transverse sections for each point. The plan uses three proton PBS fields: anterior, posterior oblique, and right oblique. Patient example courtesy of Dr. Bernard Eden

3.6.5 Patient Field QA

- Patient field QA establishes that:
    - The dose in the patient is correct.
    - The dose as delivered is correct.
- The dose in patient can only be validated by an independent dose calculation method. Monte Carlo is assumed to be most accurate and even in excess compared to the dose calculation. The use of Monte Carlo, however, requires careful validation of the Monte Carlo itself.
- The delivered dose validation is established by tracing the field and dose information from its origin in the TPS, its transfer to the delivery system, and its measurement by an independent, traceable to standards, measuring device:
    - The measurements require an equivalent dose representation in the TPS and on the delivery system. This is achieved most easily in a water-equivalent phantom.

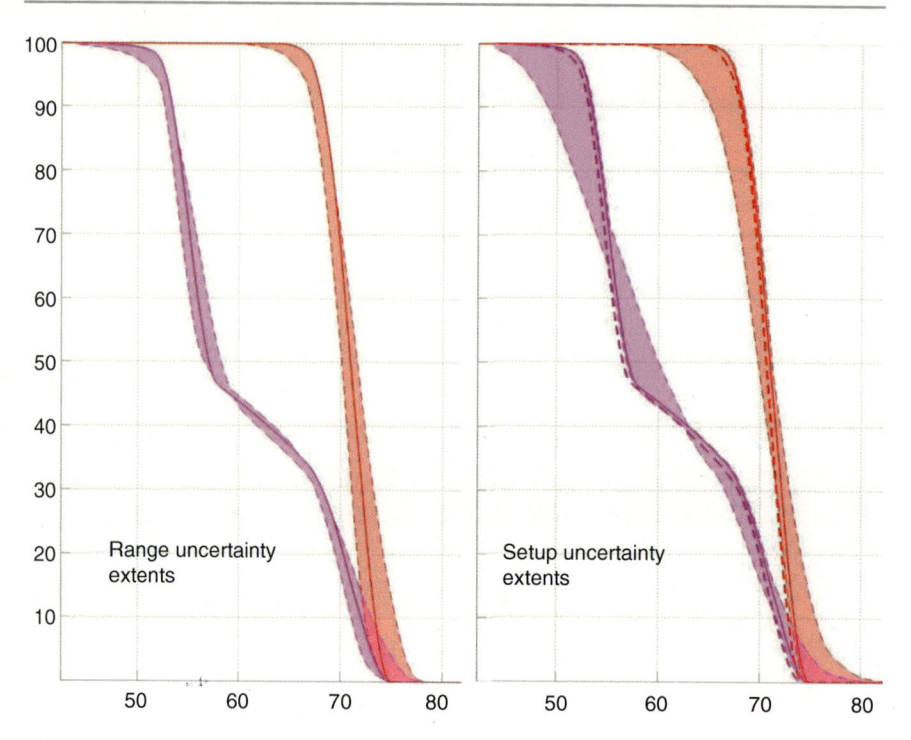

Fig. 3.30 DVHs for nominal case (*solid line*) and maximum extents given range uncertainty (*left*) and setup uncertainty (*right*). Note that the setup uncertainty has a larger effect. The setup uncertainty, if random over multiple treatment fractions N, will be reduced by approximately $\sqrt{N}$ and thus become much smaller

- Note that such a measurement may not validate consequences of inpatient heterogeneities which can only be validated through Monte Carlo.
- The measurement should quantify the three-dimensional features of the dose distribution which typically requires the measurement in at least two planes.
- The measurement should include field specific devices such as range shifter or aperture.
- Dose equivalence is established by a spatially/dosimetrically sensitive algorithm. Most commonly, the γ-index is applied. Of particular relevance is the 3D γ-index [67].

3.7 SRS Treatment Planning

- Stereotactic radiosurgery is a proven treatment modality in photon clinics with both cobalt (Gamma Knife) and traditional, gimbaled, and robotic linear accelerator systems. As opposed to traditional fractionation schedules that are generally accepted to increase the therapeutic ratio based upon the four Rs of radiobiology, photon SRS treatments rely upon a single fraction of high dose delivered to a highly localized region that achieves a therapeutic ratio by the geometric avoidance of healthy tissue. With proton SRS, the therapeutic ratio is identically determined by the localization of a high dose delivered to a targeted region and the dosimetric sparing of healthy tissues.

- In the case of proton-based SRS treatments, the dose delivered to the target is prescribed to the same level as photon therapies. The normalization level is institution specific and controls the amount of dose heterogeneity inside the targeted region.
- Proton SRS can generally achieve greater dose homogeneity due to the specifics of the dose delivery techniques compared (scattered or scanned beams) to linear accelerator-based treatments (cones and small MLC shapes).
- For smaller treatment targets, the proton-beam profiles are dominated by penumbra due to the lateral scattering of the protons as they pass through tissue. Similar to photons, the size of the penumbra increases with depth in tissue. Unlike photons, the penumbra of the proton fields is dependent more on depth and field size. For proton SRS, the penumbra is affected by field size, depth, range, apertures, range compensators, air gap, effective source position (beam optics), and tissue heterogeneities (Fig. 3.31).

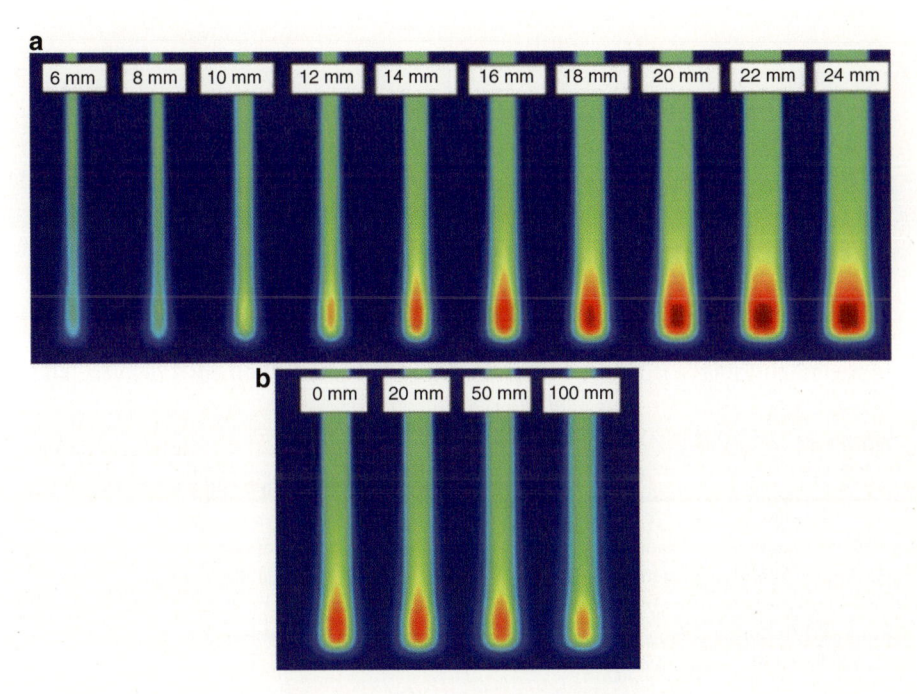

Fig. 3.31 Two factors that affect the penumbra: field size (**a**) and air gap (**b**)

3.7.1 Treatment Planning Considerations for Proton SRS

The above issues must be addressed in the commissioning of a proton SRS program and properly modeled in the treatment planning system or corrected prior to beam delivery. Additionally, treatment planning protocols can reduce the effects of scattering and penumbra through the use of beam angle optimization, limits on the minimum field sizes or target sizes, and the use of multiple treatment beams (Table 3.10). Such planning protocols will increase dose conformality to the GTV, reduce delivery uncertainty effects, and increase treatment robustness.

3.7.2 Proton SRS with Scattered Beam

- Current state-of-the-art proton SRS utilizes scattering delivery systems since scanning systems are only recently becoming more available. Treatment planning protocols employ apertures and range compensators to increase conformality in the lateral and distal directions.
- Planning for cranial SRS always includes at least two treatment beams and frequently three or more to increase conformality and plan robustness.
- The air gap is minimized to sharpen the penumbra, both geometric penumbra and scattering penumbra; and beam angles are selected to minimize tissue heterogeneities and distal edge sparing of critical organs.

3.7.3 Proton SRS with Scanned Beam

- While scanning is not widely utilized in proton SRS programs, it is expected to increase as more scanning rooms enter clinical use and proton SRS programs are commissioned in new treatment rooms.
- Scanned beam proton SRS will increase the proximal conformality of proton SRS treatments.
- There may be clinical scenarios wherein physical apertures may sharpen the penumbra and increase conformality for scanned beam proton SRS delivery and

Table 3.10 A summary of common uncertainties that can be minimized with planning protocols

Effect	Treatment planning mitigation technique
Scattering and penumbra reduce target dose	Minimum field size for treatments
Range variation increases dose to organs	Avoid distal sparing of organs
Scattering from tissue heterogeneities	Avoid beam angles parallel to tissue boundaries
Lack of dose conformality	Increase number of beams
Large dose uncertainty from a single beam angle	Increase number of beams
Range uncertainties	Beam-specific margins and/or robust optimization

should be considered in the treatment planning process if apertures are available at the institution. Range compensators may also increase the distal conformality of the scanned delivery.
- Since many SRS treatment targets are small, SFUD planning techniques are often the first option for treatment planning unless there is desire to incorporate a simultaneous integrated boost (SIB) for a GTV/CTV.
- Proton SRS can provide the clinical tools to treat more complicated target geometries that are not possible with traditional photon SRS tools. Examples which lend themselves to proton SRS as opposed to photon are indicated in Sect. 7.5. In these cases, IMPT may be considered but may introduce additional delivery uncertainties and reduced plan robustness that cannot be compensated with fractionation.

3.7.4 Commissioning and QA Considerations Specific for Proton SRS

- Commissioning of a proton SRS program must include percent depth dose (PDD) and profile measurements of small proton fields and single pencil beams.
- Some treatment planning systems only allow for an integrated depth dose (IDD) measurement which does not capture the penumbral variations, instead relying upon a deconvolution model to determine the penumbra (Fig. 3.32). While the deconvolution method can model small proton fields and single pencil beams, the model must be validated against measurements.
- The measurements must use appropriate detectors that minimize volume averaging and LET affects.
- Additional considerations for commissioning should include uncertainty analysis of all isocenters (beam, mechanical, imaging, patient positioner, etc.), specifically the coincidence of all isocenters to the radiation isocenter.
- A final component for commissioning an SRS program must include a robust end-to-end test utilizing one of the many SRS phantoms currently available. The phantom should allow for the testing of various treatment depths and target sizes

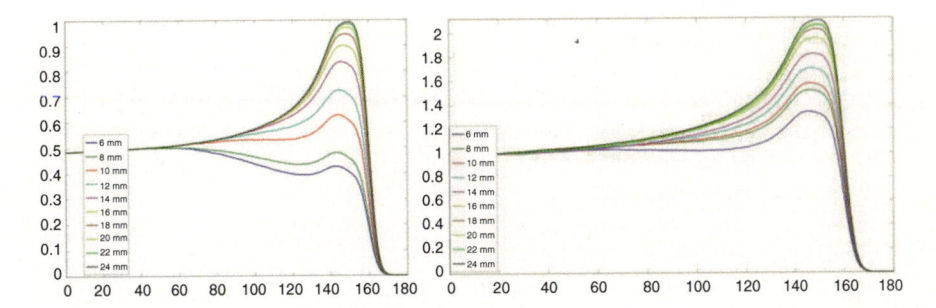

Fig. 3.32 A comparison of a PDD (*left*) and an IDD (*right*) for an SOBP with identical range and modulation but for different field sizes

and not introduce additional treatment delivery uncertainties such as SPR uncertainties from unknown plastics or oversimplified geometries that fail to test the image guidance systems.

3.7.5 Clinical Benefits of Physical Dose Properties of Proton SRS

- Given a commissioned proton SRS treatment program, the clinical benefits of proton SRS can be considered from two patient cohorts: benign and metastatic. The physical dose delivery advantage of protons versus photons is well documented in the integral dose delivered to healthy tissues.
- For superficial targets in the cranial cavity such as meningiomas near the outer surface of the cranial cavity, the integral dose to healthy tissues is zero after the distal falloff which is generally within millimeters from the distal edge of the target.
- For more centrally located targets, the integral dose difference between protons and photons is most pronounced below the 40% isodose level, assuming identical prescription doses.
- The high-dose regions, above the 40% isodose levels, are generally very similar, except that the higher dimensional planning variables of proton therapy optimization can allow for better shaping of high-dose regions when a target is in close proximity to a critical structure, especially in the case of complicated target geometries in close proximity to critical structures.

3.7.6 Benign Lesions

For benign lesions, the effects of the integral dose should be considered in the clinical evaluation of the patient's treatment options and may affect the risk of late effects of the radiation treatment. Additionally, the ability of proton therapy to increase the conformality of high-dose regions in complicated target geometries, especially when the target is in close proximity to a critical structure, should be considered in the evaluation of treatment options (Fig. 3.33).

3.7.7 Metastatic Lesions

- The benefits of reduced integral dose are not well documented for patients with metastatic lesions, and the differences of proton SRS versus photon SRS for metastatic patients can be physically described in two scenarios, regardless of the clinical benefit or need.
- There are some cases where proton SRS can reduce the high dose to critical organs for cases when the target is in close proximity to the critical organ or has a complex geometric relationship with the critical organ. The other physical difference is the reduction of brain integral dose for multiple metastatic lesions (Fig. 3.34). The clinical necessity for these physical differences is outside the scope of this section.

3 Proton Treatment Planning   95

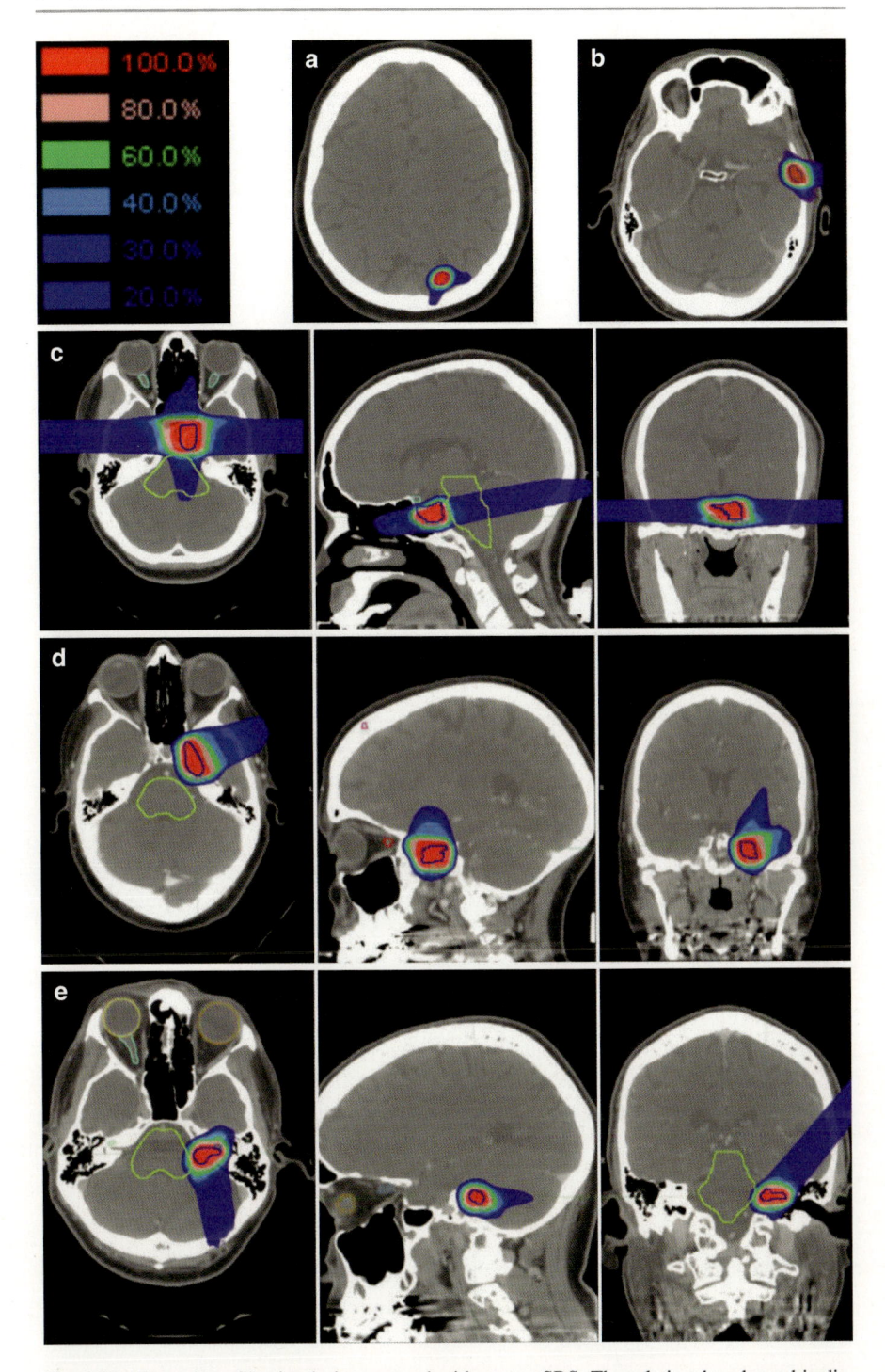

Fig. 3.33 Examples of benign lesions treated with proton SRS. The relative dose legend is displayed in the top row for all images. Displayed are axial images of an AVM (**a**) and a meningioma (**b**). Axial, sagittal, and coronal images are supplied for a pituitary target (**c**), a more central meningioma (**d**), and a cerebellopontine angle lesion (**e**)

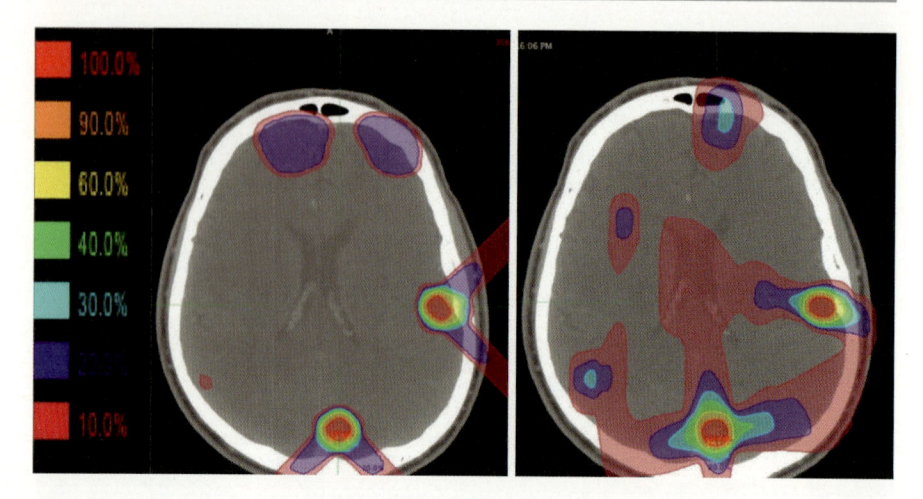

Fig. 3.34 A comparison of a proton SRS (*left*) and a photon SRS (*right*) plan for a patient with multiple metastatic lesions. The difference of integral dose to the brain can be observed

3.8 Image Guided Radiation Therapy (IGRT)

3.8.1 Purpose

IGRT generally refers to frequent, serial imaging of some kind performed in the treatment room prior to delivery of RT. The main purpose of IGRT is better localization of target and normal tissue volumes and thereby reducing uncertainty (PTV margins) and avoiding missing the tumor or overexposing OARs. For protons, it is also essential to verify the path length of proton beams.

IGRT strategies can be broadly divided into online and offline approaches. Online patient position verification and correction is *standard* in particle therapy. Setup correction protocols are routinely used. The most recent information is used in the process in order to ensure accurate delivery of treatment.

In the past 15 years, IGRT for X-ray therapy has evolved and matured with the advances in electronic portal imaging devices, kV radiographic systems, CBCT, and MR linacs. In contrast, proton therapy IGRT has lagged behind.

A summary of imaging techniques for proton therapy has been presented in Chap. 2. The relevance of various modalities to IGRT is discussed in this section.

3.8.2 In-Room Digital Radiography

- In-room digital radiography and orthogonal pair of X-ray tubes and digital flat panel imagers are the minimum requirements for proton therapy.
- 2D-2D alignment based on DRRs and comparison of anatomical landmarks (e.g., bony anatomy) is still the most commonly used IGRT technique in proton therapy.

3 Proton Treatment Planning

- Alignment algorithms can be automatic or interactive.
- The system may support the real-time monitoring and verification of the patient during fluoroscopy and respiratory gated treatment.

3.8.3 Out-of-Room CT

- Out-of-room CT is based on the use of a remote positioning and imaging system.
- Saves valuable room time for irradiation of patients.
- Some patient motion may be induced because of the transportation system.

3.8.4 Radiopaque Markers [68]

- Allows for patient setup with respect to the tumor itself instead of bony anatomy.
- Gold helical markers (10 mm length; 0.35 mm, 0.75 mm, 1.15 mm diameters).
- Dose perturbations of 31% (1.15 mm diameter) versus 23% (0.75 mm diameter) for typical lateral-opposed beams.
- Dose perturbation is not observed for 0.35 mm markers; however, they are deemed too fragile for implantation.
- Magnitude of dose perturbation depends on marker size, orientation, and distance from the beam's end of range.

3.8.5 In-Room CT [69]

- Necessary for target positioning and range verification.
- Used in vertical position for seated patients.
- Used in conjunction with a treatment couch robot on a six-axis robot.
- In-room robotic couch can transport the patient between the beam gantry and CT scanner.
- Portable large bore CT scanners are available as well.

3.8.6 CBCT

- It is expected that 2D radiography will continue to be used for proton IGRT in the foreseeable future.
- CBCT is now starting to be employed at some centers and is expected to be installed in most new installations in the next few years mostly for more precise patient positioning and adaptive radiotherapy [70].
- CBCT has the added advantage of visualizing soft tissue changes, which is important for adaptive proton RT, especially for head and neck tumors
- CBCT is, however, not accurate enough for proton plan assessment before treatment.

3.8.7 CT on Rails

- CT on rails can provide diagnostic quality imaging and has recently been installed in several proton centers.
- A robot moves the patient to imaging isocenter.
- The CT scanner translates over patient for imaging.
- A robot moves patient back to treatment position, while CT reconstruction/registration is performed.
- CT on rails will have use in adaptive replanning, particularly for head and neck cases.

3.8.8 Other Auxiliary Methods

3.8.8.1 Ultrasound
- In-room ultrasound pretreatment alignment is used for some prostate, lung, abdominal, and breast tumor sites. The most experience exists with interfractional tracking for prostate cancer
- AAPM TG 154: QA of US-guided EBRT for prostate cancer

3.8.8.2 Optical Systems
- Optical systems allow surface tracking with ceiling-mounted camera systems in the simulation and treatment rooms.
- These systems can detect intrafractional motion.
- They use rigid body transformations in combination with a least-square fit to minimize the difference between the actual expected surface.
- There are currently two commercial systems available (AlignRT and C-RAD sentinel).
- AAPM TG 147: QA of nonradiographic RT localization and positioning systems.

3.8.8.3 Radio-frequency Systems
- Only one commercial system (Calypso) available
- Currently not used in proton therapy due to potential interference of transponder beacons with proton dose distribution

3.8.8.4 Prompt Gamma Imaging
- Elemental prompt gamma (PG) rays arise during proton irradiation of tissue.
- PG ray lines are specific for the excited nucleus.
- The intensity and profile of the PG ray emission are strongly correlated to delivered dose and Bragg peak position.
- Compton cameras for PG detection and intratreatment beam range verification are under development.

3.8.8.5 Proton Radiography and CT [16]
- Proton radiography and proton CT traverse the patient with a proton beam and measure residual energy at exit.
- Proton radiography and proton CT are emerging technologies with promising properties.
- Proton radiography could track lung tumors in real time providing accurate validations of tumor motion models.
- Proton CT would provide a direct map of stopping power.
- Proton CT would provide accurate 3D maps of the patient just before treatment, opening the possibility of low-dose daily imaging for adaptive proton RT.
- First clinical systems are under development and should become available in the coming years.

3.8.8.6 PET
- PET of proton-activated isotopes has been shown to be valuable for range verification during and after treatment.
- In soft tissues, the most important radionuclide species are 11 C (half-life 20 min), 13 N (half-life 10 min), and 15 O (half-life 122 s), of which 15 O is dominant but decays fastest.
- The PET-detected activation can be compared with the expected radioactivity distribution.
- This method may serve as an in vivo, noninvasive range validation method of the entire chain of treatment planning and delivery.
- Three operational modalities are currently in use:
    - In-beam PET with modified detectors to synchronize acquisition with beam delivery during treatment
    - In-room portable PET, posttreatment
    - Offline detection of residual activation from long-lived emitters shortly after treatment, taking into consideration the physical and biological decay

3.8.8.7 Repeated 4D CT Scanning
- Treatment planning CT is just a snapshot in time before the actual treatment course.
- The patient may breathe differently or have varying breathing amplitudes over the treatment course.
- Tumor growth or shrinkage, atelectasis, radiation pneumonitis, and pericardial effusion may further change the anatomy, resulting in an altered dose distribution.
- Repeated 4D CT scanning minimizes the probability of severe geometric misses.
- 4D CTs are typically done every other week.

3.8.9 Impact of Anatomical Changes and Adaptive Radiotherapy

- Proton plans are sensitive to intrafractional variations, even with proper image-guided setup:
  - Tumor growth can cause underdosing of tumor.
  - Tumor shrinkage can cause protons to overshoot into an OAR.
  - Weight gain can cause under dosing of a distal target.
- Proton plans are more sensitive than photon plans since dose distribution can change significantly, intrinsically due to the 3D modulation of proton beam, as opposed to 2D modulation of photon beam.
- ART (adaptive radiotherapy) can correct the dosimetric effect of nonrigid anatomical changes, complementing the ability of image-guided setup to correct for rigid body translation and rotation.
- Frequency of treatment adaptation is limited by technological availability of (in-room) volumetric imaging as well as time and resources.

3.9 Emerging Technologies and Future Developments

There are two aims that drive innovation and new technologies in proton radiotherapy:

1. Leveraging the unique properties of proton (and ion) radiation
2. Decreasing the effective cost of proton radiotherapy:
   The unique properties of proton (and ion) radiation allow for:
   (a) New in vivo imaging techniques by using the proton pencil beam itself as a measurement probe. Examples include:
      - Prompt γ detection to determine the range penetration in patient and perhaps a certain level of elemental tissue composition because different atoms release different γ energies.
      - Proton radiography to image stopping power changes in the patient and to improve stopping power determination in the patient:
        - Proton tomography, by itself, may not emerge as an effective imaging means due to inpatient scattering of the proton beam. Techniques that use a combination of high-resolution CT and a limited set of proton radiographs may, in fact, be better.
        - Continued advances in CT such as multispectral analysis may be more practical and even more accurate.
   (b) Biological treatment modulation. We currently assume a constant RBE = 1.1 throughout the dose distribution. For protons, the LET effect occurs at the distal falling edge of the dose distribution. Its effect, however, is believed to be of significance. Analysis of the LET distribution may yield some clinical considerations.

It must be noted that the proton delivery system is a fully electronic system where the scanning magnet moves the beam in the lateral dimension and proton energy changes the depth of penetration. Thus, compared to a mechanical MLC system, the delivery system is:

1. Faster
2. More reliable
3. Easier to control in real time to adapt the pattern to match the patient state during treatment

   In addition, the proton spot map specifies each spot in terms of energy, location, and intensity. The control system directly (i.e., commutatively) uses these parameters to control the delivery and directly measures the same parameters. Thus, the feedback loop between delivery, measure, and adapt does not suffer from intermediate conversion. In contrast, an MLC uses leaf positions to specify MU which is certainly neither an obvious nor unique (i.e., commutative) translation. This is a clear technological advantage for proton radiotherapy in consideration of dynamic delivery requirements.

   The effective cost of proton radiotherapy may be reduced when considering desired advances in radiotherapy in general. These include:

1. IGRT—Image-guided radiotherapy and synchronized dynamic beam delivery:
   (a) The ability to use the proton beam, itself, as a direct measure of where the beam is in the patient's anatomy, creates new opportunities to control the motion.
2. ART to correct for changes in the patient:
   (a) ART primarily requires novel software architectures to allow for continuous data communication in response to patient changes. These architectures must implement DICOM second generation to address the temporal synchronization of the flow of data.
   (b) Proton ART will benefit from the superior delivery technology which will allow the adaptation to occur within the treatment session.
3. SBRT—Increase in fraction dose with concomitant reduction in treatment course length:
   (a) Clearly, the reduction in the dose bath (by approximately 1/2) will favor dose escalation with protons. Thus, proton SBRT should effectively compete and should allow a cost reduction in patient treatment length.

References

1. Bortfeld T. An analytical approximation of the Bragg curve for therapeutic proton beams. Med Phys. 1997;24(12):2024–33.
2. ICRU. ICRU Report 78: prescribing, recording, and reporting proton-beam therapy. J ICRU. 2007;7(2):1–210.
3. Khan FM, Gerbi BJ. Treatment planning in radiation oncology. Philadelphia: Wolters Kluwer Health/Lippincott Williams & Wilkins; 2012.
4. Moyers MF, Miller DW, Bush DA, Slater JD. Methodologies and tools for proton beam design for lung tumors. Int J Radiat Oncol Biol Phys. 2001;49(5):1429–38.

5. Moyers MF, Sardesai M, Sun S, Miller DW. Ion stopping powers and CT numbers. Med Dosim. 2010;35(3):179–94.
6. Yang M, Zhu XR, Park PC, Titt U, Mohan R, Virshup G, Clayton JE, Dong L. Comprehensive analysis of proton range uncertainties related to patient stopping-power-ratio estimation using the stoichiometric calibration. Phys Med Biol. 2012;57(13):4095.
7. Wu R, Amos R, Sahoo N, Kornguth D, Bluett J, Gillin M, Zhu X. SU-GG-J-80: effect of CT truncation artifacts to proton dose calculation. Med Phys. 2008;35(6):2697.
8. Moyers MF, Miller DW. Range, range modulation, and field radius requirements for proton therapy of prostate cancer. Technol Cancer Res Treat. 2003;2(5):445–7.
9. Yu Z, Bluett J, Zhang Y, Zhu X, Lii M, Mohan R, Dong L. SU-GG-T-470: impact of daily patient setup variation on proton beams passing through the couch edge. Med Phys. 2010;37(6):3294.
10. Paganetti H, Niemierko A, Ancukiewicz M, Gerweck LE, Goitein M, Loeffler JS, Suit HD. Relative biological effectiveness (RBE) values for proton beam therapy. Int J Radiat Oncol Biol Phys. 2002;53(2):407–21.
11. Paganetti H. Relative biological effectiveness (RBE) values for proton beam therapy. Variations as a function of biological endpoint, dose, and linear energy transfer. Phys Med Biol. 2014;59(22):R419.
12. Woodward WA, Amos RA. Proton radiation biology considerations for radiation oncologists. Int J Radiat Oncol Biol Phys. 2016;95(1):59–61.
13. Schneider U, Pedroni E, Lomax A. The calibration of CT Hounsfield units for radiotherapy treatment planning. Phys Med Biol. 1996;41(1):111.
14. Schaffner B, Pedroni E. The precision of proton range calculations in proton radiotherapy treatment planning: experimental verification of the relation between CT-HU and proton stopping power. Phys Med Biol. 1998;43(6):1579.
15. van Elmpt W, Landry G, Das M, Verhaegen F. Dual energy CT in radiotherapy: current applications and future outlook. Radiother Oncol. 2016;119(1):137–44.
16. Testa M, Verburg JM, Rose M, Min CH, Tang S, Bentefour EH, Paganetti H, Lu H-M. Proton radiography and proton computed tomography based on time-resolved dose measurements. Phys Med Biol. 2013;58(22):8215.
17. ICRP. ICRP Publication 23: Report of the Task Group on Reference Man. 1975.
18. ICRU. ICRU Report 44: Tissue substitutes in radiation dosimetry and measurement. 1989.
19. Schneider W, Bortfeld T, Schlegel W. Correlation between CT numbers and tissue parameters needed for Monte Carlo simulations of clinical dose distributions. Phys Med Biol. 2000;45(2):459.
20. Hansen DC, Seco J, Sørensen TS, Petersen JBB, Wildberger JE, Verhaegen F, Landry G. A simulation study on proton computed tomography (CT) stopping power accuracy using dual energy CT scans as benchmark. Acta Oncol. 2015;54(9):1638–42.
21. Hünemohr N, Paganetti H, Greilich S, Jäkel O, Seco J. Tissue decomposition from dual energy CT data for MC based dose calculation in particle therapy. Med Phys. 2014;41(6):061714.
22. Taasti VT, Høye EM, Hansen DC, Muren LP, Thygesen J, Skyt PS, Balling P, Bassler N, Grau C, Mierzwińska G, Rydygier M, Swakoń J, Olko P, Petersen JBB. Technical note: improving proton stopping power ratio determination for a deformable silicone-based 3D dosimeter using dual energy CT. Med Phys. 2016;43(6):2780–4.
23. Zhu J, Penfold SN. Dosimetric comparison of stopping power calibration with dual-energy CT and single-energy CT in proton therapy treatment planning. Med Phys. 2016;43(6):2845–54.
24. Wertz H, Jäkel O. Influence of iodine contrast agent on the range of ion beams for radiotherapy. Med Phys. 2004;31(4):767–73.
25. Hanley J, Debois MM, Mah D, Mageras GS, Raben A, Rosenzweig K, Mychalczak B, Schwartz LH, Gloeggler PJ, Lutz W, Ling CC, Leibel SA, Fuks Z, Kutcher GJ. Deep inspiration breath-hold technique for lung tumors: the potential value of target immobilization and reduced lung density in dose escalation. Int J Radiat Oncol Biol Phys. 1999;45(3):603–11.
26. Mah D, Hanley J, Rosenzweig KE, Yorke E, Braban L, Ling CC, Leibel SA, Mageras G. Technical aspects of the deep inspirational breath-hold technique in the treatment of thoracic cancer. Int J Radiat Oncol Biol Phys. 2000;48(4):1175–85.

27. Paoli J, Rosenzweig KE, Yorke E, Hanley J, Mah D, Ma jeras GS, Hunt MA, Braban LE, Liebel SA, Ling CC. Comparison of different respiratory levels in the treatment of lung cancer: implications for gated treatment. Int J Radiat Oncol Biol Phys. 1999;45(3):386–7.
28. Mageras GS, Yorke E. Deep inspiration breath hold and respiratory gating strategies for reducing organ motion in radiation treatment. Semin Radiat Oncol. 2004;14:65–75. Elsevier.
29. DeLaney TF, Kooy HM, editors. Proton and charged particle radiotherapy. Philadelphia: Lippincott Williams & Wilkins; 2008.
30. Olch AJ, Gerig L, Li H, Mihaylov I, Morgan A. Dosimetric effects caused by couch tops and immobilization devices: report of AAPM task group 176. Med Phys. 2014;41(6):061501.
31. Wang P, Yin L, Zhang Y, Kirk M, Song G, Ahn PH, Lin A, Gee J, Dolney D, Solberg TD, Maughan R, McDonough J, Teo B-KK. Quantitative assessment of anatomical change using a virtual proton depth radiograph for adaptive head and neck proton therapy. J Appl Clin Med Phys. 2016;17(2):5819.
32. Both S, Shen J, Kirk M, Lin L, Tang S, Alonso-Basanta M, Lustig R, Lin H, Deville C, Hill-Kayser C, Tochner Z, McDonough J. Development and clinical implementation of a universal bolus to maintain spot size during delivery of base of skull pencil beam scanning proton therapy. Int J Radiat Oncol Biol Phys. 2014;90(1):79–84.
33. Shen J, Liu W, Anand A, Stoker JB, Ding X, Fatyga M, Herman MG, Bues M. Impact of range shifter material on proton pencil beam spot characteristics. Med Phys. 2015;42(3):1335–40.
34. Both S, Wang KK, Plastaras JP, Deville C, Ad VB, Tochner Z, Vapiwala N. Real-time study of prostate intrafraction motion during external beam radiotherapy with daily endorectal balloon. Int J Radiat Oncol Biol Phys. 2011;81(5):1302–9.
35. Wang KK, Vapiwala N, Deville C, Plastaras JP, Scheuermann R, Lin H, Bar. Ad V, Tochner Z, Both S. A study to quantify the effectiveness of daily endorectal balloon for prostate intrafraction motion management. Int J Radiat Oncol Biol Phys. 2012;83(3):1055–63.
36. Taku N, Yin L, Teo B, Lin LL. Quantifying vaginal motion associated with daily endorectal balloon during whole pelvis radiation therapy for gynecologic cancers. Int J Radiat Oncol Biol Phys. 2014;90(1):S506.
37. Zou W, Lin H, Plastaras JP, Wang H, Bui V, Vapiwala N, McDonough J, Touchner Z, Both S. A clinically feasible method for the detection of potential collision in proton therapy. Med Phys. 2012;39(11):7094–101.
38. Brock K. TU-E-BRB-03: overview of proposed TG-132 recommendations. Med Phys. 2015;42(6):–3618.
39. Graves YJ, Smith A-A, Mcilvena D, Manilay Z, Lai YK, Rice R, Mell L, Jia X, Jiang SB, Cervinõ L. A deformable head and neck phantom with in-vivo dosimetry for adaptive radiotherapy quality assurance. Med Phys. 2015;42(4):1490–7.
40. Dice LR. Measures of the amount of ecologic association between species. Ecology. 1945;26(3):297–302.
41. Huttenlocher DP, Klanderman GA, Rucklidge WJ. Comparing images using the Hausdorff distance. IEEE T Pattern Anal. 1993;15(9):850–63.
42. Christensen GE, Johnson HJ. Invertibility and transitivity analysis for nonrigid image registration. J Electron Imaging. 2003;12(1):106–17.
43. Saleh ZH, Apte AP, Sharp GC, Shusharina NP, Wang Y, Veeraraghavan H, Thor M, Muren LP, Rao SS, Lee NY, Deasy JO. The distance discordance metric—a novel approach to quantifying spatial uncertainties in intra-and inter-patient deformable image registration. Phys Med Biol. 2014;59(3):733.
44. Schreibmann E, Pantalone P, Waller A, Fox T. A measure to evaluate deformable registration fields in clinical settings. J Appl Clin Med Phys. 2012;13(5):3829.
45. Varadhan R, Karangelis G, Krishnan K, Hui S. A framework for deformable image registration validation in radiotherapy clinical applications. J Appl Clin Med Phys. 2013;14(1):4066.
46. Brock KK. Results of a multi-institution deformable registration accuracy study (MIDRAS). Int J Radiat Oncol Biol Phys. 2010;76(2):583–96.

47. Nielsen MS, Østergaard LR, Carl J. A new method to validate thoracic CT-CT deformable image registration using auto-segmented 3D anatomical landmarks. Acta Oncol. 2015;54(9):1515–20.
48. B. Rigaud, A. Simon, J. Castelli, M. Gobeli, J.-D. Ospina Arango, G. Cazoulat, O. Henry, P. Haigron, and R. De Crevoisier. Evaluation of deformable image registration methods for dose monitoring in head and neck radiotherapy. Biomed Res Int, 2015;2015.
49. Yazdia M, Gingras L, Beaulieu L. An adaptive approach to metal artifact reduction in helical computed tomography for radiation therapy treatment planning: experimental and clinical studies. Int J Radiat Oncol Biol Phys. 2005;62(4):1224–31.
50. Axente M, Paidi A, Von Eyben R, Zeng C, Bani-Hashemi A, Krauss A, Hristov D. Clinical evaluation of the iterative metal artifact reduction algorithm for CT simulation in radiotherapy. Med Phys. 2015;42(3):1170–83.
51. Dietlicher I, Casiraghi M, Ares C, Bolsi A, Weber DC, Lomax AJ, Albertini F. The effect of surgical titanium rods on proton therapy delivered for cervical bone tumors: experimental validation using an anthropomorphic phantom. Phys Med Biol. 2014;59(23):7181.
52. Kang Y, Zhang X, Chang JY, Wang H, Wei X, Liao Z, Komaki R, Cox JD, Balter PA, Liu H, Zhu XR, Mohan R, Dong L. 4D proton treatment planning strategy for mobile lung tumors. Int J Radiat Oncol Biol Phys. 2007;67(3):906–14.
53. Dowdell S, Grassberger C, Sharp GC, Paganetti H. Interplay effects in proton scanning for lung: a 4D Monte Carlo study assessing the impact of tumor and beam delivery parameters. Phys Med Biol. 2013;58:4137–56.
54. Park PC, Zhu XR, Lee AK, Sahoo N, Melancon AD, Zhang L, Dong L. A beam-specific planning target volume (PTV) design for proton therapy to account for setup and range uncertainties. Int J Radiat Oncol Biol Phys. 2012;82(2):e329–36.
55. Goitein M. Compensation for inhomogeneities in charged particle radiotherapy using computed tomography. Int J Radiat Oncol Biol Phys. 1978;4(5):499–508.
56. Urie M, Goitein M, Wagner M. Compensating for heterogeneities in proton radiation therapy. Phys Med Biol. 1984;29(5):553.
57. Strom EA, Amos RA, Shaitelman SF, Kerr MD, Hoffman KE, Smith BD, Tereffe W, Stauder MC, Perkins GH, Amin MD, Wang X, Poenisch F, Ovalle V, Buchholz TA, Babiera G, Woodward WA. Proton partial breast irradiation in the supine position: treatment description and reproducibility of a multibeam technique. Pract Radiat Oncol. 2015;5(4):e283–90.
58. Giebeler A, Newhauser WD, Amos RA, Mahajan A, Homann K, Howell RM. Standardized treatment planning methodology for passively scattered proton craniospinal irradiation. Radiat Oncol. 2013;8(1):1.
59. Stoker J, Amos R, Li Y, Liu W, Park P, Sahoo N, Zhang X, Zhu X, Gillin M. SU-E-T-693: comparison of discrete spot scanning and passive scattering craniospinal proton irradiation. Med Phys. 2013;40(6):365.
60. Lin H, Ding X, Kirk M, Liu H, Zhai H, Hill-Kayser CE, Lustig RA, Tochner Z, Both S, McDonough J. Supine craniospinal irradiation using a proton pencil beam scanning technique without match line changes for field junctions. Int J Radiat Oncol Biol Phys. 2014;90(1):71–8.
61. Li Y, Zhang X, Dong L, Mohan R. A novel patch-field design using an optimized grid filter for passively scattered proton beams. Phys Med Biol. 2007;52(12):N265.
62. Li Y, Kardar L, Li X, Li H, Cao W, Chang JY, Liao L, Zhu RX, Sahoo N, Gillin M, Liao Z, Komaki R, Cox JD, Lim G, Zhang X. On the interplay effects with proton scanning beams in stage III lung cancer. Med Phys. 2014;41(2):021721.
63. Zeng C, Plastaras JP, Tochner ZA, White BM, Hill-Kayser CE, Hahn SM, Both S. Proton pencil beam scanning for mediastinal lymphoma: the impact of interplay between target motion and beam scanning. Phys Med Biol. 2015;60:3013–29.
64. Clasie B, Depauw N, Fransen M, Gomà C, Panahandeh HR, Seco J, Flanz JB, Kooy HM. Golden beam data for proton pencil-beam scanning. Phys Med Biol. 2012;57(5):1147.
65. Paganetti H. Dose to water versus dose to medium in proton beam therapy. Phys Med Biol. 2009;54(14):4399.

66. Trofimov A, Unkelbach J, DeLaney TF, Bortfeld T. Visualization of a variety of possible dosimetric outcomes in radiation therapy using dose-volume histogram bands. Pract Radiat Oncol. 2012;2(3):164–71.
67. Clasie BM, Sharp GC, Seco J, Flanz JB, Kooy HM. Numerical solutions of the γ-index in two and three dimensions. Phys Med Biol. 2012;57(21):6981.
68. Giebeler A, Fontenot J, Balter P, Ciangaru G, Zhu R, Newhauser W. Dose perturbations from implanted helical gold markers in proton therapy of prostate cancer. J Appl Clin Med Phys. 2009;10(1):2875.
69. Devicienti S, Strigari L, D'Andrea M, Benassi M, Dimiccoli V, Portaluri M. Patient positioning in the proton radiotherapy era. J Exp Clin Cancer Res. 2010;29(1):1.
70. Veiga C, Janssens G, Teng C-L, Baudier T, Hotoiu L, McClelland JR, Royle G, Lin L, Yin L, Metz J, Solberg TD, Tochner Z, Simone CB, Mcdonough J, Teo B-KK. First clinical investigation of cone beam computed tomography and deformable registration for adaptive proton therapy for lung cancer. Int J Radiat Oncol Biol Phys. 2016;95(1):549–59.

Tumors of the Nasopharynx

4

Jeremy Setton, Pamela Fox, Kevin Sine, Nadeem Riaz, and Nancy Y. Lee

Contents

4.1	Introduction	107
4.2	Simulation, Target Delineation, and Radiation Dose-Fractionation	108
4.3	Patient Positioning, Immobilization, and Treatment Verification	111
4.4	Proton Beam Treatment Planning	111
4.5	Proton Therapy for NPC: Clinical Outcomes	113
4.6	Discussion and Future Directions	114
References		116

4.1 Introduction

- Nasopharyngeal carcinoma (NPC) is the most common cancer originating in the nasopharynx, most commonly in the pharyngeal recess known as the fossa of *Rosenmüller*. NPC is a rare malignancy in most populations but is endemic in several well-defined populations, including natives of southern China, Southeast Asia, and the Middle East/North Africa.
- The nasopharynx is a cuboidal chamber which extends from the base of the skull to the upper surface of the soft palate. It is bounded posteriorly by the clivus and C1-C2 vertebral bodies and anteriorly communicates with the nasal cavity through the posterior choanae. The eustachian tube is located in the lateral wall

---

J. Setton • N. Riaz • N.Y. Lee (✉)
Memorial Sloan-Kettering Cancer Center, New York, NY, USA
e-mail: leen2@mskcc.org

P. Fox • K. Sine
ProCure Proton Therapy Center, Somerset, NJ, USA

© Springer International Publishing Switzerland 2018
N. Lee et al. (eds.), *Target Volume Delineation and Treatment Planning for Particle Therapy*, Practical Guides in Radiation Oncology,
https://doi.org/10.1007/978-3-319-42478-1_4

and bounded by a prominence known as the torus tubarius which lies anterior to the fossa of *Rosenmüller*.
- The nasopharynx is adjacent to a number of dose-limiting critical structures, including the temporal lobes of the brain, brainstem, optic pathways, auditory structures, salivary glands, pharyngeal constrictor muscles, and oral mucosa. Potential toxicities of treatment include temporal lobe necrosis, optic neuropathy, hearing loss, dysphagia, trismus, xerostomia, and osteoradionecrosis [1].
- The transition from conventional 2D and 3D conformal radiotherapy techniques to intensity-modulated radiotherapy (IMRT) has resulted in improvement in dose conformality and decreases in both acute and late toxicity for patients with NPC [2]. This has led to the adoption of IMRT as the standard definitive treatment for nasopharyngeal carcinoma over the past 15 years. Despite the incremental improvement relative to 2D or 3D techniques, IMRT is limited by the inherent physical limitations of megavoltage photons, as entrance and exit dose must necessarily be more widely distributed to achieve improved conformality in the high-dose regions.
- The physical properties of high-energy protons, namely, the characteristic sharp dose falloff, have led to interest in employing proton beam radiotherapy for nasopharyngeal cancer to more effectively spare nearby critical structures and decrease the toxicities of treatment while maintaining or improving tumor coverage. Comparative dosimetric analyses have demonstrated the feasibility of attaining improved conformality with proton beam radiotherapy compared to IMRT [3, 4]. There is, however, a relative paucity of clinical data reporting outcomes after proton RT for NPC [5].
- Recent improvements in delivery and treatment planning, including increased availability of pencil beam scanning technology, hold promise for further improvements in clinical outcomes for patients with NPC.

4.2 Simulation, Target Delineation, and Radiation Dose-Fractionation

- CT simulation with ≤3 mm slice thickness with and without IV contrast should be performed. The simulation scan should extend from the top of the head to the carina. The non-contrast CT should be acquired prior to the contrast scan, as treatment planning calculations must be performed using the non-contrast CT scan to avoid significant range errors. The CT must include all immobilization equipment and any additional materials potentially in the beam's path.
- The gross tumor volume (GTV) is contoured on simulation CT/MRI images and co-registered diagnostic scans. PET and MRI scans obtained for target delineation are ideally obtained in the treatment position and should be fused to the regions of interest encompassing the GTV, skull base, brainstem, and optic structures (Fig. 4.1). MRI imaging should at the minimum include T1-weighted images before and after contrast enhancement, as well as T2-weighted images.

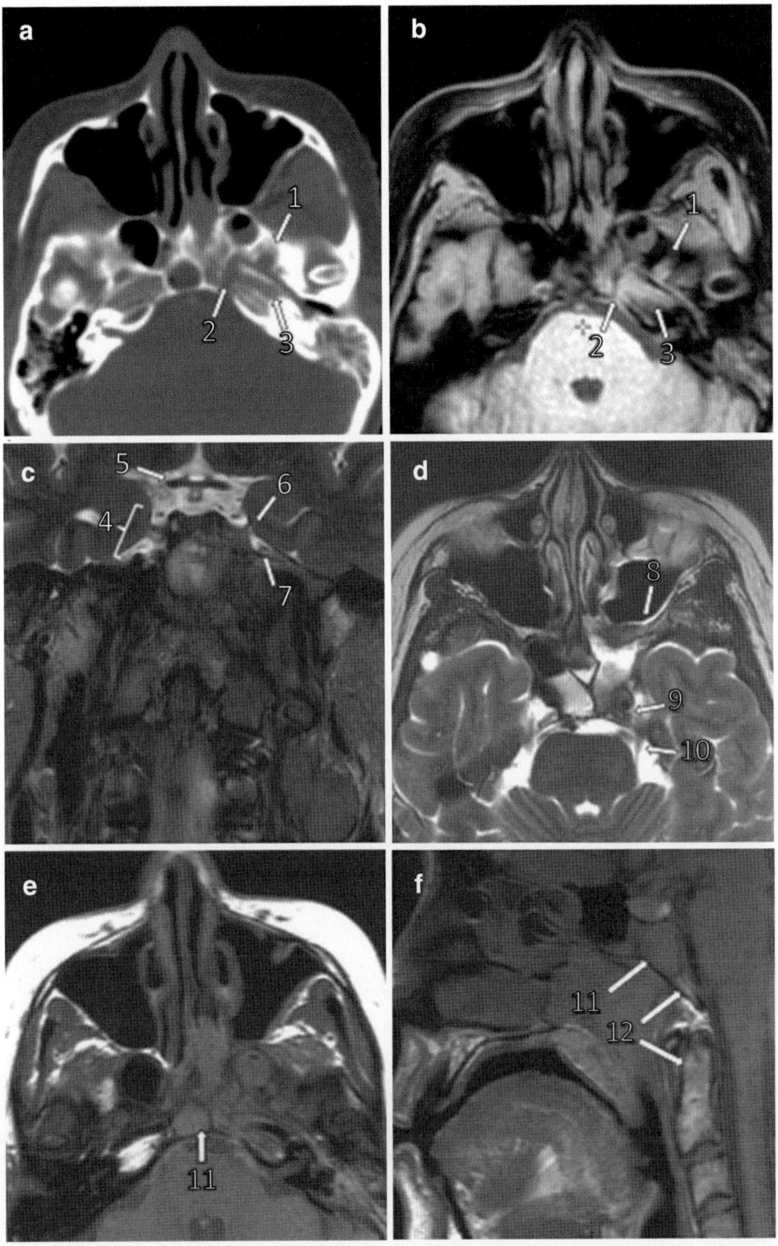

Fig. 4.1 Preoperative simulation CT and MRI imaging for T4 nasopharyngeal carcinoma with skull base invasion. (**a**) Axial CT. (**b**) Axial MRI (dual echo two-point Dixon sequence). (**c**) Coronal T2W MRI. (**d**) Axial T2W MRI. (**e**) Axial T1W MRI (precontrast). (**f**) Sagittal T1W MRI (precontrast). *1* Infiltration of foramen ovale and involvement of V3. *2* Invasion of the petrous apex. *3* Encasement of the petrous carotid artery. *4* Cavernous sinus. *5* Optic chiasm. *6* Invasion of cavernous sinus. *7* Maxillary division of trigeminal nerve (V2). *8* Invasion into pterygopalatine fossa. *9* Encasement of cavernous internal carotid artery adjacent to Meckel's cave. *10* Cisternal portion of trigeminal nerve. *11* Invasion of clivus; replacement of normal bone marrow with T1 hypointense tumor. *12* Normal marrow with T1 hyperintense fat

Table 4.1 Suggested target volumes for nasopharyngeal carcinoma

Volume	Target	Dose
GTV	All gross disease identified on imaging and physical examination	70 Gy (RBE)
High-risk clinical tumor volume (CTV_{70})	GTV + 3 mm margin. At the interface with critical dose-limiting structures, a 1 mm margin is acceptable	70 Gy (RBE)
High-risk clinical tumor volume ($CTV_{59.4}$)	CTV_{70} + 5 mm margin + regions at risk for microscopic disease: • Entire nasopharynx • Parapharyngeal space • Anterior 1/3 of clivus (entire clivus if involved) • Skull base (including coverage of foramen ovale and foramen rotundum) • Posterior 1/4 of nasal cavity and maxillary sinuses (ensuring coverage of pterygopalatine fossa) • Inferior sphenoid sinus (entire sphenoid sinus if involved) • Pterygoid fossa • Soft palate • Retropharyngeal LN + retrostyloid space • Bilateral nodal levels IB through V • Cavernous sinus should be covered for advanced (T3-T4) lesions	59.4 Gy (RBE)

Notes: (1) PTV_{70} is treated to 70 Gy in 33 fractions (2.12 Gy/fraction). $PTV_{59.4}$ is treated to 59.4 Gy in 33 fractions (1.80 Gy/fraction). A low-risk clinical tumor volume (CTV_{54}; 54 Gy in 33 fractions at 1.64 Gy/fraction) may be considered in the N0 and/or low neck (levels IV and V) at the discretion of the treating physician. (2) An intermediate dose level (PTV_{63}) may be considered for the treatment of small lymph nodes (~1 cm or less) that are suspected to be grossly involved. (3) In select cases, level IB may be omitted in the node-negative neck and/or the lower-risk node-positive neck (isolated retropharyngeal and/or isolated level IV adenopathy), at the discretion of the treating physician

    MRI fusion is especially useful for delineation of GTV at the skull base, whereas CT plays an important role in the assessment of cortical bone invasion. PET can help in the determination of whether borderline lymph nodes are grossly involved with disease. Given the propensity for nodal spread, however, a low index of suspicion is required in the clinical assessment of potentially involved lymph nodes.
- In contrast to photon treatment planning, where a standard margin may be employed for the PTV to account for day-to-day variation in setup margin, the PTV for proton therapy must account for both the setup error and a field-specific dosimetric margin. The field-specific dosimetric margin is dependent on the water equivalent range from a specific beam angle relative to the distal and proximal edges of the CTV.
- Suggested guidelines for gross and clinical target volumes based on the RTOG/NRG Nasopharyngeal Cancer Trials are detailed in Table 4.1 [6].

4 Tumors of the Nasopharynx

4.3 Patient Positioning, Immobilization, and Treatment Verification

- Proton treatment delivery can be more severely affected by variation in factors that affect radiologic depth than photon treatment delivery. Accounting for heterogeneities and the factors that affect their day-to-day variation is therefore of crucial importance in proton beam therapy. While many heterogeneities can be corrected for in treatment planning, optimization of patient positioning and immobilization is vital to ensuring correct delivery of the intended dose distribution.
- A five-point thermoplastic mask should be used for immobilization of the head, neck, and shoulders. An oral obturator or bite block may be used to depress the tongue and displace oral mucosa away from the treatment field. Immobilization devices should be radiologically thin in order to minimize lateral penumbra, and should be indexed to ensure setup reproducibility. At some centers, a board that elevates the head and neck off the treatment table is employed to minimize the air gap between the snout and patient. Control of the air gap between the snout and patient is also an important consideration as minimization of this parameter is critical to determining spot size. At the same time, careful consideration must also be given to avoiding collisions between snout and the patient or treatment table.
- For daily treatment verification, most patients undergo daily kV imaging to monitor daily reproducibility of treatment. Patients also typically undergo at least one verification simulation during the course of treatment to monitor for potential changes in anatomy resulting from weight loss or tumor regression. As noted above, relatively minor changes in patient anatomy/radiologic depth can significantly affect the delivered dose distribution due to the increased conformality and smaller number of treatment beams typically employed in proton beam treatment planning.

4.4 Proton Beam Treatment Planning

- Definitive treatment of nasopharyngeal cancer will typically require pencil beam scanning (PBS) because the added complexity of treating the bilateral neck with passively scattered beams often requires a prohibitively excessive number of beams and treatment time. Pencil beam scanning also affords the ability to achieve conformality at the proximal edge of the treatment volume, whereas passive scanning delivery cannot produce proximally conformal fields. PBS fields are composed of individual small proton "pencil" beams of uniform energy which can be deflected magnetically to the desired location or "spot." Each spot can be individually modulated in energy and intensity. Spots at a constant energy are referred to as a "spot layer"; multiple layers are typically stacked across the depth of the target to achieve coverage. Margins in the beam direction are used

to allow for range uncertainty, distal dose equilibrium, and setup error. Lateral margins are additionally employed to account for lateral dose equilibrium and setup error.
- PBS treatment planning can be achieved using either single-field optimization (SFO), in which each set of PBS fields achieves a uniform dose to the entire target, or multi-field optimization (MFO), where each field delivers a heterogeneous dose to the target and only the composite dose from all fields achieves the desired dose shape. Multiple fields can be employed in the SFO-based technique to achieve coverage of the target volume; all fields are, however, geometrically decoupled and considered independently in uncertainty mitigation. In the MFO technique, each field delivers a heterogeneous dose to the target, and only the composite dose from all fields covers the entire target and achieves the desired dose shape. MFO fields are strongly coupled and optimized as a single set.
- Beam orientation should be chosen to (1) minimize path length, (2) maximize homogeneity of tissue in the beam path, and (3) avoid directions that point toward critical organs at risk. As a result of range uncertainties and increased LET at the end of range, proton field lateral edge is often employed for penumbral separation between target and critical structure. In the nasopharynx, this often means that lateral and/or posterior beams are often employed in the treatment of the primary site to avoid ranging into the brainstem (Fig. 4.2). Moreover, anterior beam angles traversing the nasal sinuses or oral cavity are generally undesirable due to the heterogeneity of these structures and potential variation in sinus filling.

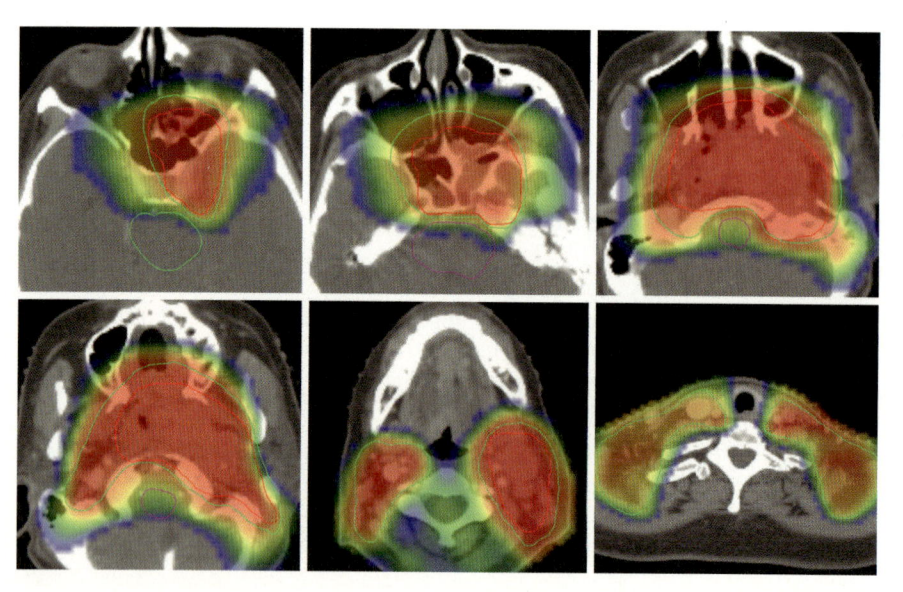

Fig. 4.2 Example PBS plan (SFO optimized) for patient with T4N2 nasopharyngeal carcinoma whose anatomy is depicted in Fig. 4.1. *Red contour* = PTV_{70}. *Green contour* = $PTV_{59.4}$

- For SFO-based plans, an optimization structure can be created to account for range uncertainty resulting from the conversion of Hounsfield units to proton stopping power. At our institution, this structure is typically created by adding a margin of 2.5% of the beam range plus an additional 2 mm. This margin is added to the distal and proximal edges of the CTV during treatment planning; the margin in the beam direction may therefore differ from the lateral margin.
- MFO can produce highly conformal plans but can be highly sensitive to motion and setup error. Uncertainty mitigation is critical to reducing this sensitivity and typically involves an explicit computation of individual factors that may potentially contribute uncertainty to the deposited dose. MFO fields are strongly coupled and are considered as a single set in the uncertainty mitigation. Robustness optimization allows for incorporation of range uncertainty into the treatment optimization process and can help ensure the dose distribution to target, and OARs remain acceptable after taking into account both setup and range uncertainties. Robustness can be visualized within a DVH using uncertainty bands that account for potential worst-case scenarios.
- Dental hardware, surgical clips, and other foreign materials often create CT artifact and can contribute to significant range uncertainty if necessary to treat through. The standard practice to deal with metal CT artifacts is to delineate such regions and to reset the Hounsfield units within these regions to average soft tissue or bone values measured in similar areas of the body where no artifacts are present. High-Z materials present in the treatment field should be contoured and assigned a CT number consistent with the proton stopping power of the material. Practically speaking, however, beam angles should be selected that minimize the need to traverse high-Z materials. HU override for such materials should be carefully evaluated on case-by-case basis as inappropriate override can lead to significant dose errors.
- Pencil beam spot size is highly dependent on the air gap present between the snout and patient. The patient should be set up and immobilized in a manner that minimizes the air gap to the greatest extent possible while still preventing collisions. Universal and/or patient-specific bolus can also be employed to minimize air gap and ensure spot size integrity.

4.5 Proton Therapy for NPC: Clinical Outcomes

- The first published report describing clinical outcomes for proton therapy in the treatment of nasopharyngeal carcinoma was from Loma Linda University Medical Center, where patients with recurrent NPC were re-irradiated with passively scattered proton therapy [7]. Sixteen patients who received prior photon-based definitive radiotherapy were treated to additional doses of 59.4–70.2 CGE. Two-year locoregional control was 50%; those who received 90% or more of the prescribed dose to 90% or more of the target volume had a 2-year local control rate of 83% compared with 17% for those with suboptimal coverage ($p = 0.006$).

- Chan et al. reported, in abstract form, early treatment outcomes for 23 patients with nasopharyngeal carcinoma who received proton-based chemoradiation on a phase II prospective study [8]. The prescription dose was 70 CGE in 35 fractions delivered with three cycles of concurrent cisplatin (100 mg/m^2) followed by adjuvant cisplatin (80 mg/m^2) and fluorouracil (1000 mg/m^2/day) for three cycles. At median follow-up of 28 months, no patient experienced local or regional relapse of disease. There was no acute or late grade 4 or 5 radiation-related adverse event. At 6 and 12 months after treatment, one patient was G-tube dependent. The most common grade ≥3 late adverse events were hearing loss in 29% of patients and weight loss in 38% of patients.
- In a case control study from MD Anderson Cancer Center, 10 NPC patients treated with IMPT were matched to 20 IMRT-treated controls, all of whom received concurrent ± adjuvant chemotherapy. IMPT was associated with significantly lower mean dose to the oral cavity, brainstem, whole brain, and mandible [4]. Patients treated with IMPT had a lower rate of G-tube insertion (20% vs. 65%), which was hypothesized to result from improved sparing of the oral cavity. The rate of grade 3 mucositis was lower (11%) than commonly reported in the IMRT literature. Of note, however, two patients in the IMPT cohort (as well as two in the IMRT-treated cohort) developed temporal lobe necrosis, including one patient who developed neurologic symptoms requiring bevacizumab.

4.6 Discussion and Future Directions

- Proton beam therapy holds significant potential for improving treatment outcomes for nasopharyngeal tumors, especially those with skull base and/or orbital invasion in which photon-based therapy will exceed dose-limiting constraints (Fig. 4.3). As the clinical implementation of pencil beam scanning technology matures, the dosimetric gains afforded by proton beam therapy have rapidly improved. Further improvements in dose conformality for PBS-based proton therapy are likely to be achievable through clinical implementation of strategies to minimize spot size (Fig. 4.4). Current spot sizes in clinical use can be as large as 9 mm, resulting in a penumbral width of up to 10 mm. Minimization of spot size and sharpening of penumbra with the addition of apertures are likely to result in significant target conformality improvements, with the potential to translate into clinically meaningful benefits for patients with NPC. Clinical implementation of three-dimensional image guidance for proton therapy is also currently under development at several centers and may lead to improved treatment accuracy and reduced dose uncertainty. Efforts to improve proton range calculation via novel imaging platforms, including PET, DECT, and prompt gamma imaging, also hold significant promise.

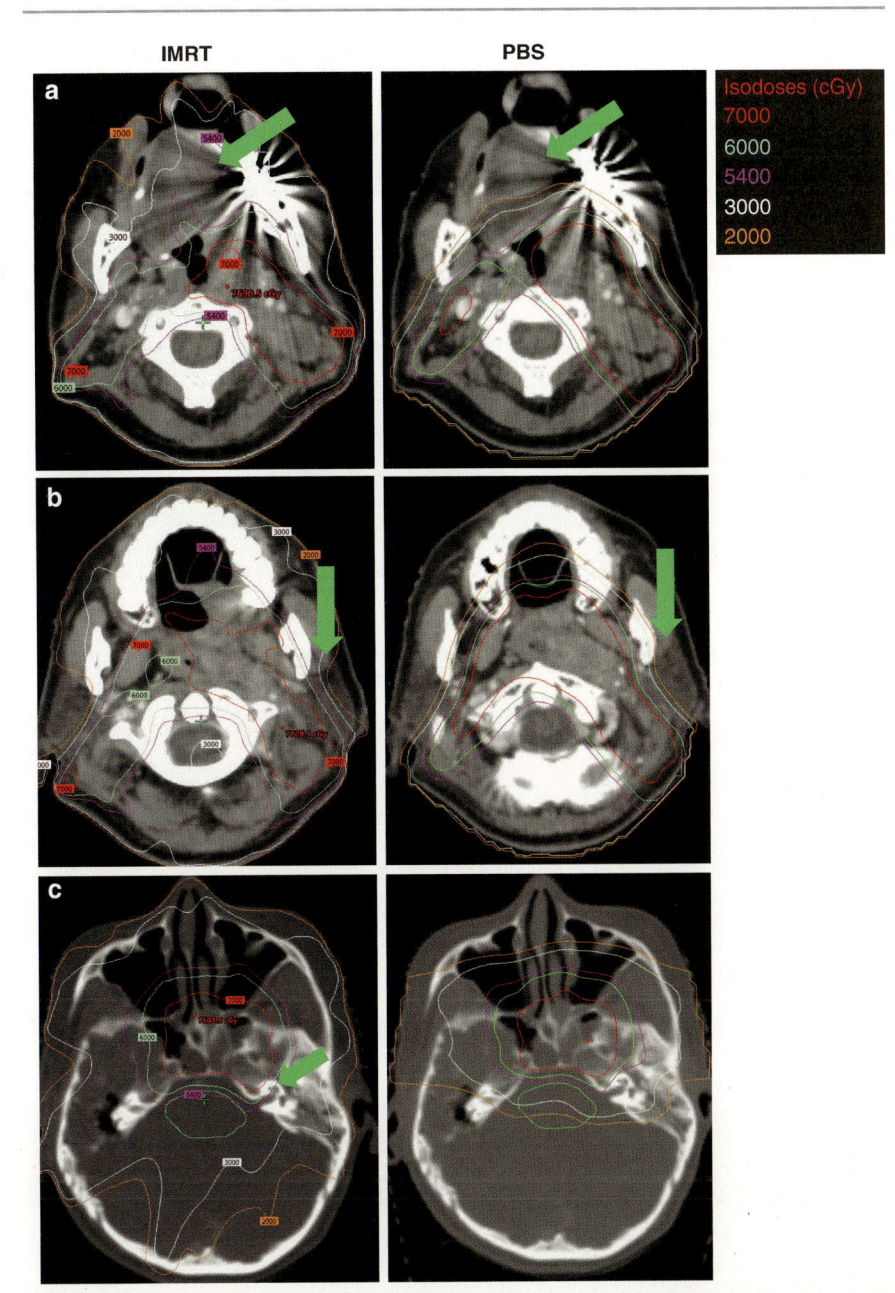

Fig. 4.3 PBS vs. IMRT dosimetric comparison for patient with T4N2 nasopharyngeal carcinoma. (**a**) Improved sparing of oral mucosa with PBS. (**b**) Increased sparing of ipsilateral parotid gland with PBS. (**c**) Cochlea and brainstem dosimetry are improved with PBS compared to IMRT, especially in cases with base of skull invasion

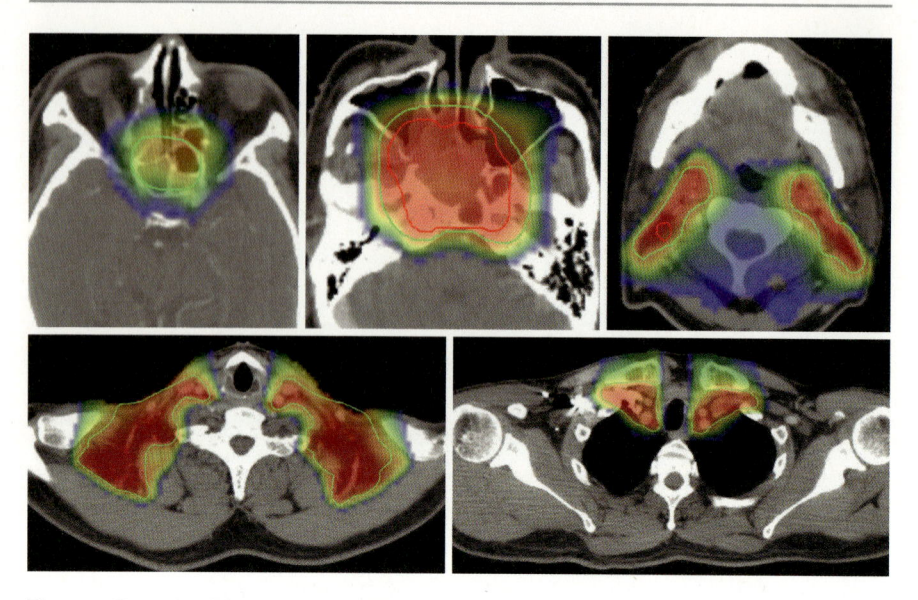

Fig. 4.4 Example PBS plan (SFO optimized) for patient with T3N2 nasopharyngeal carcinoma. *Red contour* = PTV$_{70}$. *Green contour* = PTV$_{59.4}$

References

1. Rosenthal DI, Chambers MS, Fuller CD, et al. Beam path toxicities to non-target structures during intensity-modulated radiation therapy for head and neck cancer. Int J Radiat Oncol Biol Phys. 2008;72:747–55.
2. Kuang WL, Zhou Q, Shen LF. Outcomes and prognostic factors of conformal radiotherapy versus intensity-modulated radiotherapy for nasopharyngeal carcinoma. Clin Transl Oncol. 2012;14:783–90.
3. Taheri-Kadkhoda Z, Bjork-Eriksson T, Nill S, et al. Intensity-modulated radiotherapy of nasopharyngeal carcinoma: a comparative treatment planning study of photons and protons. Radiat Oncol. 2008;3:4.
4. Lewis GD, Holliday EB, Kocak-Uzel E, et al. Intensity-modulated proton therapy for nasopharyngeal carcinoma: decreased radiation dose to normal structures and encouraging clinical outcomes. Head neck. 2016;38(Suppl 1):E1886–95.
5. Holliday EB, Frank SJ. Proton radiation therapy for head and neck cancer: a review of the clinical experience to date. Int J Radiat Oncol Biol Phys. 2014;89:292–302.
6. Lee N, Harris J, Garden AS, et al. Intensity-modulated radiation therapy with or without chemotherapy for nasopharyngeal carcinoma: radiation therapy oncology group phase II trial 0225. J Clin Oncol. 2009;27:3684–90.
7. Lin R, Slater JD, Yonemoto LT, et al. Nasopharyngeal carcinoma: repeat treatment with conformal proton therapy—dose-volume histogram analysis. Radiology. 1999;213:489–94.
8. Chan AT. A phase II trial of proton radiation therapy with chemotherapy for nasopharyngeal carcinoma. Int J Radiat Oncol Biol Phys. 2012;84:S151–2.

Oral Cavity Tumors

5

Jennifer Ma, Benjamin H. Lok, Kevin Sine, and Nancy Y. Lee

Contents

5.1	Introduction	117
5.2	Simulation, Target Delineation, and Radiation Dose/Fractionation	118
5.3	Patient Positioning, Immobilization, and Treatment Verification	121
5.4	Three-Dimensional (3D) Proton Treatment Planning	121
	5.4.1 Passive Scattering (PS)	121
5.5	Pencil-Beam Scanning (PBS)	124
	5.5.1 Passive Scattering vs. Pencil Beam-Scanning Comparisons	124
	5.5.2 Critical Structures	125
5.6	Future Developments	125
References		130

5.1 Introduction

Oral cavity and pharynx cancers account for 2.9% of all cancers in the United States. The most common sites of oral cavity cancer are the oral tongue and floor of the mouth. There are over 45,000 new cases of oral cavity and pharynx cancers diagnosed each year, with over 8500 deaths annually [1]. Known risk factors for oral cavity cancer include tobacco and alcohol use, infection with human papillomavirus, and chewing of betel nut leaves. Oral cavity cancers are often initially managed surgically, followed by radiation ± chemotherapy. Locoregionally advanced oral cavity cancers are treated with a combination of surgery and

---

J. Ma • B.H. Lok • N.Y. Lee (✉)
Memorial Sloan Kettering Cancer Center, New York, NY, USA
e-mail: leen2@mskcc.org

K. Sine
ProCure Proton Therapy Center, Somerset, NJ, USA

© Springer International Publishing Switzerland 2018
N. Lee et al. (eds.), *Target Volume Delineation and Treatment Planning for Particle Therapy*, Practical Guides in Radiation Oncology,
https://doi.org/10.1007/978-3-319-42478-1_5

RT ± chemotherapy, due to the high risk of local recurrence compared to other head and neck squamous cell carcinoma sites [2]. Risk factors for recurrence of oral cavity cancers include the presence of extracapsular nodal spread, positive resection margins, N2 or N3 nodal disease, perineural invasion, and vascular invasion [3, 4].

Oral cavity cancers are often grouped with oropharyngeal cancers; therefore, there are no published clinical studies evaluating proton therapy in oral cavity cancers alone. There are few published clinical studies assessing the role of protons for oropharyngeal cancers, which demonstrated improved locoregional control [5, 6]. The efficacy and toxicity of protons in oropharyngeal cancers are currently being further evaluated in a clinical trial setting, with patients randomized to IMRT or IMPT [7]. A previous study of IMPT in oral cavity cancers demonstrated a 2-year rate of local control of 91% and 2-year locoregional progression-free survival of 84% [6]. Incidence of late Grade 3 toxicity has not been known to increase significantly despite the higher doses administered via proton therapy, with xerostomia and mucositis being the most commonly observed adverse events [6, 7].

The RTOG 8502 regimen of photon radiotherapy has been shown to be effective for the treatment of advanced head and neck cancers. The regimen is colloquially referred to as "Quad Shot" and consists of 3.7 Gy fractions delivered twice daily over 2 consecutive days for 4 week intervals, for a total of three cycles [8]. A recent study of the RTOG8502 regimen as a hypofractionated proton radiotherapy regimen has also been shown to demonstrate a favorable palliative response in patients with incurable recurrent metastatic malignancies of the head and neck and is used at our institution for the treatment of appropriate oral cavity cancers (unpublished data).

Tumors with lower risk of lymph node metastasis (retromolar trigone, hard palate, gingiva) should be treated to the tumor bed with consideration of ipsilateral lymph nodes. For tumors with higher risk of lymph node metastasis (buccal mucosa), coverage of bilateral cervical lymph nodes should be considered. Tumors with high risk of spread to surrounding musculature and glands (oral tongue, floor of mouth) should include bilateral neck coverage and consideration for lymph node coverage in the radiation fields.

Proton therapy allows for delivery of higher radiation doses to the oral cavity with lower exposure to surrounding critical structures and without evidence of worsening toxicity. "The anterior location of oral cavity tumors along with the high risk of local recurrence offers a potential opportunity to improve outcomes with proton dose escalation, although this remains to be explored."

5.2 Simulation, Target Delineation, and Radiation Dose/Fractionation

CT can be used for initial determination of soft tissue and bony involvement (including the pterygopalatine fossa, mandible, and hard palate). Dental panoramas can determine mandibular involvement if CT cannot be obtained. For the purposes of dose calculation, a non-contrast CT needs to be employed in planning proton therapy.

MRI is critical for determination of perineural spread and primary tumor delineation, particularly if dental artifacts complicate CT visualization.

5 Oral Cavity Tumors

PET imaging is superior to CT and MRI in detection of occult nodal metastasis, although it is limited in the detection of small metastasis.

The patient should be supine with the neck in slight hyperextension for simulation. A five-point mask should be used for immobilization of the head, neck, and shoulders. A bite block can be used for oral tongue cancers to decrease dose to the superior or inferior oral cavity, as appropriate. Custom bite blocks can be fabricated to immobilize the oral tongue laterally in order to reduce unnecessary dose (Fig. 5.1).

PET and MR images should be registered to the planning CT for accurate target delineation. Uncertainties related to image fusion should be considered in the treatment planning process (Chap. 3).

Radiation dosing and fractionation varies depending on the clinical scenario (Tables 5.1, 5.2, 5.3, and 5.4).

Fig. 5.1 Uniform scanning plan demonstrating use of a custom mouth guard to offset the ipsilateral tongue to minimize the dose to the oral tongue. Bite block indicated by *red arrows* above

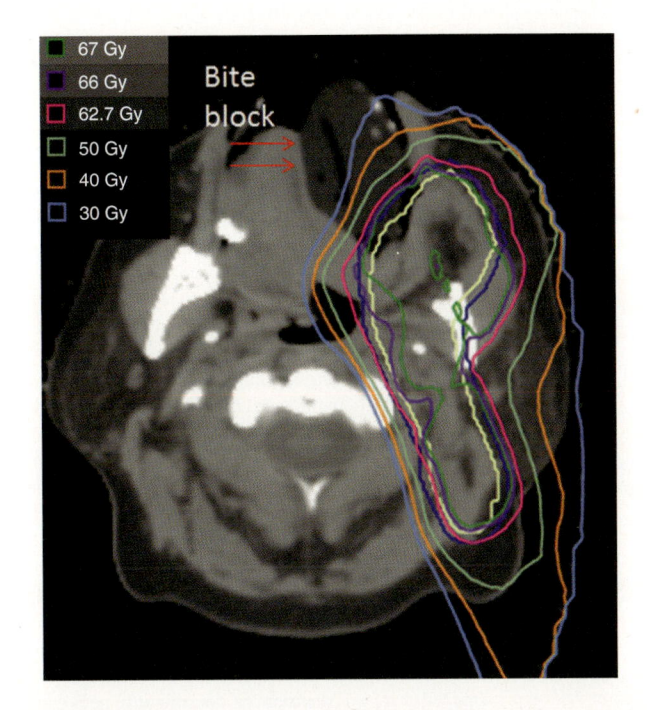

Table 5.1 Recommended target volumes and radiation doses for definitive treatment of oral cavity cancers

Volume	Target	Dose
GTV	Gross disease, involved nerves, and regional lymph nodes	70 Gy (RBE)
High-risk clinical tumor volume (CTV_{70})	Include margin of 5 mm if there is uncertainty of gross disease extent	70 Gy (RBE)
High-risk clinical tumor volume ($CTV_{59.4}$)	Include up to a 10 mm margin for positive nodes and high-risk ipsilateral or contralateral nodes	59.4 Gy (RBE)
Low-risk clinical tumor volume (CTV_{54})	Include ipsilateral and contralateral nodes at low-risk for subclinical disease	54 Gy (RBE)

Table 5.2 Recommended target volumes and radiation doses for adjuvant treatment of oral cavity cancers

Volume	Target	Dose
High-risk clinical tumor volume (CTV_{66})	Include preoperative target volume and regions of extracapsular nodal extension, soft tissue invasion, bone invasion, and positive margins	66 Gy (RBE)
High-risk clinical tumor volume (CTV_{60})	Include preoperative tumor volume and nodal disease, operative bed, and ipsilateral or contralateral nodes at high risk for subclinical disease	60 Gy (RBE)
Low-risk clinical tumor volume (CTV_{54})	Include uninvolved ipsilateral and contralateral lymph nodes at low risk for subclinical disease	54 Gy (RBE)

Table 5.3 Site-specific recommendations for clinical target delineation of oral cavity cancers

Tumor site	Stage	Clinical treatment volume
Oral tongue, floor of the mouth	T1—T4N0	Include tumor bed, base of the tongue, and entire oral tongue. Consider including the alveolar ridge for floor of the mouth lesions. Treat both sides of the neck, even for well-lateralized T1—T2N0 lesions if depth of invasion is >4 mm; inclusion in low- or high-risk CTV is up to physician discretion. Ipsilateral and/or contralateral levels I–IV can be considered
	T1—T4N1-3	Include tumor bed, base of the tongue, and entire oral tongue. Consider including the alveolar ridge for floor of the mouth lesions. Treat both sides of the neck; inclusion in low- or high-risk CTV is up to physician discretion. Ipsilateral and/or contralateral levels I–IV can be considered
Buccal mucosa	T1—T4N0	Target volume for the inner cheek should be generous and include the preoperative tumor bed, entire buccal mucosa, and ipsilateral lymph nodes. Extend coverage posteriorly to retromolar trigone and superiorly to near the inferior orbital rim. If well-lateralized, the tumor can be treated at ipsilateral levels I–IV alone. Otherwise, bilateral cervical lymph node coverage can be considered
	T1—T4N1-3	Target volume for the inner cheek should be generous and include the preoperative tumor bed, entire buccal mucosa, and ipsilateral lymph nodes. Extend coverage posteriorly to retromolar trigone and superiorly to near the inferior orbital rim. Ipsilateral levels I–IV should be treated within the neck. Treatment of contralateral neck can be considered depending on pathologic findings and discussions with the surgeon
Retromolar trigone, hard palate, gingiva	T1—T4N0	Include the preoperative target volume and postoperative tumor bed. Ipsilateral levels I–IV can be considered for all cases, with treatment of contralateral neck at physician discretion. Hard palate tumors are generally minor salivary gland tumors; "Chap. 8" can be used for treatment guidelines for coverage of lymph node regions
	T1—T4N1-3	Include the preoperative target volume and postoperative tumor bed. Treat the ipsilateral levels I–IV for all cases, and consider treatment of the contralateral neck. Hard palate tumors are generally minor salivary gland tumors; "Chap. 8: Major Salivary Glands" can be used for treatment guidelines for coverage of lymph node regions

Table 5.4 Recommended dose constraints for organs at risk in bilateral cases

Organ at risk	Recommended dose constraint
Oral cavity (excluding PTV)	Mean dose <10 Gy (RBE)
Larynx	Mean dose <20 Gy (RBE)
Ipsilateral parotid gland (for non-parotid cases)	Mean dose <26 Gy (RBE) (ideally lower)
Ipsilateral submandibular gland (for non-submandibular cases)	Mean dose <39 Gy (RBE)
Contralateral submandibular and parotid glands	Mean dose 0 Gy (RBE)
Esophagus	Max dose < Rx dose Mean dose ≤ 40 Gy (RBE) V60 ≤ 17% (ideally lower)
Brachial plexus	No hot spots
Brainstem	0.05 cc < 60 Gy (RBE) Max surface dose ≤64 Gy (RBE)
Optic nerves and optic chiasm	0.05 cc < 60 Gy (RBE)
Spinal cord	1.0 cc < 50 Gy (RBE) Surface max ≤64 Gy (RBE)

5.3 Patient Positioning, Immobilization, and Treatment Verification

CT simulation should be performed using a slice thickness of 3 mm or less. Intravenous contrast should be used for target delineation, particularly for cervical lymph node detection. The CT should span from the top of the head to the carina, with the isocenter just superior to the arytenoids.

Setup accuracy should ideally be ascertained with daily orthogonal X-ray imaging or volumetric imaging, if available, in order to confirm setup accuracy.

In-room CT imaging (i.e., cone beam CT) is ideally used for treatment verification. When in-room 3D imaging is not available, verification CT scans with the patient in treatment position are recommended during the course of treatment to assess for potential changes in anatomy such as weight loss, tumor shrinkage, and potential changes in the accuracy of the dose distribution. Currently at our center, we generally rescan every other week for definitive cases and once during treatment for postoperative cases, though there are exceptions depending on the clinical scenario.

5.4 Three-Dimensional (3D) Proton Treatment Planning

5.4.1 Passive Scattering (PS)

Three field plans are typically utilized (two to four beams) in planning oral cavity cases. With all proton planning, care must be taken not to overlap the distal end of more than two beams and no more than one beam ranging out into an organ at risk (OAR). With proton planning, air gap between the compensator and patient surface is also an important consideration. Minimizing the air gap reduces penumbra and scatter while increasing conformality. When using smaller air gaps, be mindful of collisions between the compensator and the patient or treatment table.

Worst and best case scenarios should be evaluated with relevant range uncertainties (2.5%*range + 2 mm), based on physical and biological uncertainties.

With proton planning, artifacts, dental hardware, surgical clips, and other foreign materials must be contoured and assigned the proper forced densities in order to ensure accurate beam calculation.

Special care should be taken to avoid beams traversing through dental hardware and air cavities that can change during the course of treatment (Fig. 5.2).

While planning with uniform scanning (US) or passive scattering (PS), compensators should be created with the dental filling at a lower electron density. This will maintain a smoother compensator with less ridges and pylons. After the compensator is calculated, apply appropriate forced density, and evaluate the beam coverage and OARs.

If it is necessary for the beam path to treat through the fillings, there will be a cold spot distal to the filling. This effect can be minimized by using multiple beam angles.

Patching field technique can be used to keep the parotid dose and other OARs below tolerance. Patched fields are two orthogonal beams in which the distal 50% isodose line of one beam is abutting the 50% lateral penumbra line of the other

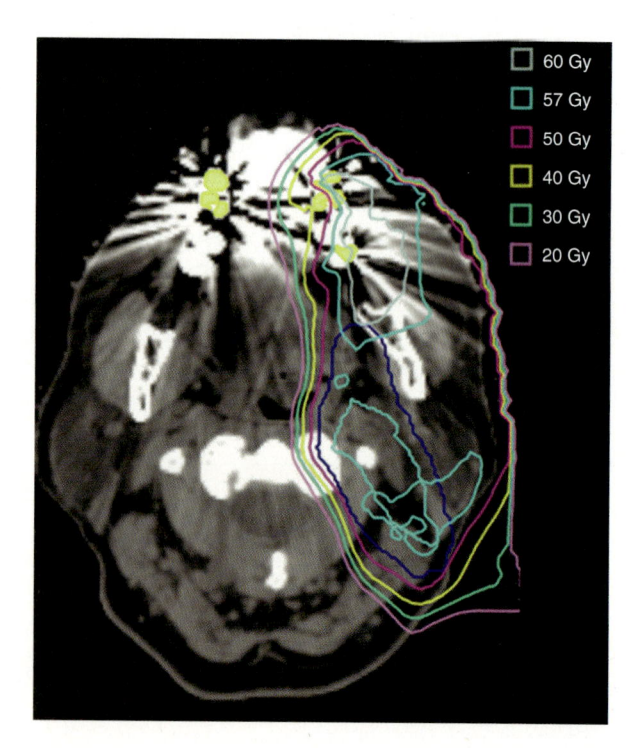

Fig. 5.2 Example of a uniform scanning plan demonstrating contouring of a dental filling artifact

5 Oral Cavity Tumors

beam. When possible, use a minimum of two patched pairs to minimize the hot spots along the patch lines. Maintain a 15–20% hot spot at the match line to allow for over and under range uncertainties (Fig. 5.3).

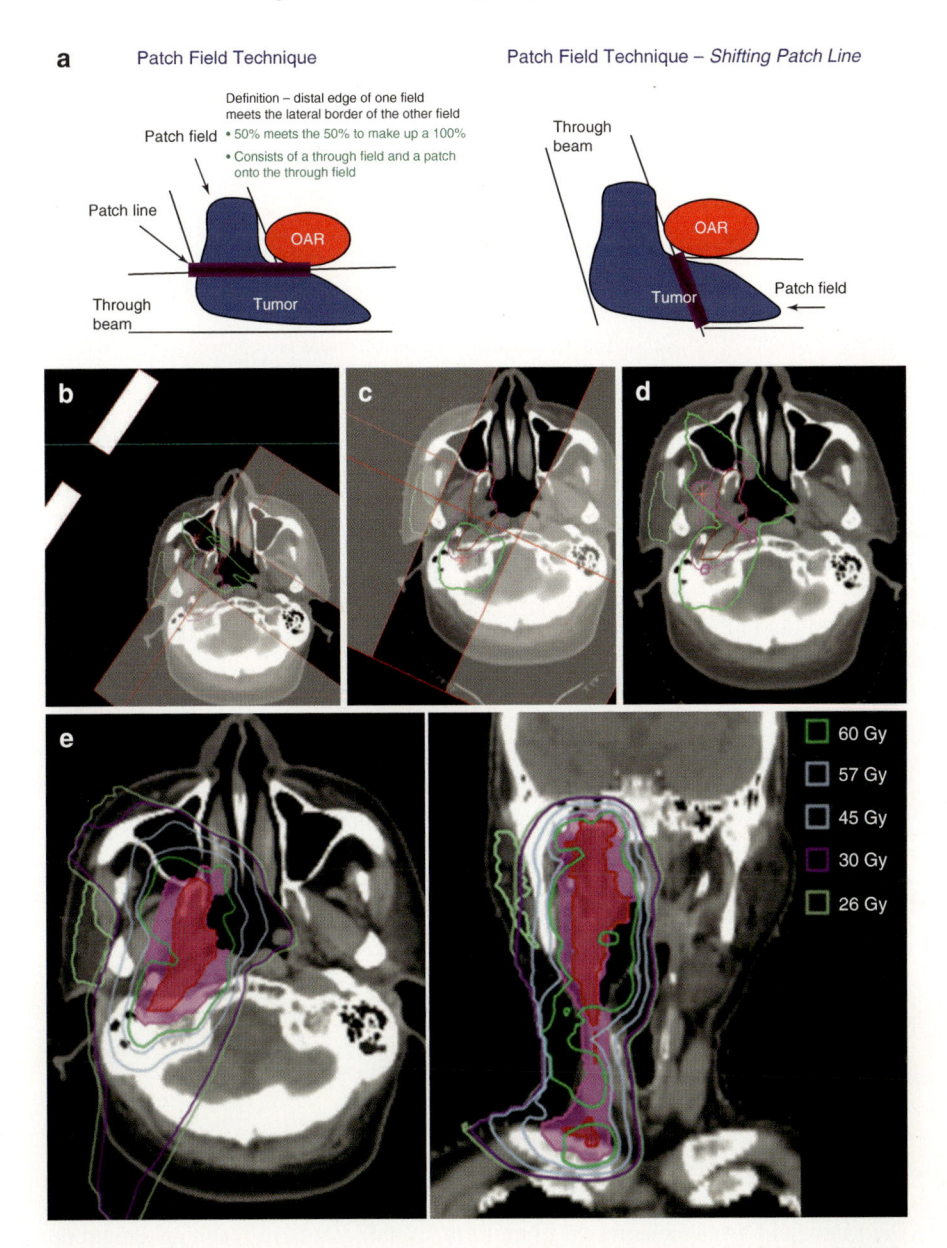

Fig. 5.3 Passive scattering plan illustrating a patch technique to avoid the parotid gland, for the treatment of a recurrent squamous cell carcinoma of the right lateral oral tongue, status post right partial glossectomy and radical resection of the right tonsil and right base of the tongue. (**a**) Illustrates the patch field technique; (**b**) demonstrates a through beam; (**c**) is the patch field abutting the 50% lateral isodose line of (**b**); (**d**) demonstrates the patch pair isodose distribution. The through beam plus patch field yields one patch pair; the 15% hot spot is represented by the *purple line*; (**e**) is the composite plan with isodose distribution of all fields

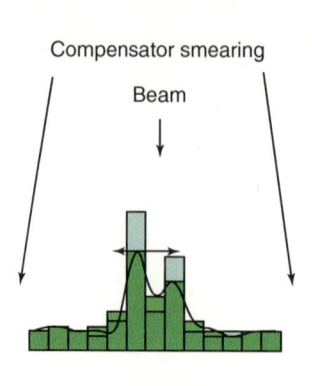

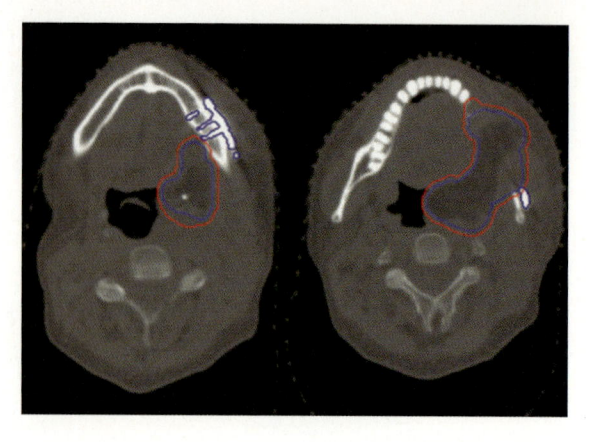

Fig. 5.4 Example of compensator smearing and plan for hardware present within the radiation field

There are times when hardware might be present in the field, such as titanium screws and surgical clips. Avoid traversing through the hardware whenever possible, although this may be unavoidable in certain cases.

Screws and clips should be overridden while creating compensators. An increase in smearing should also be utilized to increase robustness of the plan and reduce pylons in the compensator. Smearing should be at minimum ≥ PTV margin and the Moyer's formula should be considered: Smear = [(3% or range)2 + (3 mm)2 + (motion)2] ½] as a minimum (Fig. 5.4).

The following rules should be followed when performing patch fields:

- Maintain a hot spot between 15% and 20% at the intersection of the patched fields.
- The 95% isodose line should not completely break up when all beams are summed; the 90% isodose line should encompass the target.
- No more than 30% of total dose should be delivered via patched fields (exceptions are made when planning is particularly difficult due to re-treatment limitations; in these cases, a physician and physicist should be consulted).
- End of range effects should be minimized particularly in the brain or near OARs; no more than 30% of beams should end range on an OAR.

5.5 Pencil-Beam Scanning (PBS)

5.5.1 Passive Scattering vs. Pencil Beam-Scanning Comparisons

The same field arrangement used in uniform scanning/passive scanning should be used in PBS, although the number of fields may be decreased.

For oral cavity cases, single field uniform dose optimization (SFUD) should ideally be used as it results in delivery of the most robust treatment plan. Each beam should be optimized using the target and OAR constraints/objectives set by your institution. Each beam should be evaluated individually to ensure adequate target coverage and then compositely to evaluate OAR constraints and possible hot spots. As robust optimization matures in the clinical environment, intensity-modulated proton therapy (IMPT) may be more extensively used. Even though IMPT may generate a more conformal dose distribution, plan robustness must be carefully evaluated especially when robust optimization is not available on your treatment planning system (Fig. 5.5).

Robust optimization can be achieved when creating optimization constraints and objectives for the targets and OARs. The robustness optimization should be used when clinically needed and available. Each institution will set their robustness optimization parameters based upon the estimated setup tolerances and estimated range uncertainties. Robust optimization will compute, considering the over and under range, isocenter shifts, set up uncertainties, and restrict hot spots if there is over lapping of fields.

Without robust optimization, another option to ensure robustness is to create planning organ at risk volumes (PRVs) and target optimization structures to account for the uncertainties. When possible, planning should be carried out with SFUD as it is currently the most robust option available. As robust optimization is just emerging in the clinical setting, it should be carefully evaluated.

5.5.2 Critical Structures

The ipsilateral parotid gland is a critical avoidance structure, and care should be taken to minimize exposure, reducing the mean dose to <26 Gy (RBE) or, ideally, lower (Fig. 5.6).

The spinal cord should also be taken into account during the planning process. With the unique characteristics of protons, the doses are usually held to a minimum. Due to the beam stopping power of protons, the laryngeal dose can also be significantly lowered to try to maintain a mean dose of ≤15 GyE or lower (Figs. 5.7, 5.8, 5.9, 5.10).

The sharp dose falloff of protons allows for optic nerve sparing.

5.6 Future Developments

As IMPT use becomes more prevalent, additional data on the role of IMPT in oral cavity cancers will become available. The efficacy and toxicity of protons in oropharyngeal cancers is currently being further evaluated in a clinical trial setting, with patients randomized to IMRT or IMPT. The ongoing clinical trial of IMPT vs. IMRT in oropharyngeal cancers will illuminate the differences in efficacy and toxicity.

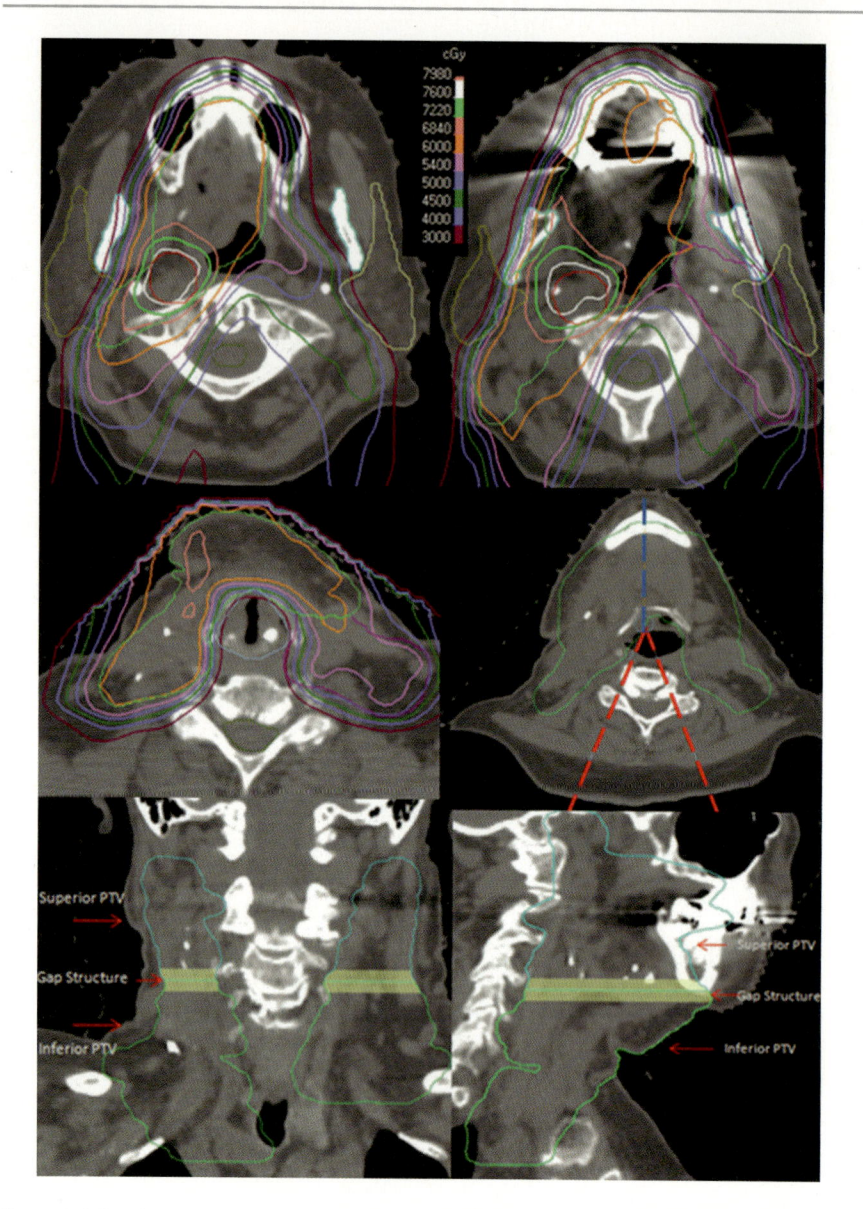

Fig. 5.5 PBS plan of a 72-year-old woman with stage T3N1 SCC of the oral tongue, status post-hemiglossectomy and cervical lymphadenectomy with modified radical neck dissection. Bilateral oral cavity cases are treated using a three-beam approach: AP (*blue dashed line*) and RPO and LPO (*red dashed lines*). The lower anterior neck is treated with the AP and is matched with the posterior oblique beams treating the upper neck and oral cavity. Although counterintuitive, treating the superior PTV with the posterior obliques is more robust than an anterior approach as slight movement in the mandible will adversely affect the beam path. The posterior approach is less susceptible to this variation in setup. This approach also maximizes parotid sparing. The target volume is divided into two parts (superior and inferior PTV), which are treated with independent dose objectives. At the match line, we create a dose gradient using a "gap structure." The structure is 1 cm superior and inferior to the match line defined by PTV volume. The gradient over 2 cm is 5% per mm, so changes in setup in between fields of up to 2 mm would only result in 10% changes in daily delivered dose, thereby reducing excessive hot or cold spots at the match line

5 Oral Cavity Tumors   127

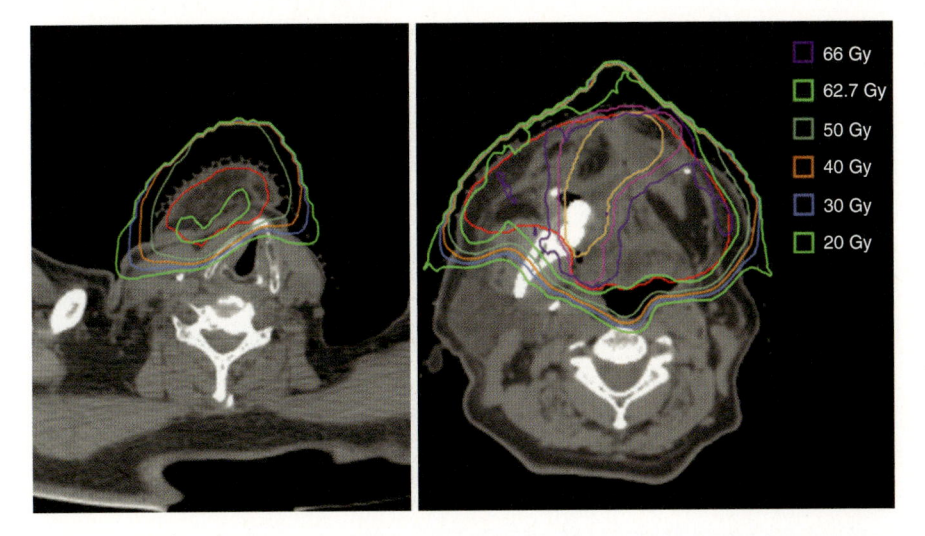

Fig. 5.6 Uniform scanning plan for the treatment of a multiply recurrent squamous cell carcinoma of the oral cavity, status post-multiple resections and postoperative radiation therapy to a total dose of 6300/5400/5000 cGy. Plan illustrates treatment to a recurrence of the gingiva and hard palate post-surgical resection with positive margins, with sparing of the larynx, parotid glands, and spinal cord

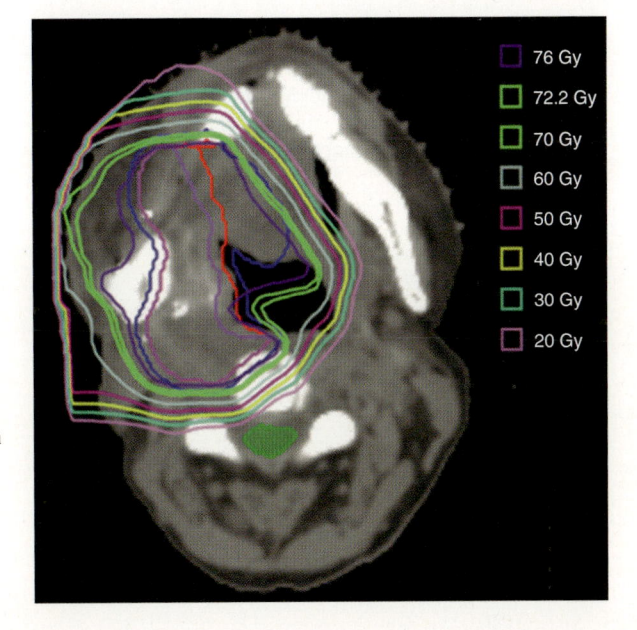

Fig. 5.7 Example of cord sparing in an initial pT1N0 right oral tongue cancer with a large right retromolar trigone recurrence, status post-surgical resection with postoperative RT to 66 Gy and surgery for a pT4aNx recurrence

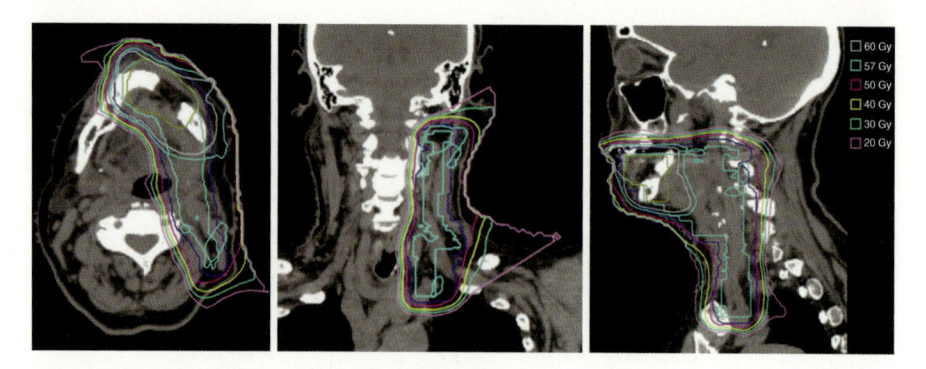

Fig. 5.8 Example of a treatment plan for a pT1N0 spindle cell SCC with 6 mm invasion and perineural invasion, status post-resection with a marginal mandibulectomy and left neck dissection. High-risk primary CTV$_{60}$ is contoured in gold

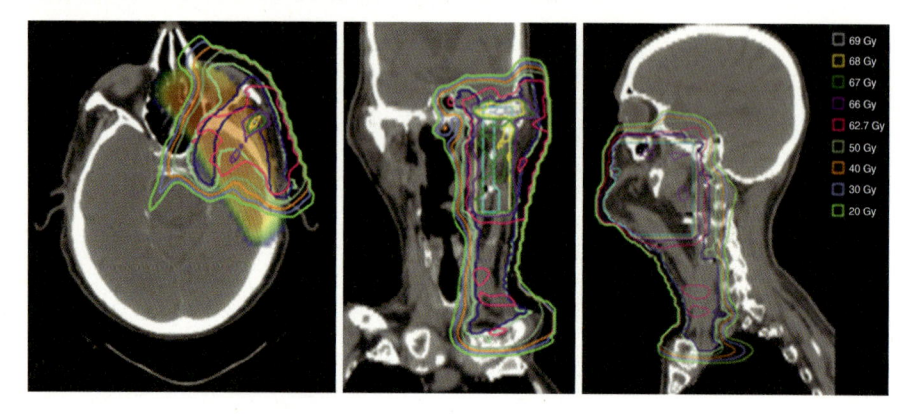

Fig. 5.9 Example of a treatment plan for a rpT4N0M0R0 SCC of the left buccal mucosa, status post-resection with positive margins and recurrent disease resected with extensive PNI, invasive islands, and tumor in the floor of the mouth and palate. Plan demonstrates ophthalmic nerve coverage tracing back to Meckel's cave; the CTV$_{50}$ is contoured in *dark blue*

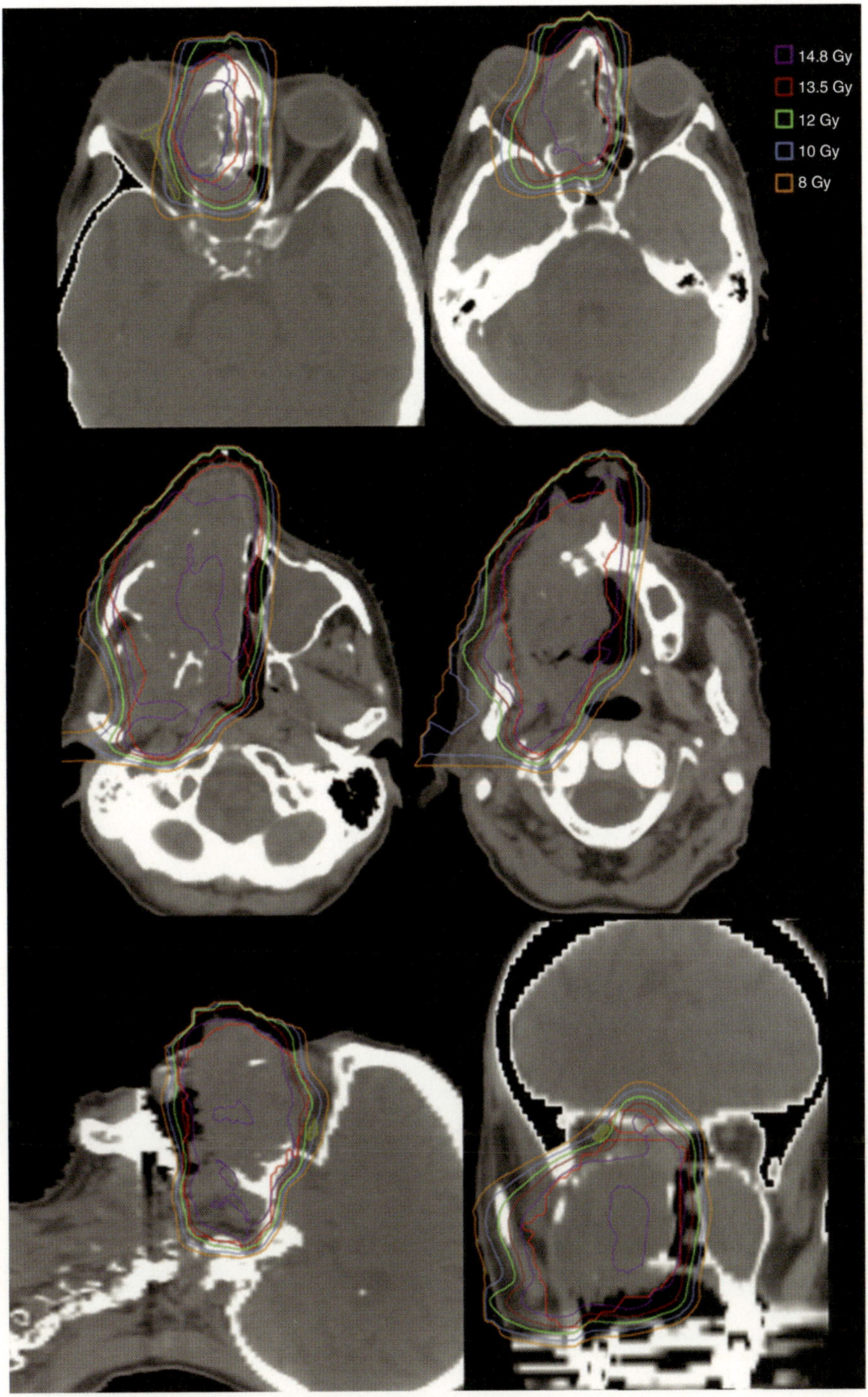

Fig. 5.10 Example of optic nerve sparing in a verrucous carcinoma of the right alveolar ridge extending up to the maxillary sinus, treated with "Quad Shot," status post-maxillectomy with re-resection of recurrence with positive margins that were treated with adjuvant RT to 66 Gy, with bulky local recurrence in the right maxilla

References

1. Gadner H. A randomized trial of treatment for multisystem Langerhans' cell histiocytosis. J Pediatr. 2001;138(5):728–34.
2. Oliver R, et al. Interventions for the treatment of oral and oropharyngeal cancers: surgical treatment. Cochrane Database Syst Rev. 2007;(4):CD006205.
3. Bernier J, Domenge C, Ozsahin M, Matuszewska K, Lefèbvre JL, Greiner RH, Giralt J, Maingon P, Rolland F, Bolla M, Cognetti F, Bourhis J, Kirkpatrick A, van Glabbeke M, European Organization for Research and Treatment of Cancer Trial 22931. Postoperative irradiation with or without concomitant chemotherapy for locally advanced head and neck cancer. N Engl J Med. 2004;350(19):1945–52.
4. Cooper JS, Pajak TF, Forastiere AA, Jacobs J, Campbell BH, Saxman SB, Kish JA, Kim HE, Cmelak AJ, Rotman M, Machtay M, Ensley JF, Chao KS, Schultz CJ, Lee N, Fu KK, Radiation Therapy Oncology Group 9501/Intergroup. Postoperative concurrent radiotherapy and chemotherapy for high-risk squamous-cell carcinoma of the head and neck. N Engl J Med. 2004;350(19):1937–44.
5. Slater JD, Yonemoto L, Mantik DW, Bush DA, Preston W, Grove RI, Miller DW, Slater JM. Proton radiation for treatment of cancer of the oropharynx: early experience at Loma Linda University Medical Center using a concomitant boost technique. Int J Radiat Oncol Biol Phys. 2005;62:494–500.
6. Frank SJ, Cox JD, Gillin M, Mohan R, Garden AS, Rosenthal DI, Gunn GB, Weber RS, Kies MS, Lewin JS, Munsell MF, Palmer MB, Sahoo N, Zhang X, Liu W, Zhu XR. Multifield optimization intensity modulated proton therapy for head and neck tumors: a translation to practice. Int J Radiat Oncol Biol Phys. 2014;89:846–53.
7. Steven J, Frank MD. Phase II/III randomized trial of intensity-modulated proton beam therapy (IMPT) versus intensity-modulated photon therapy (IMRT) for the treatment of oropharyngeal cancer of the head and neck. 24 April 2016. https://clinicaltrials.gov/show/NCT01893307.
8. Lok BH, Jiang G, Gutiontov S, Lanning RM, Sridhara S, Sherman EJ, Tsai CJ, SM MB, Riaz N, Lee NY. Palliative head and neck radiotherapy with the RTOG 8502 regimen for incurable primary or metastatic cancers. Oral Oncol. 2015;51(10):957–62.

Oropharyngeal Cancer

6

Suchit H. Patel, Amy J. Xu, Kevin Sine, Nancy Y. Lee, and Pamela Fox

Contents

6.1	Introduction	131
6.2	Simulation, Target Delineation, and Radiation Dose/Fractionation	132
6.3	Patient Positioning, Immobilization, and Treatment Verification	133
6.4	Three-Dimensional (3D) Proton Treatment Planning	133
	6.4.1 Passive Scattering (PS)	133
6.5	Pencil Beam Scanning (PBS)	135
6.6	Dosimetry and Toxicity Characteristics	137
Conclusion		139
References		139

6.1 Introduction

Oropharynx tumors (OPC) comprise 24% of all head and neck malignancies, of which the majority arise from the base of the tongue or tonsils [1–4]. Smoking and alcohol use continue to be major risk factors but the prevalence of human papillomavirus (HPV)-associated oropharyngeal cancer has steadily increased by over 200% since the late 1980s [5]. Definitive management involves surgery or radiation therapy (RT) alone for node-negative early-stage tumors or concurrent chemoradiotherapy (CRT) for nodal involvement or locally advanced disease. In surgically

S.H. Patel • A.J. Xu • N.Y. Lee (✉)
Memorial Sloan Kettering Cancer Center, New York, NY, USA
e-mail: leen2@mskcc.org

K. Sine • P. Fox
ProCure Proton Therapy Center, Somerset, NJ, USA

© Springer International Publishing Switzerland 2018
N. Lee et al. (eds.), *Target Volume Delineation and Treatment Planning for Particle Therapy*, Practical Guides in Radiation Oncology,
https://doi.org/10.1007/978-3-319-42478-1_6

managed cases, adjuvant RT or CRT is also often indicated for extracapsular extension or positive surgical margins.

Dosimetry studies dating back nearly 15 years ago have consistently demonstrated the ability of proton RT to reduce the dose to critical structures, including the spinal cord, salivary glands, oral cavity, larynx, mandible, and esophagus [6]. More recent work has focused on the ability of intensity-modulated proton therapy (IMPT) to further enhance the therapeutic ratio by providing homogeneous target coverage with further sparing of normal structures, particularly in locally advanced tumors [7, 8]. Potential reductions in toxicity achieved with proton therapy are of paramount importance in the era of HPV-related OPC in which many young patients are cured of disease and will suffer effects of treatment for decades.

Despite the theoretical benefits of proton dosimetry, experience with proton RT in OPC treatment is limited. Loma Linda University Medical Center reported a 5-year actuarial locoregional control of 84% and grade 3 late toxicity in 11% of patients treated with passively scattered proton fields to deliver concomitant proton boost along with photon treatment during the last 3.5 weeks of treatment [9].

Recent experience with IMPT and more contemporary techniques at M.D. Anderson in which bilateral neck irradiation was pursued for nearly all OPC patients with a three-field technique showed a 2-year PFS of 89% and grade 3 acute mucositis and late dysphagia rates of 58% and 12%, respectively [10].

6.2 Simulation, Target Delineation, and Radiation Dose/Fractionation

CT simulation with intravenous iodinated contrast, when not contraindicated, is crucial to facilitate anatomical delineation. For the purposes of dose calculation, a non-contrast CT needs to be included during simulation as well.

Positron emission tomography (PET) is often helpful for identification of metabolically active gross disease and involved lymph nodes. Large necrotic nodes may not show activity on PET but should be encompassed within high-dose target volumes, especially in HPV-positive cases. Likewise, small nodes that are borderline on PET may represent disease in alcohol- and smoking-related HPV-negative cases and need to be evaluated carefully. Biopsy to show evidence of gross nodal involvement is not always needed in practice, particularly in HPV-related malignancies.

Magnetic resonance imaging (MR) is recommended for accurate delineation of the extent of gross tumor in soft tissue, especially in cases in which artifact from dental amalgam limits evaluation of the tonsils. When possible, MR should be obtained in the treatment position.

PET and MR images should be registered to the planning CT for accurate target delineation. Uncertainties related to image fusion should be considered in the treatment planning process (Chap. 3).

The recommended dosing and fractionation vary:

- For definitive cases, gross tumor volume (GTV), including gross primary tumor and involved regional lymph nodes, should be treated to 70 Gy (RBE). Typically,

6 Oropharyngeal Cancer

an extra CTV margin is used only to outline areas of uncertainty in the extent of the GTV.
- Both the primary tumor site and the involved levels of the ipsilateral neck (levels II–IV) should be treated to 60 Gy (RBE). In postoperative cases, areas of surgical margin positivity or extracapsular extension can be treated to 66 Gy (RBE). Lateral retropharyngeal nodes (up to the level of the first cervical vertebra) are usually included in this target, and level Ib is not included unless there is involvement or tumor extension into the oral cavity.
- A low-risk clinical tumor volume can be treated to 50–54 Gy (RBE) that includes the uninvolved and nonsurgically violated ipsilateral neck.
- For HPV-positive disease, lower subclinical dosing may be considered, such as 54 Gy and 45 Gy to the high-risk and low-risk clinical target volumes, respectively.

Target volumes should be expanded according to institutional standards, typically by 3–5 mm, to create a planning target volume (PTV) to account for setup variation and range uncertainties.

Consultation with a medical oncologist regarding concurrent radiosensitizing chemotherapy should be considered, especially for large primary tumors, margin positivity, extensive nodal involvement, and/or suspected or confirmed extracapsular extension.

6.3 Patient Positioning, Immobilization, and Treatment Verification

Simulation and treatment should be conducted in the supine position with a 5-point mask for optimal immobilization of the head, neck, and shoulders.

Setup accuracy should be ascertained with daily orthogonal X-ray imaging or volumetric imaging, if available, to confirm setup accuracy.

When in-room 3D imaging (e.g., cone beam CT) is not available, weekly verification CT scans with the patient in treatment position are recommended during the course of treatment to assess for potential changes in anatomy (i.e., due to weight loss, tumor shrinkage, etc.) and resultant changes in the accuracy of the dose distribution. This is especially relevant for HPV-positive nodal disease, in which large necrotic nodes shrink early in the course of treatment. Replanning should be considered to reduce errors in true dosimetry in this setting.

6.4 Three-Dimensional (3D) Proton Treatment Planning

6.4.1 Passive Scattering (PS)

Generally, two or three field plans are used for ipsilateral coverage of the primary or postoperative site and regional nodes. Fields should be arranged for short depths and homogeneous coverage, which is often best achieved by anterior oblique and superior oblique beams. For large targets that are well lateralized (i.e., large primary

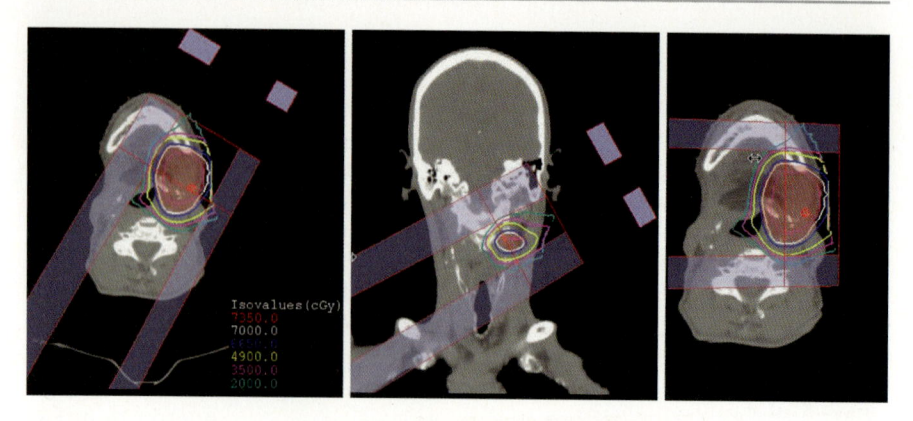

Fig. 6.1 A sample passive scattering proton plan for a patient with cT2N1 squamous cell carcinoma of the left base of tongue treated with chemoradiation followed by total glossectomy for a recurrence who then presented with a left lateral oropharyngeal wall recurrence. A three-beam passive scattering technique was utilized with a left lateral (*left panel*), left superior oblique (*center*), and an anterior oblique (*right*) beam

tumor or postoperative reconstruction), a lateral beam may also offer dosimetric advantages (Fig. 6.1).

It is not optimal to overlap the distal edge of more than two beams, and in particular, any critical organs at risk should not receive distal range out dose from more than one beam to avoid hotspots where true dose may be uncertain.

Dental artifacts can be addressed by contouring the high atomic number material and correcting for the density. Treatment planning systems should allow for manual corrections that can be determined based upon the material. If the material is not known, conservative estimates using gold or amalgam can be substituted. Additionally, the artifacts must be contoured and forced to the appropriate densities or stopping powers.

Large tumors that respond early in the treatment course should be managed with adaptive replanning to avoid off target dosimetry.

For cases requiring only unilateral treatment, passive scattering can achieve optimal coverage of the ipsilateral primary and neck and should allow minimal dose to the contralateral neck with excellent sparing of the contralateral salivary glands, oral cavity, larynx, brainstem, and spinal cord (Fig. 6.2).

6 Oropharyngeal Cancer

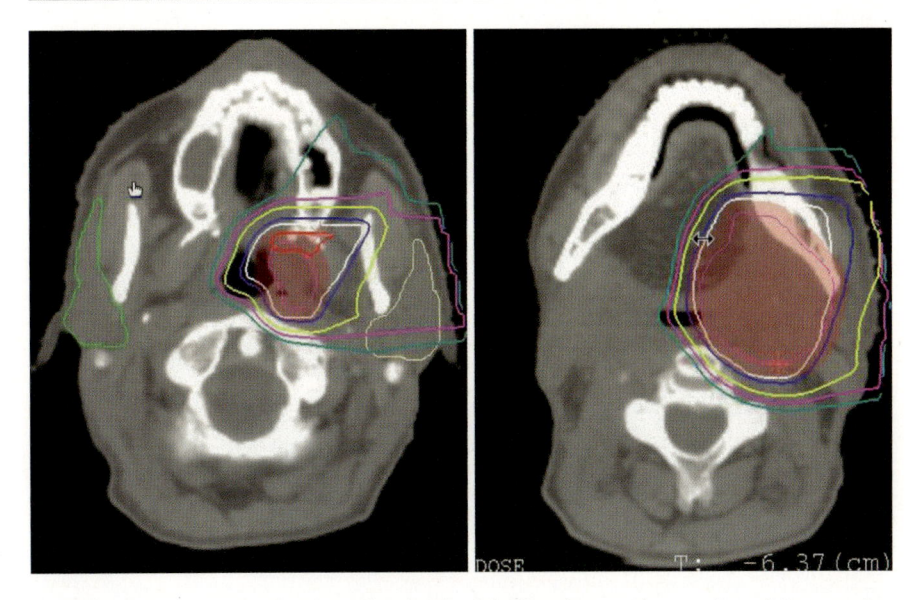

Fig. 6.2 Dose distribution for the patient in Fig. 6.1. Note the complete sparing of the contralateral submandibular and parotid glands, as well as considerable sparing of the contralateral oral cavity. Isodose lines are color-coded same as in Fig. 6.1

6.5 Pencil Beam Scanning (PBS)

Unlike other sites of the head and neck in which the skin is part of the target, for definitive cases of OPC, PBS can provide conformal plans that can better spare the skin due to greater control over the proximal dose distribution. This can be achieved through the use of explicit avoidance structures where appropriate.

While the same two to four beam arrangement that is used with PS can be used with PBS, the use of PBS allows for careful delivery of radiation to the contralateral neck while still sparing critical organs (Figs. 6.3 and 6.4).

OPC cases needing bilateral neck irradiation typically utilize bilateral oblique beams and a single midline opposing beam. Addition of extra fields does not seem to confer an advantage as it does for IMRT [11].

Care should be taken to ensure that all artifact and dental hardware are accurately contoured and proper mass density/electron density is applied prior to calculation. Use beams that avoid going through hardware, though in OPC, this is sometimes not possible.

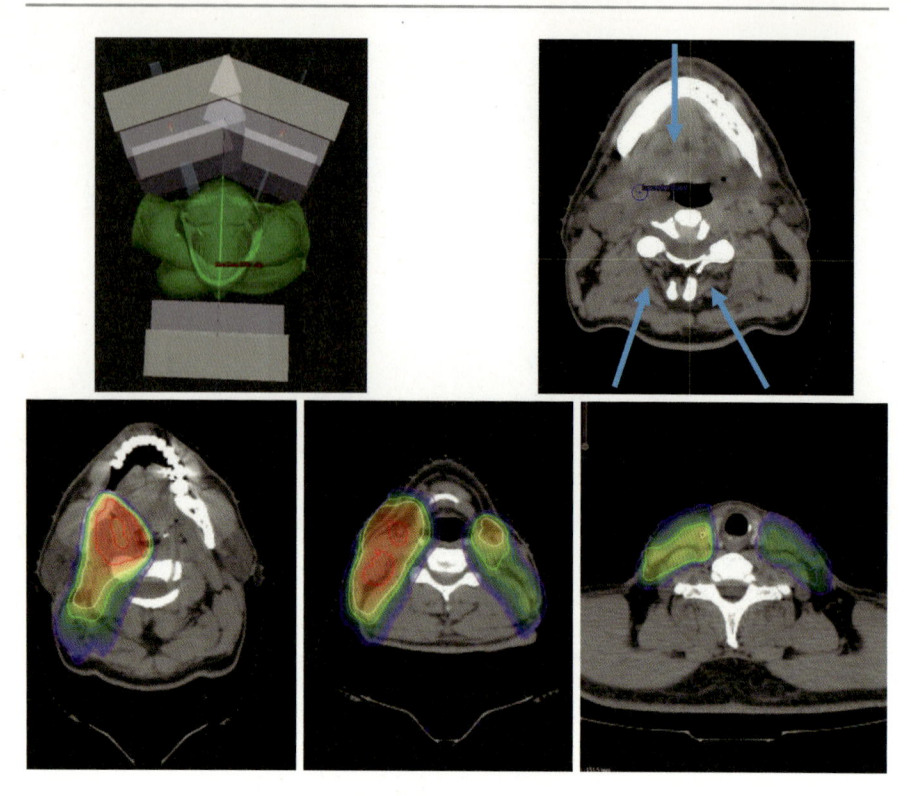

Fig. 6.3 An IMPT beam arrangement for a patient with cT2N2b SCC of the right tonsil to obtain bilateral neck treatment, utilizing bilateral posterior oblique beams and a single anterior midline beam (*upper panels*) to obtain conformal coverage of targets while sparing the larynx and oral cavity (*lower panels*). Color wash spans 40–75 Gy, and isodose lines highlight 40 Gy (*violet*), 50 Gy (*blue*), 54 Gy (*green*), 60 Gy (*yellow*), and 70 Gy (*red*)

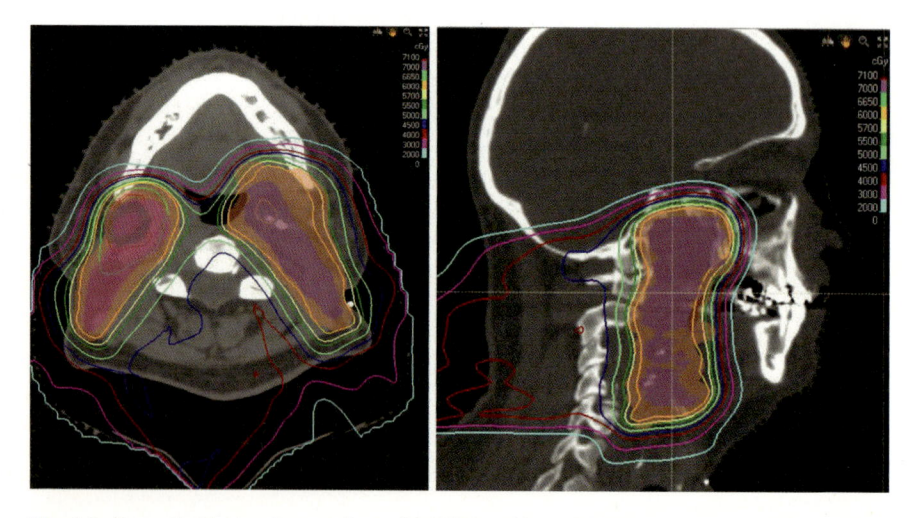

Fig. 6.4 Dose distribution for a patient with HPV-positive, pT2N2b squamous cell of left tonsil, treated with postoperative chemoradiation with proton therapy following transoral robotic resection and neck dissection. Note sparing of the anterior oral cavity, even with bilateral neck treatment

Table 6.1 OPC dose constraints guidelines at MSKCC

OAR	Constraint	Dose
Oral cavity	Mean dose	35–40 Gy
Spinal cord	Dose to 0.1 cc	<50 Gy RBE[a]
	Surface max	64 Gy RBE[b]
Brainstem	Dose to 0.05 cc	< 60 Gy RBE[a]
	Core max	53 Gy RBE
	Surface max	64 Gy RBE[b]
Cochlea[c]	Max dose	<50 Gy RBE
Parotid	Mean dose	25 Gy RBE ALARA
Larynx	Mean dose	<35 Gy RBE

[a]For plans with prescription dose ≤60 Gy RBE
[b]Isodose line may touch structure surface
[c]If ipsilateral hearing is absent, contralateral cochlea constraint is <35 Gy RBE

For the majority of cases in which bilateral neck irradiation is needed, single field optimization (SFUD) or multi-field optimization IMPT or rarely, a mix of the two techniques can be used in order to meet currently recommended dose constraints. Sample constraints are noted in Table 6.1 for OPC planning that are typically employed at MSKCC, but each center should establish their own set of dose constraints based on their clinical experience.

Modeling work has also suggested that reducing the spot size for PBS may translate into further dosimetric advantages in reducing normal tissue exposure, in particular that of the sublingual glands [12].

6.6 Dosimetry and Toxicity Characteristics

In case-matched control analysis of comparing the dosimetry of IMRT and IMPT plans for OPC patients undergoing definitive RT or CRT at MDACC, IMPT allowed for reduced dose to several critical structures when compared to IMRT plans generated on the same target volumes, particularly those related to acute oral toxicity and nausea (Table 6.2). Comparing these to additional matched patients that underwent IMRT treatment further corroborated this dosimetric benefit [7]. Similar studies have been reported elsewhere as well, specifically for OPC patients, with significant reduction in parotid, sublingual gland, and oral cavity dose [8].

Prospective OPC patients undergoing IMPT at MDACC experienced relatively favorable acute toxicities, with grade 3 dermatitis of 46%, mucositis in 58%, and dysphagia of 24%. Late grade 3 dysphagia was 12%. Median weight loss was 7.4%. One of 50 patients developed oropharyngeal mucosal ulceration 16 months after treatment completion, with stabilization of the ulcer and improvement in symptoms after hyperbaric oxygen therapy [10]. Furthermore, retrospective cohort and case-matched analyses of toxicity suggest lower rates of xerostomia, weight loss, taste and appetite changes, and reduced need for gastrostomy tubes with proton therapy for OPC, though patient-reported outcomes apparently do not reflect this fully [13, 14].

Table 6.2 Dosimetric comparison of mean dose to critical structures for 25 patients [7]

Structure	IMPT plan for IMPT-treated patients (Gy ± SD)	IMRT plan for IMPT-treated patients (Gy ± SD)	P value	IMRT plan for matched cohort of IMRT-treated patients (Gy ± SD)	P value
Anterior oral cavity	8.3 ± 5.9	31.0 ± 7.2	<0.001	30.5 ± 7.9	<0.001
Posterior oral cavity	40.5 ± 15.3	54.3 ± 8.1	<0.001	50.6 ± 8.0	0.011
Esophagus	20.9 ± 12.2	33.6 ± 14.4	0.002	18.6 ± 9.7	0.543
Inferior PC	32.8 ± 10.7	45.6 ± 10.4	<0.001	28.8 ± 15.8	0.068
Middle PC	48.2 ± 17.8	57.0 ± 14.4	0.046	54.6 ± 9.4	0.543
Superior PC	55.3 ± 13.0	58.1 ± 11.0	0.305	58.0 ± 11.3	0.511
Brainstem	7.7 ± 3.7	14.4 ± 6.4	<0.001	18.6 ± 8.8	<0.001
Cerebellum	12.6 ± 4.3	18.8 ± 4.8	<0.001	18.9 ± 7.6	<0.001
Area postrema	14.6 ± 9.0	24.5 ± 7.2	<0.001	30.7 ± 6.5	<0.001

The first two columns show the dose for IMRT and IMPT plans for the same cohort, and the rightmost column shows the mean dose for the case-matched cohort. Only selected rows shown for clarity

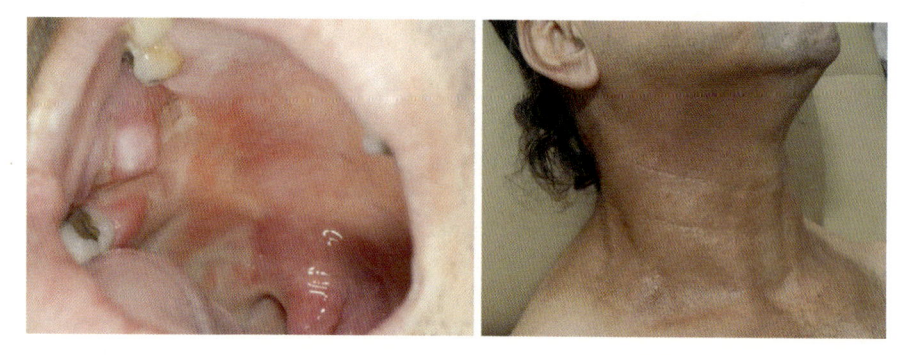

Fig. 6.5 Minimal oral cavity mucositis (*left*) and dermatitis (*right*) 1 week after completing definitive chemoradiation for the patient treated with IMPT to the bilateral neck from Fig. 6.3

While no randomized data exist to demonstrate the reduced toxicities that have been reported in case series with PBS, the anecdotal and single institution data seem promising, and patients do well with carefully planned treatment (Fig. 6.5).

Ongoing trials will further help to define the role of proton RT in the treatment of OPC. An observational study at Mayo Clinic is open to evaluate local control at 2 years, as well as quality of life measures, of mucosal sparing proton beam therapy after resection of favorable risk OPC (NCT02736786). Another observational cohort study is ongoing at MDACC to evaluate functional patient-reported outcomes following low-risk OPC treated with either definitive transoral resection or definitive IMPT (NCT02663583). Lastly, a multi-institutional randomized phase II/

III trial is ongoing to evaluate severe toxicity following IMRT vs. IMPT for locally advanced OPC (NCT01893307).

Conclusion

Reported data on the use of proton RT for patients with OPC are promising in delivering safe and effective treatment while limiting normal tissue exposure with potentially significant quality of life improvements (e.g., in reduction of mucositis, nausea, and long-term xerostomia). As technological advances with IMPT continue to grow (i.e., routine use of small spot sizes), additional benefits may be gained yet, though ongoing prospective randomized trials are ongoing to further outline the role of proton RT.

References

1. Cohan DM, Popat S, Kaplan SE, Rigual N, Loree T, Hicks WL Jr. Oropharyngeal cancer: current understanding and management. Curr Opin Otolaryngol Head Neck Surg. 2009;17(2):88–94.
2. Siegel RL, Miller KD, Jemal A. Cancer statistics, 2015. CA Cancer J Clin. 2015;65(1):5–29.
3. Gunn GB, Debnam JM, Fuller CD, et al. The impact of radiographic retropharyngeal adenopathy in oropharyngeal cancer. Cancer. 2013;119(17):3162–9.
4. Viens LJ, Henley SJ, Watson M, et al. Human papillomavirus-associated cancers—United States, 2008–2012. MMWR Morb Mortal Wkly Rep. 2016;65(26):661–6.
5. Chaturvedi AK, Engels EA, Pfeiffer RM, et al. Human papillomavirus and rising oropharyngeal cancer incidence in the United States. J Clin Oncol. 2011;29(32):4294–301.
6. Cozzi L, Fogliata A, Lomax A, Bolsi A. A treatment planning comparison of 3D conformal therapy, intensity modulated photon therapy and proton therapy for treatment of advanced head and neck tumours. Radiother Oncol. 2001;61(3):287–97.
7. Holliday EB, Kocak-Uzel E, Feng L, et al. Dosimetric advantages of intensity-modulated proton therapy for oropharyngeal cancer compared with intensity-modulated radiation: a case-matched control analysis. Med Dosim. 2016;41:189–94.
8. van de Water TA, Lomax AJ, Bijl HP, et al. Potential benefits of scanned intensity-modulated proton therapy versus advanced photon therapy with regard to sparing of the salivary glands in oropharyngeal cancer. Int J Radiat Oncol Biol Phys. 2011;79(4):1216–24.
9. Slater JD, Yonemoto LT, Mantik DW, et al. Proton radiation for treatment of cancer of the oropharynx: early experience at Loma Linda University Medical Center using a concomitant boost technique. Int J Radiat Oncol Biol Phys. 2005;62(2):494–500.
10. Gunn GB, Blanchard P, Garden AS, et al. Clinical outcomes and patterns of disease recurrence after intensity modulated proton therapy for oropharyngeal squamous carcinoma. Int J Radiat Oncol Biol Phys. 2016;95(1):360–7.
11. Steneker M, Lomax A, Schneider U. Intensity modulated photon and proton therapy for the treatment of head and neck tumors. Radiother Oncol. 2006;80(2):263–7.
12. van de Water TA, Lomax AJ, Bijl HP, Schilstra C, Hug EB, Langendijk JA. Using a reduced spot size for intensity-modulated proton therapy potentially improves salivary gland-sparing in oropharyngeal cancer. Int J Radiat Oncol Biol Phys. 2012;82(2):e313–9.
13. Blanchard P, Garden AS, Gunn GB, et al. Intensity-modulated proton beam therapy (IMPT) versus intensity-modulated photon therapy (IMRT) for patients with oropharynx cancer—a case matched analysis. Radiother Oncol. 2016;120(1):48–55.
14. Sio TT, Lin HK, Shi Q, et al. Intensity modulated proton therapy versus intensity modulated photon radiation therapy for oropharyngeal cancer: first comparative results of patient-reported outcomes. Int J Radiat Oncol Biol Phys. 2016;95(4):1107–14.

Sinonasal Cancers

7

Roi Dagan and Curtis Bryant

Contents

7.1	Introduction	141
7.2	Immobilization/Simulation	142
7.3	Target Volumes	143
7.4	Dose/Fractionation	146
7.5	Normal Tissue Definitions	147
7.6	Proton Modality	148
7.7	Lymph Node Management	150
References		151

7.1 Introduction

Sinonasal cancers are among the most rare and diverse malignancies. They account for less than 3% of all tumors of the upper aerodigestive tract and less than 0.5% of cancers with an incidence in the United States of approximately 1 in 200,000 individuals annually [1]. There are many histologic subtypes including squamous cell carcinoma, minor salivary gland cancers (adenoid cystic carcinoma, adenocarcinoma, adenosquamous carcinoma, polymorphous low-grade adenocarcinoma, and mucoepidermoid carcinoma), neuroendocrine tumors (olfactory neuroblastoma, neuroendocrine carcinoma, sinonasal undifferentiated carcinoma, and small cell carcinoma), mucosal melanoma, lymphomas, and other cancers of mesenchymal cell origins such as chondrosarcomas and osteosarcomas. Essentially all evidence supporting management decisions come from retrospective studies, and with the

R. Dagan (✉) • C. Bryant
University of Florida Health Proton Therapy Institute, Jacksonville, FL, USA
e-mail: rdagan@floridaproton.org

exception of lymphomas, surgery and radiotherapy is the mainstay of local therapy, which is guided by the following principles:

1. Cancers of sinonasal region are typically diagnosed at a locally advanced stage and are highly infiltrative with a high propensity for involvement of adjacent sinonasal cavities, orbit(s), skull base bones/foramina, or the intracranial compartment. At least 50% of patients will have tumors involving more than one anatomic subsite, and orbital invasion has been reported in 10–37% [2, 3]; cranial nerves are involved in as many as a third of patients [4], and intracranial invasion in up to 45% [3]. The locally invasive nature of these cancers underscores the importance of adequate wide-field local therapy to achieve optimal outcomes.
2. Combined modality therapy including gross total resection, via either an endoscopic or open approach, with postoperative radiotherapy has resulted in the best outcomes. However, the ability to use radical surgery and radiotherapy to eradicate local disease is limited by the tolerance of adjacent critical normal tissues (eyes, visual pathways, cranial nerves, brain stem, and brain). Serious visual pathway toxicities have been reported in over one-third of patients treated with conventional radiotherapy [5]. Many patients with intracranial disease extension will be at risk for developing radiographic and possibly symptomatic CNS effects from radiotherapy. Nevertheless, treatment intensification with dose escalation, and/or radiosensitizing chemotherapy, can potentially improve outcomes and has grown in use.
3. Local disease control is the major determinant of morbidity and mortality. Local-control rates historically ranged from 50 to 60% at 5 years with conventional radiotherapy and minimally improved to 68–75% with intensity modulated radiotherapy (IMRT). These rates closely approximate disease free and overall survival rates. Distant metastatic spread of tumors is rare with continuous local-regional control of disease occurring in 15–20% of patients, and thus, continuous local tumor control has been shown to be associated with a fourfold decrease in the risk of death [3].

Because of the challenges of delivering aggressive doses with conventional radiotherapy, proton therapy has been used extensively at centers worldwide for sinonasal cancers. The physical advantages of particle therapy can serve as a means of facilitating treatment intensification [6]. Recently reported outcomes, including a systematic review and meta-analysis, have demonstrated that proton therapy improves disease control compared with conventional RT and IMRT. The following chapter will guide readers through the treatment planning considerations for proton therapy.

7.2 Immobilization/Simulation

Patients are immobilized supine, typically on a board such as a base of skull frame, with a moldable cushion supporting the neck and helping reproduce neck extension, and a thermoplastic mask. This allows the neck and head to be extended off of the treatment table, which minimizes the potential for collisions even when treating with oblique angles, and it minimizes the air gap between the snout and the patients which reduces the lateral beam penumbra. Oral obturators/stents can be used to depress the tongue and displace a significant amount of oral cavity mucosa from the treatment field. Treatment planning CT images should include the vertex through the shoulders, which can sometimes be a source of potential collisions, and the primary treatment planning images should be free from any material that could affect the dose modeling by altering the stopping power of the native tissues. For example, IV contrast, while helpful in target and organ at risk (OAR) delineation, should not be included in the primary image set. If possible, patients should have their sinonasal region cleared of all postoperative secretions and debris, and this should be maintained throughout the treatment course.

7.3 Target Volumes

Treatment planning should be based on pre- and postoperative imaging (CT and MRI) and operative/endoscopic findings. MRI should include high-resolution, contrast-enhanced T1-weighted imaging including fat suppression, and T2-weighted imaging is also very helpful in differentiating benign mucosal secretions and mucoperiosteal thickening from tumor involvement. Dedicated coronal images can also be very helpful. CT imaging for both diagnostic and treatment planning studies should be acquired with and without IV contrast and dedicated high-resolution bone imaging can aid in accurate target definition.

In both the primary and postoperative setting, the primary site is considered at high risk for recurrence regardless of the extent of resection. We recommend targeting two separate clinical target volumes (CTVs) based on the risk of residual disease. These targets can be treated with either a sequential boost approach or an integrated boost approach. The latter approach is facilitated by the use of pencil-beam scanning intensity modulated proton therapy (IMPT). However, if a hyperfractionated dose-fractionation schedule is preferred, then a two-phase sequential boost is recommended. Either way, the following approach is used to define the target volumes:

1. The gross tumor volume (GTV) is contoured on simulation CT/MR images and co-registered diagnostic scans, and in the setting of prior resection, a pre-opGTV is contoured on co-registered preoperative CT and/or MRI. Incorporating all available information from endoscopic evaluations, diagnostic CT and MR imaging, and operative findings is critical for accurate delineation of the GTV or pre-opGTV. Examples of pre-opGTV are shown in Figs. 7.1 and 7.2.

The initial target, standard-risk clinical target volume (CTV SR), includes an expansion of the GTV or pre-opGTV. For the most common scenario of a nasal/ethmoid primary tumor, we recommend including the entire nasal cavity, the contiguous involved paranasal sinus tissues, adjacent skull base, and the adjacent

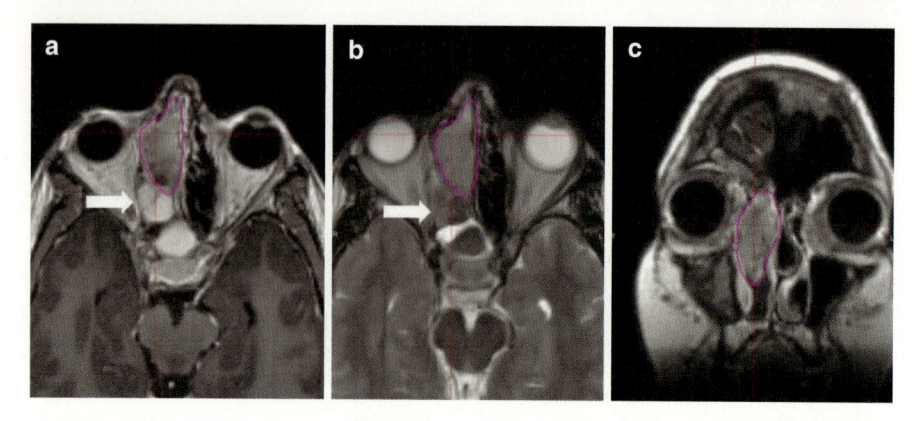

Fig. 7.1 Diagnostic preoperative MRI of a T3 N0 M0 right naso-ethmoidal sinonasal intestinal-type adenocarcinoma. (**a**) Contrast-enhanced axial T1-weighted image. (**b**) Axial T2-weighted image. (**c**) Contrast-enhanced coronal T1-weighted image. Note that both T1- and T2-weighted images are useful in distinguishing tumor from benign mucosal secretions (*arrows*), which is often characterized by high-intensity T2 signal. However, in this case, these secretions contain proteinaceous material and also appear low intensity on T2. The pre-opGTV is outlined in the *magenta contour*

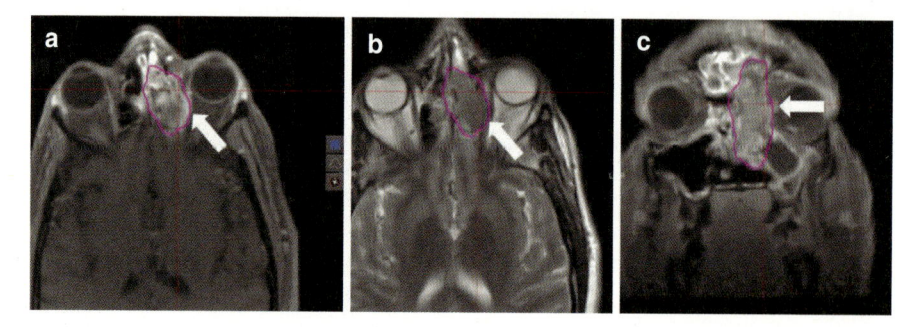

Fig. 7.2 Diagnostic preoperative MRI of a left naso-ethmoidal T4a N0 M0 high-grade adenocarcinoma with invasion of the frontal sinus and left orbit. (**a**) Contrast-enhanced axial T1-weighted fat-suppressed image. (**b**) Axial T2-weighted image. (**c**) Contrast-enhanced coronal T1-weighted fat-suppressed image. Note the minimal intraorbital invasion (*arrows*) resulting in mild left proptosis. Invasion of the periorbita is best demonstrated on fat-suppressed images. The pre-opGTV is outlined in the *magenta contour*

periorbita and dura in cases where there is intraorbital or intracranial extension, respectively (Fig. 7.3). The CTV SR expansion varies based on the extent and location of the GTV or pre-opGTV, but for a lateralized naso-ethmoidal tumor or maxillary sinus primary tumors, this volume usually does not extend to the contralateral maxillary sinus or superior 1/2 of the frontal sinuses in tumors that do not cross midline or grossly extend into the frontal sinuses. This expansion will also vary widely with respect to the GTV/pre-opGTV on any given axial slice ranging from as low as 0 mm when the target volume approaches but does not invade the intracranial or intraorbital compartments to as wide as an entire maxillary sinus (2–4 cm)

7 Sinonasal Cancers

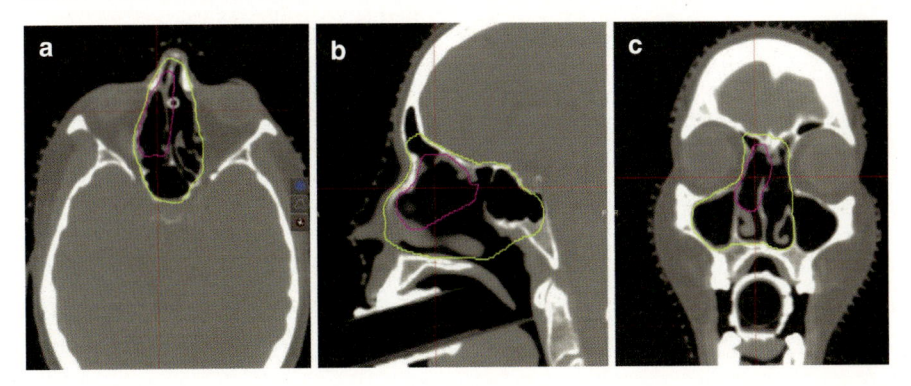

Fig. 7.3 Planning CT of a T3 N0 M0 right naso-ethmoidal sinonasal intestinal-type adenocarcinoma. The pre-opGTV is outlined in the *magenta contour*. The CTV SR (*yellow contour*) includes the entire nasal cavity, the contiguous involved paranasal sinus tissues, and adjacent skull base. Since there was no orbital or intracranial invasion, there is a minimal CTV margin along these boundaries. Since the right middle meatus was involved, there is a generous margin including the entire right maxillary sinus

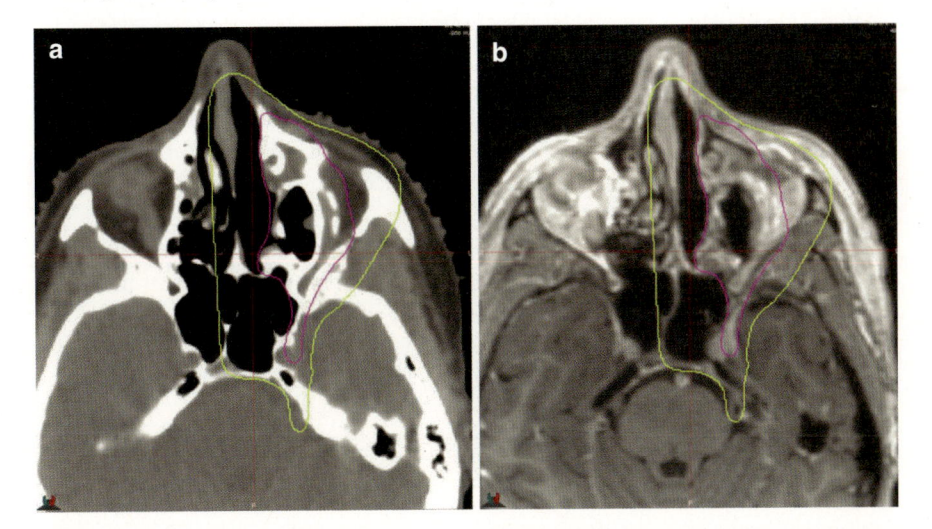

Fig. 7.4 Planning CT and MRI of a left maxillary sinus squamous cell carcinoma with clinical and radiographic perineural invasion of right V2 to the cavernous sinus. The GTV is outlined in the *magenta contour*. The CTV SR is outlined in the *yellow contour* and includes the entire cavernous sinus, trigeminal nerve root as it enters the brain stem, and the retroantral space

when covering an adjacent but uninvolved maxillary sinus with a primary naso-ethmoidal cancer.

In cases, where there is clinical or pathologic perineural spread, we recommend treatment of potentially affected skull base foramina, the cavernous sinus, and nerve roots to the brain stem (Fig. 7.4). In cases where nodal irradiation is indicated (discussed later), then the upper neck nodal regions (uppermost retropharyngeal and retrostyloid nodes) are incorporated in the CTV SR. Lastly, in the postoperative

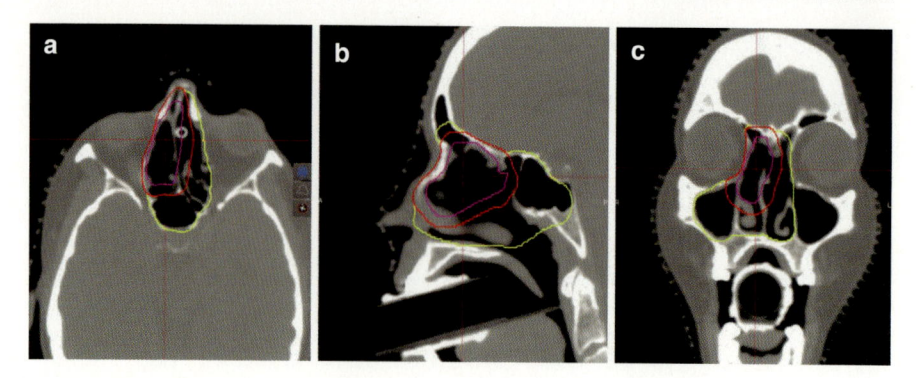

Fig. 7.5 Planning CT of a T3 N0 M0 right naso-ethmoidal sinonasal intestinal-type adenocarcinoma. The pre-opGTV is outlined in the *magenta contour*. The CTV HR (*red contour*) is a 5–10 mm expansion of the pre-opGTV confined to the CTV SR (*yellow contour*)

setting, when an open surgical approach is used, then the surgical scars should be incorporated in the CTV SR. This includes the bicoronal craniotomy incision in patients who undergo craniofacial resection.

2. The boost volume or high-risk clinical target volume (CTV HR) is defined as a customized 0–10 mm expansion of the GTV/pre-opGTV and is limited to the CTV SR. This expansion will depend on the risk of subclinical disease in the region, whether the expansion region is extended along tissue at risk for invasion or into a non-invaded compartment (Fig. 7.5).
3. PTV margins will vary among institutions based on equipment specification and immobilization and image-guidance modalities. Typically margins of 3 mm are applied to create the final target volumes.
4. Additional proximal and distal margins are applied based on beam-specific parameters.

7.4 Dose/Fractionation

Currently, there is no standard dose/fractionation regimen for sinus and nasal cavity cancers. Generally, the PTV HR is prescribed 66–70 Gy (RBE) at 2 CGE per fraction, and 45–50 Gy (RBE) are prescribed to the PTV SR. In many cases, one or both visual pathways are intimately associated with the PTV HR, placing patients at significant risk for vision loss from retinopathy or optic neuropathy. In these cases, we prefer to use hyperfractionated therapy. In this scenario we prescribe 45.6–50.4 Gy (RBE) to the PTV SR and 69.6–74.4 Gy (RBE) to the PTV HR. Hyperfractionation accomplishes two goals that may improve outcomes. First, hyperfractionation can be used to accelerate RT to combat accelerated repopulation of tumor cells after surgery and during RT [7]. Second, using a lower dose per fraction allows for dose intensification while reducing the risk of visual pathway toxicity [8, 9]. Plans are typically normalized to ensure coverage of 95% PTV SR with

100% of the prescribed dose ensuring that 99% of the PTV receives 93% of the prescription dose to minimize any potential cold spots. The boost phase is normalized independently with the goal of covering 100% of the PTV HR with 95% of the prescription dose; however, when necessary, either the number or fractions or coverage should be reduced using best clinical judgment in order to ensure normal tissue sparing.

7.5 Normal Tissue Definitions

Organs at risk (OARs) are defined on treatment planning CTs and co-registered postoperative MRIs. We recommend defining the following structures: retinas/globes, optic nerves, optic chiasm, lenses, lacrimal glands, brain stem, spinal cord, brain, temporal lobes, hippocampi, hypothalamus, pituitary, salivary glands, mandible, oral cavity, larynx, pharyngeal constrictors, and upper esophagus (Table 7.1).

Table 7.1 Dose-volume histogram planning objectives for sinonasal proton therapy plans

Structure	DVH point	Limit	Minor deviation	Major deviation
PTV	Relative dose at 95% volume	100%	D95% ≤ 100%	–
PTV	Relative dose at 99% volume	93%	D99% ≤ 93%	–
PTV	Relative volume at 110% dose	20%	V110 ≥ 20%	–
Brain stem	Absolute dose at 0.1 cc	55 Gy	55 ≤ D0.1 cc < 64 Gy	D0.1 cc ≥ 64 Gy
Brain stem	Maximum absolute dose	60 Gy	60 ≤ Dmax <67 Gy	Dmax ≥67 Gy
Brain stem surface	Absolute dose at 0.1 cc	55 Gy	55 ≤ D0.1 cc < 64 Gy	D0.1 cc ≥ 64 Gy
Brain stem core	Absolute dose at 0.1 cc	50 Gy	50 ≤ D0.1 cc < 60 Gy	D0.1 cc ≥ 60 Gy
Spinal cord	Absolute dose at 0.1 cc	50 Gy	50 ≤ D0.1 cc < 55 Gy	D0.1 cc ≥ 55 Gy
Optic chiasm	Absolute dose at 0.1 cc	55 Gy	55 ≤ D0.1 cc < 60 Gy	D0.1 cc ≥ 60 Gy
Optic chiasm	Maximum absolute dose	57 Gy	57 ≤ Dmax <62 Gy	Dmax ≥62 Gy
Optic nerve (left)	Absolute dose at 0.1 cc	55 Gy	55 ≤ D0.1 cc < 60 Gy	D0.1 cc ≥ 60 Gy
Optic nerve (right)	Absolute dose at 0.1 cc	55 Gy	55 ≤ D0.1 cc < 60 Gy	D0.1 cc ≥ 60 Gy
Retina (left)	Absolute dose at 0.1 cc	50 Gy	50 ≤ D0.1 cc < 60 Gy	D0.1 cc ≥ 60 Gy
Retina (right)	Absolute dose at 0.1 cc	50 Gy	50 ≤ D0.1 cc < 60 Gy	D0.1 cc ≥ 60 Gy
Larynx	Mean absolute dose	36 Gy	–	Dmean ≥36 Gy
Cochlea (left)	Mean absolute dose	36 Gy	36 ≤ Dmean <45 Gy	Dmean ≥45 Gy
Cochlea (right)	Mean absolute dose	36 Gy	36 ≤ Dmean <45 Gy	Dmean ≥45 Gy
Parotid (left)	Mean absolute dose	26 Gy	Dmean ≥26 Gy	–
Parotid (right)	Mean absolute dose	26 Gy	Dmean ≥26 Gy	–
Submandibular gland (left)	Mean absolute dose	40 Gy	Dmean ≥40 Gy	–

(continued)

Table 7.1 (continued)

Structure	DVH point	Limit	Minor deviation	Major deviation
Submandibular gland (right)	Mean absolute dose	40 Gy	Dmean ≥40 Gy	–
Cervical esophagus	Mean absolute dose	50 Gy	Dmean ≥50 Gy	–
Oral cavity	Mean absolute dose	36 Gy	Dmean ≥36 Gy	–
Temporal lobe (left)	Relative volume at 20Gy	10%	V20 ≥ 10%	–
Temporal lobe (left)	Absolute volume at 74Gy	2 cc	V74 ≥ 2 cc	–
Temporal lobe (right)	Relative volume at 20Gy	10%	V20 ≥ 10%	–
Temporal lobe (right)	Absolute volume at 74Gy	2 cc	V74 ≥ 2 cc	–
Hippocampus tail (left)	Mean absolute dose	20 Gy	Dmean ≥20 Gy	–
Hippocampus tail (right)	Mean absolute dose	20 Gy	Dmean ≥20 Gy	–
Hippocampus head (left)	Mean absolute dose	5 Gy	Dmean ≥5 Gy	–
Hippocampus head (right)	Mean absolute dose	5 Gy	Dmean ≥5 Gy	–
Pharyngeal constrictors	Mean absolute dose	50 Gy	50 ≤ Dmean <60 Gy	Dmean ≥60 Gy
Lacrimal gland (left)	Mean absolute dose	34 Gy	34 ≤ Dmean <41 Gy	Dmean ≥41 Gy
Lacrimal gland (right)	Mean absolute dose	34 Gy	34 ≤ Dmean <41 Gy	Dmean ≥41 Gy
Hypothalamus	Mean absolute dose	5 Gy	Dmean ≥5 Gy	–
Pituitary	Mean absolute dose	30 Gy	Dmean ≥30 Gy	–
Mandible	Mean absolute dose	40 Gy	–	Dmean ≥40 Gy
Mandible	Relative volume at 70Gy	10%	–	V70 ≥ 10%
Brain	Absolute volume at 74Gy	2 cc	V74 ≥ 2 cc	–
Lens (right)	Maximum absolute dose	15 Gy	Dmax ≥15 Gy	–
Lens (left)	Maximum absolute dose	15 Gy	Dmax ≥15 Gy	–

7.6 Proton Modality

Both scattered beams and spot-scanning beams can be used, and preferences on modality will depend on the experience of the center, provider, equipment specifications, and most importantly plan quality and robustness. The potential advantages of scanning beams include efficiency of delivery, dose homogeneity, and ability to conform high-dose volumes to concave/convex target volumes. Conversely, it is noteworthy that most of the published outcomes with proton therapy are with the use of passive scattering techniques. The lateral dose gradient will usually be sharper in a passively scattered beam shaped with a beam aperture especially when compared with pencil-beam systems with larger spot sizes. Also, in scattered proton beams, compensator smearing can be used to yield extremely robust plans despite significant variations in stopping power in areas of bone and air interfaces in the sinus cavities.

For passively scattered beams, aperture margins are customized for each patient to maximize target volume coverage and normal tissue sparing. Typically, 3–5 fields are used per plan (Fig. 7.6). Range modulation is used to ensure that the spread-out Bragg peak (defined as 90% of the mid-spread-out Bragg peak dose) covered the entire radiographic depth of the target volume. An additional distal and proximal margin is added to the CTV if larger than the PTV to account for range uncertainties [10]. Field matching can be used to reduce dose to uninvolved regions and OARs. Through/patch combinations are typically not needed and can be problematic in sinonasal cancer because the target volume and adjacent tissues will inherently involve air cavities which are unsuitable for through/patch junctions. In general, we recommend minimizing the number of field junctions, paying careful attention to uncertainties at junction lines and avoiding/minimizing the number of fields whose distal Bragg peaks end on critical normal tissues such as the spinal cord, brain stem, or visual pathways. The distal dose fall-off of each field is shaped by beam compensators, which can be edited to modify coverage goals or OAR sparing. These compensators also reduce the effects of tissue heterogeneity on the dose distribution. Compensator smoothing/smearing can be used to mitigate the effect of geometric uncertainties on radiographic depth/proton range.

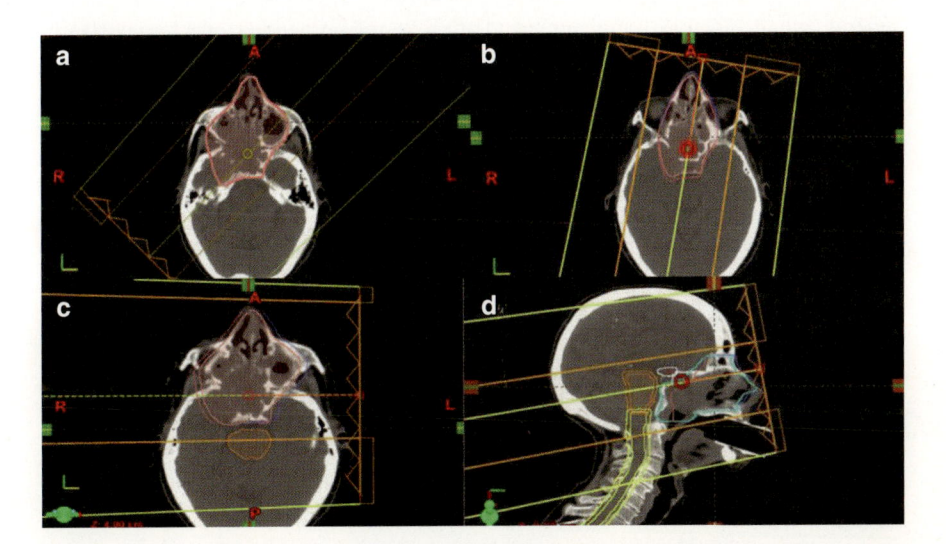

Fig. 7.6 Example of passively scattered proton therapy plan beam arrangement for a T4b N0 M0 nasal cavity squamous cell carcinoma with intracranial invasion. The beam arrangement includes a right posterior oblique field (**a**), left anterior oblique field (**b**), left lateral field (**c**), and left superior-anterior oblique field (**d**). Fields **a** and **d** cover the entire target volume, while **b** and **c** are matched fields, which can be used to reduce the dose to the eyes

In IMPT plans, typically 3–4 beams are selected, and spot placement and weighting are optimized using inverse planning software. Single-field uniform dose (SFUD) and multi-field optimized (MFO) treatment planning modes can both be used with the former delivering more robust plans, and the latter resulting in improved plan conformality and OAR sparing in plans with PTV convexities/concavities. Plan optimization, similar to IMRT, will be based on objectives for target coverage, OAR sparing, and dose uniformity and their relative weighting within a cost function. Recent advances in treatment planning software now allow for robust plan optimization and plan robustness analysis, which can reduce the impact of geometric/physical uncertainties in the optimization process.

7.7 Lymph Node Management

Elective neck irradiation remains a controversial topic in the management of sinonasal cancers. Unlike other more common mucosal cancers of the head and neck, the sinonasal region is relatively devoid of submucosal lymphatic, and lymph node metastases are far less common. Staging evaluation should include imaging of the neck, and clinically and radiographically suspicious lymph nodes, which occur in approximately 10% of patients, should be biopsied to confirm disease [3]. These nodes should be managed with gross total excision and elective dissection of the involved neck and treated with postoperative radiotherapy in a similar manner to other head and neck primary mucosal tumors. The decision to electively irradiate an uninvolved neck is far more controversial and beyond the scope of this chapter. In general, when elective lymphatic irradiation is recommended, we target lymph nodes in the retropharyngeal, retrostyloid regions, and the following cervical lymph node stations: 1b, 2a/b, 3, 4, 5a/b, and the supraclavicular lymph nodes. With well-lateralized tumors that do not invade the nasal septum or cross midline, targeting ipsilateral lymph nodes may be an appropriate volume reduction strategy to minimize potential toxicity.

Different planning strategies for elective lymph node irradiation can be incorporated with proton therapy. Whole neck radiotherapy will typically require IMPT, because the added complexity of treating the neck with passively scattered beam requires prohibitively excessive number of beams and treatment time. We advocate a more simple approach of treating the neck with conventional photon irradiation which can be dosimetrically matched to proton therapy of the primary site and upper neck or with a dosimetric gap to avoid potential hot spots (Fig. 7.7).

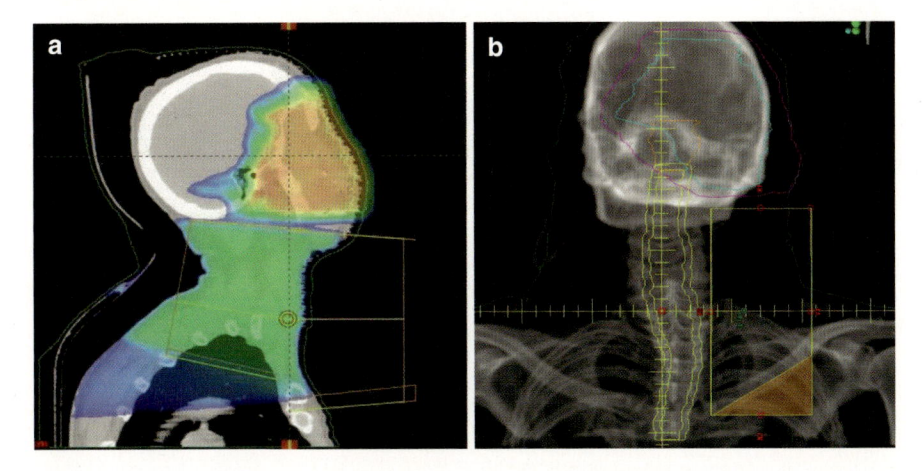

Fig. 7.7 Photon elective neck irradiation matched to passively scattered proton therapy to the primary site. The 50% isodose level from the proton therapy to the primary site is transferred to the photon treatment planning system in order to create a dosimetric match and avoid hot spot in potential overlap region

References

1. Turner JH, Reh DD. Incidence and survival in patients with sinonasal cancer: a historical analysis of population-based data. Head Neck. 2012;34(6):877–85.
2. Chu Y, Liu HG, Yu ZK. Patterns and incidence of sinonasal malignancy with orbital invasion. Chin Med J. 2012;125(9):1638–42.
3. Dagan R, Bryant CM, Li Z, et al. Outcomes of sinonasal cancer treated with proton therapy. Int J Rad Biol Phys. 2016;95(1):377–85.
4. Gil Z, Carlson DL, Gupta A, et al. Patterns and incidence of neural invasion in patients with cancers of the paranasal sinuses. Arch Otolaryngol Head Neck Surg. 2009;135(2):173–9.
5. Mendenhall WM, Amdur RJ, Morris CG, Kirwan J, Malyapa RS, Vaysberg M, et al. Carcinoma of the nasal cavity and paranasal sinuses. Laryngoscope. 2009;119(5):899–906.
6. Patel SH, Wang Z, Wong WW, et al. Charged particle therapy versus photon therapy for paranasal sinus and nasal cavity malignant diseases: A systematic review and meta-analysis. Lancet Oncol, 2014:15, pp. 1027–1038.
7. Cannon DM, Geye HM, Hartig GK, Traynor AM, et al. Increased local failure risk with prolonged radiation treatment time in head and neck cancer treated with concurrent chemotherapy. Head Neck. 2014;36(8):1120–5.
8. Mayo C, Martel MK, Marks LB, Flickinger J, Nam J, Kirkpatrick J. Radiation dose-volume effects of optic nerves and chiasm. Int J Radiat Oncol Biol Phys. 2010;76(3 Suppl):S28–35.
9. Monroe AT, Bhandare N, Morris CG, Mendenhall WM. Preventing radiation retinopathy with hyperfractionation. Int J Radiat Oncol Biol Phys. 2005;61(3):856–64.
10. Moyers MF, Miller DW, Bush DA, et al. Methodologies and tools for proton beam design for lung tumors. Int J Radiat Oncol Biol Phys. 2001;49:1429–38.

Salivary Gland Tumors

8

Jonathan E. Leeman, Paul Romesser, James Melotek, Oren Cahlon, Kevin Sine, Stefan Both, and Nancy Y. Lee

Contents

8.1	Introduction	154
8.2	Simulation, Target Delineation, and Radiation Dose/Fractionation	154
8.3	Patient Positioning, Immobilization, and Treatment Verification	155
8.4	Three-Dimensional (3D) Proton Treatment Planning	157
	8.4.1 Passive Scattering (PS)	157
	8.4.2 Pencil Beam Scanning (PBS)	158
8.5	Passive Scattering Versus Pencil Beam Scanning Comparisons	160
8.6	Dosimetric and Toxicity Comparison	162
8.7	Future Developments	162
References		162

J.E. Leeman • P. Romesser • O. Cahlon • N. Lee (✉)
Memorial Sloan Kettering Cancer Center, New York, NY, USA
e-mail: leen2@mskcc.org

J. Melotek
Department of Radiation and Cellular Oncology, University of Chicago Medicine, Chicago, IL, USA

K. Sine
Procure Proton Therapy Center, Somerset, NJ, USA

S. Both
Department of Radiation Oncology, University Medical Center Groningen, Groningen, The Netherlands
e-mail: s.both@umcg.nl

© Springer International Publishing Switzerland 2018
N. Lee et al. (eds.), *Target Volume Delineation and Treatment Planning for Particle Therapy*, Practical Guides in Radiation Oncology,
https://doi.org/10.1007/978-3-319-42478-1_8

8.1 Introduction

Salivary gland malignancies are uncommon, representing 1–6% of head and neck malignancies and 0.3% of all cancers (55% occur in parotid gland, 30% in submandibular gland, 10–15% in the sublingual and minor salivary glands). The majority of salivary gland tumors are primarily managed surgically followed by radiation ± chemotherapy. Indications for postoperative radiation include intermediate-high grade tumor, close/positive margins, lymph node metastases, and lymphovascular invasion as well as T3/T4 tumors or recurrent disease in some circumstances. The role of postoperative chemoradiation for high-risk salivary tumors is currently the subject of the ongoing RTOG 10-08 trial (NCT01220583). Unresectable cases are often managed with radiation therapy, preferably with concurrent systemic therapy.

Particle therapy, with the use of protons, neutrons, or carbon ions, has been applied to the treatment of salivary gland tumors, most frequently adenoid cystic carcinoma, with locoregional control rates ranging from 57 to 93% [1–9]. Results with proton therapy (PBRT) demonstrate encouraging efficacy in comparison with photon-based treatment. Even in modern series of photon irradiation for unresectable salivary tumors, 5-year locoregional control rates are <50% [10]. Clinical studies assessing particle therapy for salivary tumors have demonstrated skull base involvement [1], larger tumor size, unresectable disease, [2] and involvement of the sphenoid sinus and clivus [8] to be associated with lower rates of disease control. This treatment tends to be very well tolerated with low rates of severe toxicities [4, 9].

The estimated risk of positive findings in the neck is based on multiple factors including T-stage, tumor location, and histology. Risk is lowest for acinic cell, adenoid cystic carcinoma, and carcinoma ex pleomorphic adenoma, intermediate for mucoepidermoid carcinoma, and highest for squamous cell, undifferentiated, and salivary duct carcinomas. Risk estimation tables [11] are useful for predicting the risk of nodal involvement. Elective treatment of the neck is generally indicated for a risk greater than 15–20%. For histologies with high risk of perineural spread (adenoid cystic carcinoma), treatment to the adjacent cranial nerves and skull base is recommended as well. Major salivary gland tumors have low rates of contralateral neck involvement.

Proton therapy can improve the therapeutic ratio for patients with salivary gland tumors by preserving target coverage, maintaining high local control rates and simultaneously lowering normal tissue exposure [9, 12]. There is evidence that this reduces acute toxicity and therefore would also be expected to lower late toxicity. When available, PBRT should be strongly considered for administration of ipsilateral salivary gland irradiation. In cases of perineural spread or skull base involvement, PBRT may also provide a crucial benefit in sparing of the brainstem, allowing for dose escalation in this critical location [8, 13].

8.2 Simulation, Target Delineation, and Radiation Dose/Fractionation

Computed tomography (CT) simulation should be performed with intravenous iodinated contrast, when not contraindicated, to facilitate anatomical delineation. For the purposes of dose calculation, a non-contrast CT needs to be employed in planning proton therapy.

8 Salivary Gland Tumors

Table 8.1 Recommended target volumes and radiation doses

Volume	Target	Dose
Gross tumor volume (GTV)	Gross unresected disease including primary tumor, involved nerves, and regional lymph nodes	70 Gy (RBE)
High-risk clinical tumor volume (CTV$_{66}$)	Includes areas of extranodal extension or surgical margin positivity	66 Gy (RBE)
High-risk clinical tumor volume (CTV$_{60}$)	Includes the postoperative bed, both at the primary tumor site and the ipsilateral neck (levels Ib–IV). Retropharyngeal and level V lymph nodes are typically not covered due to low risk of involvement and can be omitted at the physician's discretion	60 Gy (RBE)
Low-risk clinical tumor volume (CTV$_{50-54}$)	Includes the undissected ipsilateral neck and should be treated based on estimated risk from risk factors (described in introduction)	50–54 Gy (RBE)
Contralateral neck	Treatment of the contralateral neck should be considered in cases where tumor approaches midline (typically sublingual or minor salivary gland primaries) or when involved or suspicious lymph nodes are evident in the contralateral neck. In cases of large-volume ipsilateral nodal disease, where crossing lymphatic drainage to the opposite neck is possible, treatment of the contralateral neck can be considered as well. The decision to include the undissected node negative neck should be based on risk estimation for occult metastases (described in introduction)	50–54 Gy (RBE)

Positron emission tomography (PET) is helpful for identification of metabolically active gross disease and identification of involved or suspicious lymph nodes.

Magnetic resonance imaging (MRI) is recommended for accurate delineation of the extent of gross tumor in soft tissue as well as radiographic assessment of perineural spread.

PET and MR images should be registered to the planning CT for accurate target delineation. Uncertainties related to image fusion should be considered in the treatment planning process.

The recommended dosing and fractionation vary depending on the clinical scenario (Table 8.1):

Target volumes should be expanded according to institutional standard, typically by 3–5 mm, to create a planning target volume (PTV), employed for reporting purposes [14].

Consultation with a medical oncologist for consideration of concurrent radiosensitizing chemotherapy is recommended in the setting of margin positivity, extranodal extension, or treatment of gross disease.

8.3 Patient Positioning, Immobilization, and Treatment Verification

Simulation and treatment should be conducted in the supine position with a three-point mask. A five-point mask can be considered in cases involving treatment of cervical lymph nodes.

Setup accuracy should ideally be ascertained with daily orthogonal X-ray imaging or volumetric imaging, if available.

In-room CT imaging (i.e., cone-beam CT) is ideally used for treatment verification. When in-room 3D imaging is not available, verification CT scans with the patient in treatment position are recommended during the course of treatment to assess for potential changes in anatomy (i.e., due to weight loss, tumor shrinkage, etc.) and potential changes in the accuracy of the dose distribution (Fig. 8.1). Currently at our center, we generally rescan every other week for definitive cases and once during treatment for postoperative cases, though there are exceptions to this depending on the clinical scenario.

Caution should be used when treating anterior targets with superior oblique fields as variation in daily setup and chin movement can result in skin flash with unnecessary dose to the skin of the chest wall (Fig. 8.2). In such cases, bolus can be placed on the chest to absorb stray dose).

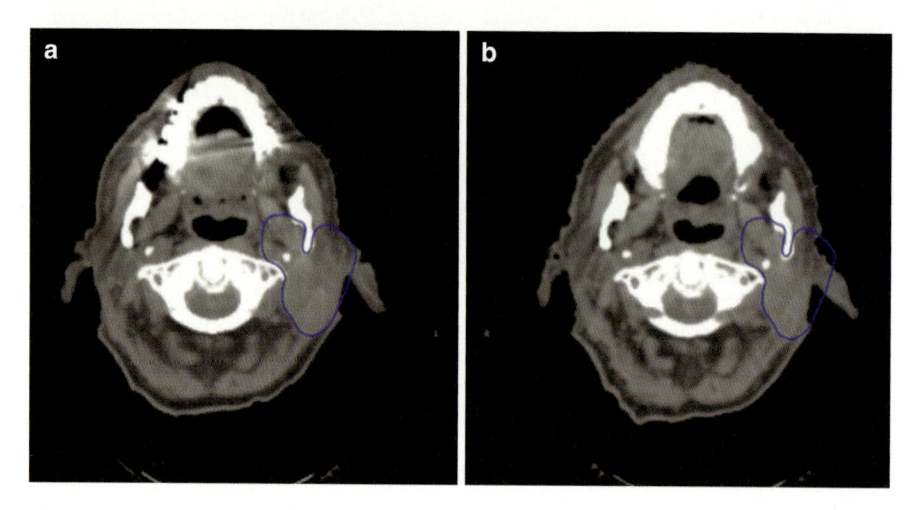

Fig. 8.1 Anatomical changes during proton treatment. (**a**) Planning simulation scan of a left auricular target. (**b**) Verification scan 2 weeks into treatment demonstrating significant tissue loss as result of treatment. This required replanning for accurate delivery of the intended plan

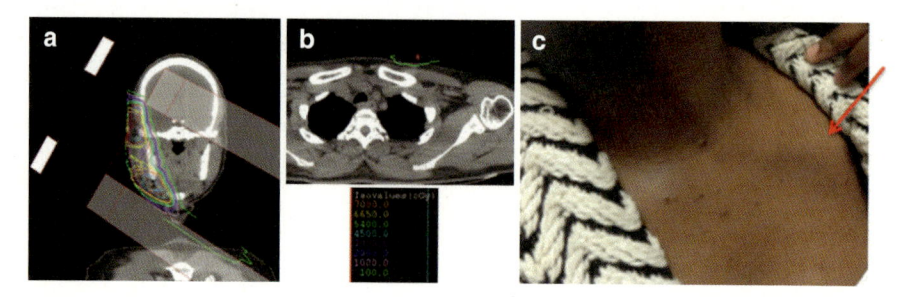

Fig. 8.2 A patient with pleomorphic adenoma of the right parotid gland treated with a superior oblique field using proton passive scattering uniform scanning (**a**). Skin flash resulted in dose to the contralateral chest (**b**). Following 42 Gy (RBE), wedge-shaped dermatitis was noted on the contralateral chest (**c**). Following this, 4 cm of bolus was placed on the chest for the remainder of treatment to absorb dose from skin flash, which resulted in rapid resolution of dermatitis

8.4 Three-Dimensional (3D) Proton Treatment Planning

8.4.1 Passive Scattering (PS)

Three field plans are typically utilized (2–4 beams, Fig. 8.3), preferably with the shortest and most homogeneous radiologic depths.

In the planning process, care should be taken to avoid the overlapping of the distal ends of more than two beams. No more than one beam should range out into an organ at risk (OAR), especially at levels of serial structures. If the distal ends overlap, alternate beam angles or range feathering can be examined (Fig. 8.4).

When treating the cervical lymph nodes in addition to the parotid/parotid bed, matched fields are typically required to cover the field in the longitudinal dimension due to potential field size limitations. When covering the skull base, matched fields are typically used for a modulation match to reduce proximal dose to skin and surrounding normal tissue, particularly the temporal lobe. Care should be taken to avoid placing match lines on OAR structures. Match line feathering can be utilized to reduce excessive hot spots at the match line level.

Over- and under-range plans should be evaluated with relevant range uncertainties as determined by each center.

In the process of beam selection, special care should be taken to avoid beams traversing through dental hardware and air cavities that can change during the course of treatment. Consult your physics team when traditional beam orientations need to be altered or when a patient has any dental hardware. In general, dental fillings as well as artifact created in adipose and muscle tissue should be contoured and assigned a predetermined density or HU value in the treatment planning system. Compensators should be created with dental fillings at a lower electron density/mass density in order to maintain a smoother compensator with fewer ridges and pylons. For plan evaluation, apply appropriate forced density/mass density. If it is necessary for the beam path to traverse dental fillings, a cold spot should be expected distally. This effect can be mitigated with the use of multiple beam angles.

For unilateral cases, uniform scanning or passive scattering can be used with excellent results. The target volume for most salivary tumor cases extends superficially, often just below the skin, resulting in little opportunity for skin sparing. The

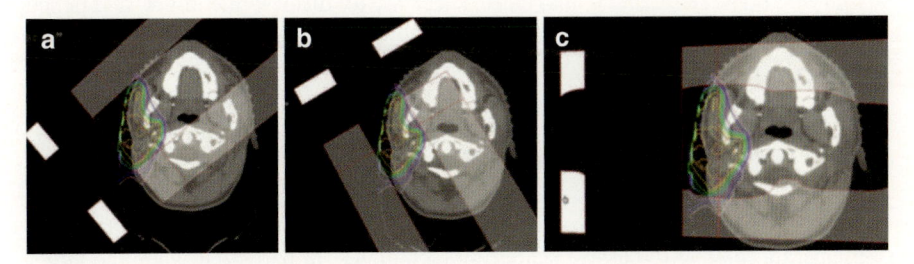

Fig. 8.3 Passive scattering uniform scanning plan for treatment of a parotid field with typical three-beam arrangement including (**a**) posterior oblique, (**b**) anterior oblique, and (**c**) superior oblique

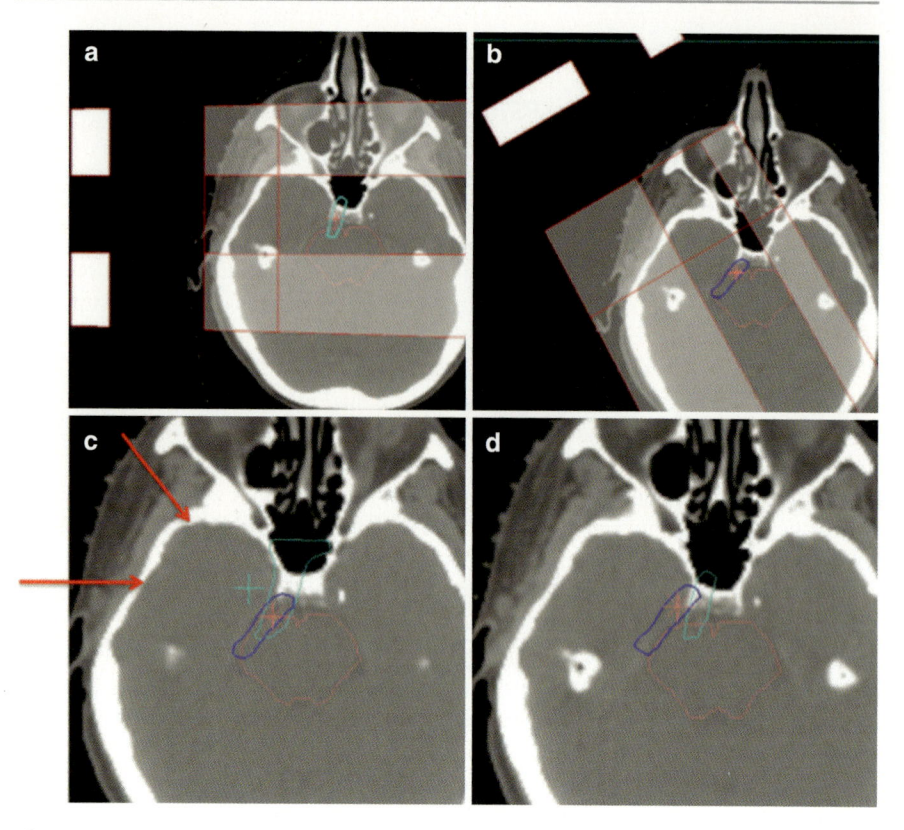

Fig. 8.4 Passive scattering uniform scanning treatment of a skull base target using lateral (**a**) and anterior oblique (**b**) beams. Distal end structures, shown in *blue* and *cyan*, were found to overlap at the brain stem (**c**). Range feathering (**d**) can be used to minimize overlap. Beam angles are indicated by *red arrows*

skin dose with uniform scanning (US/PS) is similar to the prescription dose, likely slightly higher than with intensity-modulated radiation therapy (IMRT) and similar to IMRT with bolus.

For parotid cases, the goal is to spare the contralateral salivary glands, oral cavity, larynx, brain stem, and spinal cord. These are all distal to the target, and hence comparable normal tissue sparing may be achieved with passive or scanned proton beams (Fig. 8.5).

8.4.2 Pencil Beam Scanning (PBS)

For parotid cases, PBS will provide conformal plans with an advantage in terms of skin sparing relative to passive scattering techniques, in particular when the target volume is not entirely abutting the external surface. With PBS, there is greater

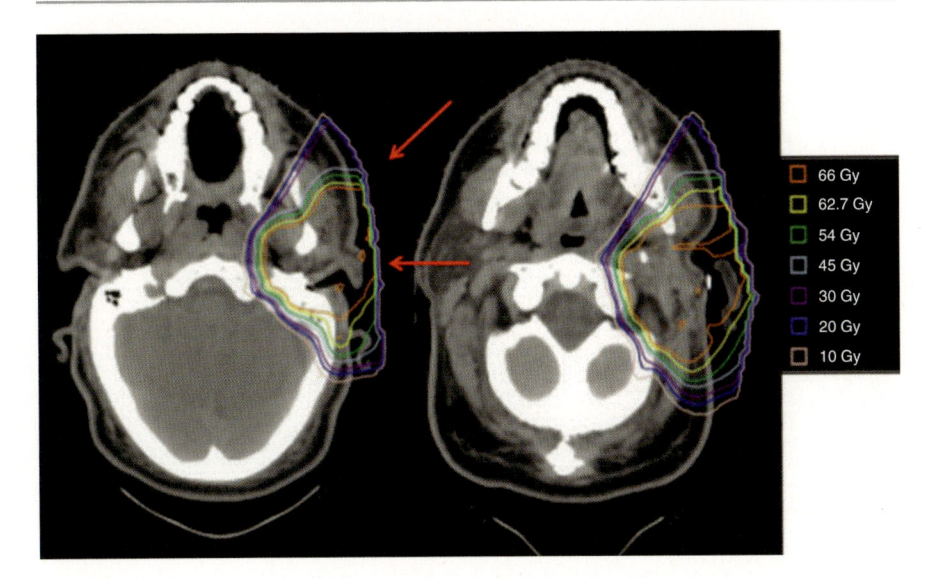

Fig. 8.5 Uniform scanning plan for treatment of a pleomorphic adenoma of the left parotid with sparing of distal OARs. Beam angles are indicated with *red arrows*

control over the proximal portion of the beam, and avoidance structures can be created to decrease the skin dose. However, in many instances, the volume will extend to the patient surface, and the advantage of PBS may be diminished.

The same two- to four-beam arrangement that is used with US/PS (Fig. 8.3) may be used with PBS as well. More often, only two fields need to be employed if the distal edges of the two beams do not overlap, due to the ability of PBS to create a 3D dose distribution with a single field. Care should be taken to ensure all artifact and dental hardware are accurately contoured and proper mass density/electron density is applied prior to calculation. If possible, use beams that avoid going through hardware. Consult your physics team at the time of volume delineation and beam orientation determination.

PBS plan optimization is performed based on the optimization volume(s) created by the planner for single field uniform dose (SFUD) treatment planning technique.

For parotid cases, SFUD should ideally be used as it results in delivery of the most robust plan. Each beam should be evaluated individually to ensure adequate coverage then compositely to evaluate OAR constraints and hot spots. As robust optimization matures in the clinical environment, IMPT may become more extensively used.

For submandibular cases, the ipsilateral parotid gland is a critical avoidance structure, and care should be taken to minimize exposure, reducing the mean dose to <26 Gy (RBE) and ideally lower (Table 8.2). This can be challenging to do with US/PS since the OAR is proximal to the target, and the target essentially wraps around the parotid gland. PBS can ideally be used to carve the dose around the parotid in these cases, using either SFUD or IMPT. However, even though IMPT may generate a more conformal dose distribution, plan robustness must be

Table 8.2 Recommended dose constraints to organs at risk when using proton beam therapy for ipsilateral treatment of salivary gland tumors

Organ at risk	Recommended dose constraint
Oral cavity excluding PTV	Mean dose <3 Gy (RBE) (<10 Gy (RBE) if covering level Ib)
Larynx	Mean dose <15 Gy (RBE)
Ipsilateral parotid gland (for non-parotid cases)	Mean dose <26 Gy (RBE) (ideally lower)
Ipsilateral submandibular gland (for non-submandibular cases)	Mean dose <39 Gy (RBE)
Contralateral submandibular and parotid glands	Mean dose 0 Gy (RBE)
Esophagus	Mean dose <10 Gy (RBE)
Brachial plexus	No hot spots
Brain stem	<5 Gy (RBE) when not covering cranial nerves/skull base when skull base is covered, maintain standard dose constraints
Optic nerves and optic chiasm	<5 Gy (RBE)
Spinal cord	<5 Gy (RBE)

These recommendations are adapted from institutional photon/IMRT treatment planning. As additional data is accumulated, these constraints will continue to be refined. In clinical practice, the planner should make every effort to achieve the lowest dose possible for all normal tissues while maximizing coverage

carefully evaluated especially when robust optimization is not available. This can be achieved by creating an optimization constraint on the external structure to a max dose of 110% with robustness optimization turned on when clinically tested and available. This will factor in over- and under-range as well as isocenter shifts and will not allow for hot spots if the fields overlap. Without robust optimization, another option is to create gradient structures to control the dose falloff. When possible, planning should be carried out with SFUD as it is currently the most robust option available. The same field arrangement should be used as would be with US/PS (ipsilateral anterior oblique, lateral and posterior oblique), although the number of fields may be decreased. As robust optimization is just emerging in the clinical setting, it should be carefully evaluated and discussed with the physics team.

8.5 Passive Scattering Versus Pencil Beam Scanning Comparisons

For cases requiring bilateral neck irradiation, PBS is the method of choice for optimal normal tissue sparing and treatment efficiency. For the majority of these cases, SFUD is possible; however, some cases might require IMPT or a combination of the two techniques in order to meet currently recommended dose constraints (Table 8.2). Planning comparisons between PS and PBS techniques are shown in Figs. 8.6 and 8.7.

8 Salivary Gland Tumors 161

Uniform scanning,
mean parotid dose 23.1 Gy(RBE)

Pencil beam scanning,
mean parotid dose 18.7 Gy(RBE)

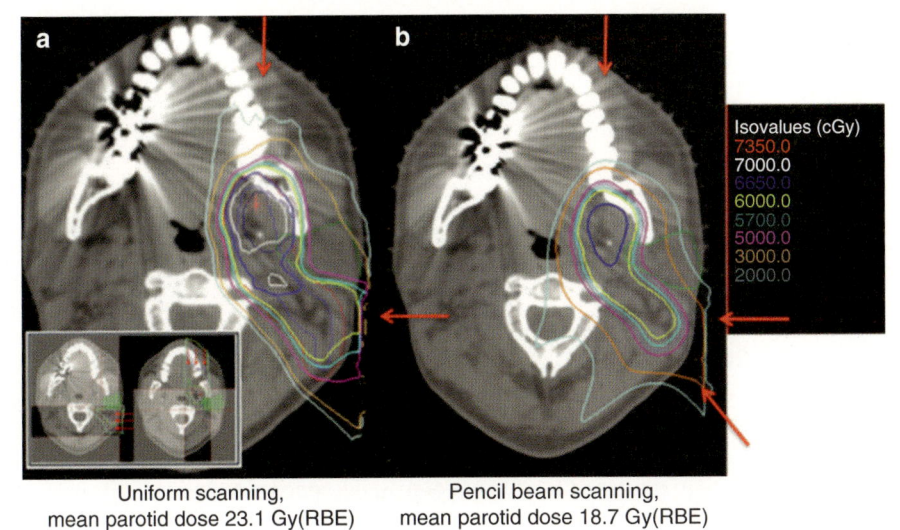

Fig. 8.6 Example of coverage of the submandibular region and cervical lymph node basins with sparing of the ipsilateral parotid gland using (**a**) passive scattering patched fields technique with patched fields indicated (inset) versus (**b**) IMPT pencil beam scanning technique. Beam directions are indicated by *red arrows*

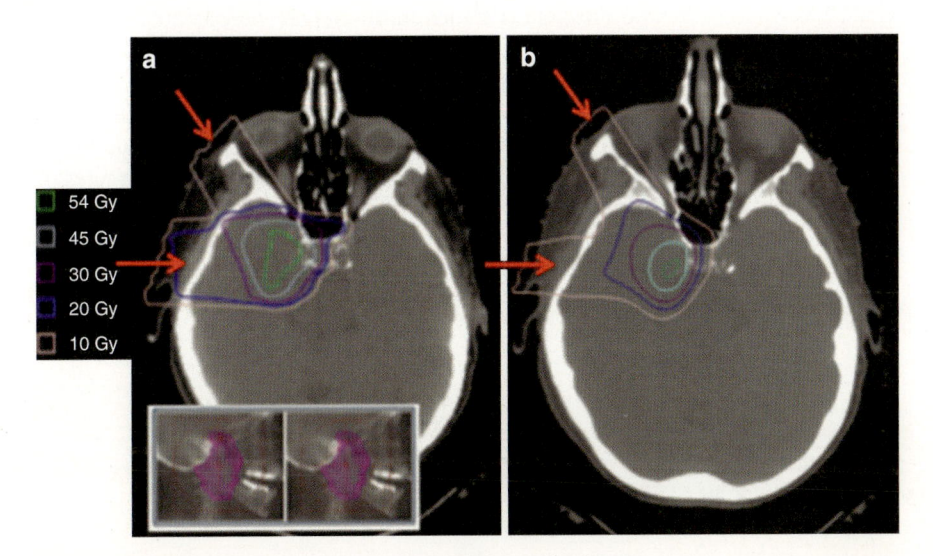

Fig. 8.7 Example of coverage of a skull base target using (**a**) passive scattering with a modulation match technique versus (**b**) PBS with SFUD technique. In such cases, PBS often offers an advantage in sparing of the proximal temporal lobe. Beam directions are indicated by *red arrows*

Table 8.3 Dosimetric comparison of IMRT versus uniform scanning PBRT for the treatment of ipsilateral major salivary gland tumors, median doses presented (Adapted from [9])

Characteristic	IMRT ($n = 23$)	PBRT ($n = 18$)	p-value
Brain stem (max dose)	29.7 Gy	0.62 Gy (RBE)	<0.001
Spinal cord (max dose)	36.3 Gy	1.9 Gy (RBE)	<0.001
Oral cavity (mean dose)	20.6 Gy	0.94 Gy (RBE)	<0.001
Contralateral parotid gland (mean dose)	1.4 Gy	0.00 Gy (RBE)	<0.001
Contralateral submandibular gland (mean dose)	4.1 Gy	0.00 Gy (RBE)	<0.001
Larynx (mean dose)	21.4 Gy	10.3 Gy (RBE)	0.182

8.6 Dosimetric and Toxicity Comparison

The use of PBRT, primarily with PS, for ipsilateral head and neck target volumes has been shown to result in significant reduction in dose to many OARs as well as reduction in acute toxicities of treatment compared to photon techniques [9, 15].

A comparison of dosimetry among patients treated with ipsilateral IMRT or PBRT for major salivary gland tumors demonstrated significantly lower maximum brain stem dose, maximum spinal cord dose, mean oral cavity dose, and contralateral parotid and submandibular doses with the use of PBRT [9]. This translated to lower rates of acute toxicity with PBRT including mucositis, nausea, dysgeusia, and fatigue. Of note, the rate of acute grade 2 dermatitis was higher with PBRT, but grade 3 dermatitis was no different. Patients in this report were treated with US/PS. No patients experience grade 4 dermatitis. With clinical deployment of IMPT, dermatitis rates are expected to decline.

Minor salivary glands lining the oral cavity are responsible for basal levels of salivation and are critical to maintenance of oral health and hygiene. Reduction in oral cavity dose is a major advantage afforded by PBRT, resulting in lower rates of mucositis and expected reduced rates of chronic xerostomia and improvements in dental health, though long-term data is not yet available. Larynx sparing may be further improved using smaller spot size and/or apertures (Table 8.3).

8.7 Future Developments

As PBS technology matures and IMPT can be more routinely and robustly deployed, projected dosimetric gains may further increase the benefits of PBS for salivary gland malignancies requiring radiation treatment.

References

1. Douglas JG, et al. Treatment of locally advanced adenoid cystic carcinoma of the head and neck with neutron radiotherapy. Int J Radiat Oncol Biol Phys. 2000;46(3):551–7.
2. Douglas JG, et al. Neutron radiotherapy for the treatment of locally advanced major salivary gland tumors. Head Neck. 1999;21(3):255–63.

3. Jensen AD, et al. Combined treatment of adenoid cystic carcinoma with cetuximab and IMRT plus C12 heavy ion boost: ACCEPT [ACC, Erbitux(R) and particle therapy]. BMC Cancer. 2011;11:70.
4. Schulz-Ertner D, et al. Therapy strategies for locally advanced adenoid cystic carcinomas using modern radiation therapy techniques. Cancer. 2005;104(2):338–44.
5. Schulz-Ertner D, et al. Feasibility and toxicity of combined photon and carbon ion radiotherapy for locally advanced adenoid cystic carcinomas. Int J Radiat Oncol Biol Phys. 2003;56(2):391–8.
6. Griffin TW, et al. Neutron vs photon irradiation of inoperable salivary gland tumors: results of an RTOG-MRC cooperative randomized study. Int J Radiat Oncol Biol Phys. 1988;15(5):1085–90.
7. Laramore GE, et al. Neutron versus photon irradiation for unresectable salivary gland tumors: final report of an RTOG-MRC randomized clinical trial. Radiation therapy oncology group. Medical Research Council. Int J Radiat Oncol Biol Phys. 1993;27(2):235–40.
8. Pommier P, et al. Proton beam radiation therapy for skull base adenoid cystic carcinoma. Arch Otolaryngol Head Neck Surg. 2006;132(11):1242–9.
9. Romesser PB, et al. Proton beam radiation therapy results in significantly reduced toxicity compared with intensity-modulated radiation therapy for head and neck tumors that require ipsilateral radiation. Radiother Oncol. 2016;118(2):286–92.
10. Spratt DE, et al. Results of photon radiotherapy for unresectable salivary gland tumors: is neutron radiotherapy's local control superior? Radiol Oncol. 2014;48(1):56–61.
11. Terhaard CH, et al. The role of radiotherapy in the treatment of malignant salivary gland tumors. Int J Radiat Oncol Biol Phys. 2005;61(1):103–11.
12. Grant SR, et al. Proton versus conventional radiotherapy for pediatric salivary gland tumors: acute toxicity and dosimetric characteristics. Radiother Oncol. 2015;116(2):309–15.
13. Chan AW, Liebsch NJ. Proton radiation therapy for head and neck cancer. J Surg Oncol. 2008;97(8):697–700.
14. NCT01220583. Radiation therapy with or without chemotherapy in treating patients with high-risk malignant salivary gland tumors that have been removed by surgery. https://clinicaltrials.gov/ct2/show/NCT01220583. Accessed September 28, 2017.
15. Stromberger C, et al. Unilateral and bilateral neck SIB for head and neck cancer patients: intensity-modulated proton therapy, tomotherapy, and RapidArc. Strahlenther Onkol. 2016;192(4):232–9.

Thyroid Cancer

9

Mauricio Gamez, Aman Anand, and Samir H. Patel

Contents

9.1	Introduction	165
9.2	Simulation, Target Delineation, and Radiation Dose/Fractionation	166
9.3	Patient Positioning, Immobilization, and Treatment Verification	167
9.4	Three-Dimensional (3D) Proton Treatment Planning	168
	9.4.1 Passive Scattering (PS)	168
	9.4.2 Pencil Beam Scanning (PBS)	169
9.5	Dosimetric and Toxicity Comparison	173
9.6	Future Developments	173
References		174

9.1 Introduction

Thyroid cancer is uncommon and only represents 1% of all diagnosed malignancies and 0.2% of cancer deaths in the USA. The incidence is increasing in part due to a better detection of subclinical disease with imaging studies in the past years. Papillary cancer is the most common thyroid malignancy and represents approximately 80% of all thyroid cancers. Follicular cancer represents approximately 10%, and the remaining 10% of thyroid tumors are medullary, anaplastic, and others. Most commonly, it affects females rather than males with a 3:1 relationship. The majority of thyroid tumors are primarily managed with surgery followed by ± radioactive iodine (RAI) in those with a differentiated thyroid cancer (DTC). Patients with anaplastic carcinoma should be immediately referred and

---

M. Gamez • A. Anand • S.H. Patel (✉)
Department of Radiation Oncology, Mayo Clinic Arizona, Phoenix, AZ, USA
e-mail: Patel.Samir@mayo.edu

© Springer International Publishing Switzerland 2018
N. Lee et al. (eds.), *Target Volume Delineation and Treatment Planning for Particle Therapy*, Practical Guides in Radiation Oncology, https://doi.org/10.1007/978-3-319-42478-1_9

have multidisciplinary management in a tertiary cancer center due to the dismal prognosis of the disease [1–3].

The role of external beam radiation therapy (EBRT) in the treatment of DTC is controversial because of a lack of prospective trials and conflicting results in the existing retrospective data [4–6].

The Endocrine Surgery Committee of the American Head and Neck Society recommends EBRT for locoregional control in DTC for patients with gross residual or unresectable locoregional disease, except for patients <45 years old with limited gross disease that is RAI avid. After complete resection, EBRT may be considered in selected patients >45 years old with high likelihood of microscopic residual disease and low likelihood of responding to RAI. EBRT should not be routinely used as adjuvant therapy after complete resection of gross disease or for cervical node involvement [1, 3].

Previously published data have shown the importance of radiation sparing midline structures (i.e., upper larynx, pharyngeal constrictors, esophagus) and other organs at risk (i.e., parotids, submandibular, and minor salivary glands) and the dose correlations of these structures with toxicity [7–10].

Proton beam therapy is a promising modality for the definitive and adjuvant treatment of thyroid cancer. Pencil beam scanning (PBS) using intensity-modulated proton therapy (IMPT) is an emerging technique allowing for conformal dose delivery [11, 12].

The goal of proton therapy is to improve locoregional control by optimizing target coverage while sparing dose to organs at risk (oral cavity, upper larynx, pharyngeal constrictors, uninvolved esophagus, brachial plexus, and lung apices) thereby limiting treatment toxicity.

9.2 Simulation, Target Delineation, and Radiation Dose/Fractionation

The physical exam, diagnostic imaging studies (CT, MRI, PET), and the operative findings should be used for treatment planning.

Fluorodeoxyglucose positron emission tomography (FDG-PET) can be helpful for identification of metabolically active gross disease and for the delineation of target volumes in patients with anaplastic and RAI-refractory differentiated carcinomas.

CT simulation should be performed to help guide the delineation of the primary tumor/surgical bed and lymph node volumes and for the purpose of dose calculation. Typically we recommend 3 mm or less slice thickness.

The use of IV contrast is typically avoided in case that the patient would subsequently need radioactive iodine administration, and it can be only justified in very particular clinical situations such as in undifferentiated or RAI-refractory thyroid cancers.

The different diagnostic imaging studies should be registered to the planning CT for more accurate target delineation. Uncertainties related to image fusion should be considered in the treatment planning process.

9 Thyroid Cancer

Table 9.1 Recommended target volumes and radiation doses

Target volume	Target coverage	Dose
Gross tumor volume (GTV)	Gross primary tumor, involved surrounding structures, regional lymph nodes	70 Gy (RBE)
High-risk clinical tumor volume (CTV$_{66}$)	Areas of positive surgical margin or shave excision or extranodal extension	66 Gy (RBE)
At risk clinical tumor volume (CTV$_{54-60}$)[a]	Areas at risk of microscopic disease primary include tracheoesophageal groove and >5 mm around GTV and CTV$_{66}$ In the postoperative setting, include surgical bed. If tracheostomy is performed, include tracheostomy stoma. Neck: in node-positive disease, include nodal levels II–VII and upper mediastinum to the level of the carina. Level V should be covered in the node-positive neck. Consider coverage of level I and retropharyngeal nodes in the setting of bulky neck disease	54–60 Gy (RBE)

[a]Uninvolved nodal regions may be treated to 54 Gy(RBE) at the discretion of treating physician. In select cases, the lateral necks can be omitted despite having pathologic lymph nodes. Please consult your surgeon

The target volumes and doses are customized for each patient according to the risks of local and regional recurrence [13, 14]. Suggested doses and target volumes are shown in (Table 9.1).

The target volumes should be expanded typically between 3 and 7 mm depending upon institutional image guidance capabilities and range uncertainty criteria selected by physics. At our institution, proton-based planning target volumes are usually comprised of 5 mm setup margin in all directions, with additional 2 mm of radial margin to account for penumbra laterally and range margins in the direction of the beam determined by the physics team.

The recommended fractionation size of the CTVs is 1.8–2.0 Gy(RBE).

9.3 Patient Positioning, Immobilization, and Treatment Verification

Simulation and treatment should be conducted in the supine position.

To allow for strict immobilization of the head, neck, and shoulder regions, a thermoplastic mask should be used.

At our institution we have selected a base of skull (Qfix® Systems, BoS™) frame assembly with a five-point mask made out of kevlar (Fig. 9.1).

Daily position setup verification should be done with orthogonal X-rays or if available with volumetric imaging.

During the course of the treatment, we recommend a verification CT scan to assess changes in the anatomy of the patient (due to tumor shrinkage, weight loss, etc.). Significant changes may necessitate treatment replanning. These scans are usually ordered during the middle of these treatments around the onset of the fourth week followed by another one in the fifth week.

Fig. 9.1 Example of our patient immobilization setup

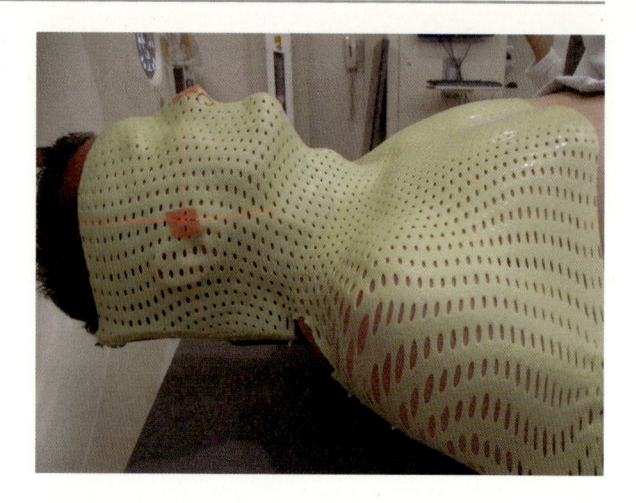

9.4 Three-Dimensional (3D) Proton Treatment Planning

9.4.1 Passive Scattering (PS)

In cases where scanning beam delivery is not available to treat thyroid cancers, passive scatter treatments can be planned with use of apertures and compensators and beam arrangements consisting of combinations of posterior and anterior oblique requiring craniocaudal tilts. This is to avoid any overlaps or patch within air cavities or in any critical structures such as larynx and esophagus regions. Field size limitations should be kept in mind when creating match fields. Some machines, depending upon the small, medium, or large snout size capabilities, will require either multiple isocentric treatments or larger couch kicks. In either case, match line feathering would be necessary to reduce sharp gradients at the junctions. Additionally, whenever planning with a posterior beam angles, care should be taken with placement of the isocenter in order to avoid potential collisions with the nozzle. One must avoid going through heterogeneities and any high atomic number material present in dental hardware if any. Material-specific relative stopping power value needs to be assigned to the CT value of the material [15]. A routine practice being followed in our clinic is to obtain the sample from surgery and determine the material type and components from the vendors. This is oftentimes then also followed by actual measuring of the relative stopping power in our proton beamline, and thereafter a proper Hounsfield unit gets assigned as depicted in Fig. 9.2. Instances which may/will require CT HU data to be overridden include:

- Tumor margin extending into the lung or deep air pockets that are surrounded by tissue
- Surgical clips (or foreign objects in general)
- Streaking artifacts resulting from high-density artifacts

Design of compensators and apertures is a crucial task for planning these cases as there are significant amounts of midline structures that need to be spared. And due to heterogeneities with the air cavities and bone, there are difficulties maintaining good distal end coverage. This oftentimes requires border smoothing. Care must be taken

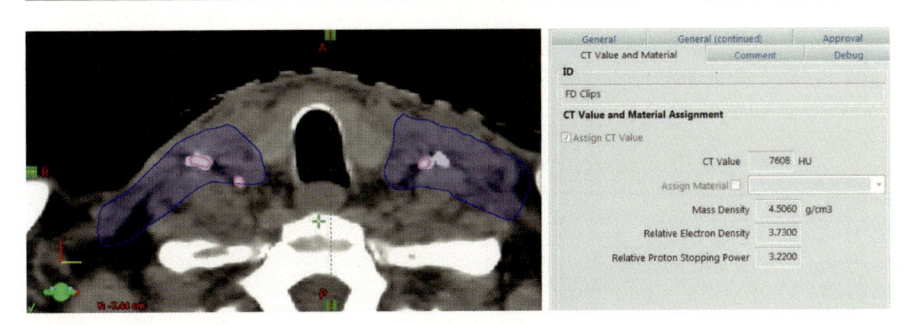

Fig. 9.2 Contouring of high-density structures in proton planning

when applying any border smoothing as it usually reduces dose conformity. To mitigate this, one would then require additional beams which depend on individual cases being planned. Aperture designs should account for air gaps and snout positions in cases of movable snouts. Compensators should be carved out with an appropriate smearing radius (SR) that will allow smooth SOBPs and few perturbations due to conical ridges. Smearing radius can ensure distal coverage; however, it can lead to reduced dose conformity, as discussed, and can be mitigated with additional beam angles.

Ideally one should use less than five beams. In general the workflow of a passive scattered beam line is much more complicated and requires very careful pre-planning preparations as listed below.

9.4.2 Pencil Beam Scanning (PBS)

With modern-day accelerators offering smaller spot sizes and use of range shifters, it has become possible to design highly conformal 3D proton plans without need for multiple beams, compensators, and apertures. The air gap between the patient and the treatment nozzle should be minimized allowing for a smaller spot size. Various methods include the use of a range shifter and/or bolus.

Usually for most of the head and neck cases, we tend to maintain the air gap as small as possible. There are different proton delivery solutions available with some allowing snout movements, while others are some sort of fixed nozzle solutions or patient-related range shifters. However, irrespective of the solution employed, one must try to minimize the air gap between the patient's external and the surface of any energy absorbers in order to keep the spot sizes small.

Scanning beam allows a greater degree of control of the dose distributions in both lateral and proximal distances. With the advent of scanning-based treatment delivery systems, one can perform unique dose painting thereby conforming therapeutic doses to tumor volumes while offering significant sparing of normal tissues. In thyroid cancer, oftentimes, the submandibular glands, oral cavity, parotids, pharyngeal constrictors, and upper larynx can be spared to a greater extent. Since the regions of interest are both distal and lateral to the tumor volumes, it is necessary to choose beam angles and lateral margins judiciously. In most of the cases, a good dose distribution can be achieved with a combination of an anterior-posterior beam angles. This approach requires the physics planning team to design beam-specific optimization target volumes as they apply to each clinical case. At our institution, in addition to the lateral margins and the range

Fig. 9.3 Sub-target volume cropping

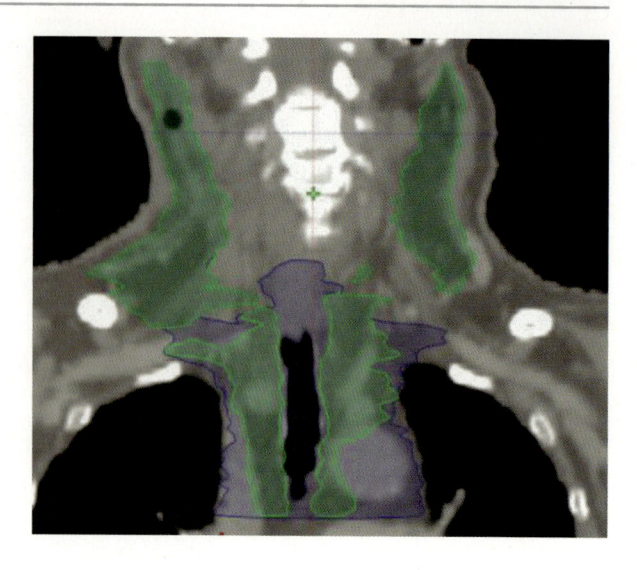

margins in the direction of the beam, one spot sigma lateral margin is added to the optimization volume in the beam properties. From our planning studies, we observed a pair of anterior and posterior beam angles suffice achieving highly conformal dose distributions with IMPT. When optimizing to more than one target volume to different dose levels, care must be taken to not have any overlapping margins within the target structures. For an example, if a plan involves two targets, CTV1 and CTV2, where the dose to CTV1 > CTV2, then Boolean operations will have to be used:

CTV1 (high-risk volume) = no Boolean operation needed
CTV1sub = CTV2 − CTV1

where CTV1sub is a new structure as seen in Fig. 9.3 on the right in *blue*. Care must be taken to not alter physician-drawn CTVs as the final dose assessments should be made to the original CTVs.

Generating a robust plan without any computer-assisted robust optimization requires precise preparation of planning structures through which the fluence can be shaped and spot placements can be controlled within and around the target volumes. In our clinic this was achieved by generating optimization target volume (OTV) structures which were beam specific and were carved out around the parotid, submandibular gland (SMG), and the oral cavity. An example shown on Fig. 9.4 is a typical 2 mm cropping of our OTV from the SMG. Typically with these arrangements, one is able to achieve adequate target coverage with robust organ at risk (OAR) sparing. In order to obtain adequate robustness, our OTVs consisted of 3% of the range compounded with 2–3 mm of setup errors which have been established based on our clinical experience and image guidance capabilities. Criteria for evaluating robustness are mostly institutional dependent. For our clinic we evaluate all our head and neck tumors against a setup uncertainty of 3 mm compounded with 3% CT to relative stopping power-based range errors [16]. As an example, based on Eclipse™ (Varian Medical Systems, Palo Alto, CA) Treatment Planning System Ver. 13.6 at our institution, we are able to achieve conformal and robust target coverages. The robustness of our plans is measured as D95 and V95 target doses under worst case scenarios (setup and range).

9 Thyroid Cancer

Fig. 9.4 Cropping of OTV from the left submandibular gland (2 mm)

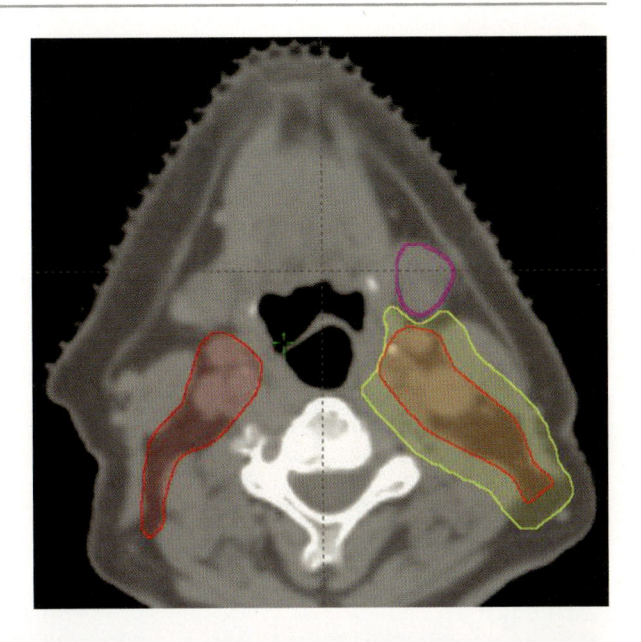

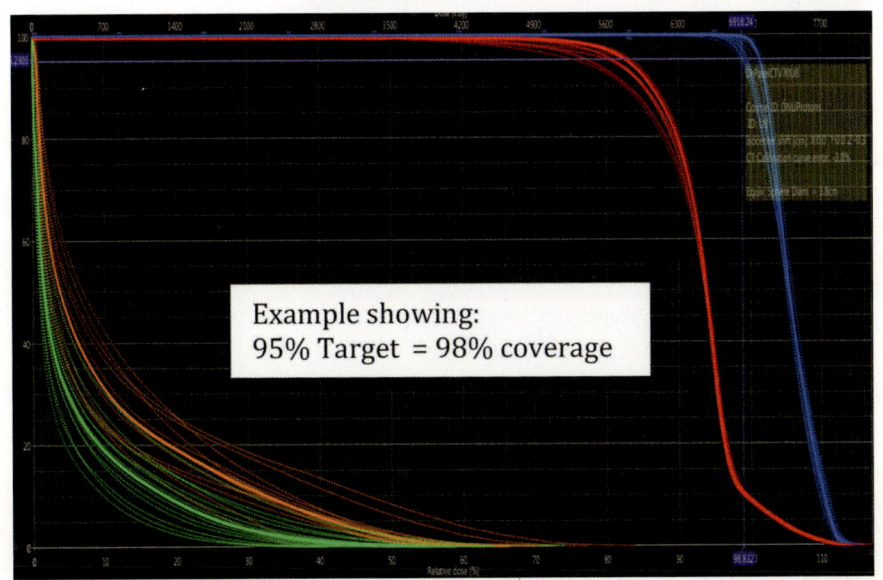

Fig. 9.5 Thyroid plan robustness. DVH band indicates 95% of the target is receiving 98% of the prescription dose

An example of one of the thyroid plan's robustness (Fig. 9.5) is displayed in the DVH band indicating 95% of the target receiving 98% of the prescription dose with 3% and 3 mm setup and range uncertainties. Also, with any opposite beam arrangements, it is important to evaluate inter-field robustness. Essentially, the field tapering and the gradients produced at match lines should be evaluated very carefully for any cold or hot spots shown in Fig. 9.6. We evaluate all our match lines for smooth dose falloffs. It

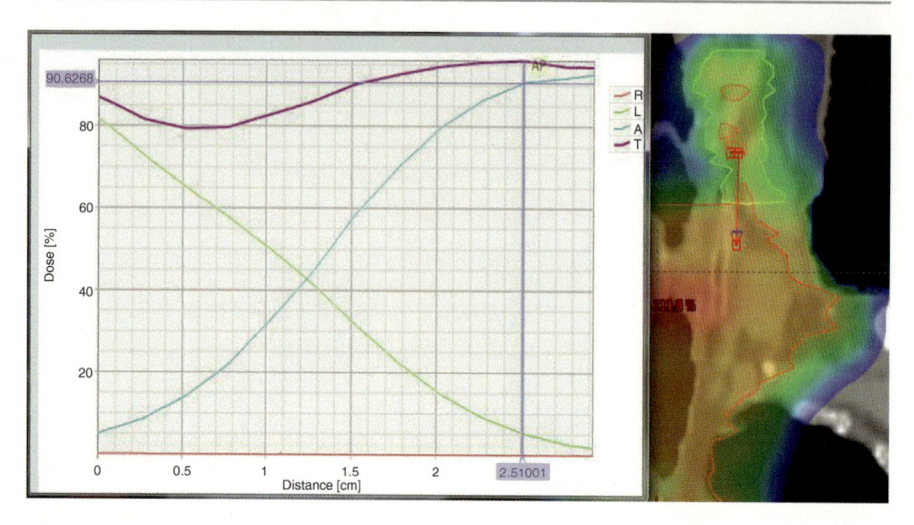

Fig. 9.6 Match lines for smooth dose falloffs

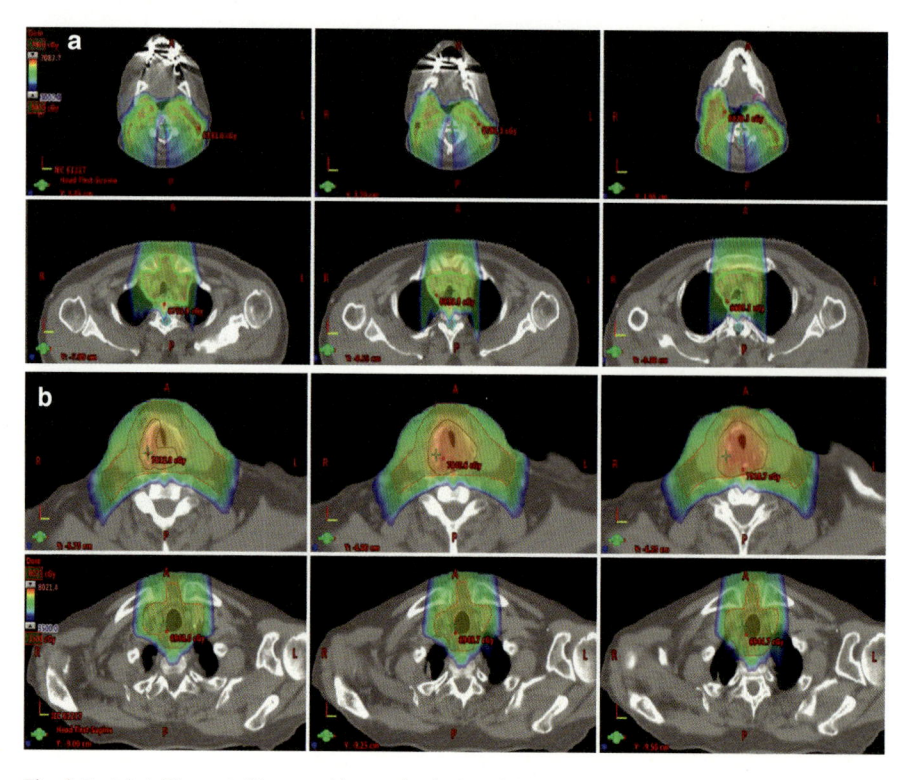

Fig. 9.7 (**a**) A 70-year-old man with anaplastic thyroid cancer involving the right neck, s/p total thyroidectomy, and right modified radical neck dissection. Postoperative chemoradiation therapy was recommended to the thyroid bed, central compartment, cervical neck levels II–VII, and mediastinal lymph nodes to the carina (CTV$_{60}$). (**b**) A 79-year-old man with recurrent Hurthle cell cancer, s/p total thyroidectomy, and subsequent radioactive iodine documented with local recurrence was recommended definitive radiation therapy to the area of gross disease, central compartment, and bilateral cervical neck levels II–VII (CTV$_{70}$ and CTV$_{56}$)

9 Thyroid Cancer

Table 9.2 Recommended dose constraints to OARs when using proton beam therapy with PBS technique for treatment of thyroid cancer

Organ at risk	Recommended dose constraint
Oral cavity	Mean < 39 Gy (RBE)
Parotid	Mean < 26 Gy (RBE)
Submandibular gland	Mean < 39 Gy (RBE)
Larynx	Mean < 44 Gy (RBE)
Constrictors	Mean < 55 Gy (RBE)
Esophagus	Mean < 34 Gy (RBE)
Spinal cord	Max point dose <45 Gy (RBE)
Brachial plexus	Max point dose <65 Gy (RBE)
Lung	Mean < 20 Gy (RBE), V20 < 37%

These recommendations are adapted from photon/IMRT treatment planning data

should also be noted, since these are mono-isocentric treatments and do not require moving patient support systems between the deliveries of two fields, we can ensure robust intrafractional dose delivery with the immobilization system discussed earlier. Overall, we are able to reach highly conformal target coverage with significant sparing of healthy tissues. Scanning beam offers greater flexibility in calculating a simultaneous integrated boost volume plan with both SFUD and IMPT planning techniques. Shown below in Fig. 9.5a and b, we have dose color wash for cases planned to 60 Gy(RBE) in 30 Fx to a single target (Fig. 9.7a) and dose painting to multiple targets (CTV 70 and CTV 56) in Fig. 9.7b.

9.5 Dosimetric and Toxicity Comparison

The use of proton beam radiation therapy (PBRT), particularly with PBS, for definitive or postoperative cases of thyroid cancer can result in a significant reduction in the dose delivered to different organs at risk (OARs) and potentially translates to a reduction of treatment toxicities compared to photon techniques (Table 9.2) [14].

Efforts should be made by the planner to achieve the lowest dose possible for all normal tissues after maximizing the target coverage.

Dose volumetric comparisons of treatment plans with IMRT or PBRT done at our institution have demonstrated significant dose reduction to the oral cavity, parotids, submandibular glands, upper larynx, pharyngeal constrictors, spinal cord, and lung. With this emerging technique, we hope this will translate in lower rates of acute toxicity including oral mucositis, xerostomia, dysgeusia, and dysphagia and decreased late toxicity such as radiation pneumonitis, brachial plexopathy, and secondary malignancy.

9.6 Future Developments

As proton therapy becomes more available and with better imaging quality verification, the use of PBS with IMPT can be more routinely used for the treatment for thyroid cancers when clinically indicated with the dosimetric advantages of this modality and the benefit of reduced toxicity.

References

1. Kiess AP, Agrawal N, Brierley JD, et al. External-beam radiotherapy for differentiated thyroid cancer locoregional control: a statement of the American Head and Neck Society. Head Neck. 2016;38:493–8.
2. Harrison LB, Sessions SB, Kies MS, editors. Head and neck cancer: a multidisciplinary approach. 4th ed. New York: Lippincott Williams & Wilkins; 2014.
3. Shindo ML, Caruana SM, Kandil E, et al. Management of invasive well-differentiated thyroid cancer: an American Head and Neck Society consensus statement. AHNS consensus statement. Head Neck. 2014;36:1379–90.
4. Schwartz DL, Lobo MJ, Ang KK, et al. Postoperative external beam radiotherapy for differentiated thyroid cancer: outcomes and morbidity with conformal treatment. Int J Radiat Oncol Biol Phys. 2009;74:1083–91.
5. Terezakis SA, Lee KS, Ghossein RA, et al. Role of external beam radiotherapy in patients with advanced or recurrent nonanaplastic thyroid cancer: Memorial Sloan-Kettering Cancer Center experience. Int J Radiat Oncol Biol Phys. 2009;73:795–801.
6. Rosenbluth BD, Serrano V, Happersett L, et al. Intensity-modulated radiation therapy for the treatment of nonanaplastic thyroid cancer. Int J Radiat Oncol Biol Phys. 2005;63:1419–26.
7. Levendag PC, Teguh DN, Voet P, et al. Dysphagia disorders in patients with cancer of the oropharynx are significantly affected by the radiation therapy dose to the superior and middle constrictor muscle: a dose-effect relationship. Radiother Oncol. 2007;85:64–73.
8. Eisbruch A, Kim HM, Feng FY, et al. Chemo-IMRT of oropharyngeal cancer aiming to reduce dysphagia: swallowing organs late complication probabilities and dosimetric correlates. Int J Radiat Oncol Biol Phys. 2011;81:e93–9.
9. Eisbruch A, Ten Haken RK, Kim HM, et al. Dose, volume, and function relationships in parotid salivary glands following conformal and intensity-modulated irradiation of head and neck cancer. Int J Radiat Oncol Biol Phys. 1999;45:577–87.
10. Eisbruch A, Kim HM, Terrell JE, et al. Xerostomia and its predictors following parotid-sparing irradiation of head-and-neck cancer. Int J Radiat Oncol Biol Phys. 2001;50:695–704.
11. Holliday EB, Frank SJ. Proton radiation therapy for head and neck cancer: a review of the clinical experience to date. Int J Radiat Oncol Biol Phys. 2014;89:292–302.
12. Metz JM, editor. Proton therapy. Radiation medicine rounds. New York: Demos Medical; 2010.
13. Lee NY, Lu JJ, editors. Target volume delineation and field setup: a practical guide for conformal and intensity-modulated radiation therapy. New York: Springer; 2012.
14. Lee NY, Riaz N, Lu JJ, editors. Target volume delineation for conformal and intensity-modulated radiation therapy. New York: Springer; 2015.
15. Ma C, Lomax T, editors. Proton and carbon ion therapy. Florida: CRC Press; 2012.
16. DeLaney TF, Kooy HM, editors. Proton and charged particle radiotherapy. New York: Lippincott Williams & Wilkins; 2007.

Non-melanoma Skin Cancer with Clinical Perineural Invasion

10

Curtis Bryant and Roi Dagan

Contents

10.1	Introduction	175
10.2	Immobilization/Simulation	177
10.3	Target Delineation and Dose	177
10.4	Elective Radiation Therapy to Regional Nodal Stations	179
10.5	Radiation Dose and Fractionation	180
10.6	Target Coverage	180
10.7	Normal Tissue Definition	181
10.8	Three-Dimensional (3D) Proton Treatment Planning	182
	10.8.1 Passive Scattering Versus Spot Scanning	182
10.9	Planning with Passive Scattering	182
	10.9.1 Planning with Spot Scanning	184
References		184

10.1 Introduction

Non-melanoma skin cancer (NMSC) is the most common cancer in the USA and includes cutaneous basal cell and squamous cell carcinoma [1]. Although these skin cancers often present as localized and resectable [2], rarely, NMSC can present or recur with clinical perineural invasion, a condition wherein tumor cells surround nearby nerve sheaths and spread proximally along the motor or sensory nerve to the base of skull [3, 4]. From there, the tumor can spread intracranially to the nerve ganglion. The hallmarks of clinical perineural invasion are radiographic evidence of

C. Bryant (✉) • R. Dagan
University of Florida Health Proton Therapy Institute,
2015 North Jefferson St., Jacksonville, FL 32206, USA
e-mail: cbryant@floridaproton.org

© Springer International Publishing Switzerland 2018
N. Lee et al. (eds.), *Target Volume Delineation and Treatment Planning for Particle Therapy*, Practical Guides in Radiation Oncology,
https://doi.org/10.1007/978-3-319-42478-1_10

nerve invasion and clinical symptoms, including paresthesia, formication, and numbness or paralysis of the involved nerve [3, 4].

NMSCs with clinical perineural invasion are challenging to treat in part because of tumor location. These NMSCs often originate from the midface, scalp, or lateral surface of the face. In these locations, branches of the fifth or seventh cranial nerve can be involved, and the disease may track to the base of skull and approach the brain, brainstem, inner ear, and/or optic structures [3, 4]. Radiographic examples of clinical perineural invasion can be seen in Figs. 10.1 and 10.2.

Surgical resection of NMSCs in these locations puts important cranial nerves and blood vessels at risk, making it difficult to obtain a gross total resection without causing major adverse effects. Radiation therapy is indicated when the expected morbidity of surgical resection is unacceptable. Because high-dose radiation therapy may also cause significant morbidity, the superior conformality of particle therapy may improve the therapeutic ratio in the management of NMSCs with clinical perineural invasion when compared to photon-based radiation therapy [5]. Proton therapy has been shown to reduce the dose to the organs at risk (OAR) significantly when compared to photon-based radiation for other head and neck and base-of-skull tumors [6–8]. Proton therapy also reduces the risk for acute and late side effects when compared to intensity-modulated radiation therapy when using ipsilateral head and neck treatment plans commonly employed for NMSCs [9]. The focus of this chapter is to describe the recommended method of proton therapy delivery for NMSC with clinical perineural invasion.

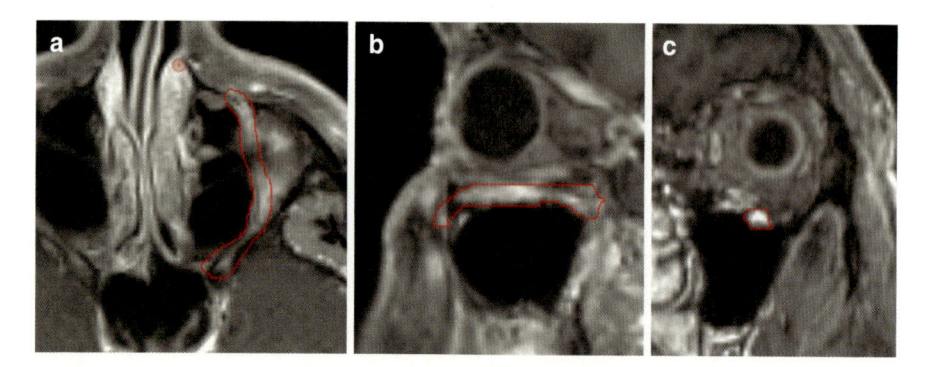

Fig. 10.1 Diagnostic preoperative magnetic resonance imaging (MRI) of a recurrent T4 N0 M0 basal cell carcinoma involving the V2 branch of the left trigeminal nerve. The patient underwent a previous resection of a cutaneous basal cell carcinoma without displaying any local recurrence on the skin. Perineural invasion is best visualized on MRI. On T1-weighted MRI images, involved nerves may be enlarged and often show abnormal contrast enhancement. There may also be enhancement and atrophy of the muscles innervated by the affected nerve. (**a**) Contrast-enhanced axial T1-weighted image. (**b**) Contrast-enhanced sagittal T1-weighted image. (**c**) Contrast-enhanced T1-weighted coronal image. Note that on T1-weighted contrast-enhanced images, tumors showing perineural invasion of major nerves usually enhance. The gross tumor volume is outlined in the red contour

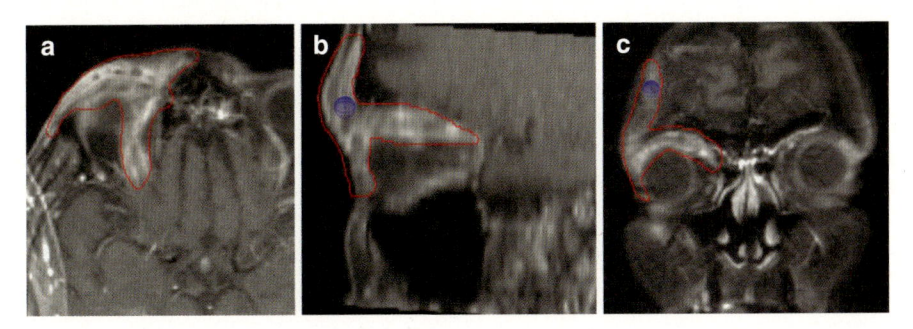

Fig. 10.2 Diagnostic magnetic resonance imaging of a patient with recurrent squamous cell carcinoma of the skin of the right forehead and upper eyelid. The tumor locally recurred after initial resection to involve the subcutaneous tissue above the right eye and the V1 branch of the trigeminal nerve. (**a**) Contrast-enhanced fat-suppressed axial T1-weighted image. (**b**) Contrast-enhanced fat-suppressed sagittal T1-weighted image. (**c**) Contrast-enhanced fat-suppressed coronal T1-weighted image. The gross tumor volume is outlined in the *red contour*

10.2 Immobilization/Simulation

Immobilization is performed with the patient positioned supine and the head and neck in a base-of-skull frame. The neck is extended with an Aquaplast mask fitted over the patient's head and neck. A neck cushion is used to minimize air gaps behind the neck. The base-of-skull frame allows for the patient's head and neck to be extended beyond the table, which minimizes the air gap between the treatment head and reduces the lateral penumbra of the beam. Oral stents may be placed in the mouth to push the tongue out of the treatment volume, particularly if the maxilla is being treated. If there is gross cancer on the skin that must be treated, its location and extent are marked with a wire at the time of simulation. Computed tomography (CT) scans are obtained with and without intravenous contrast. The primary image set is the non-contrasted CT scan to ensure that the introduction of contrast, which has a high stopping power, does not falsely affect proton dosimetry when planning. The CT scans are obtained from the vertex of the skull to the upper chest. Obtaining T1- and T2-weighted multiplanar magnetic resonance imagings (MRI) with 1- to 2-mm-thick slices is critical for treatment planning. These images help define the primary tumor and the route of perineural spread.

10.3 Target Delineation and Dose

The target volumes and OARs are delineated on the planning CT scan according to the guidelines of the International Commission on Radiation Units and Measurements [10]. The gross tumor volume (GTV) is contoured on the CT planning scan. The registered MRI scans should aid in the visualization of the areas of gross perineural involvement. If systemic therapy was delivered or surgery performed before radiation therapy, a pretreatment GTV is created and outlined on the treatment planning CT. The standard-risk clinical target volume (CTV SR) should include the GTV and the involved nerve from its distal end to its ganglion due to the potential for skip lesions extending from the proximal to the distal end of the involved nerve. Depending on the tumor location, the CTV SR may also include other nerve branches if they are at risk of involvement, and a contouring atlas has recently been published to guide the development of the CTV [11]. Examples of target volumes are included in Figs. 10.3 and 10.4.

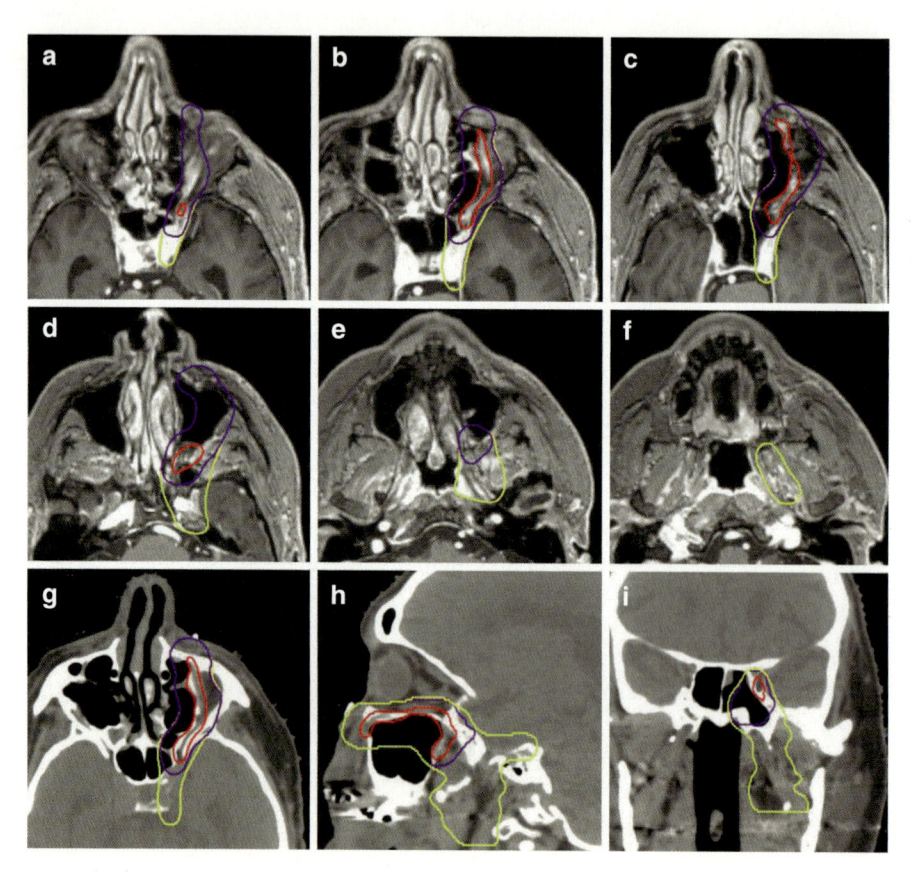

Fig. 10.3 (a–f) Planning magnetic resonance imaging fused to the planning computed tomography of a patient with a recurrent basal cell carcinoma with clinical perineural invasion of the V2 branch of the trigeminal nerve. The gross tumor volume is outlined in the *red contour*. The high-risk clinical target volume (CTV HR; *purple*) includes the gross tumor with a 5-mm margin edited for anatomic boundaries. The standard-risk CTV (*yellow contour*) includes the CTV HR and areas at risk for microscopic tumor spread, including the entire cavernous sinus, trigeminal ganglion, and the proximal aspect V3 branch of the trigeminal nerve. (g–i) The planned computed tomography in the axial, sagittal, and coronal views

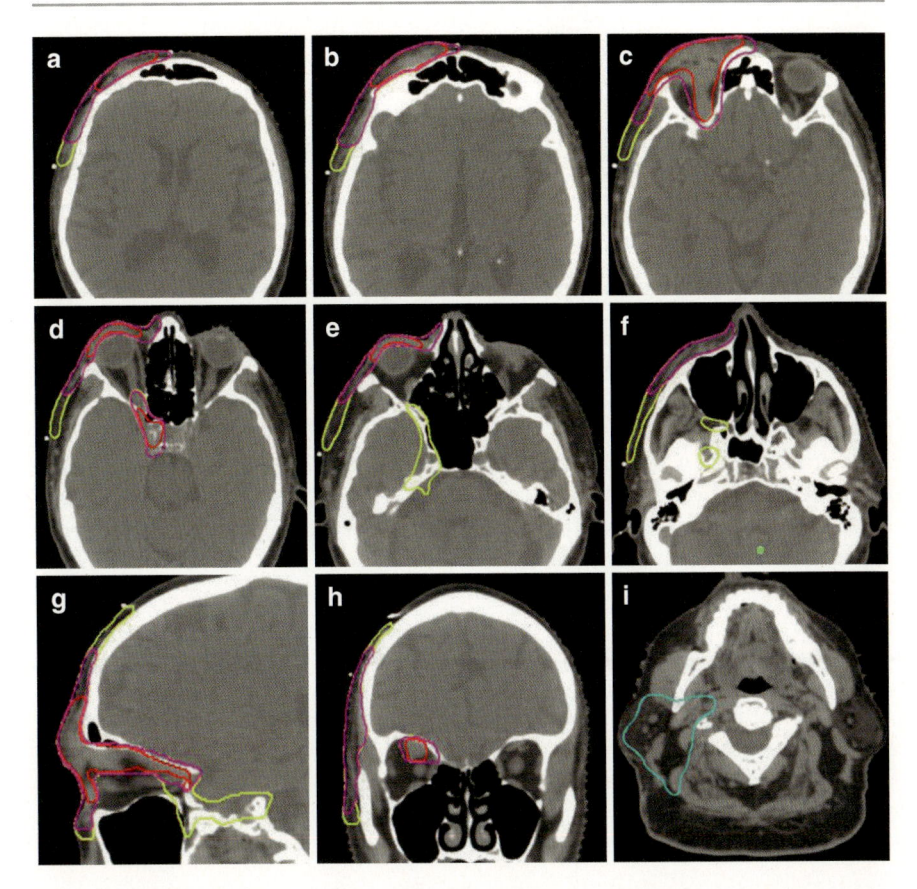

Fig. 10.4 Planned computed tomography of a patient with recurrent squamous cell carcinoma of the skin of the right forehead and upper eyelid. The tumor locally recurred after initial resection to involve the subcutaneous tissue above the right eye and the V1 branch of the trigeminal nerve. The pre-gross tumor volume is outlined in the red contour. The standard-risk clinical target volume (CTV; *yellow contour*) is highlighted in yellow, and it includes the skin of the right forehead, the ipsilateral cavernous sinus, and the trigeminal ganglion. The high-risk CTV (*pink contour*) includes the gross cancer involving V1, the subcutaneous tissue of the forehead, the upper eyelid, and the grossly involved aspect of the cavernous sinus. The right parotid and regional nodal stations in the ipsilateral neck are included in a separate standard-risk CTV (*blue contour*), and it too is treated with proton therapy

10.4 Elective Radiation Therapy to Regional Nodal Stations

For patients with clinical perineural invasion, the risk for regionally involved lymph nodes is greater than 15%; consequently, elective nodal radiation should be performed [5]. For lesions involving the midface, the lymph nodes at risk for microscopic disease include the ipsilateral lateral retropharyngeal nodes as well as levels IB, II, III, and IV. For tumors that involve the ears, scalp, temple, preauricular region, forehead, or cheek, the parotid is also at risk for regional nodal spread and should be treated with elective radiation therapy.

10.5 Radiation Dose and Fractionation

When delivering proton therapy with a sequential boost technique, our recommendation is to treat the planning target volume (PTV) SR to 50 Gy (RBE) at 2 Gy (RBE) per fraction. A boost dose should be provided to the high-risk PTV (PTV HR) of 16–20 Gy (RBE) at 2 Gy (RBE) per fraction (to a total 66–70 Gy [RBE]). If the optic chiasm, optic nerve, or retina is in close proximity to the PTV HR, the patient will be at significant risk for vision loss from retinopathy or optic neuropathy. Hyperfractionated radiation therapy has been shown to reduce the risk for visual deficits after high-dose radiation while accelerating the treatment schedule and potentially increasing the potential for local control in patients with head and neck cancers [12]. Consequently, for patients at high risk for vision loss, we recommend treating the PTV SR to 50.4 Gy (RBE) at 1.2 Gy (RBE) per fraction using twice-daily fractionation with a 6-h interval between doses. The PTV HR is then treated to an additional 19.2–24 Gy (RBE) at 1.2 Gy (RBE) per fraction (to a total dose of 69.4–74.4 Gy [RBE]). Table 10.1 summarizes our recommendations for dose delivery and target volume delineation.

10.6 Target Coverage

The goals for target coverage for fractionated radiation should be explicit and followed closely. Our recommendation is to cover 95% of the PTV with the target dose. We also recommend that 99% of the target receive at least 93% of the target dose to minimize cold spots. The volume of tissue receiving more than 110% of the target dose is limited to 20% of the PTV or less. The location of hot spots is limited

Table 10.1 Recommendations for dose delivery and target volume delineation

Volume	Target	Dose
GTV	Gross disease seen on CT and/or MRI and on physical examination of a primary skin lesion	–
HR CTV	The gross disease with an isocentric 0.5-cm margin edited for anatomic boundaries to clinical spread. If a primary skin lesion is included in the target volume, a 1- to 2-cm margin on the skin surface should be provided	66–70 Gy (RBE) at 2 Gy (RBE) per fraction Or 69.4–74.4 Gy (RBE) at 1.2 Gy (RBE) per fraction using twice-daily fractionation
SR CTV	The gross disease with an isocentric margin expansion of 0.5–1 cm edited for anatomic boundaries to clinical spread. If the nerve ganglion is involved, other proximal branches of the named nerve may be included. Also the regional nodes at risk for spread should be included in this volume	50 Gy (RBE) at 2 Gy (RBE) per fraction Or 50.4 Gy (RBE) at 1.2 Gy (RBE) per fraction using twice-daily fractionation

CT computed tomography, *MRI* magnetic resonance imaging, *GTV* gross tumor volume, *HR CTV* high-risk clinical target volume, *SR CTV* standard-risk clinical target volume

to areas within the CTV. If the dose to OARs, including the brainstem or optic chiasm, is predicted to be critically high, the number or fractions or target coverage can be compromised as per the clinician's best judgment. We also take into consideration the preferences of the patient and the risks that he or she is willing to accept in hope of a cure.

10.7 Normal Tissue Definition

The OARs are contoured on the CT planning scan and on the treatment planning MRI obtained at the time of simulation. The following normal structures are contoured at the time of planning: retinas, optic nerves, optic chiasm, lenses, lacrimal glands, brainstem, spinal cord, temporal lobes, hippocampi, hypothalamus, pituitary gland, parotid glands, larynx, submandibular glands, pharyngeal constrictors, and lenses. The radiation dose to these target structures are calculated at the time of treatment planning and kept as low as possible. A recommended dose constraint guideline is listed in Table 10.2.

Table 10.2 Dose constraint guideline

Structure	DVH point	Limit	Minor deviation	Major deviation
PTV	Relative dose at 95% volume	100%	D95% ≤ 100%	–
PTV	Relative dose at 99% volume	93%	D99% ≤ 93%	–
PTV	Relative volume at 110% dose	20%	V110 ≥ 20%	–
Brainstem	Absolute dose at 0.1 cm^3	55 Gy	55 ≤ D0.1 cm^3 < 64 Gy	D0.1cm^3 ≥ 64 Gy
Brainstem	Maximum absolute dose	60 Gy	60 ≤ Dmax <67 Gy	Dmax ≥67 Gy
Brainstem surface	Absolute dose at 0.1 cm^3	55 Gy	55 ≤ D0.1 cm^3 < 64 Gy	D0.1cm^3 ≥ 64 Gy
Brainstem core	Absolute dose at 0.1 cm^3	50 Gy	50 ≤ D0.1 cm^3 < 60 Gy	D0.1cm^3 ≥ 60 Gy
Spinal cord	Absolute dose at 0.1 cm^3	50 Gy	50 ≤ D0.1 cm^3 < 55 Gy	D0.1cm^3 ≥ 55 Gy
Optic chiasm	Absolute dose at 0.1 cm^3	55 Gy	55 ≤ D0.1 cm^3 < 60 Gy	D0.1cm^3 ≥ 60 Gy
Optic chiasm	Maximum absolute dose	57 Gy	57 ≤ Dmax <62 Gy	Dmax ≥62 Gy
Optic nerve, left	Absolute dose at 0.1 cm^3	55 Gy	55 ≤ D0.1 cm^3 < 60 Gy	D0.1cm^3 ≥ 60 Gy
Optic nerve, right	Absolute dose at 0.1 cm^3	55 Gy	55 ≤ D0.1 cm^3 < 60 Gy	D0.1cm^3 ≥ 60 Gy
Retina, left	Absolute dose at 0.1 cm^3	50 Gy	50 ≤ D0.1 cm^3 < 60 Gy	D0.1cm^3 ≥ 60 Gy
Retina, right	Absolute dose at 0.1 cm^3	50 Gy	50 ≤ D0.1 cm^3 < 60 Gy	D0.1cm^3 ≥ 60 Gy
Larynx	Mean absolute dose	36 Gy	–	Dmean ≥36 Gy
Cochlea, left	Mean absolute dose	36 Gy	36 ≤ Dmean <45 Gy	Dmean ≥45 Gy
Cochlea, right	Mean absolute dose	36 Gy	36 ≤ Dmean <45 Gy	Dmean ≥45 Gy
Parotid, left	Mean absolute dose	26 Gy	Dmean ≥26 Gy	–
Parotid, right	Mean absolute dose	26 Gy	Dmean ≥26 Gy	–

(continued)

Table 10.2 (continued)

Structure	DVH point	Limit	Minor deviation	Major deviation
Submandibular gland, left	Mean absolute dose	40 Gy	Dmean ≥40 Gy	–
Submandibular gland, right	Mean absolute dose	40 Gy	Dmean ≥40 Gy	–
Cervical esophagus	Mean absolute dose	50 Gy	Dmean ≥50 Gy	–
Oral cavity	Mean absolute dose	36 Gy	Dmean ≥36 Gy	–
Pharyngeal constrictor	Mean absolute dose	50 Gy	50 ≤ Dmean <60 Gy	Dmean ≥60 Gy
Lacrimal gland, left	Mean absolute dose	34 Gy	34 ≤ Dmean <41 Gy	Dmean ≥41 Gy
Lacrimal gland, right	Mean absolute dose	34 Gy	34 ≤ Dmean <41 Gy	Dmean ≥41 Gy
Hypothalamus	Mean absolute dose	5 Gy	Dmean ≥5 Gy	–
Pituitary	Mean absolute dose	30 Gy	Dmean ≥30 Gy	–
Mandible	Mean absolute dose	40 Gy	–	Dmean ≥40 Gy
Mandible	Relative volume at 70 Gy	10%	–	V70 ≥ 10%
Brain	Absolute volume at 74 Gy	2 cm³	V74 ≥ 2 cm³	–
Lens, right	Maximum absolute dose	15 Gy	Dmax ≥15 Gy	–
Lens, left	Maximum absolute dose	15 Gy	Dmax ≥15 Gy	–

DVH dose-volume histogram, *PTV* planned target volume

10.8 Three-Dimensional (3D) Proton Treatment Planning

10.8.1 Passive Scattering Versus Spot Scanning

Proton therapy can be delivered using passive scattering or spot scanning. Each technique has its unique advantages and disadvantages. For example, because passive-scattering proton therapy uses brass apertures to shape the edges of the beam, the lateral dose gradient will usually be sharper than that of some pencil beam systems, particularly those with larger spot sizes. Passive-scattering planning also utilizes compensator smoothing and smearing, which helps to improve plan robustness. In spot-scanning intensity-modulated proton therapy (IMPT) plans, the beam is scanned magnetically to cover the target. Spot placement and weighting are optimized using inverse planning software, which is a more efficient process than planning passive-scattering proton therapy. Additionally, spot scanning delivered using IMPT usually improves conformality in plans featuring PTVs with convexities.

10.9 Planning with Passive Scattering

Typically, 3–5 fields are used to deliver passive-scattering proton therapy to non-melanoma skin cancers with clinical perineural invasion. For each field, range modulation is used to ensure that the spread-out Bragg peak covers the entire radiographic depth of the CTV. Range uncertainty is accounted for by adding to the distal margin a distance calculated as 2.5–3% of the expected range plus 1.5–2 mm. Field-specific apertures conform the beam laterally to the target, and the distal dose falloff of each field is shaped by custom beam compensators. Compensator smearing can be performed to account for geometric uncertainties in proton range caused by patient motion or setup inaccuracies.

Examples of block design and beam angles used for typical plans are included in Figs. 10.5 and 10.6. In general, we recommend minimizing the number of fields for

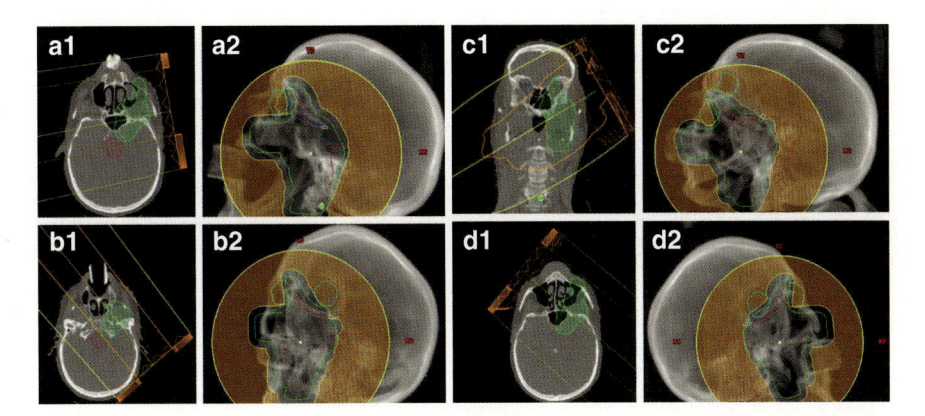

Fig. 10.5 Example of a passive-scatter proton therapy plan in the management of a patient with an rT4 N0 M0 squamous cell carcinoma of involving the V2 branch of the left trigeminal nerve. The standard-risk planned target volume is shown in green. (**a**1, 2) A 4-field proton plan is displayed with the left-anterior oblique, (**b**1, 2) left-posterior oblique, (**c**1, 2) left-posterior superior-posterior oblique, and (**d**1, 2) right-superior-anterior oblique fields. Each field uses block margins and angles to treat the target and spare organs at risk

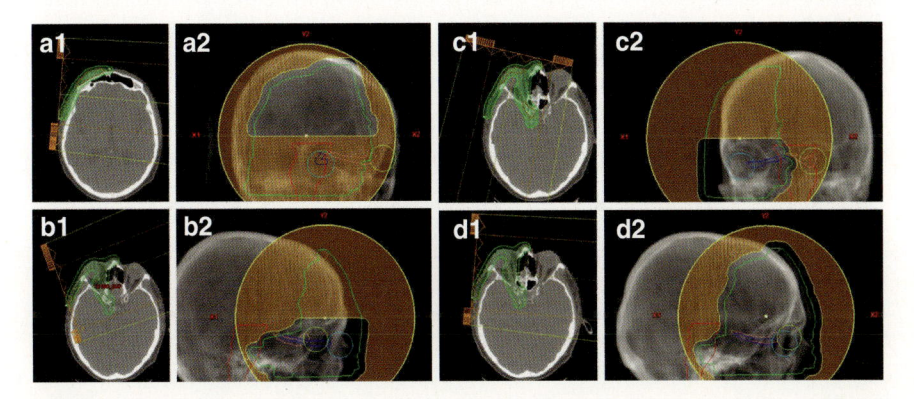

Fig. 10.6 An example of a passive-scattered proton therapy plan in the management of a patient with recurrent squamous cell carcinoma of the skin of the right forehead and upper eyelid. The tumor locally recurred after initial resection to involve the subcutaneous tissue above the right eye and the V1 branch of the trigeminal nerve. The planned target volume (PTV) is shown in green. (**a**1, 2) A 4-field proton plan is displayed with the right-anterior-superior oblique field functioning as a match field and treating the upper aspect of the PTV. (**b**1, 2) A right-posterior-oblique field treats the inferior aspect of the PTV. (**c**1, 2) A left-anterior-oblique field treats the inferior PTV. (**d**1, 2) A right-anterior-oblique field treats the entire PTV

which the spread-out Bragg peak ends on an OAR—such as the brainstem or optic chiasm—because of concerns that the radiobiological equivalence (RBE) of the beam in this location could exceed 1.1. Our general rule is that no more than one-third of the fraction dose is delivered using a field that ends on a critical structure. We also try to minimize the number of beams that overlap on the skin because there is relatively little skin sparing with proton therapy. Noncoplanar beams can be used to avoid delivering dose to the OARs, like the optic structures, but the number of such fields should be minimized to reduce the treatment time and to improve setup accuracy since performing a couch kick introduces uncertainty. In most cases, we minimize the use of patch-and-through fields to eliminate the potential for under- and overdosage at the dosimetric matchlines. Field matching can be used to reduce the dose to OARs near the PTV and also to improve conformality when the target volume sharply changes shape and depth as seen in Fig. 10.5a1–b1.

Delivering elective nodal radiation can be challenging with passive-scattering proton therapy when attempting to use the same fields as those designed for the primary site. We treat the neck with conventional photon irradiation, which can be dosimetrically matched to fields treating the clinical target volume at the primary site. A dosimetric gap of 5 mm can be used to avoid potential hot spots between the two plans.

10.9.1 Planning with Spot Scanning

With spot scanning, the proton beam is magnetically scanned to cover the target in three dimensions. The beam can be delivered using one of two treatment planning modes: single-field uniform dose (SFUD) mode or multi-field uniform dose (MFUD) mode. In SFUD, the scanning pattern and beam intensity are optimized for each field, but the dose distribution is uniform over the target volume. In MFUD, all of the fields are optimized together to provide a uniform dose to the target with each individual field providing a heterogeneous intensity of radiation to the target volume. MFUD is often described as IMPT and can provide better conformality than SFUD plans. Similar to passive scattering, most proton plans with spot scanning will include 3–5 proton beams. Similar to intensity-modulated radiation therapy, plan optimization is based on objectives for target coverage, OAR sparing, dose uniformity, and their relative weights in the planning algorithm. With MFUD, apertures and compensators are unnecessary, and a spread-out Bragg peak is not created so that the uncertainties associated with spot-scanning proton therapy plans are different. Although concerns about the robustness of IMPT plans are a subject of controversy, recent advancements in the analysis of plan robustness have alleviated some concerns, making MFUD an excellent choice in the management of NMSCs with clinical perineural invasion.

References

1. American Cancer Society. Key statistics for basal and squamous cell skin cancers. 2016. http://www.cancer.org/cancer/skincancer-basalandsquamouscell/detailedguide/skin-cancer-basal-and-squamous-cell-key-statistics.

2. Mendenhall WM, Million RR, Mancuso AA, Cassisi NJ, Flowers FP. Carcinoma of the skin. In: Million RR, Cassisi NJ, editors. Management of head and neck cancer: a multidisciplinary approach. 2nd ed. Philadelphia, PA: J. B. Lippincott Company; 1994. p. 643–91.
3. Feasel AM, Brown TJ, Bogle MA, Tschen JA, Nelson BR. Perineural invasion of cutaneous malignancies. Dermatol Surg. 2001;27(6):531–42.
4. Geist DE, Garcia-Moliner M, Fitzek MM, Cho H, Rogers GS. Perineural invasion of cutaneous squamous cell carcinoma and basal cell carcinoma: raising awareness and optimizing management. Dermatol Surg. 2008;34(12):1642–51.
5. Mendenhall WM, Amdur RJ, Hinerman RW, et al. Skin cancer of the head and neck with perineural invasion. Am J Clin Oncol. 2007;30(1):93–6.
6. Mendenhall NP, Malyapa RS, Su Z, et al. Proton therapy for head and neck cancer: rationale, potential indications, practical considerations, and current clinical evidence. Acta Oncol. 2011;50(6):763–71.
7. Mock U, Georg D, Bogner J, Auberger T, Potter R. Treatment planning comparison of conventional, 3D conformal, and intensity-modulated photon (IMRT) and proton therapy for paranasal sinus carcinoma. Int J Radiat Oncol Biol Phys. 2004;58(1):147–54.
8. Lomax AJ, Goitein M, Adams J. Intensity modulation in radiotherapy: photons versus protons in the paranasal sinus. Radiother Oncol. 2003;66(1):11–8.
9. Romesser PB, Cahlon O, Scher E, et al. Proton beam radiation therapy results in significantly reduced toxicity compared with intensity-modulated radiation therapy for head and neck tumors that require ipsilateral radiation. Radiother Oncol. 2016;118(2):286–92.
10. Definition of volumes. J ICRU. 2010;10(1):41–53.
11. Ko HC, Gupta V, Mourad WF, et al. A contouring guide for head and neck cancers with perineural invasion. Pract Radiat Oncol. 2014;4(6):e247–58.
12. Bhandare N, Monroe AT, Morris CG, Bhatti MT, Mendenhall WM. Does altered fractionation influence the risk of radiation-induced optic neuropathy? Int J Radiat Oncol Biol Phys. 2005;62(4):1070–7.

Head and Neck Reirradiation

Carl DeSelm, Upendra Parvathaneni, and Kevin Sine

Contents

11.1 Introduction 187
11.2 Simulation, Target Delineation, and Radiation Dose/Fractionation 188
11.3 Patient Positioning, Immobilization, and Treatment Verification 188
11.4 Target Delineation 189
11.5 Proton Treatment Planning 191
11.6 Critical Structure Constraints 193
11.7 Toxicity 195
11.8 Future Developments 195
References 196

11.1 Introduction

- Treatment of locoregional failure, recurrence, or second primary tumor after prior exposure to high-dose (>50 Gy) RT in the head and neck is difficult. If left untreated, the prognosis is very poor, with a median survival of only 5 months [1]. Surgical resection and reirradiation are the only two curative options, and surgical resection is only possible in roughly 20% of patients [2–4]. When

---

C. DeSelm
Memorial Sloan Kettering Cancer Center, New York, NY, USA

University of Washington Medical Center, Seattle, WA, USA

U. Parvathaneni (✉)
University of Washington Medical Center, Seattle, WA, USA
e-mail: Upendra@Uw.edu

K. Sine
ProCure Proton Therapy Center, Somerset, NJ, USA

© Springer International Publishing Switzerland 2018
N. Lee et al. (eds.), *Target Volume Delineation and Treatment Planning for Particle Therapy*, Practical Guides in Radiation Oncology,
https://doi.org/10.1007/978-3-319-42478-1_11

feasible, surgery achieves a 5-year overall survival rate of roughly 16–36% [5, 6], and adjuvant radiation is often recommended.
- Although the timing is sometimes debated, PFS is improved with immediate compared to delayed postoperative reirradiation [7].
- Many head and neck cancer-related deaths result from persistent or recurrent locoregional disease, even in the setting of metastatic disease, exemplifying the continued importance of local control [8, 9].
- In addition, uncontrolled locoregional disease in the H&N is extremely detrimental to patients' QOL due to pain, bleeding, foul odor, and unsightly fungating masses.
- One-year LRC and OS for proton reirradiation from the largest reported series are 70% and 67%, respectively [10]. This compares favorably to photon reirradiation, where retrospective comparison from the same institution showed 1 year LRC and OS of 55% and 59%, respectively [11].
- ≤60 Gy is associated with a greater hazard ratio for local failure in the setting of reirradiation [12].
- For patients who are poor candidates for full-dose reirradiation, a less aggressive radiation regimen may be offered, known as the "Quad Shot" (3.7 Gy twice daily × 2 days, followed by a 4-week break, repeated up to 3–4 cycles) [13]. This regimen carries less risk and fewer side effects as it allows for response and symptom assessment between courses and provides palliative benefit and potentially local control benefit over no reirradiation [13].

11.2 Simulation, Target Delineation, and Radiation Dose/Fractionation

- CT simulation should be performed, ideally with IV contrast for target delineation and without contrast to be used for proton planning.
- If the tumor is not well circumscribed on CT, or if there is suspicion of soft tissue infiltration or perineural infiltration, MR is recommended.
- Recurrent disease patients should undergo PET for staging, which should be used when designing the head and neck target volume.
- If multiple areas of disease are suspected, confirmational biopsy of each area is recommended (the sensitivity of the biopsy technique should also be considered when interpreting any negative results).
- Elective nodal irradiation is not performed.
- Target volumes should be expanded according to institutional standard, typically by 3–5 mm, to create a planning target volume (PTV).
- Consultation with a medical oncologist for consideration of concurrent chemotherapy is recommended in an attempt to salvage with a curative intent.

11.3 Patient Positioning, Immobilization, and Treatment Verification

- Simulation and treatment should be conducted in the supine position with a 3-point mask for a head recurrence or a 5-point mask for disease present in the neck.

11 Head and Neck Reirradiation

- Daily orthogonal X-ray imaging or volumetric imaging (typically, with cone beam CT) is recommended to confirm setup accuracy.
- For base of skull tumors, tumors near any critical structures, or in situations where tissue heterogeneity fluctuates (such as in the sinuses where secretions and inflammation change over days), daily in-room CT imaging (i.e., cone-beam CT) is ideally used for treatment verification.
  - When in-room 3D imaging is not available, verification CT scans with the patient in treatment position are recommended during the course of treatment (e.g., every other week or once mid-treatment, depending on the tumor location and potential for anatomic changes during treatment due to weight loss, tumor shrinkage, edema, etc.).

11.4 Target Delineation

- GTV: Gross tumor volume is all-known gross disease that can be seen, palpated, or imaged, by planning CT, PET, MRI, and/or other imaging studies.
- CTV: This high-risk subclinical volume will include the tumor bed for postoperative cases. In some instances, signal changes by specialized MRI sequences or by PET may be suspicious for disease but not definitive, and inclusion of these areas is subject to clinical judgment. Elective nodal regions are not included.
- PTV: Planning target volume is CTV plus margin to ensure that the prescribed dose is actually delivered to the CTV. This margin accounts for variations in treatment delivery, including variations in setup between treatments. PTV expansions are beam specific (to account for range uncertainty) and defined at the time of treatment planning (generally 3–5 mm).
- OARs: The normal anatomy to be outlined on each CT image will include all organs potentially at risk by being within three slices of the beam path. Organs that should always be considered are the parotid and submandibular glands, eyes, optic nerves, optic chiasm, lacrimal glands, lenses, brainstem, spinal cord, temporal lobes of the brain, cochlea, brachial plexus, thyroid, larynx, esophagus, and often the carotid arteries; other structures may be considered at the time of treatment planning. The spinal cord, optic nerves, and optic chiasm should be contoured on each CT slice, when anatomically in the vicinity of the target volume. For reirradiation cases, considering the carotid arteries as an avoidance structure can significantly limit dose to this critical structure (Fig. 11.1). This may help minimize the risk of the feared potential complication of carotid blowout, which is fatal in 76% of cases [14].

General target volume and dosing guidelines are shown in (Table 11.1):

Table 11.1 Recommended target volumes and radiation doses

Volume	Target	Dose
Gross tumor volume (GTV)	Gross tumor (by imaging or physical exam, including gross residual disease after resection)	66–72 Gy(RBE)
Microscopic residual disease	Positive margin or high-risk features present post-resection, with no gross residual disease apparent by imaging or exam	60–70 Gy(RBE)

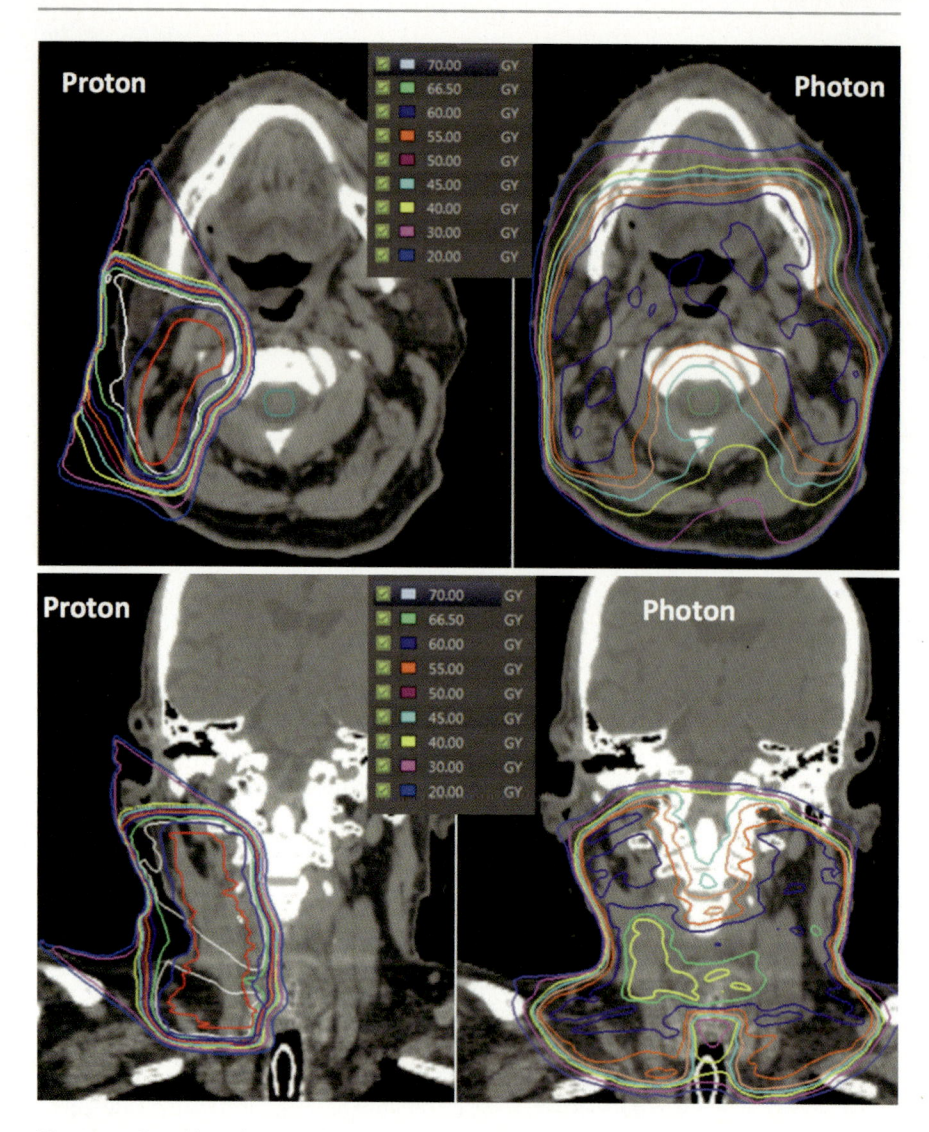

Fig. 11.1 Carotid sparing proton therapy. Proton therapy (*left plan*, *solid red* and *light green lines* in DVH) significantly limits dose to the carotid arteries compared with IMRT (*right plan*, *dotted red* and *light green lines* in DVH) and can be considered an additional avoidance structure in the reirradiation setting

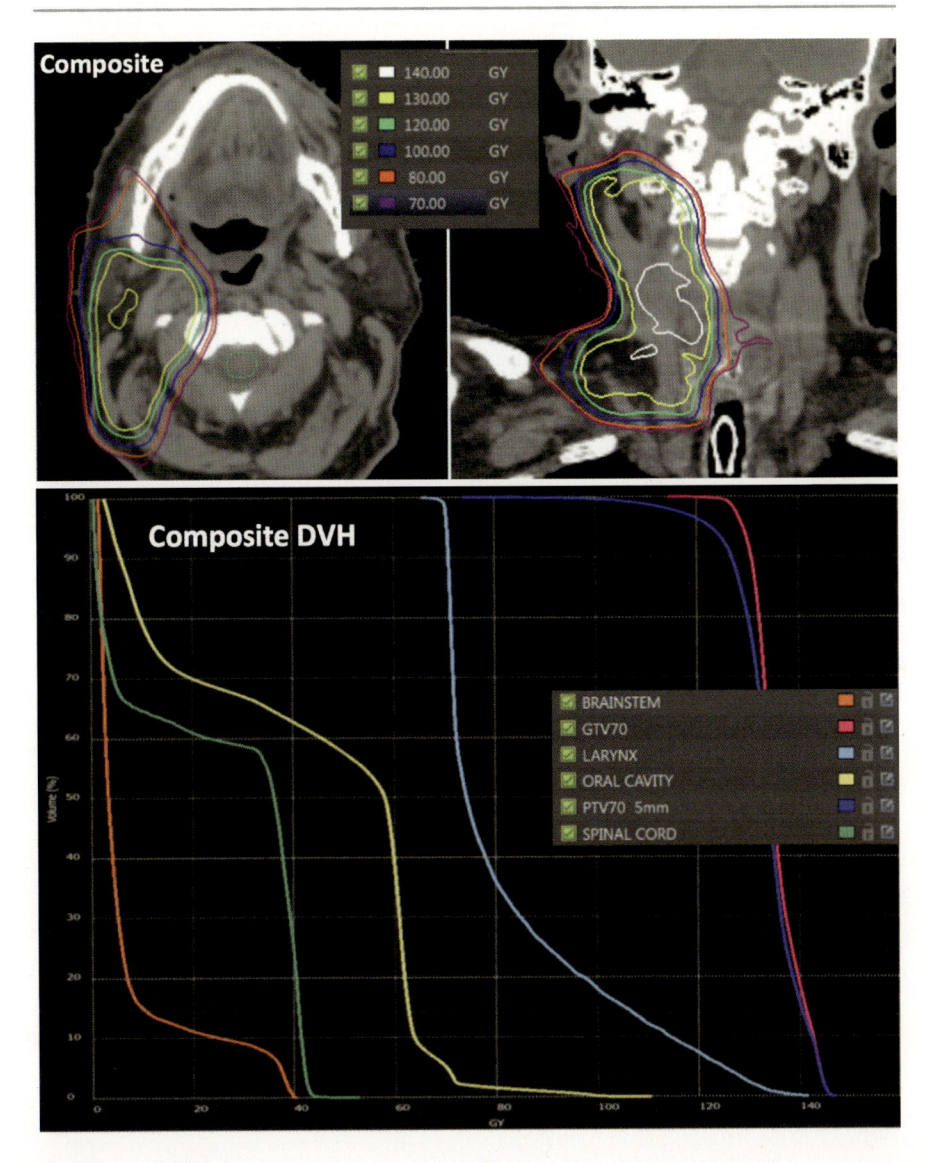

Fig. 11.1 (continued)

11.5 Proton Treatment Planning

Since recurrent tumor is often solitary and not multifocal/bilateral, either passive scattering (PS)/uniform scanning (US) or pencil beam scanning (PBS) generally provides adequate coverage and conformity. When deliberating between these options, consider:

– PBS provides greater control over the proximal portion of the beam, so skin dose or proximal OARs can be better avoided, in particular when targets are deep

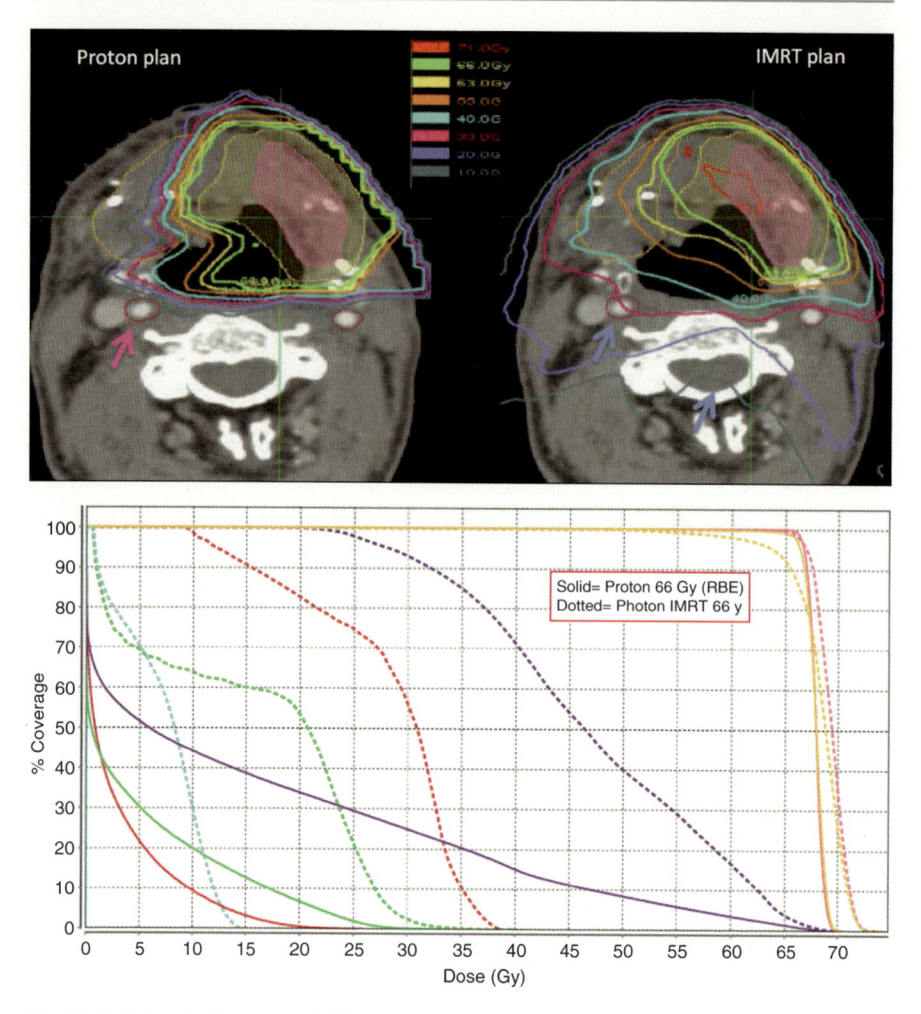

Fig. 11.2 Reirradiation proton, initial photon, and composite proton-photon plans. IMRT initially delivered 70 Gy to the GTV (*right top* and *middle*). Proton ReRT delivered an additional 70 Gy to the GTV (*left top* and *middle*). Composite plan (*lower panel*) successfully delivered a total of 140 Gy to the GTV with limited dose to normal structures (composite DVH shown)

seated and relatively small. For example, for a deep-seated tongue-base recurrence, PBS may provide more skin sparing compared to PS/US. However, the skin sparing with both modalities would be approximately similar for a superficial parotid recurrence.
- For cases with bilateral disease, PBS is the method of choice, due to the higher complexity of the case and greater control over OAR dose constraints.

Special considerations:

- The skin overlying the carotid arteries must be bolstered by a free flap after neck dissections to minimize the risk of carotid blowout.
- Be cognizant of treating anterior targets with superior oblique fields as variation in chin movement can result in skin flash with unnecessary dose to the skin of the chest wall (see Salivary chapter).
- Note when tissue heterogeneities exist, such as air pockets, dense bone, tissue density interfaces (bronchus/soft tissue), or skin surface irregularities; avoid beams through these heterogeneities if possible, especially if they have the potential to move (such as the airway near the larynx).
- Dental fillings or metal hardware, such as spinal fixation, causes loss of critical CT information needed to accurately calculate proton range. These structures can be contoured and assigned a fixed HU for treatment planning, but mixed alloy hardware or implants with materials of varying density may cause unexpected dose perturbations at the tissue/hardware interface (such as dose reduction distal to the implants, elevated dose distal to the edges of the hardware, and range degradation [15], which in the setting of reirradiation may become even more impactful. Multiple beams with varied angles relative to the hardware, the use of PS/US rather than PBS, integration of photons for a portion of the treatment, or at least metal artifact reduction algorithms are recommended.
- Dental artifacts could also be replaced by non-radiopaque composite material that minimizes the impact of the artifacts [16].
- It is possible that normal tissues that are immediately distal to the target may receive higher doses with proton therapy due to the distal end RBE effect, compared to photon therapy where the uncertainties are less; avoid placing the distal edge of more than one proton beam adjacent to a critical structure to minimize this uncertainty (Chap. 3).
- Over and under range plans should be evaluated with relevant range uncertainties as determined by each center (Chaps. 1, 3).
- Previous RT beam angles should be avoided during the ReRT planning process to avoid excessive dose along the proton beam path.
- The number of fields employed should be kept at minimum in order to decrease the volume or irradiated tissue.
- Treatment planning should include a separate review of the prior radiation plan, the current reirradiation plan, and a composite of both plans (Fig. 11.2).

11.6 Critical Structure Constraints

- Guidelines for meeting dose constraints in the primary setting are adapted below for reirradiation. In critical late responding structures, such as the brainstem and spinal canal, all attempts are made to limit the total dose from all treatments (previous and current) to the maximum described, which is the limit that would be used if only one radiation course were planned. This does not take into consideration the fact that there is a variable degree of tissue recovery between radiation courses, especially if separated by over 6 months; the length of time from prior radiation and the prior radiation dose distribution should be taken into consideration when assessing the relevance of the recommended dose constraints. Regarding reirradiation tolerance of acute responding tissue, clinical studies have shown an almost complete recovery within a few months [17]. With regard to reirradiation of late responding tissue, tolerance is dependent on the specific organ at risk.

- Attempts to obtain prior dose files and generate composite dose distributions will be made whenever possible.
- Constraining dose to the spinal cord, brainstem, and optic structures are most critical. For all other normal tissues, attempt to achieve the lowest dose possible dose (ALARA) if constraints cannot be strictly met (Fig. 11.3).

Definitive Dose (70 Gy):

Structure	Total Dose	To	Comments
Cord	53Gy	Core max	Max from current treatment
	64Gy	Surface max	
	70Gy	Dose to 0.1cc	Max from all treatments (past and present)
Optic Chiasm	60Gy	Dose to 0.05cc	Max from current treatment
	58Gy	Mean dose	
	70Gy	Dose to 0.05cc	Max from all treatments (past and present)
Optic Nerve	60Gy	Dose to 0.05cc	Max from current treatment*
	70Gy	Dose to 0.05cc	Max from all treatments (past and present)*
Brainstem	64Gy	Surface max dose	Max from current treatment; Core defined as 3mm diameter central structure within
	53Gy	Core max dose	
	70Gy	Dose to 0.05cc	Max from all treatments (past and present)
Cochlea	55Gy	Max dose	ALARA; aim for this max from all treatments (past and present)*
Retina	70Gy	Dose to 0.05cc	ALARA; aim for this max from all treatments (past and present)
Lacrimal Gland	50Gy	Mean dose	
Lens	25Gy	Max dose	
Parotid	26Gy	Mean dose	
Oral Cavity	40Gy	Mean dose	
Mandible	No hot spots	0.05 cc	
Mandible not in PTV	70Gy		
Branchial Plexus	65Gy	D95	
	70Gy	Max dose	
Esophagus	75Gy<1.5cc of partial circumference		
Submandibular Gland	39Gy		
Larynx	70Gy	0.05 cc	

*one side may be exceeded if the contralateral side is functional

Quad Shot:

Structure	Total Dose	To:	Comments
Spinal Canal, Brainstem, Chiasm, Optic Nerve	10Gy, cycle	Max point dose	Max dose from each cycle
	70Gy (max)		Total max dose from all treatments, past and present
Brachial Plexus	No hot spots		
Other normal tissues	ALARA		

Fig. 11.3 Dose volume constraints for normal critical structures. These dose values can be used as guidelines for constraining the optimization process during treatment planning; most critical are spinal cord, brainstem, and optic structures

11.7 Toxicity

Toxicity is entirely dependent on the location of the tumor and the dose to the surrounding normal structures, but for an average patient:

>20% can expect:

- Painful mucositis, dysphagia, and odynophagia
- Fatigue
- Dry mouth (xerostomia)
- Taste changes (hypogeusia)
- Thickened saliva
- Loss of appetite
- Nausea/vomiting
- Skin redness and irritation
- Weight loss

5–20% of patients will experience:

- Skin breakdown
- Dehydration requiring IV fluids
- Loss of appetite requiring nutrition supplementation
- Mouth inflammation and blisters (radioepithelitis of pharyngeal mucosa)

<5% of patients will experience:

- Carotid blowout, dysphagia, hoarseness, permanent xerostomia, trismus, nasal dryness, serous otitis media, dental decay, esophageal constriction, permanent skin changes including telangiectasias or skin breakdown (sometimes requiring a flap reconstruction), hypothyroidism, ototoxicity (especially if concurrent cisplatin is administered), and increased risk for secondary malignancies.
- Osteoradionecrosis may occur in 5% or less of patients but can be reduced by dental evaluation before radiation, as per the standard of care.
- Depending on the location of the tumor, blindness may occur if the tumor is close to or surrounding optic structures, and deafness may occur if the tumor is close to or touching the tympanic canal or CN VIII. In the vast majority of cases, this will be unilateral.

11.8 Future Developments

Many questions remain unanswered regarding proton reirradiation. For example, further knowledge of proton RBE, such as the precise effect of dose, depth, and edge effect, may further enhance our ability to plan reirradiation cases. The alpha/beta ratio of a recurrent tumor, or a tumor that has been previously reirradiated, may be significantly different from the primary tumor and from the normal surrounding tissue. Since RBE increases with decreasing alpha/beta ratio, this may impact future treatment planning. Additionally, our understanding of normal tissue tolerance to reirradiation, and the factors that influence this tolerance, such as the low-dose bath, the effect of being located at the distal edge of the beam, and the effect of initial dose and time from initial treatment, is constantly evolving.

References

1. Stell P. Survival times in end-stage head and neck cancer. Eur J Surg Oncol. 1989;15:407–10.
2. Mabanta SR, Mendenhall WM, Stringer SP, Cassisi NJ. Salvage treatment for neck recurrence after irradiation alone for head and neck squamous cell carcinoma with clinically positive neck nodes. Head Neck. 1999;21:591–4.
3. Ridge JA. Squamous cancer of the head and neck: surgical treatment of local and regional recurrence. Semin Oncol. 1993;20:419–29.
4. Taussky D, Rufibach K, Huguenin P, Allal AS. Risk factors for developing a second upper aerodigestive cancer after radiotherapy with or without chemotherapy in patients with head-and-neck cancers: an exploratory outcomes analysis. Int J Radiat Oncol Biol Phys. 2005;62:684–9.
5. Williams R. Recurrent head and neck cancer: the results of treatment. Br J Surg. 1974;61:691–7.
6. Ridge J. Squamous cancer of the head and neck: surgical treatment of local and regional recurrence. Semin Oncol. 1993;5:419–29.
7. Janot F, de Raucourt D, Benhamou E, et al. Randomized trial of postoperative reirradiation combined with chemotherapy after salvage surgery compared with salvage surgery alone in head and neck carcinoma. J Clin Oncol. 2008;26:5518–23.
8. Kotwall C, Sako K, Razack MS, Rao U, Bakamjian V, Shedd DP. Metastatic patterns in squamous cell cancer of the head and neck. Am J Surg. 1987;154:439–42.
9. Nishijima W, Takooda S, Tokita N, Takayama S, Sakura M. Analyses of distant metastases in squamous cell carcinoma of the head and neck and lesions above the clavicle at autopsy. Arch Otolaryngol Head Neck Surg. 1993;119:65–8.
10. Romesser PB, Cahlon O, Scher ED, et al. Proton beam reirradiation for recurrent head and neck cancer: multi-institutional report on feasibility and early outcomes. Int J Radiat Oncol Biol Phys. 2016;95:386–95.
11. Riaz N, Hong JC, Sherman EJ, et al. A nomogram to predict loco-regional control after re-irradiation for head and neck cancer. Radiother Oncol. 2014;111:382–7.
12. McDonald MW. Reirradiation of recurrent and second primary head and neck cancer with proton therapy. Int J Radiat Oncol Biol Phys. 2016;94:930–1.
13. Lok BH, Jiang G, Gutiontov S, et al. Palliative head and neck radiotherapy with the RTOG 8502 regimen for incurable primary or metastatic cancers. Oral Oncol. 2015;51:957–62.
14. McDonald MW, Moore MG, Johnstone PA. Risk of carotid blowout after reirradiation of the head and neck: a systematic review. Int J Radiat Oncol Biol Phys. 2012;82:1083–9.
15. Verburg JM, Seco J. Dosimetric accuracy of proton therapy for chordoma patients with titanium implants. Med Phys. 2013;40:071727.
16. Richard P, Sandison G, Dang Q, Johnson B, Wong T, Parvathaneni U. Dental amalgam artifact: adverse impact on tumor visualization and proton beam treatment planning in oral and oropharyngeal cancers. Pract Radiat Oncol. 2015;5:e583–8.
17. De Crevoisier R, Bourhis J, Domenge C, et al. Full-dose reirradiation for unresectable head and neck carcinoma: experience at the Gustave-Roussy Institute in a series of 169 patients. J Clin Oncol. 1998;16:3556–62.

Lung Cancer

12

Daniel Gomez, Heng Li, Xiaodong Zhang, and Steven Lin

Contents

12.1	Introduction	197
12.2	Simulation, Target Delineation, and Radiation Dose/Fractionation	198
12.3	Patient Positioning, Immobilization, and Treatment Verification	200
12.4	Dose Constraints	201
12.5	Proton Beam Therapy Planning	201
	12.5.1 Passive Scattering PBT Planning	201
	12.5.2 IMPT Treatment Planning	203
12.6	Clinical Outcomes of Proton Beam Therapy for Lung Cancer	206
12.7	Discussion and Future Directions	207
References		208

12.1 Introduction

Lung cancer is one of the most common malignancies, accounting for approximately 225,000 new cases and 160,000 deaths per year [1]. Treatment of lung cancer is dependent on stage, with early stages treated by surgery or radiation alone and more advanced tumors receiving bi- or trimodality therapy.

Several studies have demonstrated a dosimetric benefit of particle therapy over intensity-modulated radiation therapy (IMRT) in select cases of lung cancer [2–4]. This dosimetric superiority has been shown in cases of early-stage and locally advanced disease, as well as when comparing 3D conformal therapy and IMRT with

D. Gomez (✉) • S. Lin
Department of Radiation Oncology, MD Anderson Cancer Center, Houston, TX, USA
e-mail: dgomez@mdanderson.org

H. Li • X. Zhang
Department of Radiation Physics, MD Anderson Cancer Center, Houston, TX, USA

© Springer International Publishing Switzerland 2018
N. Lee et al. (eds.), *Target Volume Delineation and Treatment Planning for Particle Therapy*, Practical Guides in Radiation Oncology, https://doi.org/10.1007/978-3-319-42478-1_12

proton beam therapy (PBT). Notably, the improvement in normal tissue dose has primarily been present in the low-dose regions, such as the volume receiving 5 and 10 Gy(RBE) (V5 and V10, respectively). This selective benefit is due to the sharp dose buildup with PBT. The "low-dose bath" advantage of PBT is not present with advanced photon techniques.

With regard to clinical outcomes, particle therapy has been reported both for early-stage and locally advanced NSCLC [5–9]. In these studies, clinical outcomes appear to be similar to improved compared to that observed with advanced photon modalities such as IMRT and VMAT. One randomized trial has recently been reported comparing particle therapy to photons in the setting of locally advanced NSCLC. Specifically, MD Anderson Cancer Center and Massachusetts General Hospital performed a phase II randomized study comparing IMRT with passive scattered PBT in locally advanced NSCLC. The results have recently been reported in abstract form, and no statistical differences were found between the two modalities with regard to recurrence or grade ≥ 3 pneumonitis. Future analyses from this study are focusing on comparing imaging data, blood samples, further toxicity endpoints, and quality of life to determine how these factors may impact outcomes.

The dosimetric and clinical reports of particle therapy in lung cancer can thus be summarized as follows. There appears to be a dosimetric benefit for proton therapy in certain clinical scenarios, but there is not strong evidence that "all comers" with lung cancer benefit clinically from this treatment compared to advanced photon techniques. Thus, selection of patients is of critical importance, particularly when a passive scattering technique is used. These selection criteria will be discussed further below.

Small cell lung cancer (SCLC) almost always presents as locally advanced or metastatic and therefore has similar simulation, target delineation, and planning principles that apply in PBT. However, experience is very limited. In one report of six patients with a median follow-up time of 12 months, 1-year overall survival and progression-free survival rates were 83% and 66%, respectively [10]. Thus, while much of the discussion on NSCLC with regard to particle therapy techniques can be extrapolated to SCLC, more investigation is needed on outcomes with PBT, including rates of local control and the benefit of such modalities as IMPT.

12.2 Simulation, Target Delineation, and Radiation Dose/Fractionation

Patients should be simulated with their arms above their head for beam arrangement selection not dissimilar to proton techniques. An immobilization device of the upper body should be used in conjunction with 4D image acquisition to capture respiratory motion. If patients cannot raise their arms above their head, the simulation can be done with the arms at the side, though this setup may markedly limit the potential for a dosimetric benefit, particularly if passive scattering PBT is being used.

For both node-negative and node-positive disease, involved field techniques are used with 4D planning regardless of whether a photon or proton technique is utilized.

The gross tumor volume (GTV) is contoured using the CT scan of the chest with contrast and PET scan for guidance, along with histologic findings on the mediastinoscopy or endobronchial ultrasound.

There are two potential approaches for expanding on the GTV to capture both internal motion and microscopic disease. The first involves an expansion of the GTV to the CTV, followed by a further expansion to the ITV to account internal motion, followed by a PTV expansion for daily variations in patient position and movement. The second technique, which is often utilized at our institution, is performed by delineating the GTV and then assessing for internal motion. We then define a structure called the iGTV, which is then expanded to create the iCTV (which is very similar to the ITV). The advantage of the latter approach is that internal motion is being assessed on gross disease, the motion of which may be easier to delineate.

For early-stage lung cancer/SBRT, per RTOG standards, no distinct CTV margin is included, and only a PTV is delineated. For locally advanced disease, standard GTV to CTV treatment margins from the GTV (or iGTV) to CTV are 0.6–0.8 cm to control for microscopic disease, as have been defined on prior pathologic studies [11].

With regard to expansion to a planning target volume (PTV) for proton therapy, note that there is not a standard uniform PTV as exists with photon planning, which is secondary to patient setup error and is typically fixed (e.g., at 0.5–1.0 cm). Rather, the PTV includes two components: (1) *setup margin*, which takes into account day to day setup errors and is dependent on the image-guided radiation therapy (IGRT) method that is used, and (2) *dosimetric margin*, which is field-specific and encompasses proximal, distal, and lateral margins for that particular field (due to dose uncertainty in the beam path).

The PTV setup margin for PBT is 0.5 cm for photon techniques and is an extension directly from the GTV. However, this setup margin presumes that CBCT is available for daily localization. If daily CT imaging is not available, we would recommend strong consideration of fiducial placement, with daily kV imaging during treatment and a 0.5–1.0 cm PTV setup margin.

For locally advanced lung cancer (NSCLC or SCLC), the following PTV margin is utilized: 1.0–1.5 cm without daily image-guided radiation therapy (IGRT), such as kV imaging or cone-beam CT scan; 0.5–1.0 cm for either 4D CT planning or CBCT, but not both; 0.5 cm for 4D CT planning and daily kV imaging; and 0.3 cm for 4D CT planning and CBCT guidance.

The field-specific dosimetric margin is dependent on the water-equivalent range relative to the most proximal and distal points of the CTV from a specific beam angle and typically ranges from approximately 0.5 to 1.0 cm.

There are several 1–10 fraction dose regimens which have been reported and that are acceptable for PBT. In our institution, proton doses are reported with RBE = 1.1, and we routinely utilize a dose of 50 Gy in 4 fractions for peripheral disease and 70 Gy(RBE) in 10 fractions for central disease [12–14]. For locally advanced NSCLC treated with chemotherapy and radiation, the standard dose is 60 Gy(RBE) in 30 fractions, based on the recently published RTOG 0617 trial demonstrating no benefit to dose escalation to 74 Gy [15]. For SCLC, the standard-dose regimen remains 45 Gy(RBE) in 30 fractions delivered twice daily based on the results of a randomized trial comparing once daily to twice daily radiation [16]. However, the ongoing trial RTOG 0538/CALGB 30610 is currently comparing this standard regimen to a 7-week daily course of 70 Gy(RBE) in 35 fractions.

Simultaneous integrated boost regimens have been applied to the lung cancer setting as well [17–20], and multiple studies are ongoing evaluating the safety and efficacy of this approach.

12.3 Patient Positioning, Immobilization, and Treatment Verification

As noted above, patients should be simulated with the arms above their head if feasible and with upper indexed body immobilization.

For daily treatment verification, most patients undergo daily kV imaging and at least one verification simulation to ensure that there have not been substantial changes in tumor volume or differences in patient anatomy that would warrant replanning. This midtreatment verification is particularly important with particle

Table 12.1 Key definitions in PBT, dosing recommendations for locally advanced NSCLC, and SCLC

	SABR	Locally advanced NSCLC	SCLC
Prescription dose/fractions	Many 1–10 fraction regimens in use. MDACC regimen: peripheral, 12.5 Gy(RBE) × 4 fractions; central, 7Gy(RBE) × 10 fractions	Standard regimen 60 Gy(RBE) in 30 fractions with concurrent chemotherapy	Standard regimen 45 Gy(RBE) in 30 fractions twice daily with concurrent chemotherapy
iGTV to CTV margin	0 cm	0.6–0.8 cm	0.6–0.8 cm
CTV to PTV setup margin	0.5 cm (GTV to PTV) if daily CT available. If not available, 0.5–1.0 cm, ideally with fiducial placement	1.0–1.5 cm without daily IGRT 0.5 cm with daily kV imaging 0.3 cm with daily CBCT	1.0–1.5 cm without daily IGRT 0.5 cm with daily kV imaging 0.3 cm with daily CBCT
Daily treatment verification	CT scanning (e.g., CBCT, CT-on-Rails) if available and strongly recommended. If not available, strongly consider fiducial placement and then daily kV imaging with 0.5–1.0 cm setup margin	Daily kV imaging, weekly CBCT if available	Twice daily kV imaging (with each fraction), weekly CBCT if available
Verification simulation	None	At least 1 time during treatment (week 3–4), more if significant tumor changes are observed	Consider after first week of treatment if bulky disease

Table 12.2 Dosimetric constraints for PBT in standard fractionated radiation delivered once daily

Normal structure	Dose constraint
Spinal cord	Maximum dose ≤45 Gy
Heart	V30 ≤ 45 Gy(RBE), mean dose <26 Gy(RBE)
Esophagus	Mean dose < 34 Gy(RBE), V50 < 50%
Total lung	Mean dose < 20 Gy(RBE), V20 < 35%
Kidney	20 Gy(RBE) < 33% of bilateral kidney
Liver	V30 ≤ 40%

therapy, where seemingly minor differences in these parameters can have pronounced dosimetric effects.

If in-room CT capability is present, we recommend weekly cone-beam CT scans in addition to the midtreatment verification scan (Table 12.1).

12.4 Dose Constraints

Many constraints exist for PBT, which are based upon the number of fractions being delivered; constraints are from photon therapy. These constraints can be found through the National Comprehensive Cancer Network guidelines (www.nccn.org). For standard fractionated radiation delivered once daily, Table 12.2 depicts our institutional constraints. For twice daily regimens, such as that given in SCLC, similar constraints are used with the exception of the spinal cord dose, which should be limited to a maximum dose of <40 Gy(RBE).

12.5 Proton Beam Therapy Planning

12.5.1 Passive Scattering PBT Planning

12.5.1.1 Patient Selection

Patient selection for passive scattering is of importance because a non-negligible percentage of patients will have superior plans with advanced conformal techniques, such as IMRT. There are several reasons why some photon plans may be improved compared to PBT. First, there are some limitations in beam angles with passive scattering PBT due to uncertainty of dose in the beam path. Second, passive scattering PBT requires a "backstop" in order to provide much of the sharp dose falloff, which can be difficult in the context of early-stage, parenchymal lung tumors. Without high-density tissue distal to the target, dose "spikes" can occur that can then substantially affect the dosimetry. The high-dose spikes may contribute to more dose to the normal tissues than necessary and thus lead to toxicity.

With these limitations in mind, from a dosimetric standpoint, the following patients are thus good candidates for passive scattering PBT compared to IMRT: (1) location of tumor in tissue that can provide a suitable backstop that utilizes the dose falloff properties of proton therapy; (2) IMRT not feasible due to inability to meet low-dose constraints, such as V5, V10, or V20; and (3) anterior mediastinal tumors in that are proximal to the heart, lung, spinal cord, and esophagus.

12.5.1.2 Treatment Planning

A review of the passive scattering planning approach at MDACC can demonstrate several key principles of this modality, as well as its relative benefits and limitations. An example of this process is as follows. First, the physician contours the appropriate GTV and CTV and specifies the setup margin for PTV that should be used. Second, in order to provide adequate coverage of the target, all iGTV contours that overlap with lung parenchyma are overridden to represent solid tissue. If not overridden, the proton beam may "undershoot" the intended target. However, it should also be noted that doing so also creates the dosimetric disadvantage of potentially "overshooting" the tumor in certain phases of the respiratory cycle [21]. Third, the tissue in the diaphragm is overridden so that the diaphragm does not enter the treatment field, producing an inadequate distal margin (with again the risk of overshooting the target in specific cycles).

The fourth step is beam selection using several criteria. Beams are generally avoided that traverse through breast tissue, to maximize reproducibility and stability. For similar reasons, beams also aren't placed through the edge of the couch. Next, for all beams that range into the spinal cord, adequate margin is ensured through the ETV so that the spinal cord is not overdosed. At our institution, we typically utilize at least one beam that is off-cord, for similar reasons. Finally, a beam is selected that minimizes the aperture size, to reduce the dose to normal tissues. These features of beam selection are demonstrated below (Fig. 12.1).

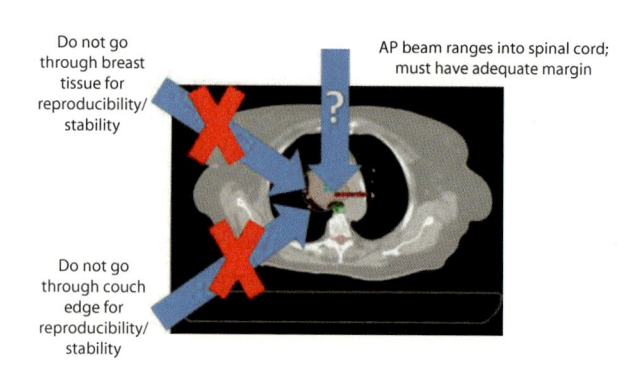

Fig. 12.1 Beam selection in passive scattering PBT

After beam selection, the compensator and aperture are edited to optimize the plan. Then, the weighting of the beam is adjusted as needed to further improve target and normal structure dose. Finally, the robustness of the plan is verified on both the T0 and T50 breathing phases. This consistency verification is again particularly important in PBT, due to the dose sensitivity to changes in tissue heterogeneity [21].

If dose constraints cannot be met at the desired dose with either photon techniques or passive scattering PBT, consideration can be given to implement pencil-beam scanning/intensity-modulated proton therapy (IMPT).

12.5.2 IMPT Treatment Planning

12.5.2.1 Patient Selection

IMPT offers the following benefits over passive scattering PBT: (1) improved conformality and (2) reduced influence of beam placement because dose can be supplemented where necessary through the technique of "patching," which also can reduce the magnitude of hot spots.

IMPT could be suitable for simultaneous integrated boost regimens because by placing the proton Bragg peak in the target, the target dose could be escalated while contributing very little dose to normal tissue. A comparative clinical trial is undergoing at our institution using IMPT and IMRT SIB techniques.

Limitations of IMPT include (1) higher dose sensitivity to changes in anatomy and tumor size due to the lower number of beams and very high conformality and (2) risk for reduced local control due to interaction between respiratory motion and spot-scanning delivery, leading to target miss through certain phases of the respiratory cycle. Two specific scenarios where this reduced dose to the target has been found in lung cancer are in the development (or reduction) of atelectasis and in changes in tumor size, the former of which is demonstrated in Fig. 12.2.

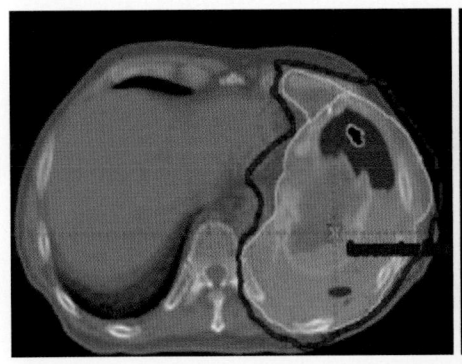

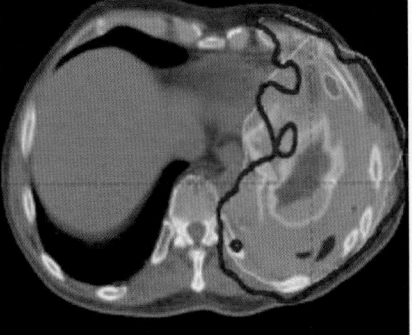

Fig. 12.2 Reduced target dose due to changes in lung volume that occurred approximately midway through a 5-week course of radiation therapy to the lung

IMPT has often been utilized in the following scenarios: (1) mediastinal but laterally displaced tumors in which there is an improved dose distribution to the lung and esophagus, (2) extremely challenging cases where the dose constraints can't be met with other techniques (e.g., large bilateral mediastinal masses), and (3) the re-irradiation setting, where the goal is to almost completely avoid dose to one or more normal structures. However, with the increased availability and experience with IMPT, more patients have been selected for this approach, particularly in locally advanced lung cancer. Several trials are ongoing examining the safety and efficacy of this approach, with particular attention being paid to local control given the concerns with respiratory motion interplay.

IMPT planning differs substantially from that of passive scattering PBT, in several ways: (1) beams are selected largely based on the minimal excursion of the proton beam path length covering the target throughout the respiratory cycle; (2) 4D treatment planning, where multiple phases from the 4DCT were used instead of the average CT, to further reduce the impact of respiratory motion on treatment planning, could be used to further reduce the impact of respiratory motion; (3) given that the technique is sensitive to changes in anatomy and tumor size, robustness optimization is often used to reduce this sensitivity; and (4) robustness evaluation of the treatment plan ensures the dose distribution and dose to target, and OARs remain acceptable with setup and range uncertainty under consideration.

Figure 12.3 shows an example of beam angle selection with water-equivalent thickness (WET) analysis, where the WET change between T0 and T50 were examine. Beam angles including one at 160° were selected for this patient because

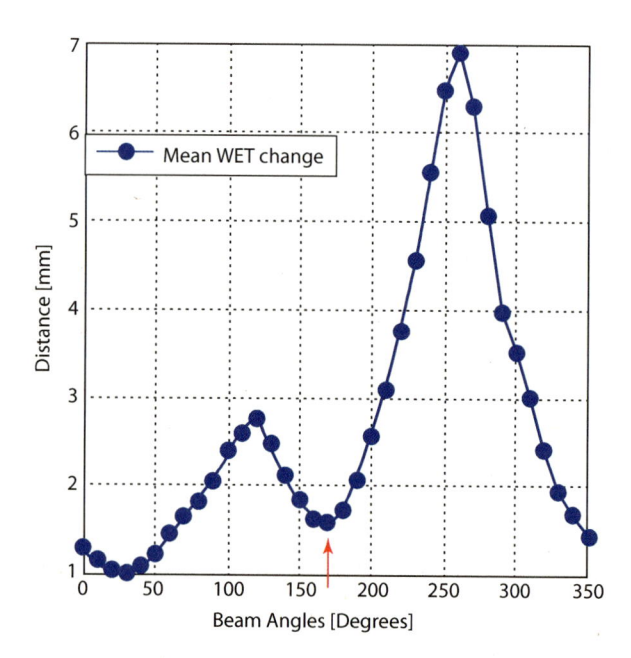

Fig. 12.3 Change in water-equivalent thickness required to cover the target volume between T0 and T50 as a function of beam angle (from Chang 2014)

of the small WET change indicating less impact from the respiratory motion, along with other considerations including patient anatomy and tumor location.

4D treatment planning [22], along with fractionation and delivery techniques such as re-scanning and optimization of the delivery sequence [23], could be used to reduce the impact of intra-fractional respiratory motion for IMPT.

Robustness optimization could lead to reduced sensitivity of the dose distribution in patient to inter-fractional setup and range uncertainties or anatomy change [24] and could be combined with 4D treatment planning [22].

The following Figs. 12.4 and 12.5 shows a sample workflow for IMPT treatment planning [25].

Robustness evaluation is crucial to IMPT planning. For lung cancer cases, we consider a difference of ≤5% between the worst-case dose distribution and the nominal dose to be acceptable [25]. If the plan was found to be not robust (quantified by a $> 5\%$ difference), then the plans are typically re-optimized.

Fig. 12.4 Procedural flow chart for intensity-modulated proton therapy (IMPT) quality assurance. 4D CT Z four-dimensional computed tomography; MFO Z multifield optimization; SFO Z single-field optimization (Chang 2014)

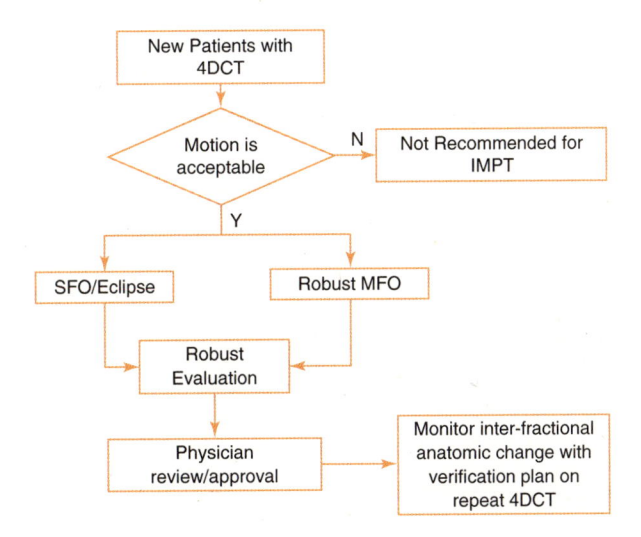

Fig. 12.5 Robustness evaluation of an IMPT plan. *Solid lines* indicate nominal DVH calculated from the time-averaged CT scan; *dotted lines*, DVH calculated from the iso- or relative stopping-power-ratio-shifted scenarios (from Chang 2014)

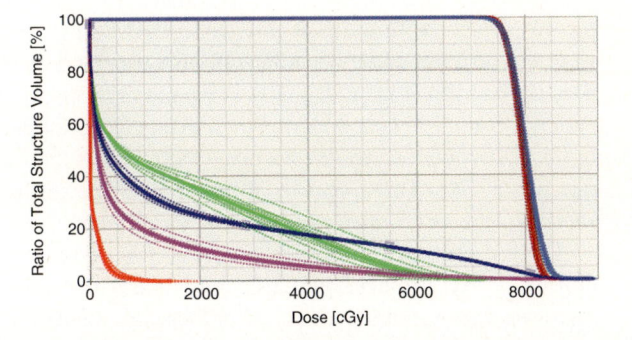

12.6 Clinical Outcomes of Proton Beam Therapy for Lung Cancer

Several retrospective and prospective single-arm studies have reported outcomes of proton beam therapy for lung cancer. With regard to early-stage cancer, several studies have been published that have demonstrated analogous results to SBRT, with high rates of local control and low toxicity [9, 26–28]. For instance, investigators from Loma Linda examined outcomes for hypofractionated radiation doses of 51–70 Gy(RBE) in 10 fractions over 2 weeks for stage T1/T2N0M0 biopsy proven NSCLC. They reported disease-specific survival rates of 88% and an overall survival of 60% at 4 years. No patient of the 111 reported required steroids for radiation pneumonitis, and central versus peripheral location did not correlate with survival outcomes. The authors therefore concluded that this regimen achieved excellent outcomes, possibly warranting the exploration of further dose escalation [28]. Of course, the primary obstacle in the setting of early-stage disease is the baseline low rate of toxicity and high local control rates with photon-based SBRT techniques, which can lead to reluctance of both physicians and patients to enroll on comparative effectiveness studies. Indeed, one recent trial from MD Anderson Cancer Center attempted to compare these two techniques in centrally located lesions and was closed due to poor accrual.

There has been more momentum for the study of proton beam therapy in the locally advanced setting, due to higher local failure rates and the common difficulty of achieving dose constraints. Therefore, several trials have reported clinical outcomes in this setting as well [29–34]. Again, in the single-arm and retrospective setting, proton beam therapy appears to hold great promise for improving the standard of care in definitive treatment. For example, investigators from Japan [35] retrospectively studied 57 patients with stage III NSCLC treated with PBT, none of whom had received concurrent chemotherapy. A median dose of 74 Gy(RBE) was administered (range 50–85 GY(RBE)) in 2-Gy(RBE) fractions (range 2–6.6 Gy(RBE)). One- and two-year OS rates were 65.5 and 39.4%. After a median follow-up interval of 22 months (for surviving patients), 2-year progression-free survival (PFS) and local control rates were 24.9 and 64.1%. Distant metastasis was the most common site of initial recurrence. In a phase II study by investigators at MD Anderson Cancer Center, [36] the authors reported outcomes with passively scattered PBT and concomitant chemotherapy (weekly carboplatin and paclitaxel) for 44 patients with unresectable stage III NSCLC. One-year OS and PFS rates were 86 and 63%, and the median OS time was 29.4. In this trial, the most common sites of recurrence were distantly (19 patients, 43%) and isolated local failures (4 patients, 9.1%). This cohort was then expanded to 84 patients by Xiang et al. [37]. In this subsequent study, the median OS time was 29.9 months, and the 3-year OS rate was 37.2%. Three-year local recurrence-free survival, distant metastasis-free survival, and a PFS rates were 34.8%, 35.4%, and 31.2%, respectively.

These outcomes compare favorably to prior studies of concurrent chemoradiation in locally advanced NSCLC, particularly the OS rate of almost 30 months. There are several possible reasons for these excellent outcomes, including improved patient selection, a higher tumor dose leading to improved disease control, and a direct correlation of reduced normal tissue dose and decreased toxicity. However, the premise of clinical superiority with protons versus photon techniques requires rigorous testing through randomized trials. Indeed, MD Anderson Cancer Center and Massachusetts General Hospital conducted a phase II Bayesian randomized trial of intensity-modulated radiation therapy versus passive scattering proton beam therapy for locally advanced lung cancer. In this trial, 149 patients with locally advanced disease were randomized to one of these two techniques at a dose of 60–74 Gy(RBE), with each patient receiving the highest dose level that could be achieved within this range without exceeding critical dose constraints. The two co-primary endpoints were local recurrence and Grade 3 or higher radiation pneumonitis. The authors found no difference in either co-primary endpoint (or when put together) between the modalities [38]. Currently, the two modalities are being tested in a larger phase III study, with OS as the primary endpoint (RTOG 1308, NCT01993810).

12.7 Discussion and Future Directions

Motion management in IMPT for lung cancer is of critical importance because of the sensitivity of the proton beam to the path length change induced by respiratory motion and the anatomy change over time. Currently most patients treated with IMPT are treated with free-breathing technique. However, due to concerns of the motion induced uncertainty, the range of the acceptable respiratory motion is usually limited. One of the reports limits the respiratory motion range to <5 mm [21, 25]. Advanced motion management techniques are being developed to make IMPT available to more patients. For example, real-time gated proton beam therapy (RGPT) system was recently developed to deliver gated treatment with high efficiency [39]. Another major concern for IMPT in lung cancer is the anatomy change over time. It has been demonstrated that adaptive therapy is necessary for a large proportion of IMPT lung cancer patients even with robustness optimization, and therefore repeating imaging and adaptive therapy is mandatory [24, 25, 40]. It is highly desirable to investigate techniques to reduce the need of or improve the efficiency of adaptive therapy for IMPT.

From a clinical outcomes standpoint, prior studies have demonstrated feasibility with respect to producing similar, if not improved, results when compared to photon-based techniques. When examining early versus locally advanced stages of disease, the most promising outcomes have been generated in the locally advanced setting, where dose constraints are more difficult to meet and locoregional failures can be as high as 50%. Disappointingly, after apparent superiority to 3D-CRT in dosimetric, retrospective, and prospective trials, the only reported prospective randomized comparative effectiveness trial demonstrated no difference in either toxicity or local control. The investigators of that trial have outlined several potential reasons for this lack of benefit, including the treatment of all patients with 3D planning techniques (rather than IMPT), as well as the fact that adequate proton delivery likely requires a learning curve, a premise that was supported by the results of this trial. And indeed, this concept is being further tested in an ongoing cooperative group trial, with OS as the primary endpoint. However, given these negative results, it is clear that the threshold for justification of proton beam therapy in "all comers" has been elevated. Therefore, future trials are likely to focus on appropriate patient selection, as well as novel delivery techniques such as spot-scanning proton arc (SPArc) therapy [41] and dynamic collimation [42], which could offer robust delivery with further reduce dose to OARs.

References

1. Larsen H, Sorensen JB, Nielsen AL, Dombernowsky P, Hansen HH. Evaluation of the optimal duration of chemotherapy in phase II trials for inoperable non-small-cell lung cancer (NSCLC). Ann Oncol. 1995;6(10):993–7.
2. Zhang X, Li Y, Pan X, et al. Intensity-modulated proton therapy reduces the dose to normal tissue compared with intensity-modulated radiation therapy or passive scattering proton therapy and enables individualized radical radiotherapy for extensive stage IIIB non-small-cell lung cancer: a virtual clinical study. Int J Radiat Oncol biol Phys. 2010;77(2):357–66.
3. Wang C, Nakayama H, Sugahara S, Sakae T, Tokuuye K. Comparisons of dose-volume histograms for proton-beam versus 3-D conformal x-ray therapy in patients with stage I non-small cell lung cancer. Strahlenther Onkol. 2009;185(4):231–4.
4. Chang JY, Zhang X, Wang X, et al. Significant reduction of normal tissue dose by proton radiotherapy compared with three-dimensional conformal or intensity-modulated radiation therapy in stage I or stage III non-small-cell lung cancer. Int J Radiat Oncol biol Phys. 2006;65(4):1087–96.
5. Nguyen QN, Ly NB, Komaki R, et al. Long-term outcomes after proton therapy, with concurrent chemotherapy, for stage II–III inoperable non-small cell lung cancer. Radiother Oncol. 2015;115(3):367–72.
6. McAvoy SA, Ciura KT, Rineer JM, et al. Feasibility of proton beam therapy for reirradiation of locoregionally recurrent non-small cell lung cancer. Radiother Oncol. 2013;109(1):38–44.
7. Ishikawa Y, Nakamura T, Kato T, et al. Dosemetric parameters predictive of rib fractures after proton beam therapy for early-stage lung cancer. Tohoku J Exp Med. 2016;238(4):339–45.
8. Hoppe BS, Henderson R, Pham D, et al. A phase 2 trial of concurrent chemotherapy and proton therapy for stage III non-small cell lung cancer: results and reflections following early closure of a single-institution study. Int J Radiat Oncol biol Phys. 2016;95(1):517–22.
9. Bush DA, Cheek G, Zaheer S, et al. High-dose hypofractionated proton beam radiation therapy is safe and effective for central and peripheral early-stage non-small cell lung cancer: results of a 12-year experience at Loma Linda University medical Center. Int J Radiat Oncol Biol Phys. 2013;86(5):964–8.
10. Colaco RJ, Huh S, Nichols RC, et al. Dosimetric rationale and early experience at UFPTI of thoracic proton therapy and chemotherapy in limited-stage small cell lung cancer. Acta Oncol. 2013;52(3):506–13.
11. Giraud P, Antoine M, Larrouy A, et al. Evaluation of microscopic tumor extension in non-small-cell lung cancer for three-dimensional conformal radiotherapy planning. Int J Radiat Oncol Biol Phys. 2000;48(4):1015–24.
12. Kelly P, Balter PA, Rebueno N, et al. Stereotactic body radiation therapy for patients with lung cancer previously treated with thoracic radiation. Int J Radiat Oncol Biol Phys. 2010;78(5):1387–93.
13. Chang JY, Roth JA. Stereotactic body radiation therapy for stage I non-small cell lung cancer. Thorac Surg Clin. 2007;17(2):251–9.

14. Chang JY, Balter PA, Dong L, et al. Stereotactic body radiation therapy in centrally and superiorly located stage I or isolated recurrent non-small-cell lung cancer. Int J Radiat Oncol Biol Phys. 2008;72(4):967–71.
15. Bradley JD, Paulus R, Komaki R, et al. Standard-dose versus high-dose conformal radiotherapy with concurrent and consolidation carboplatin plus paclitaxel with or without cetuximab for patients with stage IIIA or IIIB non-small-cell lung cancer (RTOG 0617): a randomised, two-by-two factorial phase 3 study. Lancet Oncol. 2015;16(2):187–99.
16. Turrisi AT 3rd, Kim K, Blum R, et al. Twice-daily compared with once-daily thoracic radiotherapy in limited small-cell lung cancer treated concurrently with cisplatin and etoposide. N Engl J Med. 1999;340(4):265–71.
17. Zhang W, Liu C, Lin H, et al. Prospective study of special stage II (T2b-3N0M0) non-small-cell lung cancer treated with hypofractionated-simultaneous integrated boost-intensity modulated radiation therapy. J Cancer Res Ther. 2015;11(2):381–7.
18. Weiss E, Fatyga M, Wu Y, et al. Dose escalation for locally advanced lung cancer using adaptive radiation therapy with simultaneous integrated volume-adapted boost. Int J Radiat Oncol Biol Phys. 2013;86(3):414–9.
19. Ji K, Zhao LJ, Liu WS, et al. Simultaneous integrated boost intensity-modulated radiotherapy for treatment of locally advanced non-small-cell lung cancer: a retrospective clinical study. Br J Radiol. 2014;87(1035):20130562.
20. Dirkx ML, van Sornsen De Koste JR, Senan S. A treatment planning study evaluating a 'simultaneous integrated boost' technique for accelerated radiotherapy of stage III non-small cell lung cancer. Lung Cancer. 2004;45(1):57–65.
21. Kang Y, Zhang X, Chang JY, et al. 4D proton treatment planning strategy for mobile lung tumors. Int J Radiat Oncol Biol Phys. 2007;67(3):906–14.
22. Liu W, Schild SE, Chang JY, et al. Exploratory study of 4D versus 3D robust optimization in intensity modulated proton therapy for lung cancer. Int J Radiat Oncol Biol Phys. 2016;95(1):523–33.
23. Li H, Zhu XR, Zhang X. Reducing dose uncertainty for spot-scanning proton beam therapy of moving Tumors by optimizing the spot delivery sequence. Int J Radiat Oncol Biol Phys. 2015;93(3):547–56.
24. Li H, Zhang X, Park P, et al. Robust optimization in intensity-modulated proton therapy to account for anatomy changes in lung cancer patients. Radiother Oncol. 2015;114(3):367–72.
25. Chang JY, Li H, Zhu XR, et al. Clinical implementation of intensity modulated proton therapy for thoracic malignancies. Int J Radiat Oncol Biol Phys. 2014;90(4):809–18.
26. Bush DA, Slater JD, Bonnet R, et al. Proton-beam radiotherapy for early-stage lung cancer. Chest. 1999;116(5):1313–9.
27. Chang JY, Komaki R, Wen HY, et al. Toxicity and patterns of failure of adaptive/ablative proton therapy for early-stage, medically inoperable non-small cell lung cancer. Int J Radiat Oncol Biol Phys. 2011;80(5):1350–7.
28. Do SY, Bush DA, Slater JD. Comorbidity-adjusted survival in early stage lung cancer patients treated with hypofractionated proton therapy. J Oncol. 2010;2010:251208.
29. Niho S, Motegi A, Kirita K, et al. Proton beam therapy (PBT) and concurrent chemotherapy using cisplatin (CDDP) and vinorelbine (VNR) for locally advanced non-small cell lung cancer (NSCLC). J Clin Oncol. 2015;33(15):e18525.
30. Nguyen Q, Komaki R, Liao Z, et al. The 5-year outcome for patients diagnosed with locally advanced non-small cell lung cancer treated with definitive concurrent chemotherapy and proton beam therapy. Int J Radiat Oncol. 2014;90:S19–20.
31. Lievens Y, Verhaeghe N, de Neve W, et al. Proton radiotherapy for locally-advanced non-small cell lung cancer, a cost-effective alternative to photon radiotherapy in Belgium? J Thorac Oncol. 2013;8:S839–S40.
32. Koay EJ, Lege D, Mohan R, Komaki R, Cox JD, Chang JY. Adaptive/nonadaptive proton radiation planning and outcomes in a phase II trial for locally advanced non-small cell lung cancer. Int J Radiat Oncol Biol Phys. 2012;84(5):1093–100.

33. Kesarwala AH, Ko CJ, Ning H, et al. Intensity-modulated proton therapy for elective nodal irradiation and involved-field radiation in the definitive treatment of locally advanced non-small-cell lung cancer: a Dosimetric study. Clin Lung Cancer. 2015;16(3):237–44.
34. Kesarwala AH, Ko C, O'Meara WP, et al. Feasibility of proton therapy for elective nodal irradiation in patients with locally advanced non-small cell lung cancer. Int J Radiat Oncol. 2012;84(3):S577–S8.
35. Oshiro Y, Mizumoto M, Okumura T, et al. Results of proton beam therapy without concurrent chemotherapy for patients with unresectable stage III non-small cell lung cancer. J Thorac Oncol. 2012;7(2):370–5.
36. Chang JY, Komaki R, Lu C, et al. Phase 2 study of high-dose proton therapy with concurrent chemotherapy for unresectable stage III nonsmall cell lung cancer. Cancer. 2011;117(20):4707–13.
37. Xiang ZL, Erasmus J, Komaki R, Cox JD, Chang JY. FDG uptake correlates with recurrence and survival after treatment of unresectable stage III non-small cell lung cancer with high-dose proton therapy and chemotherapy. Radiat Oncol. 2012;7:144.
38. Liao ZX, Lee JJ, Komaki R, Gomez DR, O'Reilly M, Allen P, Fossella FV, Heymach JV, Blumenschein GR, Choi NC, Delaney T, Hahn SM, Lu C, Cox JD, Mohan R. Bayesian randomized trial comparing intensity modulated radiation therapy versus passively scattered proton therapy for locally advanced non-small cell lung cancer. J Clin Oncol. 2016;34(suppl):abstr 8500.
39. Yamada T, Miyamoto N, Matsuura T, et al. Optimization and evaluation of multiple gating beam delivery in a synchrotron-based proton beam scanning system using a real-time imaging technique. Phys Med. 2016;32(7):932–7.
40. Hoffmann L, Alber M, Jensen MF, Holt MI, Moller DS. Adaptation is mandatory for intensity modulated proton therapy of advanced lung cancer to ensure target coverage. Radiother Oncol. 2017;122(3):400–5.
41. Ding X, Li X, Zhang JM, Kabolizadeh P, Stevens C, Yan D. Spot-scanning proton arc (SPArc) therapy: the first robust and delivery-efficient spot-scanning proton arc therapy. Int J Radiat Oncol Biol Phys. 2016;96(5):1107–16.
42. Smith B, Gelover E, Moignier A, et al. Technical note: a treatment plan comparison between dynamic collimation and a fixed aperture during spot scanning proton therapy for brain treatment. Med Phys. 2016;43(8):4693.

Esophagus Cancer

13

Steven H. Lin, Heng Li, and Daniel Gomez

Contents

13.1	Introduction	211
13.2	Simulation, Target Delineation, and Radiation Dose/Fractionation	212
13.3	Patient Positioning, Immobilization, and Treatment Verification	213
	13.3.1 Passive Scattering PBT Planning	214
	13.3.2 IMPT Treatment Planning	215
13.4	Dosimetric and Toxicity Comparison	217
13.5	Future Developments	218
References		219

13.1 Introduction

Worldwide, esophageal cancer (EC) is the sixth leading cause of death and is responsible for over 400,000 cases (4.9%) [1]. It is notable that the incidence differs greatly, depending on the region of the world. The highest incidence is in the Asian and Middle Eastern countries [2]. In most Western countries, such as in the United States, adenocarcinoma has eclipsed squamous cell carcinoma as the predominant histologic type and usually afflicts white males. In contrast, squamous cell carcinoma is mostly related to smoking and alcoholism in Asia and Middle Eastern countries. In addition, adenocarcinoma is largely related to the growing epidemic of obesity in the western and other developed countries and the associated reflux esophagitis and Barrett's pre-neoplasia that result [3].

Since surgical resection with or without adjuvant therapy is the standard approach, with cure rates that are approximately 20%, preoperative chemoradiation

S.H. Lin • H. Li • D. Gomez (✉)
MD Anderson Cancer Center, Houston, TX, USA
e-mail: dgomez@mdanderson.org

© Springer International Publishing Switzerland 2018
N. Lee et al. (eds.), *Target Volume Delineation and Treatment Planning for Particle Therapy*, Practical Guides in Radiation Oncology,
https://doi.org/10.1007/978-3-319-42478-1_13

is now increasingly being adopted due to the evidence showing an improvement in overall survival compared to surgery alone. The largest of the published randomized trials performed in the modern era was the phase III randomized study from the Dutch group, in which 366 evaluable patients were randomized to surgery vs. preoperative chemoradiation to 41.4 Gy with carboplatin and paclitaxel [4]. Notably, there was a significantly improved median OS in the preoperative group of 49.4 months vs. 24.0 months in the surgery alone group. The pathologic complete response (pCR) in the preoperative chemoradiation group was overall 29%. The pCR rate of squamous cell carcinoma was higher compared to adenocarcinoma (49% vs. 23%, $p = 0.008$), which also translated to an improved overall survival difference of chemoradiation relative to surgery alone in squamous tumors relative to adenocarcinomas (adjusted HR 0.42 (0.23–0.79) vs. HR 0.74 (0.54–1.02)).

Due to the location of the disease in the central mediastinum, proton beam therapy (PBT) is ideal for the treatment of EC. That is, mid- and distal esophageal tumors span posteriorly across the heart and are very close proximity to the left atrium and anteriorly to the thoracic vertebrae. Dose comparisons with 3D conformal therapy and IMRT will be described further below.

13.2 Simulation, Target Delineation, and Radiation Dose/Fractionation

Simulation—respiratory motion should be assessed using a four-dimensional (4D) scan. Note that the esophagus and surrounding structures can move substantially with respiratory motion, particularly at the GE junction. Patients should ideally be simulated with their arms above their head, to maximize the number of beam arrangements that can be used. To improve reproducibility, patients should be advised to be NPO for at least 3 h prior to the simulation and each daily treatment.

Target delineation—target delineation differs depending on the location of the tumor within the esophagus. Upper esophagus tumors are defined as those within the cervical and upper thoracic regions, and lower esophagus tumors are in the mid- and distal esophagus, including at the GE junction. Siewert type III GE junction tumors should be managed like gastric cancers, including target delineation.

Upper esophagus tumors—the GTV consists of the gross tumor. The CTV consists of a 3.5 cm margin superiorly-inferiorly and a 1 cm margin laterally, but not crossing anatomic boundaries (modified for boundaries such as vessels or the bone). However, for cervical esophagus lesions, the upper margin should be the inferior border of the cricoid cartilage. The CTV should also include elective treatment of the supraclavicular fossa bilaterally, even if not involved.

Lower esophagus tumors—the GTV consists of the gross tumor. The CTV consists of a 3.5 cm margin superiorly-inferiorly and a 1 cm margin laterally, but not crossing anatomic boundaries (modified for boundaries such as vessels or the bone). The CTV should also include the left gastric lymph nodes for patients with distal esophagus/GEJ tumors (Siewert type I/II disease). For patients with node-positive disease, the celiac axis should also be electively covered if not involved.

With particle therapy, The PTV is only used for recording and reporting purposes (ICRU 78). The PTV is generated by expanding the CTV with a patient setup margin, which is 0.5–1.0 cm, based on the image guidance that is available. At our institution, we utilize daily kV imaging and thus a 0.5 cm PTV margin.

In addition to the PTV, a dosimetric margin is also needed for particle therapy due to range uncertainties and modulation of beams, which will be described in more detail in the planning techniques below.

Radiation dose (upper esophagus tumors)—patients with upper esophagus tumors are less likely to undergo surgery. Therefore, dose escalation above 50.4 Gy can be considered (50.4–60 Gy in 1.8–2.0 Gy fractions).

Lower esophagus tumors—the standard dose remains 40–50.4 Gy in 1.8–2.0 Gy fractions. Dose escalation can be considered in the context of a clinical trial.

	Upper esophagus tumors	Lower esophagus tumors
GTV (with internal motion)	Gross tumor	Gross tumor
CTV	*Cervical*—superior to cricoid cartilage, inferior 3.5 cm, lateral 1 cm (respecting anatomic boundaries), bilateral SCV fossa *Upper thoracic*—superior-inferior 3.5 cm, lateral 1 cm (respecting anatomical boundaries)	*Middle esophagus*—superior-inferior 3.5 cm, lateral 1 cm (respecting anatomical boundaries), left gastric and celiac lymph nodes not considered unless involved *Distal esophagus/GEJ (Siewert I/II)*—superior-inferior 3.5 cm, lateral 1 cm (respecting anatomical boundaries), routinely electively cover left gastric lymph nodes, celiac nodes in node-positive disease *Siewert type III*—treat like gastric cancer
Patient setup margin	0.5–1.0 cm—0.5 cm if daily kV IGRT used	0.5–1.0 cm—0.5 cm if daily kV IGRT used
Prescription dose	50.4–60 Gy RBE in 1.8–2.0 Gy fractions	40–50.4 Gy RBE in 1.8–2.0 Gy fractions

13.3 Patient Positioning, Immobilization, and Treatment Verification

Patients should be placed supine and immobilized in a 5-point mask with indexed head, neck, and shoulder stabilization in patients with cervical tumors.

For patients with thoracic and GEJ tumors, immobilization involves the use of indexed upper vac-lok/alpha cradle, with bilateral arms up. Vac-lok deflation has to be monitored.

Isocenter is placed at the carina.

Daily kV imaging should be used for all patients. If available, weekly in-room volumetric imaging (e.g., cone-beam CT scan or CT on rails) can be obtained weekly.

Breath-holding and gating techniques are not typically done in esophagus cancer tumors; however, they have the potential to be used for target motion management.

Substantial changes in anatomy and/or tumor size during the course of treatment are rare, and thus adaptive simulations are not routinely scheduled. However, if daily or weekly imaging shows changes in normal tissue or tumor or if the patient undergoes a prolonged treatment break, then we do recommend that a verification CT study be performed as soon as possible.

13.3.1 Passive Scattering PBT Planning

Typically for patients with distal tumors, the beam arrangement is most commonly posteroanterior (PA) and left lateral oblique (LAO) (Fig. 13.1). However, optimal beam arrangements are determined on a case-by-case basis, and alternative beam arrangements can be used. For proximal to mid-esophagus tumors, an anteroposterior (AP) and PA beam arrangement could be considered, exercising caution in the AP direction because of the range uncertainty into the spinal cord.

For free-breathing treatment, in order to ensure target coverage in all breathing phases, a planning diaphragm structure is created from the T0 to T50 phases of the 4DCT. The density of the diaphragm is then overridden using the average Hounsfield unit (HU) of the maximum intensity projection (MIP) scan generated from the 4DCT. The treatment plan is then designed with the overridden average CT. This technique ensures adequate coverage to the distal end of target even with respiratory motion as shown in Fig. 13.1.

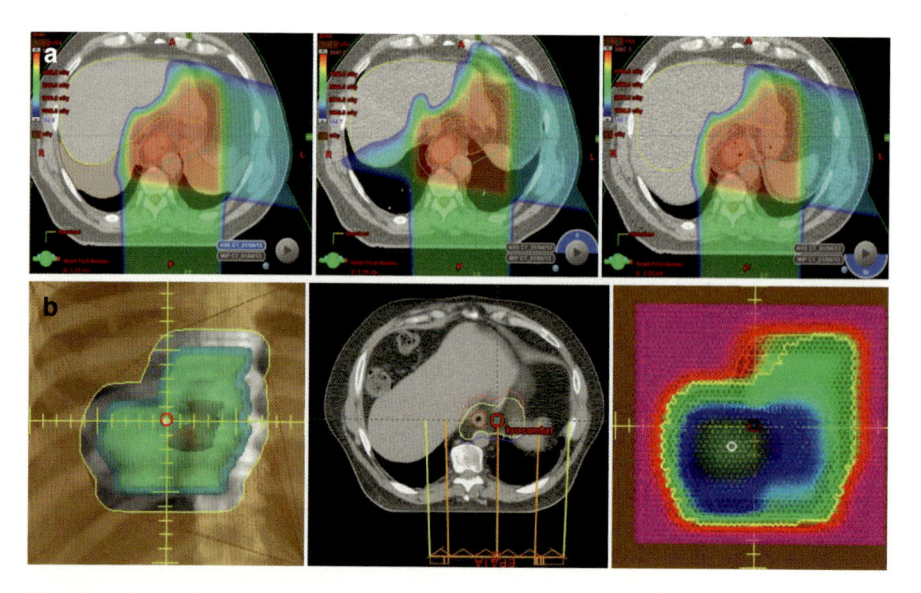

Fig. 13.1 Overriding diaphragm in treatment for esophagus cancer. (**a**) *Left*: plan dose calculated on average CT with diaphragm override. *Middle*: dose calculated on T0. *Right*: dose calculated on T50. (**b**) *Left*: aperture design with lateral margin consists of setup margin and dosimetric margin to account for beam penumbra. *Middle*: distal (*red*) and proximal (*blue*) margins. *Right*: compensator design with smearing

13 Esophagus Cancer 215

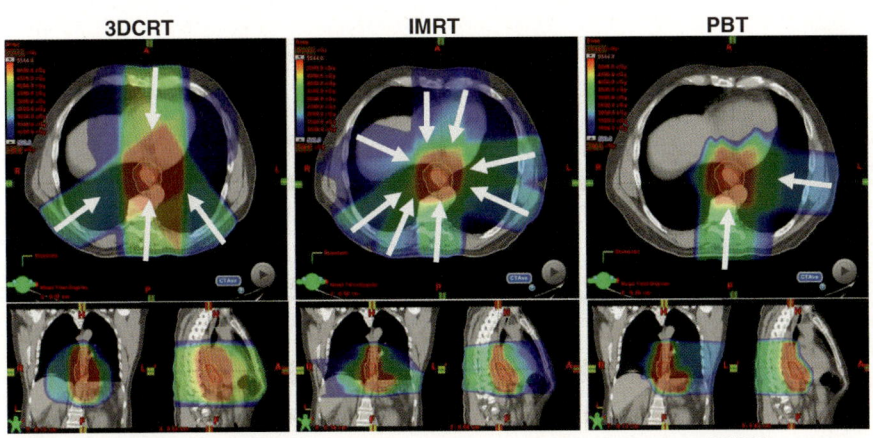

3DCRT: 4-field static photons; IMRT: 5-field modulated photons; PBT: 2-field passive scatter protons (PA/LPO)

Fig. 13.2 Beam arrangement and dosimetric comparisons of photon (3D or IMRT) and PBT plans for a distal esophageal tumor

Typical margins for passive proton beam treatment planning were used [5]: aperture design with setup margin and dosimetric margin, beamline design that includes distal and proximal margins based on beam range to account for range uncertainties, and compensator design with smear margin to ensure distal target coverage (Fig. 13.2).

13.3.2 IMPT Treatment Planning

IMPT offers superior dose conformity compared to PSPT, and it delivers less integral dose than IMRT. However, IMPT is more sensitive to respiratory motion than PSPT and therefore poses an even larger challenge in implementation of the technique. This is particularly relevant for distal esophageal tumors.

One way to assess the impact of respiratory motion is to assess the changes of water equivalent thickness (WET) of the proton beam. A study has shown that the change in WET is correlated with respiratory motion which generates dose uncertainty for distal esophageal treatment plans [6].

The same study also established that for distal esophagus, the optimal beam angles range between 150 and 210 degrees, to avoid the diaphragm motion in the beam path. Typically two to three beams could be used for the plan in this range.

Both single-field optimization (SFO), where each field is optimized to deliver the prescribed dose to target dose to target volume [7], and IMPT, where all spots from all fields are optimized simultaneously (Chap. 3), could be used for PBS planning. In general, IMPT offers more flexibility with more degrees of freedom and could result in more conformal dose distribution, but IMPT plans are also less robust compared to SFO plans due to the complex dose distribution in each fields. For esophageal tumors, SFO and IMPT plans could achieve similar quality for current dose

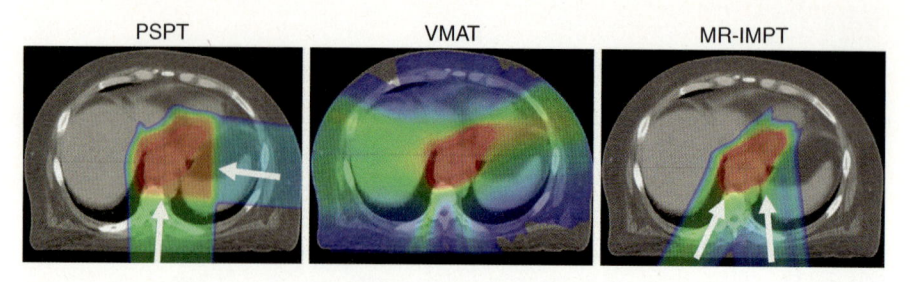

Fig. 13.3 Demonstration of benefit of IMPT compared to PSPT and VMAT in distal esophagus cancer. Note that there are improved conformality and sparing of the surrounding liver, stomach, heart, and soft tissue

Fig. 13.4 (**a**) An example of a ΔWET curve created by plotting ΔWET value against beam angle. The solid circles indicate the three beam angles that are in the approximate range of the minimum ΔWET. These are the beam angles used in plan A. The open circles correspond to the three beam angles around the maximum ΔWET, which are the beam angles used in plan B. (**b**) Beam arrangement for plan A. (**c**) Beam arrangement for plan B. The contour is ICTV (From reference [6])

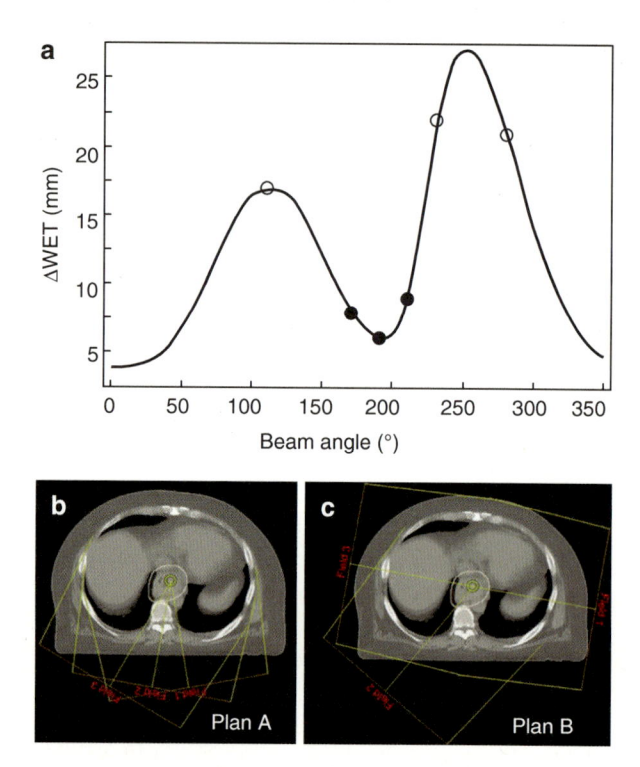

prescription levels, with the exception of slightly elevated spinal cord dose in the SFO plans but still within 45–50 GY(RBE).

4D treatment planning and robustness optimization could further reduce the impact of respiratory motion to the dose distribution, but these techniques may not be readily available [6]. However, active target motion management techniques such as breath holding could be employed (Figs. 13.3 and 13.4).

13.4 Dosimetric and Toxicity Comparison

A 3D conformal approach for esophagus cancer introduces relatively higher radiation dose to the heart, especially with an AP beam. IMRT is able to reduce the high-dose scatter across the heart by placing the entrance dose posteriorly, thereby subjecting the heart and lung dose to low exit radiation dose. Proton beam further improves the dosimetric parameters since with the Bragg peak, there is virtually no exit dose. Therefore, even with only two beams used in passive scattering proton, there is a substantial reduction in dose to the lung and heart. A number of dosimetric planning studies have been conducted that have compared proton beam with photon modalities. In a study comparing photons vs. protons using 3D planning (3DCRT vs. PSPT) in five patients, improved dosing to the spinal cord, lung, heart, and kidneys was found, with better tumor control probability by 2–23% units (mean 20%) [8].

The dosimetric benefit described above is also observed when compared to IMRT plans. This proton vs. photon comparison was done in a study comparing IMRT to two-field AP/PA or three-field AP/two posterior oblique PSPT field arrangements in 15 patients [9]. While PSBT substantially reduced the V5–V20, mean lung dose, and spinal cord dose, the dose-sparing effect was not observed in the heart. This discrepancy is likely due to the suboptimal beam arrangement that these earlier experiences reflected, as we recently demonstrated in a planning study comparing passive scattering proton therapy (PSPT) with IMRT in 55 patients with mid- to distal ECs to determine the dosimetric or anatomic factors that led to suboptimal proton dose distribution [10]. Specifically, we identified patients with "suboptimal" dosimetry compared to IMRT and then attempted to determine whether the dosimetric characteristics could be improved with alternative approaches. We found that the primary reasons for suboptimal dosimetry were (1) nonstandard beam arrangements such as AP/PA or AP/PA/left lateral approach, (2) 1:1 beam weighting of the left lateral/PA beam, and/or (3) unique patient anatomy such as the CTV wrapping around the heart.

Clinically, our institution has also compared toxicity in PBT vs. photon techniques, both from a dosimetric and clinical outcome standpoint [11]. During this period, 208, 164, and 72 patients were treated with 3D, IMRT, or PSBT, respectively. With regard to comparative dosimetry, significant differences were appreciated between each of the modalities, particularly for PBT as compared to the other modalities.

We also evaluated the incidence of postoperative pulmonary, cardiac, wound, and gastrointestinal (GI) complications in 444 patients treated with neoadjuvant chemoradiation from 1998 to 2011. On univariate analysis, a number of factors predicted for adverse events, but the radiation modality used was only associated with pulmonary and GI complications. On multivariate analysis, only radiation modality and pre-radiation diffusion capacity of the lung for carbon monoxide (D_{LCO}) were independently associated with pulmonary complications. With regard to GI complications, radiation modality trended toward statistical significance between the two techniques, with protons having a slightly improved incidence of these adverse events. When the three radiation modalities were compared, there was a significant increase in pulmonary complications of 3D vs. IMRT (odds ratio [OR], 4.10; 95% confidence interval [CI] 1.37–12.29) or 3D vs. PBT (OR 9.13; 95% CI, 1.83–45.42), but there was no difference in IMRT vs. PBT after adjusting for the pre-radiation D_{LCO} level (OR 2.23; 95% CI, 0.86–5.76) [11].

Investigators from the University of Pennsylvania recently published a prospective study of 14 patients who received PSPT for recurrent esophagus cancer over a 15-year period at their institution, to assess the outcomes and toxicity of this approach. The authors reported one grade 5 toxicity, an esophagopleural fistula that may have been related to tumor progression, as well as four grade 3 toxicities: heart failure, esophageal stricture, esophageal ulceration, and percutaneous endoscopic gastrostomy tube dependence. The median OS time was 14 months, leading the authors to conclude that this approach has an "encouraging" symptom control rate and "favorable" survival [12].

The utility of PBT (passive scattering or IMPT) vs. photon (IMRT) techniques should be further evaluated in prospective, randomized trials. MD Anderson Cancer Center is currently leading a phase IIB randomized study comparing these approaches (NCT01512589), with the co-primary endpoints being total toxicity burden and disease-free survival. Anticipated accrual is 180 patients, with approximately 50% accrual at the time of this publication.

13.5 Future Developments

Substantial progress has been made with regard to proton therapy in esophagus cancer over the past decade. Dosimetry has been compared to IMRT and 3DCRT, optimal beam arrangements have been defined, planning techniques have been refined, IMPT has been implemented, and comparative effectiveness studies have been initiated. The next 10–20 years will likely involve further refinement of IMPT in this setting, along with the standardization of planning approaches. The identification of appropriate patients for this approach will also be critical, and one substantial benefit from the completion of ongoing randomized studies will be to determine the subsets of patients that derive the greatest clinical benefit from the utilization of proton therapy. Ideally, this approach will be possible in an increasing number of patients with limited treatment options, such as those with in-field local failures. Finally, imaging studies will enhance our understanding of the differences between proton and photon techniques in the context of both tumor response and toxicity. Fields such as radiomics in combination with sensitive imaging modalities (MRI, PET) will improve our comprehension of the early effects of protons and whether these can be predictive and prognostic of ultimate outcomes.

References

1. Jemal A, Siegel R, Xu J, Ward E. Cancer statistics, 2010. CA Cancer J Clin. 2010;60(5):277–300.
2. Jemal A, Bray F, Center MM, Ferlay J, Ward E, Forman D. Global cancer statistics. CA Cancer J Clin. 2011;61(2):69–90.
3. Enzinger PC, Mayer RJ. Esophageal cancer. N Engl J Med. 2003;349(23):2241–52.
4. van Hagen P, Hulshof MC, van Lanschot JJ, et al. Preoperative chemoradiotherapy for esophageal or junctional cancer. N Engl J Med. 2012;366(22):2074–84.
5. Li H, Giebeler A, Dong L, et al. Treatment planning for passive scattering proton therapy. In: Das IJ, Paganetti H, editors. Principles and practice of proton beam therapy; 2015.
6. Yu J, Zhang X, Liao L, et al. Motion-robust intensity-modulated proton therapy for distal esophageal cancer. Med Phys. 2016;43(3):1111.
7. Zhu XR, Sahoo N, Zhang X, et al. Intensity modulated proton therapy treatment planning using single-field optimization: the impact of monitor unit constraints on plan quality. Med Phys. 2010;37(3):1210–9.
8. Isacsson U, LennernÃs B, Grusell E, Jung B, Montelius A, Glimelius B. Comparative treatment planning between proton and x-ray therapy in esophageal cancer. Int J Radiat Oncol Biol Phy. 1998;41(2):441–50.
9. Zhang X, Kl Z, Guerrero TM, et al. Four-dimensional computed tomography-based treatment planning for intensity-modulated radiation therapy and proton therapy for distal esophageal cancer. Int J Radiat Oncol Biol Phys. 2008;72(1):278–87.
10. Wang J, Palmer M, Bilton SD, et al. Comparing proton beam to intensity modulated radiation therapy planning in esophageal cancer. Int J Particle Ther. 2015;1(4):866–77.
11. Wang J, Wei C, Tucker SL, et al. Predictors of postoperative complications after trimodality therapy for esophageal cancer. Int J Radiat Oncol Biol Phys. 2013;86(5):885–91.
12. Fernandes A, Berman AT, Mick R, et al. A prospective study of proton beam Reirradiation for esophageal cancer. Int J Radiat Oncol Biol Phys. 2016;95(1):483–7.

Carbon Ion Radiation Therapy for Liver Tumors

14

Zheng Wang, Wei-Wei Wang, Kambiz Shahnazi, and Guo-Liang Jiang

Contents

14.1	Physical Dose Distribution Comparison Between Proton and Carbon Ion	222
	14.1.1 Hepatic Radiation Injury and Proliferation	222
	14.1.2 Clinical Relevance	223
14.2	Radiobiological Effect Comparison Between Protons and Carbon Ions	225
14.3	The Technical Challenges in CIRT for HCC	227
	14.3.1 Target Motion Control	227
	14.3.2 The Interplay Effect: Rescanning	228
14.4	Clinical Results for Application of CIRT for HCC	229
14.5	Practice in Shanghai Proton and Heavy Ion Center for HCC	230
	14.5.1 Target Volume	230
	14.5.2 Verification	231
Conclusion		233
References		233

Carbon ion radiation therapy (CIRT) facilities are available in Japan, Germany, and China. The National Institute of Radiological Science (NIRS) and Hyogo Ion Beam Medical Center (HIBMC), both institutions in Japan, have used CIRT to treat hepatocellular carcinoma (HCC) patients, and Heidelberg Ion Beam Therapy Center (HIT) in Germany has treated a limited number of patients. The outcomes of CIRT for HCC have been very encouraging. Shanghai Proton and Heavy Ion Center (SPHIC) has been using CIRT for HCC since 2014. In this section, we will address CIRT for HCC.

Z. Wang • W.-W. Wang • K. Shahnazi
G.-L. Jiang (✉)
Department of Radiation Oncology, Shanghai Proton and Heavy Ion Center,
4365 Kang Xin Road, Shanghai 201321, China
e-mail: guoliang.jiang@sphic.org.cn

© Springer International Publishing Switzerland 2018
N. Lee et al. (eds.), *Target Volume Delineation and Treatment Planning for Particle Therapy*, Practical Guides in Radiation Oncology,
https://doi.org/10.1007/978-3-319-42478-1_14

14.1 Physical Dose Distribution Comparison Between Proton and Carbon Ion

Similar to protons, the carbon ion beam possesses the same characteristics of physical dose distribution, such as the "Bragg peak"; however, compared to protons, the carbon ion "Bragg peak" is much steeper and the width narrower. In scan beam facilities, a ripple filter has to be used to widen the "Bragg peak" in order to decrease the number of scanned layers. In addition, the dose behind the "Bragg peak," called fragment tail dose, is slightly higher than that of proton dose tail. In other words, the carbon ion dose behind the "Bragg peak" is slightly larger than for protons (Fig. 14.1). Furthermore, the lateral penumbra of the carbon ion beam is smaller than that of the proton beam (Fig. 14.2). As a result, the carbon ion beam can deliver less dose to organs at risk (OARs), which are located laterally at the axis of the beam direction, but slightly more dose to OARs behind the target.

14.1.1 Hepatic Radiation Injury and Proliferation

For HCC irradiation, it is the consensus that the dose to uninvolved healthy liver is critical for the success of the radiotherapy. The most severe radiation complication is radiation-induced liver disease (RILD). Once RILD occurs, over 70% of patients will die of this fatal complication. Therefore the priority in HCC irradiation is to prevent RILD in these patients. Unfortunately, the majority of HCC patients are associated with hepatic cirrhosis, which is induced by hepatitis B virus in Asia, or in the western countries by hepatitis C, or alcohol abuse. Therefore, keeping the radiation dose as low as possible to the normal liver is the first priority when an HCC radiation plan is designed.

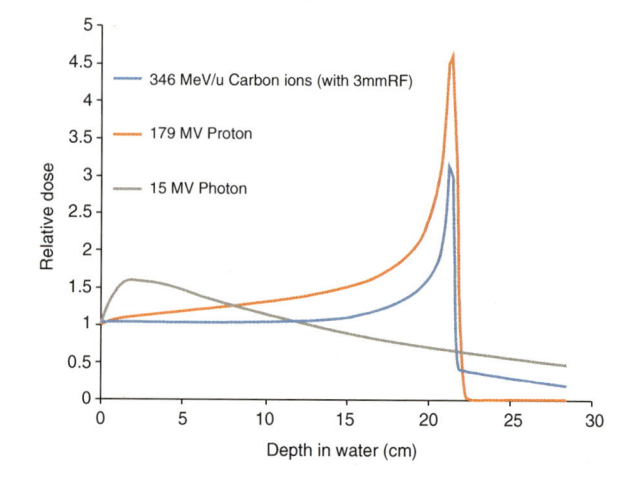

Fig. 14.1 Percentage depth dose distributions in water for 15 MV photon, 179 MeV proton, and 346 MeV/u carbon ion (with 3 mm ripple filter)

14 Carbon Ion Radiation Therapy for Liver Tumors

Fig. 14.2 The lateral penumbras of proton and carbon ion beams at the "Bragg peak" dose area

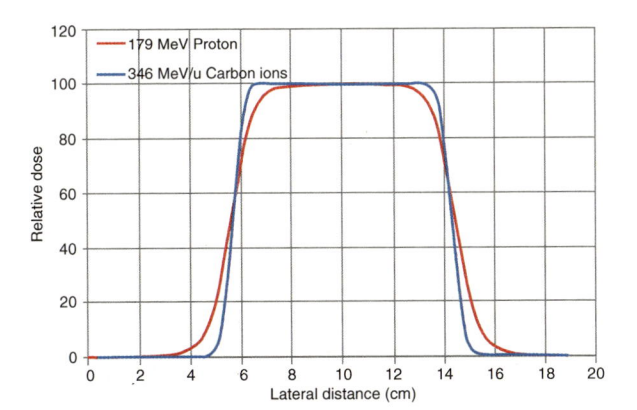

From previous photon experience reported in the literature for HCC irradiation, the mean dose to normal liver, defined as the whole liver volume minus GTV, is one of the most important parameters [1, 2]. After radiation-induced liver injury, the remaining healthy liver can be stimulated to repopulate significantly and could compensate for the lost hepatic function, which means the capability to proliferate in remaining healthy liver is also important in HCC irradiation. From animal studies on the liver, it was found that proliferation occurs after irradiation injury [3, 4, 5]:

(1) Unirradiated liver possessed a very strong capability to proliferate after hepatic radiation injury.
(2) The liver with low-dose irradiation also had the capability to proliferate, but the liver receiving higher dose had poorer capability to proliferate.
(3) The cirrhotic liver induced by chemicals could also repopulate, but its capability would be poorer than the normal liver [6].

However, in the clinic, it is very difficult to predict the hepatic capability of proliferation after different irradiation doses to different scales of cirrhosis at the current time. Therefore, a strategy should be to keep a part of the healthy liver totally unirradiated, the unirradiated healthy liver volume as much as possible, and the dose to healthy liver as low as possible. From the above considerations, protons and CIRT are superior to IMRT.

14.1.2 Clinical Relevance

Dose comparisons has been evaluated for three plans of therapy, photon intensity-modulated radiation therapy (IMRT), intensity-modulated proton therapy (IMPT), or intensity-modulated carbon ion therapy (IMCT), for each of eight HCC patients,

Fig. 14.3 Dose distribution comparison in a typical hepatocellular carcinoma patient. (**a**) Photon IMRT, (**b**) proton, and (**c**) carbon ion; (**d**) dose volume histogram for the target (ITV) (*brown line*), liver (*green line*), right kidney (*pink line*), and stomach (*blue line*). The ITV coverage, liver mean dose, kidney mean dose, and stomach maximum dose were 93.6%, 16.71 GyE, 0.20 GyE, and 1.60 GyE for proton; 90.3%, 15.23 GyE, 0.01 GyE, and 9.75 GyE for carbon ion; and 98.7%, 21.35 Gy, 4.84 Gy, and 19.57 Gy for photon IMRT, respectively

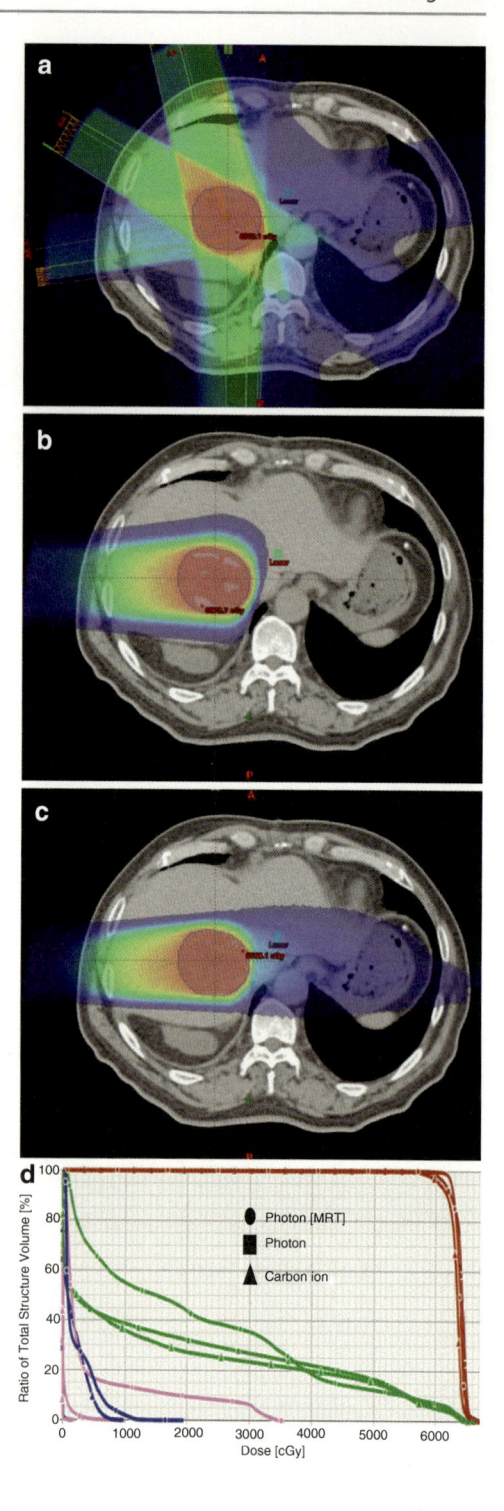

Table 14.1 Comparison of doses to the liver, right kidney, and stomach using IMRT, proton, and carbon ion beam from eight hepatocellular carcinomas

Dose parameter	Photon	Proton	Carbon
ITV coverage (V95%)	99.8 ± 3.2	99.6 ± 4.8	99.9 ± 3.7
Liver			
Mean dose (GyE)	23.17 ± 4.30*	17.00 ± 2.92#	15.49 ± 2.62$
Kidney			
Mean dose (GyE)	5.91 ± 10.7+	2.84 ± 8.46&	2.00 ± 9.41=
Stomach			
Max dose (GyE)	29.92 ± 7.10**	2.61 ± 13.55##	10.03 ± 12.79$$

t test: * vs. #, $p = 0.00$; * vs. $, $p = 0.00$; # vs. $, $p = 0.01$; + vs. &, $p = 0.02$; + vs. =, $p = 0.01$; ## vs. $$, $p = 0.01$
For all other comparisons between two parameters, p were >0.05

who were finally irradiated with CIRT in our center. Figure 14.3 shows the dose distributions from one of the eight HCC patients irradiated by IMRT, proton beam, and carbon ion beam. Table 14.1 summarizes the doses to the tumor, liver, right kidney, and stomach from 8 HCC patients. To produce the same target coverage (95% of ITV covered by 95% of prescribed dose), proton and carbon ion beams deliver lower doses to the kidney and liver compared to IMRT for the same patient. Moreover, carbon ion beam delivers lower doses to the kidney and liver compared to protons because of smaller penumbra. However, due to the tail dose behind "Bragg peak," the stomach located distal to the target receives slightly higher dose with carbon ions compared to protons. Overall, CIRT has been shown to be more advantageous compared to protons with lower mean dose to the normal liver, which is the most important issue to reduce the hepatic toxicity, although the dose to stomach is slightly higher, which is likely negligible and will not produce stomach toxicity.

Because of the sharper penumbra of the carbon ion beam (Fig. 14.2), CIRT is more suitable for HCC patients if the tumor is located close to the gastrointestinal (GI) tract. Figure 14.4 demonstrates the dose distributions of proton and carbon ion treatment plans in one HCC patient. The lesion was close to duodenum, and the colon was embedded in the concave target. The dose volume histogram (DVH) in Fig. 14.4c shows that the doses delivered to the duodenum and colon by CIRT were lower than that by protons.

14.2 Radiobiological Effect Comparison Between Protons and Carbon Ions [7, 8, 9]

The biological effect of protons is a little higher than ^{60}Cobalt with relative radiobiological effect (RBE) of 1.0–1.1, but the carbon ion is different from proton. The RBE depends on beam LET. The LET of carbon ion is mixed with low LET in the entrance plateau dose and high LET in the area of the "Bragg peak." From preclinical experiments, it has been shown that 70% of DNA damage is the result of DNA

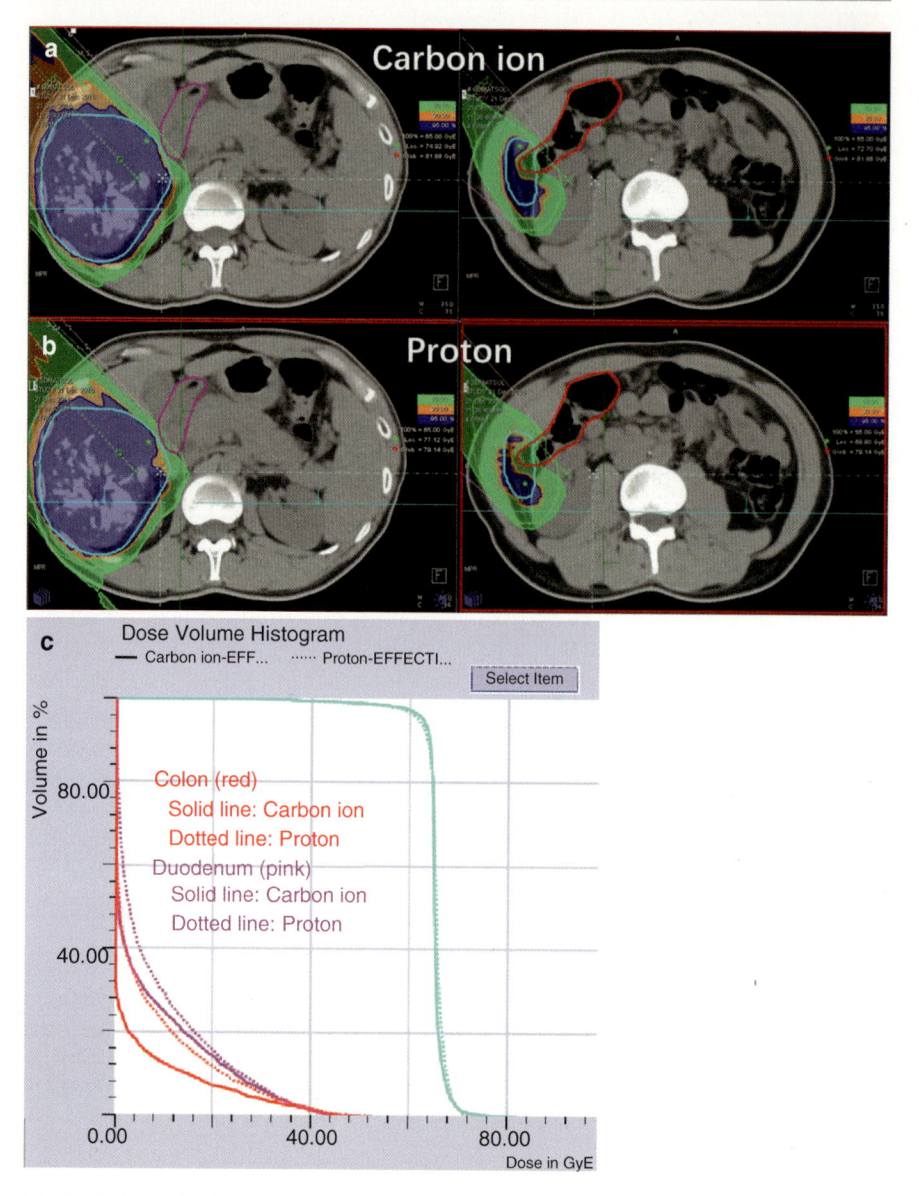

Fig. 14.4 Dose distribution for a hepatocellular carcinoma located close to the duodenum (*pink line*) and colon (*red line*), irradiated by CIRT (**a**) and proton (**b**), and dose volume histogram (**c**)

double strand breaks at the carbon ion Bragg peak. The group at the Heidelberg Ion Beam Therapy Center (HIT) in Germany performed colony formation assays in four HCC cell lines (HepG2, HuH7, Hep3B, and PLC) and found RBEs in the range of 2.1–3.3 compared with photons. From cell survival data, α- and β-values were calculated by linear-quadratic model. As shown in Table 14.2, α-values of carbon ion

14 Carbon Ion Radiation Therapy for Liver Tumors

Table 14.2 α- and β-values from colony formation assay for four hepatocellular carcinoma cell lines

Beam	Parameter	Cell line			
		HepG2	Hep3B	HuH7	PLC
Photons	α	0.1482	0.3966	0.2973	0.3817
	β	0.0927	0.02301	0.03963	0.01244
Caron ion	α	1.733	0.8659	1.892	1.531
	β	−0.1685	0.4962	−0.1272	−0.07204

Adapted from Habermehl D [10]

increased, and β-values of carbon ion decreased for all four cell lines, indicating that the loading of lethal damage increased and the sublethal damage decreased. The change of α- and β-values implies that CIRT yields more DNA double-strand breaks than photon [10]. However, in the entrance dose area, the RBE is a little higher than 1. Moreover, cell kill from carbon ions at the depth of the "Bragg peak" does not rely on the presence of oxygen [11]. Thus, hypoxic tumor cells can be killed effectively and the oxygen enhance ratio (OER) decreased to 1.5–2. Overall, carbon ions have much stronger cell killing effects than photons and protons for X-ray-resistant tumor cells, including S and G_0 phase cells, hypoxic cells, and intrinsically resistant tumor cells. At the time of diagnosis, the majority of HCCs are large in size and likely contain a large proportion of hypoxic tumor cells. Therefore, use of CIRT may potentially further improve the local control of HCC, especially for large HCCs with a significant necrotic component.

14.3 The Technical Challenges in CIRT for HCC

14.3.1 Target Motion Control

There are several ways to control for motion of liver tumors including active breathing control (ABC) and abdominal compression. Additionally, respiratory gating devices have also been used to control for target motion in particle therapy. The Anzai respiratory gating system, a Japanese product, has been used in Japan and many other centers for protons and carbon ion therapy. The patient's breathing pattern is monitored by a pressure sensor mounted on a belt, which is fastened to the patient's abdomen. When radiation is being delivered, Anzai continues to monitor the patient's breathing phases and automatically sends signals to the synchrotron to trigger the ion beam on and off according to a predetermined gating window. The patient should be trained well to cooperate with Anzai and to keep a regular breathing rate. Before starting Anzai gated irradiation, we monitor the patient's respiratory pattern using an online X-ray fluoroscopic imaging system in our treatment room to make sure that the breathing amplitude and rate detected by Anzai correspond to the internal target motion. It is critical to ensure synchronization between breathing and internal target motion. In our practice, monthly quality assurance for the Anzai device and good training of the patient can ensure optimal Anzai gating matching.

In order to decrease irradiation to the healthy liver, a narrow gating window should be chosen. From 4D-CT images, the gating window is selected, typically at the end of exhalation phase, e.g., from 40% of exhalation to 40% of inhalation, which provides a dose delivery time of 2–3 s. The ITV is formed by fusing CTVs at 40% exhalation, at end exhalation, and at 40% inhalation. When choosing the gating window, it is important to account for the interplay effect in the pencil beam scanning approach (detailed below). This experiment simulates the moving target in a phantom. A number of films were placed in a moving target to measure the target dose homogeneity. The target dose homogeneity becomes worse with increasing target motion range. However, the homogeneity was acceptable until the target motion reached 5.9 mm. Finally, we decided that the residual target motion in the gating window should be <5 mm for daily practice (Huang ZJ, et al. unpublished data).

14.3.2 The Interplay Effect: Rescanning

The technique of pencil beam scanning is the best way to deliver dose uniformly and conformally and sufficiently to protect OARs. However, it presents a great challenge for moving targets because of the so-called interplay effect, which introduces dose delivery uncertainty with poor dose homogeneity. To deal with the interplay effect, a beam rescanning technique was explored.

Mori in NIRS developed the rescanning approach for pencil beam scanning of carbon ion therapy, layered phase-controlled rescanning (PCR), and evaluated dose distribution simulated for various numbers of PCR for 30 liver cancers. It was found that PCR provided satisfactory dose homogeneity to the target. The homogeneity index (HI) decreased from 4.6 ± 1.2 (ungated) and 2.9 ± 1.5 (gated) to 0.5 ± 0.9 (ungated) and 1.2 ± 0.6 (gated), respectively, after eight rounds of PCR. In other words, a rescanning approach improved dose homogeneity, which partly accounted for the interplay effect. When the rescanning approach was used in combination with respiratory gating, HI was further improved as shown above [12].

Because it is nearly impossible to align the patient's breathing pattern with the simulation 4D-CT, Mori further studied irregular breathing. They designed a gating plan based on the first breath phase but calculated the target dose delivered by eight PCR on the irregular breathing pattern from real respiratory patterns in ten HCC patients. The study showed that D95 (lowest dose encompassing 95% of CTV) from the irregular breath treatment was 97.6 ± 0.5% and D95 from the planning dose was 98.5 ± 0.4%. Dmax/Dmin within the CTV was 1.6 ± 0.6% from the irregular breath treatment and 0.7 ± 0.2% from the planning. The above deviations can be considered acceptable. Therefore, the rescanning technique could possibly resolve the negative interplay effect for the moving target, even under irregular breathing [13].

Sometimes, PCR could not be completed within a single gating window due to the particular irradiation specifications, such as a large layer size, in which case the iso-energy layer has to be completed using the next gating window. In these situations, the effect of rescanning is effectively nullified. NIRS proposed that the dose rate was adjusted to irradiate the number of rescans within multiple gating windows repeatedly until the total prescribed dose was given within a single gating window [14].

To deal with the interplay effect, another method to increase the scanning spot was proposed by GSI and HIT in Germany. They performed 4D dose calculation for treatment plans with variable beam parameters, including lateral raster spacing, beam spot (full width at half maximum), iso-energy slice spacing, and gating window. The assessed dosimetric parameters were under- and overdose, dose homogeneity, and DVH. Their study concluded that an increased beam spot size/lateral raster spacing could significantly mitigate the dose heterogeneities induced by the interplay effect [15].

14.4 Clinical Results for Application of CIRT for HCC

NIRS is the first hospital to treat HCC with CIRT in the world. Since 1995, they have carried out a series of prospective clinical trials to find the optimal dose and fractionation of CIRT for HCC. In 2004, they reported the results of 24 HCC treated by CIRT as part of a dose escalation study. The doses were given in 15 fractions over 5 weeks. During a median follow-up of 71 months, no severe adverse effects and no treatment-related deaths occurred. The local control (LC) and overall survival (OS) rates were 92% and 92%, 81% and 50%, and 81% and 25% at 1 year, 3 years and 5 years, respectively [16]. In 2010, they again reported on 64 HCCs irradiated with carbon ion to 52.8 GyE in four fractions. The 5-year OS and LC were 22.2% and 87.8% in HCC close to the porta hepatis and 34.8% and 95.7% in HCC distant from the hepatis, respectively. No patients developed biliary stricture [17]. In their book *Carbon Ion Radiotherapy* published in 2014, they reported on 133 HCC treated by CIRT with two fractions. 92% of patients were Child-Pugh A and 8% Child-Pugh B, and 87% were UICC stage 1–2 and 23% of stage IIIa and IVa. The median maximum tumor diameter was 42 mm (14–140 mm). The carbon ion dose ranged from 32 GyE to 45 GyE in two fractions. Acute toxicity was slight with only four cases of grade 3 hepatic toxicity and no other grade 3 and grade 4–5 toxicity, including late toxicity. For the higher-dose group (45.0 GyE) and the lower-dose group ($\leq$42.8 GyE), the LC rates were 98% and 90% at 1 year and 83% and 76% at 3 years, respectively. The OS rates were 95% and 96% at 1 year and 71% and 59% at 3 years in the higher-dose group (45.0 GyE) and the lower-dose group ($\leq$42.8 GyE), respectively [18, 19].

HIBMC reported on the treatment of HCC patients with protons or carbon ion beams. There were 242 HCC patients irradiated with protons to 52.8–84.0 GyE in 4–38 fractions and 101 HCC patients treated with carbon ions to 52.8–76.0 GyE in 4–20 fractions. The 5-year LC and OS rates for all patients were 90.8% and 38.2%, respectively. The 5-year LC rates were 90.2% and 93%, and the 5-year OS were 38% and 36.3%, respectively, for proton and carbon ion. No patients died of treatment-related toxicities [20].

Heidelberg Ion Therapy Center (HIT) in Germany published their protocol of a dose escalation study of carbon RT for HCC in 2011. They planned to give a treatment scheme of 40–56 GyE with fraction size of 10–14 GyE [21]. In 2013, they reported the preliminary results of six patients from the first dose level (40 GyE in 10 fractions). No severe adverse events occurred, and the LC rate was 100% with a median follow-up time of 11 months [22].

14.5 Practice in Shanghai Proton and Heavy Ion Center for HCC

In our center, the treatment strategies for technically unresectable and medically inoperable HCC include the use of combined transcatheter arterial chemoembolization (TACE) and particle irradiation, including proton, CIRT, or combination of proton and CIRT. Particle irradiation should be started after 2–4 cycles of TACE. The advantage of TACE prior to irradiation includes the following: (1) subclinical intrahepatic spreading could be detected by arteriography and injected iodine, (2) arteriography and the deposited iodine aid in contouring GTV margin, and (3) the deposited iodine also serves as a marker for image-guided radiation. The interval between TACE and particle irradiation should be at least 1 month based on our experience. More cycles of TACE can be considered after particle therapy, if patients can tolerate it. Anti-hepatitis virus agent is strongly recommended before, during, and after particle therapy for HCC associated with hepatitis.

Management of target motion with ABC involves a breath hold after deep inspiration. However, the deviation of reproducibility of the target position under ABC should be added to form an ITV. If the patient cannot cooperate with ABC, the patient can be trained for Anzai gating. The residual motion in the gating window is limited to less than 5 mm. When both above methods fail, abdominal compression can be used, but still the residual tumor motion should be less than 5 mm after abdominal compression.

For accurate delineation of GTV, the necessary images include arteriography CT with oral GI contrast, MRI with contrast, and PET/CT. To measure target motion, a 4D-CT is needed for patients with Anzai gating and abdominal compression, and the target reproducibility should be evaluated by fluoroscopy in a conventional simulator.

14.5.1 Target Volume

The definitions for the target are:

(1) GTV includes the gross tumor shown on images.
(2) CTV includes an extra margin of 5 mm added to GTV.
(3) ITV includes CTV plus appropriate margin depending on the deviation of target reproducibility for ABC, the fused CTVs from Anzai gating windows, or the fused CTVs from the end of inhalation and the end of exhalation for abdominal compression.

(4) PTV includes 3–5 mm added to ITV with additional margin in the beam axis directions.

The deposited iodine inside tumor should be overridden with soft tissue density before dose calculation.

The deposited iodine inside the tumor can be used for image guidance. When no iodine is deposited, insertion of fiducials is necessary adjacent to the tumor. After the patient is set up, two orthogonal films by kilovoltage X-ray are taken for position verification.

14.5.2 Verification

Several verification steps are undertaken before treatment. First, it is mandatory to have the plan verified by a group of 24 ion chambers in a water phantom prior to implementing CIRT. Moreover, immediately after irradiation, the patient is moved to PET/CT for PET scanning, and it is scanned on a flatbed table, in the same position as treatment with immobilization device. Figure 14.5 shows a PET image taken about 10 min after completion of 10 GyE of CIRT in an HCC patient. The verification performed in vivo only involved a geometric dose distribution, not a real biological dose distribution.

For CIRT fractionation, although Japanese data showed the optimal dose for controlling HCC, we are not able to implement this directly from their experience because of the different biological models used to convert the physical dose to biological dose. In Japan, the microdosimetric kinetic model (MKM) is used,

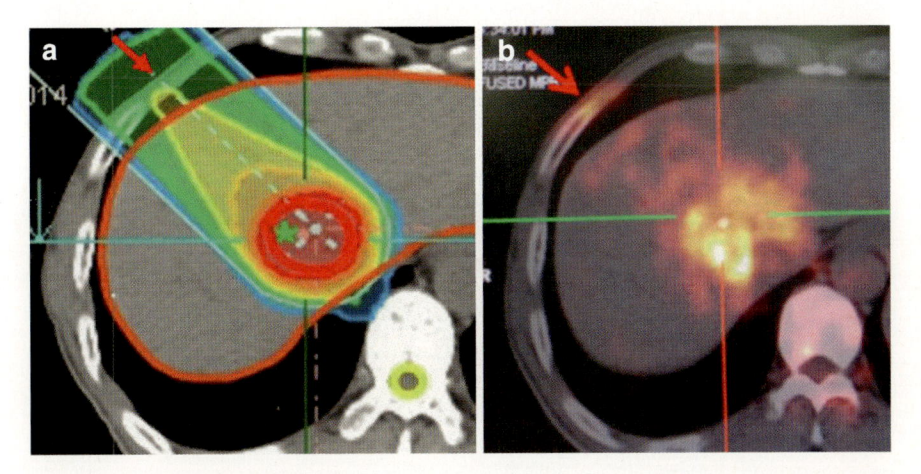

Fig. 14.5 PET image after 10 GyE of carbon ion irradiation for a hepatocellular carcinoma. (**a**) Biological dose distribution: *thick red line*, GTV; *thin red line*, 10 GyE. (**b**) PET image taken 10 min after 10 GyE of carbon ion

whereas, the local effect model (LEM) is used in HIT and our center. The same physical doses are converted to different biological doses by MKM and LEM [23, 24]. Therefore, the biological dose equivalent to ^{60}Cobalt (GyE) is really not equal using the two methods. We have carried out a dose escalation study again to find the appropriate dose/fractionation in SPHIC. Our aim is to deliver dose of BED_{10} of 100.

The following data are still under investigation in SPHIC. They are experimental and need to be confirmed. We would like to warn the readers to be very cautious in citing them for their practice.

The investigated fractionations for HCC were 5.5–6.5 GyE per fraction for ten fractions in 2 weeks for HCC ≥ 5 mm away from the GI tract and for tumors within 5 mm from the GI tract the combined proton of 50 GyE in 25 fractions and carbon ion of 15 GyE in five fractions until proton of 18 GyE in nine fractions and carbon ion of 45 GyE in 15 fractions.

For OAR dose constrains in CIRT for HCC, there has not been any clear data published yet in the literature. Our OAR dose constraints for 5.5–6.5 GyE/fraction are listed in Table 14.3, which are based on photon stereotactic body radiation (SBRT). Table 14.4 is for conventional fraction (2–3 GyE/fraction).

Table 14.3 OAR dose constrains for tumor located ≥ 5 mm away from the GI tract with 5.5–6.5 GyE per fraction

Liver	Normal liver volume of >700 mL, mean dose to normal liver[a] <15 GyE, V21 < 33%, V15 < 50%
	When normal liver volume of <700 mL, V17 < 70%
Kidney	Mean dose <12 GyE, V15 < 33%
Spinal cord	Maximum <27 GyE
Stomach	Maximum <32 GyE, V21 < 5 cm^3
Duodenum	Maximum <33 GyE
Small bowel	Maximum <34 GyE
Colon	Maximum <36 GyE

[a]Whole liver volume—GTV

Table 14.4 OAR dose constrains for tumors located <5 mm away from the GI tract with 2–3 GyE/fraction

Liver	Liver without cirrhosis, mean dose to normal liver[a] <30 GyE; liver with cirrhosis (Child-Pugh A), mean dose to normal liver <23 GyE
Stomach	V58 GyE < 0.03 mL; V50GyE < 5 mL; V45 GyE < 30 mL
Duodenum	V59 GyE < 0.03 mL; V56GyE < 5 mL; V45 GyE < 30 mL
Small bowel	V58 GyE < 0.03 mL; V50GyE < 10 mL; V45 GyE < 30 mL
Kidney	Single kidney, V18 < 80%; both kidneys, one >20 GyE and the other V18 < 10%
Spinal cord	Maximal <45 GyE, PRV V50 GyE < 1%

[a]Whole liver volume—GTV

Conclusion

(1) The clinical outcomes obtained with CIRT for HCC recently are encouraging.
(2) The technique of pencil beam scanning to treat HCC in CIRT needs further development.
(3) The optimal dose fractionation of CIRT for HCC and dose constraints for OARs should be further investigated based on biological models.
(4) CIRT to treat HCC is not yet in a fully mature stage and requires more evidence from clinical data.

References

1. Liang SX, Zhu XD, Xu ZY, et al. Radiation-induced liver disease in three-dimensional conformal radiation therapy for primary liver carcinoma: the risk factors and hepatic radiation tolerance. Int J Radiat Oncol Biol Phys. 2006;65(2):426–34.
2. Xu ZY, Liang SX, Zhu J, et al. Prediction of radiation-induced liver disease by Lyman normal-tissue complication probability model in three-dimensional conformal radiation therapy for primary liver carcinoma. Int J Radiat Oncol Biol Phys. 2006;65(1):189–95.
3. Zhao JD, Jiang GL, Hu WG, et al. Hepatocyte regeneration after partial liver irradiation in rats. Exp Toxicol Pathol. 2009;61(5):511–8.
4. Ren ZG, Zhao JD, Gu K, et al. Hepatic proliferation after partial liver irradiation in rat. Mol Biol Rep. 2012;39(4):3829–36.
5. Gu K, Lai ST, Ma NY, et al. Hepatic regeneration after sublethal partial liver irradiation in cirrhotic rats. J Radiat Res (Tokyo). 2011;52(5):582–91.
6. Gu K, Zhao JD, Ren ZG, et al. A natural process of cirrhosis resolution and deceleration of liver regeneration after thioacetamide withdrawal in a rat model. Mol Biol Rep. 2011;38(3):1687–96.
7. Fokas E, Kraft G, An H, Engenhart-Cabillic R. Ion beam radiobiology and cancer: time to update ourselves. Biochim Biophys Acta. 1796;2009:216–29.
8. Allen C, Borak TB, Tsujii H, et al. Heavy charged particle radiobiology: using enhanced biological effectiveness and improved beam focusing to advance cancer therapy. Mutat Res. 2011;711:150–7.
9. Furusawa Y. The characteristics of carbon ion radiotherapy. In: Tsujii H, Kamada T, Shirai T, Noda K, Tsuji H, Karawawa K, editors. Carbon ion radiotherapy. Japan: Springer; 2014. p. 25–37.
10. Habermehl D, Ilicic K, Dehne S, et al. The relative biological effectiveness for carbon and oxygen ion beams using the raster-scanning technique in hepatocellular carcinoma cell lines. PLoS One. 2014;9(12):e113591.
11. Bassler N, Toftegaard J, Luhr A, et al. LET-painting increases tumor control probability in hypoxic tumors. Acta Oncol. 2014;53:25–32.
12. Mori S, Zenklusen S, Inaniwa T, et al. Conformity and robustness of gated rescanned carbon ion pencil beam scanning of liver tumors at NIRS. Radiother Oncol. 2014;111:431–6.
13. Mori S, Inaniwa T, Furukawa T, et al. Amplitude-based gated phase-controlled rescanning in carbon-ion scanning beam treatment planning under irregular breathing conditions using lung and liver 4DCTs. J Radiat Res. 2014;55:948–58.
14. Ogata S, Mori S, Yasuda S. Extended phase-correlated rescanning irradiation to improve dose homogeneity in carbon-ion beam liver treatment. Phys Med Biol. 2014;59:5091–9.
15. Richter D, Graeff C, Jakel O, et al. Residual motion mitigation in scanned carbon ion beam therapy of liver tumors using enlarged pencil beam overlap. Radiother Oncol. 2014;113:290–5.

16. Kato H, Tsujii H, Miyamoto T, et al. Results of the first prospective study of carbon ion radiotherapy for hepatocellular carcinoma with liver cirrhosis. Int J Radiat Oncol Biol Phys. 2004;59(5):1468–76.
17. Imada H, Kato H, Yasuda S, et al. Conparison of efficacy and toxicity of short-course carbon ion radiotherapy for hepatocellular carcinoma depending on their proximity to the porta hepatis. Radiother Oncol. 2010;96:231–5.
18. Tsujii H, Kamada T, Shirai T, et al. Carbon-ion radiotherapy: principles, practices, and treatment planning. Japan: Springer; 2014. p. 213–8.
19. Imada H, Kato H, Yasuda S, et al. Compensatory enlargement of the liver after treatment of hepatocellular carcinoma with carbon ion radiotherapy - relation to prognosis and liver function. Radiother Oncol. 2010;96:236–42.
20. Komatsu S, Fukumoto T, Demizu Y, et al. Clinical results and risk factors of proton and carbon ion therapy for hepatocellular carcinoma. Cancer. 2011;117(21):4890–904.
21. Combs SE, Habermehl D, Ganten T, et al. Phase I study evaluating the treatment of patients with hepatocellular carcinoma (HCC) with carbon ion radiotherapy: the PROMETHEUS-01 trail. BMC Cancer. 2011;11:67.
22. Habermehl D, Debus J, Ganten T, et al. Hypofractionated carbon ion therapy delivered with scanned ion beam for patients with hepatocellular carcinoma - feasibility and clinical response. Radiat Oncol. 2013;8:59.
23. Steinstrater O, Grun R, Scholz U, et al. Mapping of RBE-weighted doses between HIMAC and LEM based treatment planning system for carbon ion therapy. Int J Radiat Oncol Biol Phys. 2012;84(3):854–60.
24. Fossati P, Molinelli S, Matsufuji N, et al. Dose prescription in carbon ion radiotherapy: a planning study for compare NIRS and LEM approaches with a clinically-oriented strategy. Phys Med Biol. 2012;57:7543–54.

Pancreatic and Stomach Malignancies

15

Pamela J. Boimel, Jessica Scholey, Liyong Lin, and Edgar Ben-Josef

Contents

15.1	Introduction	235
	15.1.1 Pancreatic Cancer	235
	15.1.2 Gastric Cancer	237
15.2	Simulation and Motion Management	239
15.3	Target Delineation and Radiation Dose/Fractionation	243
15.4	Proton Treatment Planning	245
	15.4.1 Planning Target Structures	246
	15.4.2 Contouring and Overrides	247
	15.4.3 Beam Angle Selection	248
15.5	Reirradiation	250
15.6	Dosimetric and Toxicity Comparison	250
15.7	Patient Positioning, Immobilization, and Treatment Verification	252
15.8	Discussion and Future Developments	252
References		253

15.1 Introduction

15.1.1 Pancreatic Cancer

- Pancreatic cancer is a morbid disease with a high mortality rate, and patients are often diagnosed with metastatic disease at presentation. Approximately 53,000 patients were diagnosed with pancreatic cancer in 2016, and only 7.7% of them will be alive in 5 years [1, 2]. Despite the high rate of distant dissemination, up to 30% of patients die of local disease progression [3]. While the treatment paradigm for

P.J. Boimel • J. Scholey • L. Lin • E. Ben-Josef (✉)
Department of Radiation Oncology, University of Pennsylvania, Philadelphia, PA, USA
e-mail: Edgar.Ben-Josef@uphs.upenn.edu

pancreatic cancer may change with the development of prognostic and predictive biomarkers to help determine who may benefit from local treatment versus systemic treatment, we currently utilize surgical resection when patients have resectable disease followed by adjuvant chemotherapy, with or without adjuvant chemoradiation. Patients with borderline or unresectable disease are treated with chemotherapy, and we often utilize chemoradiation for local disease control with some patients who had borderline resectable disease subsequently able to undergo surgical resection.

- Local failure occurs in about 50 percent of patients following resection and results in considerable morbidity and mortality. The use of postoperative radiation is supported by the GITSG 91-73 study, which showed an increased median survival from 11 to 20 months with chemoradiation following surgery compared to observation alone [4]. RTOG 9704 also reported on adjuvant chemoradiation, with a median survival of 20.5 months in the concurrent gemcitabine and radiation arm [5]. However, the use of adjuvant radiation has been controversial, since the CONKO-001 study of chemotherapy versus observation showed gemcitabine alone conferred a median survival of 22.8 months [6], EORTC 40891 showed no difference between chemoradiation and observation [7], and ESPAC-1 showed a benefit to chemotherapy over chemoradiation [8]. It is important to note that in the EORTC study, 45% of patients had ampullary cancer (with a better prognosis), so it was likely underpowered to detect a survival advantage in the pancreatic cancer patients, and 20% of the chemoradiation arm did not receive the prescribed regimen. There is also very strong evidence for adjuvant chemoradiation in large retrospective case series from Johns Hopkins and the Mayo Clinic showing the median survival extended from 11 to 20 months with adjuvant chemoradiation [9]. A National Cancer Database study using propensity score analysis in 11,526 patients revealed that chemoradiation was associated with improved overall survival, compared to adjuvant chemotherapy alone, when each was matched to surgery alone with a hazard ratio of 0.7–1.04, respectively [10]. The phase III RTOG 0848 trial of resected pancreatic head tumors treated with five cycles of adjuvant gemcitabine ± erlotinib and then, if free from progression, randomized to an additional cycle of chemotherapy or an additional cycle followed by chemoradiation is currently open to accrual and will help determine the optimal adjuvant regimen.
- There is evidence that for borderline resectable disease, local radiation treatment with concurrent high-dose chemotherapy offers a survival advantage, improved disease control, and the potential for a high rate of an R0 resection. A multi-institutional phase II trial of systemic dosing gemcitabine and oxaliplatin with radiation (30 Gy in 15 fractions) resulted in a 63% resection rate, 84% of which had negative margins, and a median survival of 18 months [11]. The benefit of chemoradiation compared to chemotherapy alone in unresectable disease has been controversial. The limitations in the intact setting have been toxicity to the upper abdominal structures as a result of the large radiation fields needed to cover the gross tumor volume in the 3D conformal era. The ECOG 4201 randomized phase II study of gemcitabine alone versus gemcitabine with concurrent conventional radiation (IMRT not allowed) showed an improved median survival and decreased local recurrence with radiation but with substantial grade 3 and 4 toxicities [12]. A phase I/II study from the University of Michigan evaluated high-dose conformal IMRT with concurrent gemcitabine and showed an

increased median survival of 14.8 months and an increased freedom from local progression of 60% compared to historical controls [13]. More recently, the Lap 07 trial randomized unresectable patients to gemcitabine versus gemcitabine + erlotinib, and then patients without progression were additionally randomized to chemoradiation, 54 Gy with concurrent capecitabine, versus additional chemotherapy [14]. The results showed no significant difference in overall survival between chemoradiation and chemotherapy alone but did show decreased locoregional progression in patients receiving chemoradiation. There are many patients for whom local progression results in significant morbidity and mortality. Autopsy series have reported that up to 30 percent of patients die of local disease progression which was correlated with the expression of SMAD4, indicating there are patients for whom local disease control is very important [3]. Local progression of unresected pancreatic cancer can also result in significant morbidity with obstructive symptoms, bleeding, bowel perforation, and pain necessitating palliation even in the patient with metastatic disease.
- With little improvement in survival seen in studies of chemoradiation using modest radiation doses (~50–54 Gy in 1.8–2 Gy fractions), dose escalation has been attempted with 3D conformal radiation, resulting in significant gastrointestinal toxicities [15]. Studies utilizing IMRT have reported lower rates of acute grade 3 nausea and vomiting, diarrhea, and late gastrointestinal toxicities such as duodenal ulceration compared to studies using 3D conformal radiation [16]. However, IMRT dose escalation with concurrent gemcitabine also resulted in significant toxicities, with 24% of patients experiencing grade 3 or 4 dose-limiting toxicities [13]. SBRT has been evaluated for unresectable disease with comparable median survival to conventional fractionation and with increased concern for acute gastrointestinal toxicity when the disease is in close proximity to or invading the duodenum [17]. In theory, proton radiation with its characteristic Bragg peak and rapid falloff at the distal end of the proton beam could be superior to IMRT or SBRT in sparing normal tissues. In practice, however, range uncertainties related to CT calibration, organ motion, and patient setup have necessitated an increase in margins in proton therapy. As double-scattered (DS) and uniform scanning (US) proton therapy cannot modify beam portal along their beam path, conformality is increased with pencil beam scanning (PBS) compared to DS and US.

15.1.2 Gastric Cancer

- While the incidence of gastric cancer is declining, it still contributes significantly to cancer mortality as the third leading cause of cancer-related death worldwide. In locally advanced and node-positive disease, surgery with lymphadenectomy is the mainstay of treatment. The use of perioperative chemotherapy and/or adjuvant chemoradiation has been controversial. Neoadjuvant and adjuvant chemotherapy may be offered based on results of the MAGIC trial of perioperative chemotherapy showing increased overall survival and improved progression-free survival compared to surgery alone. Alternatively, patients may proceed with surgery and then receive adjuvant chemoradiation, done frequently in the United States, based on results of the North American Intergroup 0116 trial showing a survival advantage. Practically, the decision to offer perioperative chemotherapy or adjuvant chemoradiation may depend on the local extent of disease, resectability at presentation, and pathologic risk factors after resection such as the margin status and extent of the lymph node dissection.

- The surgical approach for stomach tumors is either a total gastrectomy for proximal 1/3 and diffuse gastric malignancies or a subtotal gastrectomy for tumors of the gastric antrum (distal 2/3) [18]. Surgical margins are very important due to the infiltrative nature, and a 5 cm proximal and distal margin has historically been recommended. However, recent multi-institutional retrospective analysis of distal gastric cancers indicated that 3 cm may be adequate [19]. There are 16 lymph node stations, and the extent of their dissection is described in the surgical literature. A D1 lymph node dissection is the removal of the adjacent perigastric lymph nodes (stations 1–6) alone; a D2 dissection includes the additional dissection of the hepatic, left gastric, celiac, and splenic nodes (stations 1–11) as well as a splenectomy; and a D3 dissection additionally adds the porta hepatic and periaortic nodes (stations 1–16). In practice a D2 dissection with removal of at least 15 lymph nodes is recommended, but this is often dependent on the experience of the surgeon performing the surgery, and many patients have much more limited D1 dissections with fewer lymph nodes removed.

- Adjuvant chemoradiation is often offered based on the results of the Intergroup 0166 randomized trial of postoperative radiation with 45 Gy and fluorouracil and leucovorin versus observation. The 3-year overall survival was significantly increased to 50% in patients receiving chemoradiation from 41% with observation alone, supporting the use of adjuvant chemoradiation [20]. In this trial a D2 lymph node dissection was recommended; however, only 9.6% had a D2, 36% had a D1, and 54% had less than a D1 lymph node dissection. These results imply that chemoradiation may benefit a population without an adequate lymphadenectomy. The acute toxicity rate was also significant in this study in the 2D planning era, with 54% hematologic and 33% gastrointestinal grade 3 or greater toxicity. Seventeen percent stopped treatment due to toxicity and there was a 1% death rate. The ARTIST I trial evaluated adjuvant chemotherapy versus chemoradiation in patients who underwent a D2 lymph node dissection and found no survival or distant metastasis-free survival difference [21]. However, there was a significant decrease in local relapse rate with chemoradiation which can cause significant morbidity in this population. A subset analysis of the ARTIST I trial found a disease-free survival benefit in patients with lymph node-positive disease, and the ARTIST II trial is currently evaluating the benefit of chemoradiation in lymph node-positive disease. It is also important to note that on subset analysis of the INT-0116 trial, there appeared to be a reduced effect of chemoradiation in patients with diffuse-type histology. The ARTIST I trial had a high proportion of patients with diffuse-type histology (63% in the chemoradiation arm) which we know have worse outcomes and may have made it difficult to show a benefit.

- There are patients who benefit from adjuvant chemoradiation, and likely those with positive lymph nodes, less than a D2 lymph node dissection, and positive or inadequate surgical margins benefit more from adjuvant radiation treatment. The treatment volume encompasses the tumor bed, the remaining stomach, anastomoses, hepatogastric ligament, and at-risk and dissected lymph node volumes. With a large treatment volume, it is important that we utilize advances in radiation treatment delivery with more conformal techniques to reduce toxicity. Three-dimensional conformal treatment has been compared with IMRT and was found to increase conformality and decrease the dose to the spinal cord, kidneys, liver, and heart [22]. Proton beam radiation is promising as another treatment modality in gastric malignancy to spare dose to nearby OARs with the potential to decrease toxicity.

15.2 Simulation and Motion Management

Robust indexed immobilization is strongly recommended when treating pancreatic and gastric malignancies to minimize interfraction patient setup error. Immobilization vacuum bags can be used provided that the bag volume does not change through the course of treatment, as variation in bag volume can perturb the proton beam range. If used, bag volume should be verified with imaging prior to each treatment. Alternatively, simulation and treatment may be performed using a wing board or alpha cradle and indexed knee lock to prevent rotation in the legs and hips (Fig. 15.1). Simulation scans should be performed in the supine position with arms up and away from the treatment area. Scans should be acquired from the carina to below the iliac crest.

Non-contrast CT scans should be obtained for treatment planning for the purpose of dose calculation. A high-resolution CT scan (slice thickness of 3 mm or less) with IV contrast may be subsequently performed for improved delineation of the primary tumor, vasculature, and lymph nodes. Volumen (0.1% barium suspension),

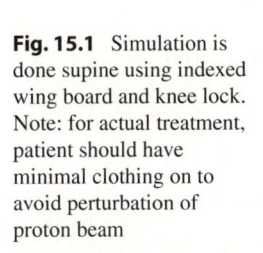

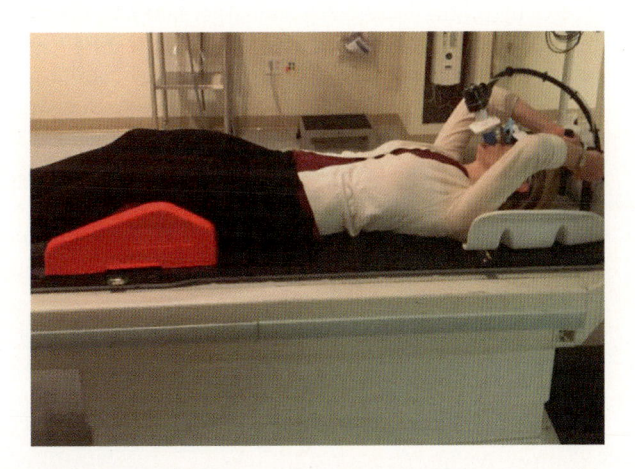

Fig. 15.1 Simulation is done supine using indexed wing board and knee lock. Note: for actual treatment, patient should have minimal clothing on to avoid perturbation of proton beam

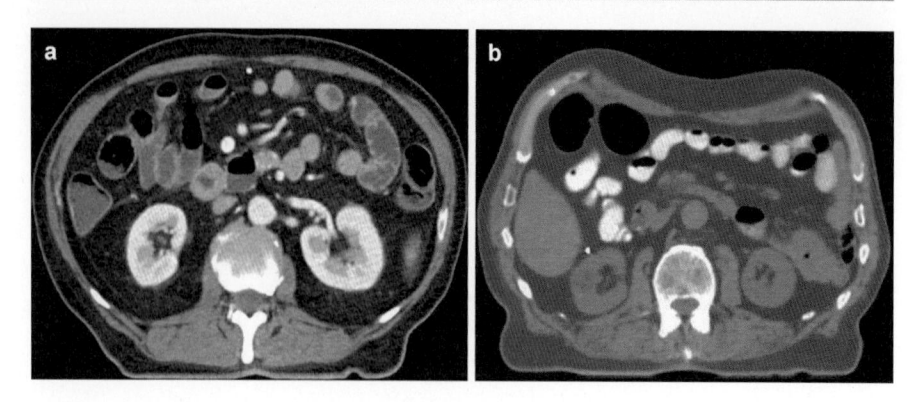

Fig. 15.2 (a) Volumen oral contrast, when used with IV contrast, allows for improved mural detail in the duodenum and bowel. (b) Barium as an oral contrast agent

a negative oral contrast agent with low attenuation (Fig. 15.2a), allows for excellent distention as well as superior visualization of mural detail of the duodenum and small intestine with CT imaging [23]. It is recommended that contrast scans be performed subsequent to scans used for treatment planning; however, if that is not possible, any material existing in the planning scan which will not be present for treatment must be overridden and assigned appropriate Hounsfield unit (HU) values. Of note, metal mash stents in the common bile duct do not perturb the proton dose distribution and do not need to be overridden. Additional imaging such as diagnostic-quality CT, PET-CT, and/or MRI may also be useful to visualize involved lymph nodes, extent of gross disease, and recurrent disease. In the case of postoperative radiation, preoperative imaging should also be used when delineating the target volume. If possible, all scans should be acquired with the patient in the same position as CT simulation for improved accuracy in image registration. Patients are instructed to not take anything by mouth (NPO) for a minimum of 3 hours prior to simulation to decrease variability in gastric volume. Patients may be given specific dietary instructions to be NPO for a few hours prior to treatment fractions as well, depending on the location of the target and its proximity to the stomach or when treating gastric cancer. For example, when treating gastric adenocarcinoma after a subtotal gastrectomy at our institution, patients are instructed to withhold food and fluid consumption for 3 hours prior to simulation and daily treatment so that stomach and bowel volumes are reproducible.

Respiratory- and gastrointestinal-induced motion management is an important component of treating thoracic and abdominal malignancies as these regions routinely exhibit significant motion [24, 25]. An in-depth analysis of motion mitigation techniques is beyond the scope of this chapter, although Task Group 76 of the American Association of Physicists in Medicine discusses a comprehensive overview of available options [26]. Several motion mitigation methods are employed at our institution when treating pancreatic and gastric targets, depending on the degree of anatomical motion exhibited by the patient. These methods include using respiratory-correlated (or 4DCT) scans and adding an ITV to account for motion,

15 Pancreatic and Stomach Malignancies

deep inspiration breath hold (DIBH), or abdominal compression. The modality of motion management is particularly important for unresected pancreatic adenocarcinoma, since the tumor and duodenum are usually in close proximity. We recommend motion management with breath hold (involuntary with Active Breathing Control, ABC, or voluntary deep inspiratory breath hold, DIBH, with SDX), when treating unresected pancreatic tumors.

Fluoroscopy can be useful in identifying the degree of a patient's anatomical motion [27–30]. At our institution, patients who are being simulated for an abdominal malignancy may undergo a pre-simulation fluoroscopy session to assess the degree of motion and determine which method may be the best option to mitigate or account for motion during treatment (Fig. 15.3). Not all abdominal lesions can be clearly visualized on fluoroscopy and should be administered on a per-patient basis. Visualization techniques may aid in delineating volumes of interest in the fluoroscopy, such as implanted markers, oral contrast to distinguish stomach volume, or nearby visible landmarks whose motion may act as a surrogate for the region of interest (for example, the liver or diaphragm). In general, patients with less than 5 mm of motion undergo 4DCT scans, with treatment planning being performed on the CT scan comprised of the average of all breathing phases. Patients with greater than 5 mm of motion may require DIBH or abdominal compression to reduce the

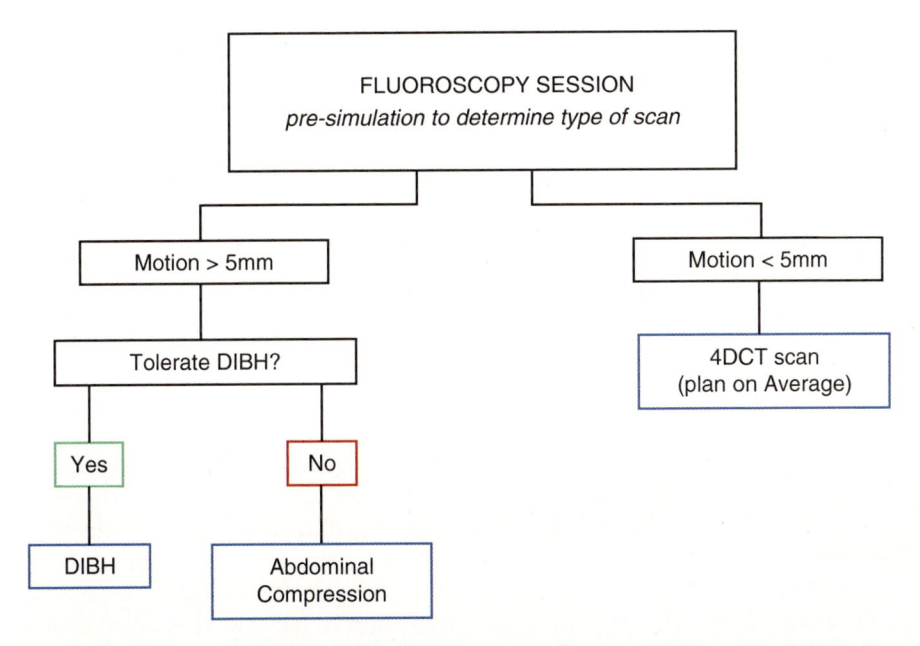

Fig. 15.3 Example of workflow diagram from pre-simulation fluoroscopy session to determine type of motion management used. General practice at our institution is that if motion is less than 5 mm, planning is performed on a free-breathing average CT scan. If motion is greater than 5 mm and DIBH is tolerated, SDX or ABC device is utilized for DIBH. If not tolerated, abdominal compression using a belt is utilized. Motion should be carefully evaluated by the treating team on a per patient basis

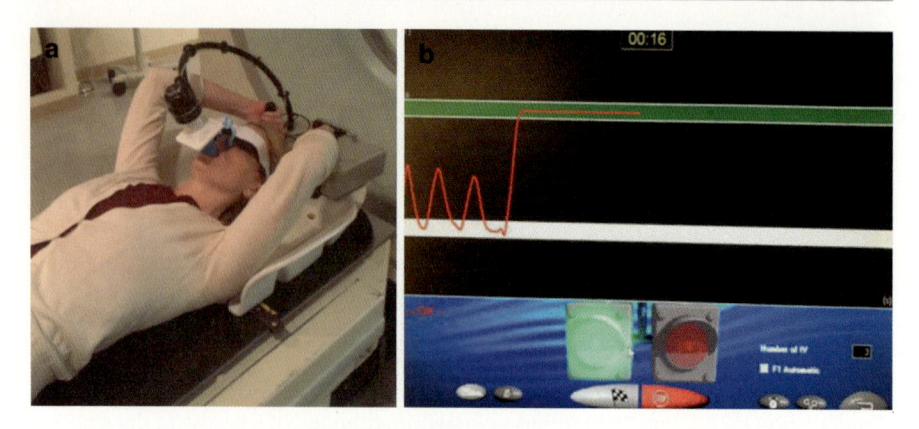

Fig. 15.4 (a) Voluntary DIBH using spirometric motion management is shown. (b) Patient interface when using voluntary breath-hold SDX system. Therapists are instructed to turn the treatment beam on during the predefined inhale region (shown in *green*)

amount of anatomical motion. DIBH may be achieved using a device such as the Active Breathing Control or ABC (Elekta Medical Systems, Stockholm, Sweden) or the Spirometric Motion Management System or SDX (Qfix, Avondale, PA), both of which have been implemented at our institution (Fig. 15.4). Because SDX requires patient compliance and the ability to hold one's breath as instructed, abdominal compression using a compression belt may be more tolerable. One advantage of the ABC device over SDX is that with ABC the time of breath hold is controlled by the therapist (rather than by the patients). This allows for correct timing of the administration of IV contrast. Contrast-enhanced scans using breath hold with the SDX device are very difficult to obtain.

An important consideration when using abdominal compression is minimizing variability in anatomical deformation caused by the belt. It is important that the belt be placed in the same position each day, including indexing and belt tightness. Positioning of the belt and abdominal anatomy can be verified using x-ray portals, verification CT scans, and/or onboard CBCT if available. In general, image guidance should be used to ensure that interfraction range variations are less than 3 mm for 95% of the target volume [31]. Additional imaging used for target delineation should employ the same compression as used for the planning CT. For example, if MRI is used for anatomical delineation, an MRI-compatible compression belt should be used. This prevents propagating differences in anatomical positioning caused by the belt. As with any system, patients should undergo training with the appropriate motion management devices to maximize their effectiveness. During simulation, care should be taken to keep devices outside of the potential treatment field.

Accurate registration between imaging sets is important. In addition to bony anatomy, we focus fusions on patient vasculature (celiac and SMA) for unresectable pancreatic head tumors. With breath-hold devices, there is variability in the position of the abdominal target, even with identical tidal volumes. To account for this reproducibility error, at our institution an additional superior and inferior margin of 2 mm is added to CTV [32, 33].

While pencil beam scanning (PBS) proton therapy can create more conformal dose distributions versus passive scattering techniques, the use of PBS in thoracic and abdominal malignancies has been limited due to the uncertain relationship between spot scanning and respiratory-related anatomical motion [34]. This complicated interplay effect between spot delivery and organ motion has made passive scattering techniques, specifically double scatter or uniform scanning, preferable when treating patients with higher levels of anatomical motion, although PBS is being increasingly adopted for more cases at our institution.

15.3 Target Delineation and Radiation Dose/Fractionation

- The gross tumor volume (GTV) for definitive chemoradiation of borderline or unresectable locally advanced pancreatic adenocarcinoma is drawn on the non-contrast-enhanced, simulation CT scan using the registered contrast-enhanced simulation CT scan and MRI/PET if available to delineate the extent of the gross tumor visible and any involved lymph nodes (≥ 1 cm). On contrast-enhanced scans, pancreatic tumors are often hypodense/hypointense compared to normal pancreatic tissue on the late arterial and venous phases, although they can rarely be isodense/isointense and harder to distinguish from the surrounding parenchyma. To assist with delineation, it can be helpful to carefully look at the biliary anatomy and follow the dilated intrapancreatic biliary duct to the point of obstruction in order to locate tumors in the pancreatic head. Pancreatic tumors often appear as hazy dark-gray soft tissue which can extend into the abdominal fat and duodenum and wrap around the vasculature. Following the celiac and SMA carefully to look for tumor wrapping around these vessels can also help delineate the GTV boarders. At our institution we do not electively treat lymph nodes based on data that when prophylactic nodal radiation was omitted, there were few peripancreatic lymph node failures and all were within the 80% isodose line [35]. The CTV is generated by adding a 5 mm margin to the GTV and a PTV by adding 5 mm to the CTV for setup errors.
- Target volumes for pancreatic cancer in the postoperative setting have been well described by consensus contouring guidelines [36]. The clinical target volume is the proximal 1–1.5 cm of the celiac artery, the proximal 2.5 cm of the superior mesenteric artery (SMA), the portal vein (PV) contoured from its junction with the superior mesenteric vein up to the bifurcation of the left and right branches, the pancreaticojejunostomy (PJ), the preoperative tumor volume and surgical bed including any clips left intraoperatively, and the aorta from the most superior structure (PJ, PV, or celiac) down to the level of the L2 vertebral body. Each of these structures is contoured separately with differential expansion to CTV as previously described. These separate CTV structures are then booleaned together into one CTV structure. An ITV is generated from the 4DCT to account for respiratory motion, and then a 5 mm PTV is added (Table 15.1).

Table 15.1 Recommended target volumes and radiation dose ranges (for an RBE = 1.1) for pancreatic and gastric cancers

Clinical scenario	Target	Dose
Definitive chemoradiation for pancreatic cancer	Pancreatic tumor and involved lymph nodes (≥ 1 cm)	5400–5940 cGy
Postoperative chemoradiation for pancreatic cancer	Proximal celiac artery, SMA, PV Pancreaticojejunostomy Preoperative tumor volume Surgical bed/clips Aorta	4500–5400 cGy May boost + margins (5940 cGy)
Adjuvant chemoradiation for gastric cancer	Anastomoses Tumor bed (including clips/gastric remnant) Hepatogastric ligament Lymph nodes • Perigastric • Suprapancreatic • Celiac • **Cardiac tumors**—add L hemidiaphragm, right and left cardiac, pancreatic body, left gastric, and hepatic and celiac arteries • **Body tumors**—porta hepatic, splenic hilum, pancreatic body, pancreaticoduodenal, left gastric, and hepatic artery • **Antrum tumors**—porta hepatic, pancreaticoduodenal, pancreatic head	4500 cGy Consider boost to 5040 (or 5400–5940 cGy for positive margins)
Reirradiation for local recurrence	Gross disease	5400–5940 cGy

- For gastric cancer, a lymph node contouring atlas has been published which nicely describes the anatomic boundaries and contouring of the 16 lymph node stations described in the literature [37]. The CTV includes the anastomoses (esophagojejunal for total gastrectomy and gastrojejunal for a subtotal gastrectomy as well as the duodenal stump), preoperative tumor bed, hepatogastric ligament, and regional lymph nodes. In general lymph node coverage should depend on the location of the tumor within the stomach. For all scenarios we would include the N1 perigastric lymph nodes and suprapancreatic and celiac lymph nodes. For tumors of the *proximal 1/3 of the stomach (cardia)*, we would additionally include lymph nodes along the left and right cardia, the lesser and greater curvature, L hemidiaphragm, and pancreatic body. The left gastric artery, hepatic artery, and celiac artery are also included in the CTV. For tumors of the *middle 1/3 of the stomach (body)*, we would include lymph nodes of the lesser and greater curvature, splenic hilum, porta hepatic, pancreaticoduodenal, and pancreatic body as well as the left gastric artery and hepatic artery. For tumors of the *distal 1/3 of the stomach (antrum)*, we would

Table 15.2 Recommended dose constraints (for an $RBE = 1.1$) to organs at risk for treatment of pancreatic and gastric cancer

Organ at risk	Dose constraints
Kidney (left and right)	$V18 \leq 50\%$
Liver	Mean ≤ 30 Gy
Stomach	D_{max} 60, $V54 \leq 2\%$, $V45 \leq 25\%$
Small bowel	D_{max} 60, $V54 \leq 2\%$, $V50.4 \leq 5\%$, $V45 \leq 25\%$
Large bowel	D_{max} 60, $V54 \leq 2\%$, $V50.4 \leq 5\%$, $V45 \leq 25\%$
Duodenum	D_{max} 60, $V55 \leq 1$ cc, $V54 \leq 5\%$
Spinal cord	Max ≤ 45 Gy

include lymph nodes of the lesser and greater curvature, porta hepatic, pancreaticoduodenal, and pancreatic head lymph nodes. For tumors near the pylorus, we would take an additional distal margin into the duodenum of about 5 cm (Table 15.1).
- Normal abdominal structures such as the liver, kidneys, spinal cord, stomach (for pancreatic cancers), and small and large bowel are contoured as organs at risk. For unresected locally advanced pancreatic cancer, it is important to carefully delineate and contour the duodenum as there can be overlap between the duodenum and target volume (Table 15.2).

15.4 Proton Treatment Planning

Because of the complicated interplay effect between anatomical motion and spot scanning, the majority of pancreatic and gastric cancer patients at our institution have been treated with passive scattering techniques (double scatter or uniform scanning). In select cases where PBS is particularly desirable (e.g., if trying to treat a target with irregular geometry or further spare nearby organs), careful evaluation of anatomical motion is required. A study from our institution investigated the dosimetric impacts of treating abdominal lesions with PBS. It was found that for small motion ($M\perp < 7$ mm anΔWET <5 mm, where $M\perp$ is the perpendicular motion amplitude and ΔWET is the change in water equivalent thickness), motion mitigation was not needed. For moderate motion ($M\perp$ 7–10 mm or ΔWET 5–7 mm), abdominal compression produced a modest improvement. For large motion ($M\perp > 10$ mm or ΔWET > 7 mm), abdominal compression and/or some other forms of mitigation strategies were required [38]. Because of anatomical variability and motion in the abdomen, our institution treats PBS using single-field uniform dose (SFUD) techniques and will be the focus of this chapter. However, future developments in robust optimization may allow for more widespread implementation of intensity-modulated proton therapy (IMPT).

15.4.1 Planning Target Structures

Proton beam range uncertainty due to conversion between CT Hounsfield units and proton stopping-power ratio must always be considered when treating with proton radiotherapy.

- Passive scattering: when treating with passive scattering at our institution, this uncertainty is mitigated by adding additional distal and proximal margins to the CTV structure which correct for range uncertainty of 3.5% (of beam range) +3 mm in the distal direction and proximal directions (Fig. 15.5). Lateral margins should also be added to account for motion and setup errors.

Compensator: when using a range compensator to modulate the dose in passive scattering, it is important to use compensator smearing to ensure that the proton beam adequately shapes target volume despite any setup errors and intrafraction motion. At our institution, the smearing parameter is derived from Moyers et al. [39] and is calculated using the following equation:

$$\sqrt{(IM+SM)^2 + \left[0.03 \times \left(CTV_{depth} + Compensator_{thickness}\right)\right]^2}$$

where IM is internal motion, SM is setup margin, and CTV_{depth} is the distal depth of the CTV. At our institution we determine internal motion on a patient-specific basis and utilize 3 mm setup error to determine the compensator smearing parameter.

- Pencil beam scanning: to account for proton beam range uncertainty in PBS, a planning optimization structure can be created when using a single-field optimization planning technique. At our institution, an optimization structure is created by adding to the CTV a margin of 3.5% of the beam range (accounting for uncertainty in the conversion from Hounsfield unit (HU) values to proton stopping power) plus an additional 1 mm margin (correcting for beam calibration uncertainty). Specific uncertainty values employed should be evaluated on an institutional basis) (Fig. 15.6).

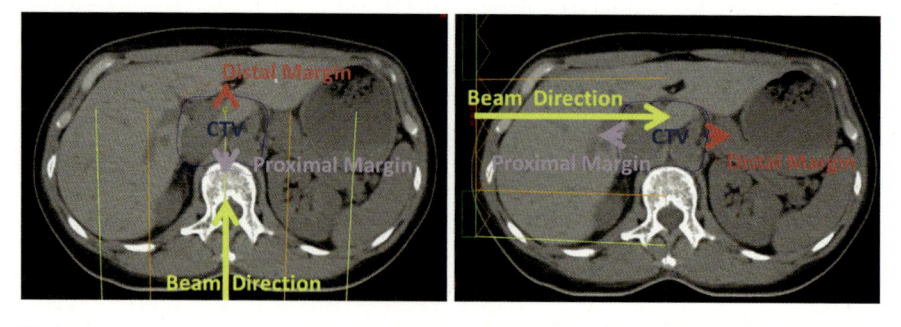

Fig. 15.5 Examples of distal (*red*) and proximal (*purple*) margins added to the CTV target along the beam direction for a patient being treated with a posterior beam (*left*) and right lateral beam (*right*) using passive scattering proton technique

15 Pancreatic and Stomach Malignancies

Fig. 15.6 Pencil beam scanning target volume (PBSTV) optimization structure (*red*) is created by adding a margin of 3.5% of the beam range plus 1 mm to CTV structure (*blue*) in the direction of the beam. A conventional PTV structure (CTV + 5 mm) is shown in green for comparison

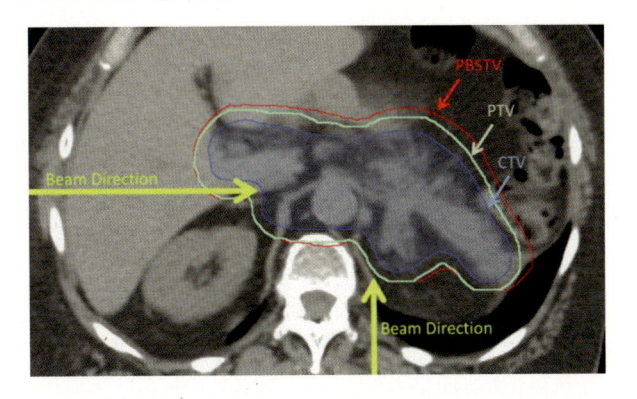

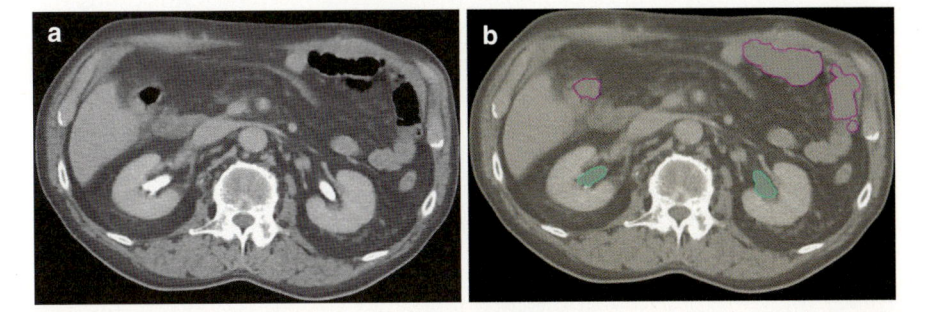

Fig. 15.7 It is recommended that contrast scans be acquired after treatment planning scans. However, if that is not possible, any contrast material appearing in the planning scan which will not be present for treatment should be overridden to the appropriate HU value. Shown are examples of HU material overrides for kidney contrast and bowel gas

15.4.2 Contouring and Overrides

- To account for changes in bowel filling, gas and stool are contoured and assigned an HU value similar to the surrounding tissues. Artifacts created by high-density material should be overridden to an appropriate HU value. It is recommended that contrast scans be performed subsequent to planning CT so that no contrast is present in planning scan; however, if that is not feasible, any high-contrast material that appears in planning scan (e.g., barium) should be assigned an appropriate density or HU value (Fig. 15.7). Manual HU overrides are not required for Volumen contrast.
- If the diaphragm is in close proximity to the target or treatment fields, a diaphragm override volume can be created by adding an additional margin to the diaphragm which is defined by the inferior borders of the lung in the exhale and inhale scans when 4DCT-based planning is employed (Fig. 15.8). The HU value of this margin should be overridden to the value determined by sampling the most superior slice containing the dome of the liver, which generally varies between −50 and +50 HUs.

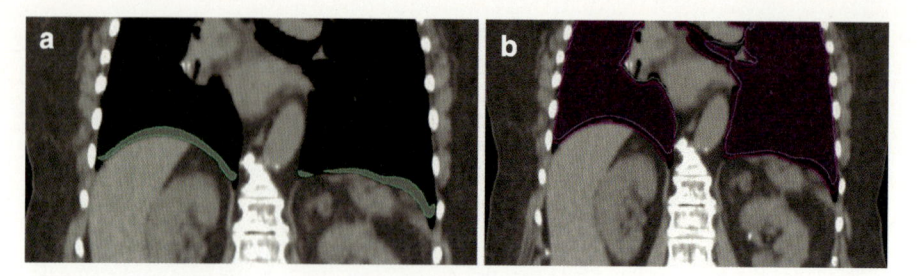

Fig. 15.8 To account for motion of the diaphragm, an additional margin can be added to the diaphragm (**a**) and is constructed by subtracting the lung contours between the inhale and exhale scans (**b**) when 4DCT is used for planning purposes

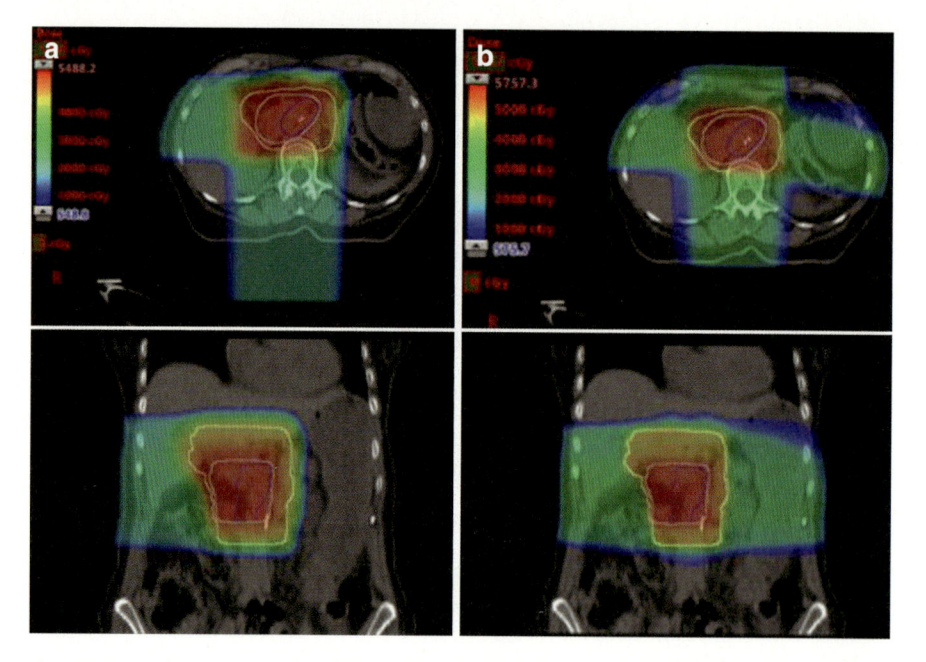

Fig. 15.9 Postoperative radiation for T3 N1 pancreatic adenocarcinoma with a close uncinate margin (4500 cGy to entire postoperative CTV; 5400 cGy to post-op bed, anastomoses, clips, and SMA; and 5940 cGy in region of close margin). (**a**) Patient was treated with a double-scatter proton plan consisting of a posterior and right lateral beam arrangement to avoid the bowel, stomach, and left kidney. (**b**) For comparison, an IMRT photon plan is shown. To achieve adequate target coverage in this case, photons deliver higher dose to the stomach, bowel, and left kidney, making protons the more desirable option

15.4.3 Beam Angle Selection

- For both passive scatter and PBS techniques, beam arrangements typically consist of 2–3 coplanar fields, which usually include a posterior beam and either a posterior oblique or right-sided beam (blocking the cord) (Figs. 15.9,

15.10 and 15.11). Gantry angles should be chosen to minimize dose to spinal cord, kidneys, skin overlap, and duodenal dose from the beam penumbra [40]. When using an abdominal compression belt, it is important to override artifacts caused by the belt and attempt to choose beam arrangements which do not shoot through the belt.
- Beams which enter anteriorly or from the patient's left side are avoided due to uncertainties created by presence of air, motion of stomach and bowel, and variability in anterior abdominal tissue.
- If treating with anterior beam arrangements provides a more desirable plan, these beams can be used and possibly given a lower weight (Fig. 15.12). A left-sided beam may be needed when covering left hemidiaphragmatic, perigastric lymph nodes, and splenic lymph nodes for adjuvant gastric cancer cases. The weight of the posterior beam may also be limited by tolerance doses to the kidneys or cord.

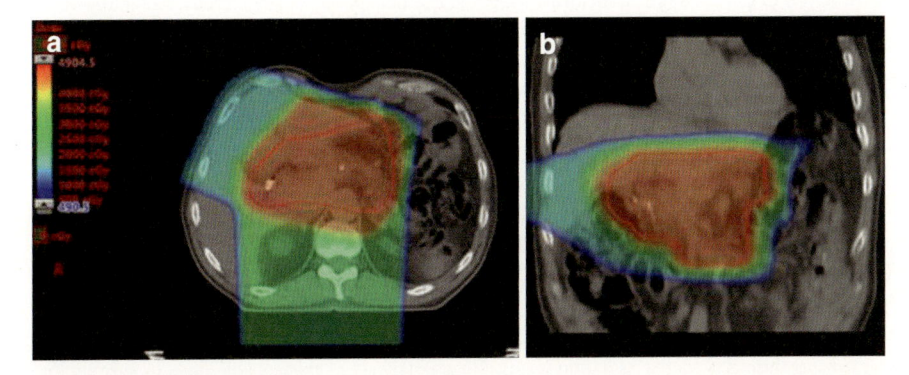

Fig. 15.10 Postoperative radiation for gastric adenocarcinoma in the antrum, treated with double-scatter proton therapy using a posterior and right anterior oblique beam to avoid proton beam traversing through the bowel. Axial (**a**) and coronal (**b**) views are shown with PTV shown in *red*

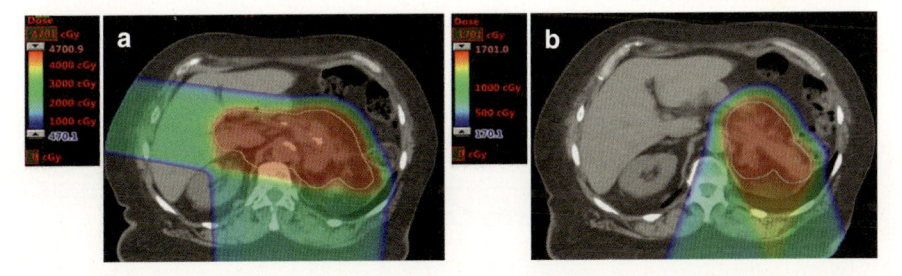

Fig. 15.11 Pancreatic cancer patient (post distal pancreatectomy) with surgical bed recurrence was treated using PBS proton therapy at our institution. (**a**) To achieve lateral coverage on the right side of the target, a right anterior oblique beam was used with a posterior beam in the plan treated to 44 Gy. (**b**) Gross residual disease received a conedown to total dose of 60 Gy using right and left posterior oblique beams. In both plans the bowel is almost completely spared, and we avoid treating through variable bowel volume

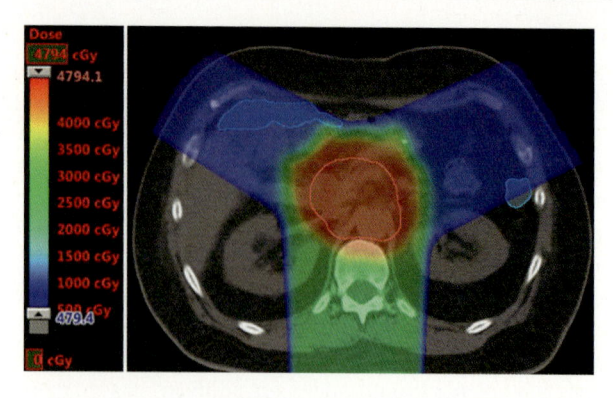

Fig. 15.12 Pancreatic patient treated with double-scatter proton technique using a posterior beam plus two anterior oblique beams. Anterior beams were chosen in this case to minimize kidney dose. To avoid large beam perturbations due to anatomical changes in anterior anatomy (e.g., fluctuations in bowel gas), anterior beams were weighted less than posterior beam (beam weighting of 0.2 for each anterior beam and 0.6 for posterior beam were used)

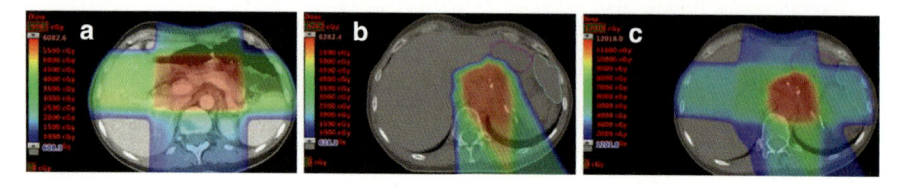

Fig. 15.13 (**a**) Pancreatic case originally treated with photons after Whipple procedure. (**b**) Patient had local recurrence which was treated with double-scatter proton therapy using posterior beams to avoid dose overlap of lateral and anterior organs. (**c**) Sum total of photon and proton treatments indicates higher radiation dose to disease sites and manageable dose to surrounding healthy organs

15.5 Reirradiation

Both PBS and passive scatter techniques can be used for treating pancreatic and gastric malignancies which have received prior radiation to help limit dose to normal tissue that has already been irradiated (Fig. 15.13).

15.6 Dosimetric and Toxicity Comparison

- We have previously reported on a dosimetric study comparing IMRT versus double-scattering (DS) and pencil beam scanning (PBS) proton radiation for unresected pancreatic head cancers [40]. This study demonstrated that both DS and PBS decreased duodenum, stomach, and small bowel dose in the low-dose region. The V20 Gy to the stomach was reduced from about 20% with IMRT to 10% with proton beam radiation, and for the small bowel, V20 was 6.5% with PBS, 9.8% with DS, and 19.7% with IMRT. However, dose to the duodenum, stomach, and

15 Pancreatic and Stomach Malignancies

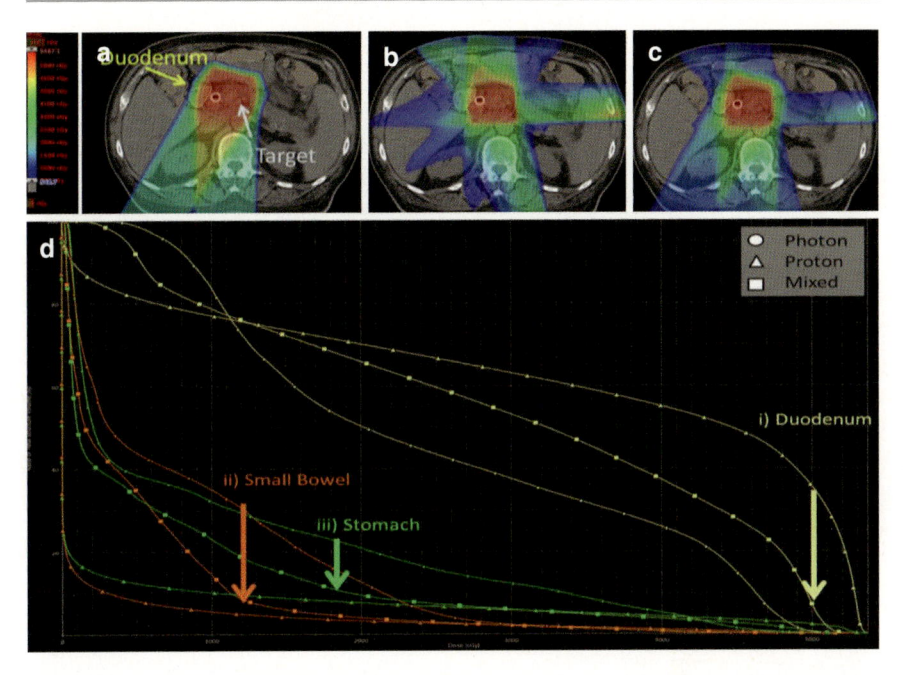

Fig. 15.14 (**a**) In some cases, a proton plan (using posterior and right posterior oblique beams) may result in a larger volume of tissue going to D_{max} in critical organs near the PTV or if overlapping the PTV (e.g., the duodenum). (**b**) An IMRT plan may decrease the volume of high dose to the OAR due to increased conformality, at the expense of increased low-dose spread to other OARs. (**c**) A combined proton (*double-scatter*)/photon plan was administered to this patient to achieve an optimal balance between high- and low-dose sparing. (**d**) DVH comparison for photon-only plan (*circle*), proton-only plan (*triangle*), and mixed proton-photon plan (*square*). In this case, the benefit of a mixed proton-photon plan included significant decrease in (i) high dose to duodenum versus proton-only plan, (ii) low dose to small bowel versus photon-only plan, and (iii) low dose to stomach versus photon-only plan

small bowel in the high-dose region (>40 Gy) showed IMRT to be superior followed by PBS and finally DS. This study highlighted that in unresected pancreatic head tumors, in close proximity to or invading the duodenum, there is a need for high conformality which may not be met by DS or PBS plans alone. The quality of life and toxicity outcomes for this comparison have not yet been evaluated. It is unknown how a large volume of duodenum/stomach/small bowel getting a low-dose bath from IMRT may impact the toxicity or quality of life of patients compared to a mid- to high-dose point near the tumor as long as maximum dose constraints to OARs are met. As our proton beam radiation techniques advance and we improve motion management techniques as previously described and begin to utilize IMPT, we may potentially achieve the optimal combination of high conformality combined with minimal integral dose to nearby OARs. In the meantime, our institution has routinely used mixed photon/proton plans to decrease the volume of duodenum in the high-dose region while still achieving lower integral dose to the abdomen than a photon plan alone (Fig. 15.14).

- A unique and rare presentation of pancreatic cancer is the local-regional recurrence, with or without minimal metastatic burden. These tumors may be characterized by intact expression of SMAD4 [3]. We have previously enrolled patients with locally recurrent pancreatic adenocarcinoma on a proton beam reirradiation registry and reported on 15 of these patients [41]. Proton reirradiation was generally well tolerated with a median survival of 15.7 months and minimal grade 1 and 2 non-hematologic acute toxicities, grade 3 fatigue in 2 patients, and no grade 2 or higher late toxicities [41]. There was one duodenum ulceration in a patient treated to progression of unresected locally advanced adenocarcinoma with duodenum abutting the PTV. We recommend patients are treated to the gross disease alone with minimal CTV expansions (the median CTV in our reirradiation cohort was 71 cc) and try to avoid beam angles which overlap with the prior radiation fields.

15.7 Patient Positioning, Immobilization, and Treatment Verification

Treatment positioning should be performed using the same immobilization techniques as used in simulation. Localization should be performed daily by matching bony anatomy in orthogonal x-ray imaging. If volume of stomach will impact treatment delivery, oral contrast can be administered to more clearly delineate gastric volume in kV imaging. If available, onboard volumetric imaging (CBCT) can be used to verify soft tissue anatomy. For proton patients we perform biweekly verification scans to check for changes in anatomy, such as weight loss, and variation in bowel gas and gastric filling.

15.8 Discussion and Future Developments

- The utilization of protons for treating pancreatic and gastric cancers can be useful to decrease integral dose to stomach, bowel, kidney, and liver depending on the location of the PTV and beam arrangement chosen. In the case of adjuvant chemoradiation for resected pancreatic and gastric cancers, where field sizes are often large, proton radiation can reduce dose to OARs sparing kidney, liver, and a large amount of bowel, improving the toxicity profile. Advances in co-registration software for image fusions, incorporating cone beam CT into IGRT for proton delivery, gating for motion management, and better understanding of the range uncertainty (allowing margins to be decreased) would help us advance proton planning and treatment.
- Delivering radiation with limited motion (e.g., using breath hold) is of great importance as it allows delivery of higher doses to target, lower doses to OARs, and more treatment reproducibility. Motion management is particularly important with proton therapy and truly critical with PBS.

15 Pancreatic and Stomach Malignancies

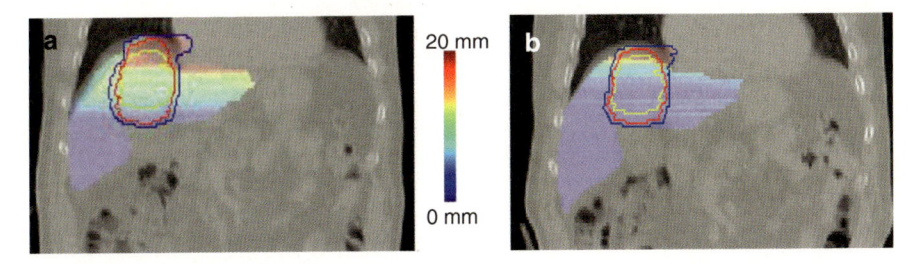

Fig. 15.15 Figure showing the difference in motion without (**a**) and with (**b**) abdominal compression. Difference of CTV (*yellow*), ITV (*red*), BSPTV (*blue*), and ΔWET (*color wash*) over CT images (Figure courtesy of Liyong Lin's oral presentation at the AAMP meeting, 2016)

- Further investigation of motion mitigation techniques will likely make treating with PBS more clinically feasible. Studies at our institution have utilized abdominal compression to decrease motion for the treatment of liver tumors with PBS [38, 42]. Abdominal compression resulted in reduction of the beam-specific PTV (PBSTV)/CTV and ITV/CTV volume ratios, less overlap of BSPTV with heart, and a clear reduction of motion, thus less variability in water equivalent thickness (WET) traversed by the proton beam. When PBS plans utilizing abdominal compression were analyzed using 4DCT for ten patients being treated to a liver tumor, this method resulted in decreased mean liver dose, smaller ITV and PBSTV margins, and a reduction in motion amplitude. Although this study focused on liver patients, the implications and conclusions can be similarly applied when treating other abdominal targets (Fig. 15.15).
- Utilizing proton beam radiation for unresected pancreatic cancer can be challenging due to larger volumes of the duodenum which may be included in the high-dose region of the PTV. Combination photon/proton plans can be used to reduce the volume of the duodenum treated to high dose, reduce the volume of the stomach and bowel in the low- to intermediate-dose range, and decrease overall integral doses. In the future, the use of PBS with abdominal compression, cone beam CT, and IMPT may allow for improved conformality and decreased margins near the duodenum.

References

1. Siegel RL, Miller KD, Jemal A. Cancer statistics, 2016. CA Cancer J Clin. 2016;66:7–30.
2. Howlader NNA, Krapcho M, Miller D, Bishop K, Altekruse SF, Kosary CL, Yu M, Ruhl J, Tatalovich Z, Mariotto A, Lewis DR, Chen HS, Feuer EJ, Cronin KA, editors. SEER Cancer Statistics Review, 1975–2013. Bethesda, MD: National Cancer Institute. https://seer.cancer.gov/csr/1975_2014/, based on November 2015 SEER data submission, posted to the SEER web site
3. Iacobuzio-Donahue CA, Fu B, Yachida S, Luo M, Abe H, Henderson CM, Vilardell F, Wang Z, Keller JW, Banerjee P, et al. DPC4 gene status of the primary carcinoma correlates with patterns of failure in patients with pancreatic cancer. J Clin Oncol. 2009;27:1806–13.

4. Kalser MH, Ellenberg SS. Pancreatic cancer. Adjuvant combined radiation and chemotherapy following curative resection. Arch Surg. 1985;120:899–903.
5. Regine WF, Winter KA, Abrams R, Safran H, Hoffman JP, Konski A, Benson AB, Macdonald JS, Rich TA, Willett CG. Fluorouracil-based chemoradiation with either gemcitabine or fluorouracil chemotherapy after resection of pancreatic adenocarcinoma: 5-year analysis of the U.S. intergroup/RTOG 9704 phase III trial. Ann Surg Oncol. 2011;18:1319–26.
6. Oettle H, Neuhaus P, Hochhaus A, Hartmann JT, Gellert K, Ridwelski K, Niedergethmann M, Zulke C, Fahlke J, Arning MB, et al. Adjuvant chemotherapy with gemcitabine and long-term outcomes among patients with resected pancreatic cancer: the CONKO-001 randomized trial. JAMA. 2013;310:1473–81.
7. Smeenk HG, van Eijck CH, Hop WC, Erdmann J, Tran KC, Debois M, van Cutsem E, van Dekken H, Klinkenbijl JH, Jeekel J. Long-term survival and metastatic pattern of pancreatic and periampullary cancer after adjuvant chemoradiation or observation: long-term results of EORTC trial 40891. Ann Surg. 2007;246:734–40.
8. Neoptolemos JP, Stocken DD, Friess H, Bassi C, Dunn JA, Hickey H, Beger H, Fernandez-Cruz L, Dervenis C, Lacaine F, et al. A randomized trial of chemoradiotherapy and chemotherapy after resection of pancreatic cancer. N Engl J Med. 2004;350:1200–10.
9. Hsu CC, Herman JM, Corsini MM, Winter JM, Callister MD, Haddock MG, Cameron JL, Pawlik TM, Schulick RD, Wolfgang CL, et al. Adjuvant Chemoradiation for pancreatic adenocarcinoma: the Johns Hopkins Hospital-Mayo Clinic collaborative study. Ann Surg Oncol. 2010;17:981–90.
10. Kooby DA, Gillespie TW, Liu Y, Byrd-Sellers J, Landry J, Bian J, Lipscomb J. Impact of adjuvant radiotherapy on survival after pancreatic cancer resection: an appraisal of data from the national cancer data base. Ann Surg Oncol. 2013;20:3634–42.
11. Kim EJ, Ben-Josef E, Herman JM, Bekaii-Saab T, Dawson LA, Griffith KA, Francis IR, Greenson JK, Simeone DM, Lawrence TS, et al. A multi-institutional phase 2 study of neoadjuvant gemcitabine and oxaliplatin with radiation therapy in patients with pancreatic cancer. Cancer. 2013;119:2692–700.
12. Loehrer PJ Sr, Feng Y, Cardenes H, Wagner L, Brell JM, Cella D, Flynn P, Ramanathan RK, Crane CH, Alberts SR, Benson AB 3rd. Gemcitabine alone versus gemcitabine plus radiotherapy in patients with locally advanced pancreatic cancer: an eastern cooperative oncology group trial. J Clin Oncol. 2011;29:4105–12.
13. Ben-Josef E, Schipper M, Francis IR, Hadley S, Ten-Haken R, Lawrence T, Normolle D, Simeone DM, Sonnenday C, Abrams R, et al. A phase I/II trial of intensity modulated radiation (IMRT) dose escalation with concurrent fixed-dose rate gemcitabine (FDR-G) in patients with unresectable pancreatic cancer. Int J Radiat Oncol Biol Phys. 2012;84:1166–71.
14. Hammel P, Huguet F, van Laethem JL, Goldstein D, Glimelius B, Artru P, Borbath I, Bouche O, Shannon J, Andre T, et al. Effect of Chemoradiotherapy vs chemotherapy on survival in patients with locally advanced pancreatic cancer controlled after 4 months of gemcitabine with or without Erlotinib: the LAP07 randomized clinical trial. JAMA. 2016;315:1844–53.
15. Ceha HM, van Tienhoven G, Gouma DJ, Veenhof CH, Schneider CJ, Rauws EA, Phoa SS, Gonzalez Gonzalez D. Feasibility and efficacy of high dose conformal radiotherapy for patients with locally advanced pancreatic carcinoma. Cancer. 2000;89:2222–9.
16. Bittner MI, Grosu AL, Brunner TB. Comparison of toxicity after IMRT and 3D-conformal radiotherapy for patients with pancreatic cancer - a systematic review. Radiother Oncol. 2015;114:117–21.
17. Chang DT, Schellenberg D, Shen J, Kim J, Goodman KA, Fisher GA, Ford JM, Desser T, Quon A, Koong AC. Stereotactic radiotherapy for unresectable adenocarcinoma of the pancreas. Cancer. 2009;115:665–72.
18. Gouzi JL, Huguier M, Fagniez PL, Launois B, Flamant Y, Lacaine F, Paquet JC, Hay JM. Total versus subtotal gastrectomy for adenocarcinoma of the gastric antrum. A French prospective controlled study. Ann Surg. 1989;209:162–6.
19. Squires MH 3rd, Kooby DA, Poultsides GA, Pawlik TM, Weber SM, Schmidt CR, Votanopoulos KI, Fields RC, Ejaz A, Acher AW, et al. Is it time to abandon the 5-cm margin

rule during resection of distal gastric adenocarcinoma? A multi-institution study of the U.S. gastric cancer collaborative. Ann Surg Oncol. 2015;22:1243–51.
20. Smalley SR, Benedetti JK, Haller DG, Hundahl SA, Estes NC, Ajani JA, Gunderson LL, Goldman B, Martenson JA, Jessup JM, et al. Updated analysis of SWOG-directed intergroup study 0116: a phase III trial of adjuvant radiochemotherapy versus observation after curative gastric cancer resection. J Clin Oncol. 2012;30:2327–33.
21. Park SH, Sohn TS, Lee J, Lim DH, Hong ME, Kim KM, Sohn I, Jung SH, Choi MG, Lee JH, et al. Phase III trial to compare adjuvant chemotherapy with Capecitabine and Cisplatin versus concurrent Chemoradiotherapy in gastric cancer: final report of the adjuvant Chemoradiotherapy in stomach tumors trial, including survival and subset analyses. J Clin Oncol. 2015;33:3130–6.
22. Ringash J, Perkins G, Brierley J, Lockwood G, Islam M, Catton P, Cummings B, Kim J, Wong R, Dawson L. IMRT for adjuvant radiation in gastric cancer: a preferred plan? Int J Radiat Oncol Biol Phys. 2005;63:732–8.
23. Megibow AJ, Babb JS, Hecht EM, Cho JJ, Houston C, Boruch MM, Williams AB. Evaluation of bowel distention and bowel wall appearance by using neutral oral contrast agent for multi-detector row CT. Radiology. 2006;238:87–95.
24. Suramo I, Paivansalo M, Myllyla V. Cranio-caudal movements of the liver, pancreas and kidneys in respiration. Acta Radiol Diagn (Stockh). 1984;25:129–31.
25. Bryan PJ, Custar S, Haaga JR, Balsara V. Respiratory movement of the pancreas: an ultrasonic study. J Ultrasound Med. 1984;3:317–20.
26. Kissick MW, Mackie TR. Task group 76 report on 'The management of respiratory motion in radiation oncology' [med. Phys. 33, 3874-3900 (2006)]. Med Phys. 2009;36:5721–2.
27. Kubo HD, Hill BC. Respiration gated radiotherapy treatment: a technical study. Phys Med Biol. 1996;41:83–91.
28. Minohara S, Kanai T, Endo M, Noda K, Kanazawa M. Respiratory gated irradiation system for heavy-ion radiotherapy. Int J Radiat Oncol Biol Phys. 2000;47:1097–103.
29. Ford EC, Mageras GS, Yorke E, Rosenzweig KE, Wagman R, Ling CC. Evaluation of respiratory movement during gated radiotherapy using film and electronic portal imaging. Int J Radiat Oncol Biol Phys. 2002;52:522–31.
30. Ozhasoglu C, Murphy MJ. Issues in respiratory motion compensation during external-beam radiotherapy. Int J Radiat Oncol Biol Phys. 2002;52:1389–99.
31. Veiga C, Janssens G, Teng CL, Baudier T, Hotoiu L, McClelland JR, Royle G, Lin L, Yin L, Metz J, et al. First clinical investigation of cone beam computed tomography and deformable registration for adaptive proton therapy for lung cancer. Int J Radiat Oncol Biol Phys. 2016;95:549–59.
32. Wong JW, Sharpe MB, Jaffray DA, Kini VR, Robertson JM, Stromberg JS, Martinez AA. The use of active breathing control (ABC) to reduce margin for breathing motion. Int J Radiat Oncol Biol Phys. 1999;44:911–9.
33. Dawson LA, Brock KK, Kazanjian S, Fitch D, McGinn CJ, Lawrence TS, Ten Haken RK, Balter J. The reproducibility of organ position using active breathing control (ABC) during liver radiotherapy. Int J Radiat Oncol Biol Phys. 2001;51:1410–21.
34. Grassberger C, Dowdell S, Lomax A, Sharp G, Shackleford J, Choi N, Willers H, Paganetti H. Motion interplay as a function of patient parameters and spot size in spot scanning proton therapy for lung cancer. Int J Radiat Oncol Biol Phys. 2013;86:380–6.
35. Murphy JD, Adusumilli S, Griffith KA, Ray ME, Zalupski MM, Lawrence TS, Ben-Josef E. Full-dose gemcitabine and concurrent radiotherapy for unresectable pancreatic cancer. Int J Radiat Oncol Biol Phys. 2007;68:801–8.
36. Goodman KA, Regine WF, Dawson LA, Ben-Josef E, Haustermans K, Bosch WR, Turian J, Abrams RA. Radiation therapy oncology group consensus panel guidelines for the delineation of the clinical target volume in the postoperative treatment of pancreatic head cancer. Int J Radiat Oncol Biol Phys. 2012;83:901–8.
37. Wo JY, Yoon SS, Guimaraes AR, Wolfgang J, Mamon HJ, Hong TS. Gastric lymph node contouring atlas: a tool to aid in clinical target volume definition in 3-dimensional treatment planning for gastric cancer. Pract Radiat Oncol. 2013;3:e11–9.

38. Lin LSS, Kang M, et al. Evaluation of motion mitigation using abdominal compression in the clinical implementation of pencil beam scanning proton therapy of liver tumors. Med Phys. 2017;44(2):703–12.
39. Moyers MF, Miller DW, Bush DA, Slater JD. Methodologies and tools for proton beam design for lung tumors. Int J Radiat Oncol Biol Phys. 2001;49:1429–38.
40. Thompson RF, Mayekar SU, Zhai H, Both S, Apisarnthanarax S, Metz JM, Plastaras JP, Ben-Josef E. A dosimetric comparison of proton and photon therapy in unresectable cancers of the head of pancreas. Med Phys. 2014;41:081711.
41. Boimel P, Berman Abigail, Li, Jonathan, Apisarnthanarax, Smith, Both, Stefan, Lelionis, Kristi, Larson, Gary, Lukens, J. Nicholas, Ben-Josef, Edgar, Metz, James, Plastaras, John: Proton beam reirradiation for locally recurrent pancreatic adenocarcinoma *Poster at the American Society for Therapeutic Radiology and Oncology Annual Meeting San Antonio, Tx* 2015.
42. Lin L: Implementation of Pencil Beam Scanning (PBS) Proton Therapy Treatment for Liver Patient. *AAPM 58th Annual Meeting, Washington DC* 2016.

Lower Gastrointestinal Malignancies

16

John P. Plastaras, Stefan Both, Haibo Lin, and Maria Hawkins

Contents

16.1	Introduction	258
16.2	Rectal Adenocarcinoma	258
16.3	Simulation, Target Delineation, Radiation Dose, and Fractionation	259
16.4	Passive Scattering Treatment Planning	260
16.5	Pencil Beam Scanning	262
	16.5.1 Irregular Targets	262
	16.5.2 Robustness Planning	262
16.6	Anal Cancer	264
	16.6.1 Simulation, Target Delineation, Organ at Risk Delineation, and Radiation Dose/Fractionation	264
	16.6.2 Patient Positioning, Immobilization, and Treatment Verification	265
16.7	3D Proton Passive Scattering vs Pencil Beam Scanning Planning	266
	16.7.1 Passive Scattering	266
	16.7.2 Pencil Beam Scanning	266
	16.7.3 Dosimetric and Toxicity Comparison	267
	16.7.4 Future Developments	268
References		268

J.P. Plastaras (✉) • H. Lin
Department of Radiation Oncology, University of Pennsylvania Perelman School of Medicine, Philadelphia, PA, USA
e-mail: Plastaras@uphs.upenn.edu

S. Both
Department of Radiation Oncology, University Medical Center Groningen, Groningen, The Netherlands
e-mail: s.both@umcg.nl

M. Hawkins
CRUK MRC Oxford Institute for Radiation Oncology, Gray Laboratories, University of Oxford, Oxford, UK

© Springer International Publishing Switzerland 2018
N. Lee et al. (eds.), *Target Volume Delineation and Treatment Planning for Particle Therapy*, Practical Guides in Radiation Oncology,
https://doi.org/10.1007/978-3-319-42478-1_16

16.1 Introduction

Lower GI cancers present a particular problem for multidisciplinary care. Concurrent chemoradiotherapy is the standard of care, but with it comes a host of treatment-related toxicities. For rectal cancer, preoperative chemoradiation with 5-fluorouracil- (5-FU)-based treatment followed by total mesorectal excision results in the best local control. For anal squamous cell cancer (SCC), definitive chemoradiation with two sensitizing agents has allowed curative treatment without the need for surgery.

Fortunately, lower GI cancers are curable, but survivors may face not only acute but also late toxicities including the bowel, bladder, bone marrow, and sexual function toxicities as well as an increased risk for second malignant neoplasms. Acute toxicities are significant in these diseases as they dictate how fit patients are as they head into surgery (for rectal adenocarcinomas) or the likelihood of finishing treatment within a narrow package time (for anal SCCs). One of the major treatment-limiting acute toxicities is bowel toxicity, usually manifest as diarrhea. Because 5-FU, which can cause bowel mucositis, is frequently combined with pelvic radiation, treatment-related diarrhea is common. Historically, dosimetric planning parameters for bowel have focused on the maximum radiation dose. Even as recently as the "failed" RTOG 0822 trial for rectal cancer using IMRT in combination with capecitabine and oxaliplatin, volumetric small bowel limits were set for V35, V40, and V45 [1]. However, more recent retrospective data have suggested that the volume of bowel, in particular small bowel, that receives low to medium doses of radiation is most predictive of clinically significant diarrhea during concurrent chemoradiation. Doses ranging from 15 to 25 Gy are the most predictive of acute GI toxicity regardless of how the bowel is contoured (tight individual loops or a peritoneal structure) [2–6]. Another important acute toxicity during lower GI chemoradiation is bone marrow toxicity. This is particularly important when marrow-toxic agents like mitomycin C are employed, as is standard for anal SCC. Even for rectal adenocarcinoma, most patients will proceed to adjuvant chemotherapy with regimens like FOLFOX, so marrow preservation is an important goal. Sexual function after combined modality treatment for lower GI cancers can certainly suffer. Protection of gonads, the vagina, and the external genitalia has been difficult to achieve in the 3DCRT era, but modern techniques may improve on this. Son et al. showed that mean dose (<43 Gy) and generalized equivalent uniform dose (<35 Gy) to the vagina are important predictors of vaginal stenosis [7]. Attention to vaginal dose, starting with contouring the vagina as an avoidance structure, may help reduce the negative quality of life impact of chemoradiation. The role of proton therapy (PT) in GI cancers has been reviewed [8], but there is a paucity of clinical data published for lower GI cancers.

16.2 Rectal Adenocarcinoma

PT is currently being used for rectal cancers in some centers. Early comparative dosimetry studies showed an advantage for PS PT over three-dimensional conformal radiotherapy (3DCRT) photons with respect to the small bowel, bladder, and femoral heads in the postoperative setting [9] and for unresectable rectal cancers with dose escalation [10]. More recent studies comparing IMRT and PS PT have also shown dosimetric improvements with proton therapy with respect to the bladder, bowel, testes, and bone marrow [11, 12]. In particular, passive scattering (PS) PT had lower small bowel V10–V20 volumes, which is predicted to correlate to acute diarrhea with 5FU-based chemoradiation [11]. A comparison of intensity-modulated radiation therapy (IMRT) with pencil beam scanning (PBS) PT using lateral beams in the preoperative setting showed that PBS PT could deliver much lower small bowel V15 (66 cc vs. 286 cc), lower bladder, and lower femoral head doses [13]. In a retrospective series comparing 39 patients treated with IMRT and 26 patients treated with PBS PT in the neoadjuvant setting with concurrent chemotherapy, there was significantly less grade ≥ 2 diarrhea in PBS PT patients (12% vs. 39%, $p = 0.022$) [14]. Proton therapy has also been explored in the reirradiation setting for rectal cancer with superior bowel dosimetry and feasible treatment in a small number of patients [15].

16.3 Simulation, Target Delineation, Radiation Dose, and Fractionation

The first major decision with regard to positioning is whether to simulate the patient in the supine or prone position. When using 3DCRT for rectal cancer, prone positioning with a "belly board" can displace pelvic loops of small bowel away from the target volume. However, this position is not always comfortable for the patient and is generally less stable than the supine position. Precise positioning is more critical for robust proton therapy delivery, so supine positioning has its advantages. The decision for prone versus supine positioning for rectal cancer should be individualized to the patient and the intended proton technique.

In general:

- CT simulation should be performed with a comfortably full bladder (when possible to displace small bowel from the target volume), with intravenous iodinated contrast (when not contraindicated) to facilitate elective nodal anatomical delineation. Pelvic floor immobilization is required in the supine position (knee and ankle support). For the purposes of dose calculation, a non-contrast CT needs to be employed in planning proton therapy. Standard oral contrast agents need to be overridden and can cause artifacts that can make proton planning more complicated. A negative contrast agent with Hounsfield units close to tissue, such as VoLumen®, can help with bowel definition without needing to be overridden.
- A vaginal cylinder can be used to displace the anterior vagina away from the target volume. We have found that an empty bladder is more reproducible than a variably full bladder for consistent vaginal cylinder position during treatment (personal communication, James M. Metz MD).
- MRI and/or PET/CT may be helpful for accurate delineation of the extent of the primary tumor and involved lymph nodes [16, 17].
- The GTV and involved nodes should be defined using all imaging modalities and these should be registered to planning CT for accurate delineation. Registering over the area of interest should be considered to minimize uncertainties.

- The CTV (elective nodal area) should include internal iliac lymph nodes, mesorectal, and presacral space. If appropriate, ischiorectal fossa should be included. The Radiation Therapy Oncology Group (RTOG) elective nodal anorectal atlas [18] has high-resolution pictorial details and instructions regarding elective nodal contouring.
- The PTV should be created from CTV with expansion according to institutional standard accounting for setup and delivery uncertainties and mainly used for dose recording and reporting purposes (ICRU 78).
- The following organs at risk (OAR) are segmented:
  Small bowel: Contouring should include all individual small bowel loops to at least 2 cm above the superior extent of both PTVs. It may be helpful to initially delineate the large bowel +/− endometrium to exclude these from subsequent delineation of small bowel.
  External genitalia: Delineation of the male genitalia should include the penis and scrotum. In woman it should include the clitoris and labia majora and minora out to the inguinal creases. Superior border in both sexes should lie midway through the symphysis pubis. A planning structure that defines the "perineal skin" may also be helpful to avoid inadvertent hot spots in the skin folds.
  Bladder: From dome to the neck including outer bladder wall.
  Right and left femoral heads: To be contoured separately on each side, including the ball of the femur, trochanters, and proximal shaft to the level of the bottom of ischial tuberosities.
  Vagina: Soft tissue extending from the vaginal meatus to the inferior aspect of the uterus [7].

16.4 Passive Scattering Treatment Planning

Treatment planning for anorectal cancers is complex due to concerns related to inconsistent patient positioning (especially the pelvic tilt) and varying patterns of bowel gas both in and outside of the mesorectal target. PS PT is limited by the maximum field size and the lack of proximal target conformality. The latter in particular can lead to high-skin doses, especially in the gluteal cleft which is prone to desquamation. However, compared to pencil beam scanning, PS PT is generally more robust with regard to the aforementioned uncertainties regarding positioning and bowel gas.

To account for the range uncertainties from multiple sources such as energy fluctuation of the delivery machine (~1 mm), compensator manufacturing (2 mm), and translation of the CT Hounsfield number into proton's stopping power (~3.5% of depth of CTV), distal and proximal margins are added to the CTV along beam direction to ensure sufficient target coverage. For PS technique, the distal margin is calculated by 3.5% distal CTV depth plus 3 mm, while proximal margin is 3 mm plus 3.5% of proximal CTV depth [19]. The same CTV to PTV expansions are applied to the other directions.

For patients with "simple" target volumes, namely, patients who do not have indications to treat the external iliac or inguinal nodes, high-quality PS plans can be generated that compare favorably to PBS plans with respect to avoiding OARs. In Fig. 16.1, both PS and PBS plans deliver minimal dose to the bowel, in part due to favorable bowel anatomy even in the supine position.

16 Lower Gastrointestinal Malignancies

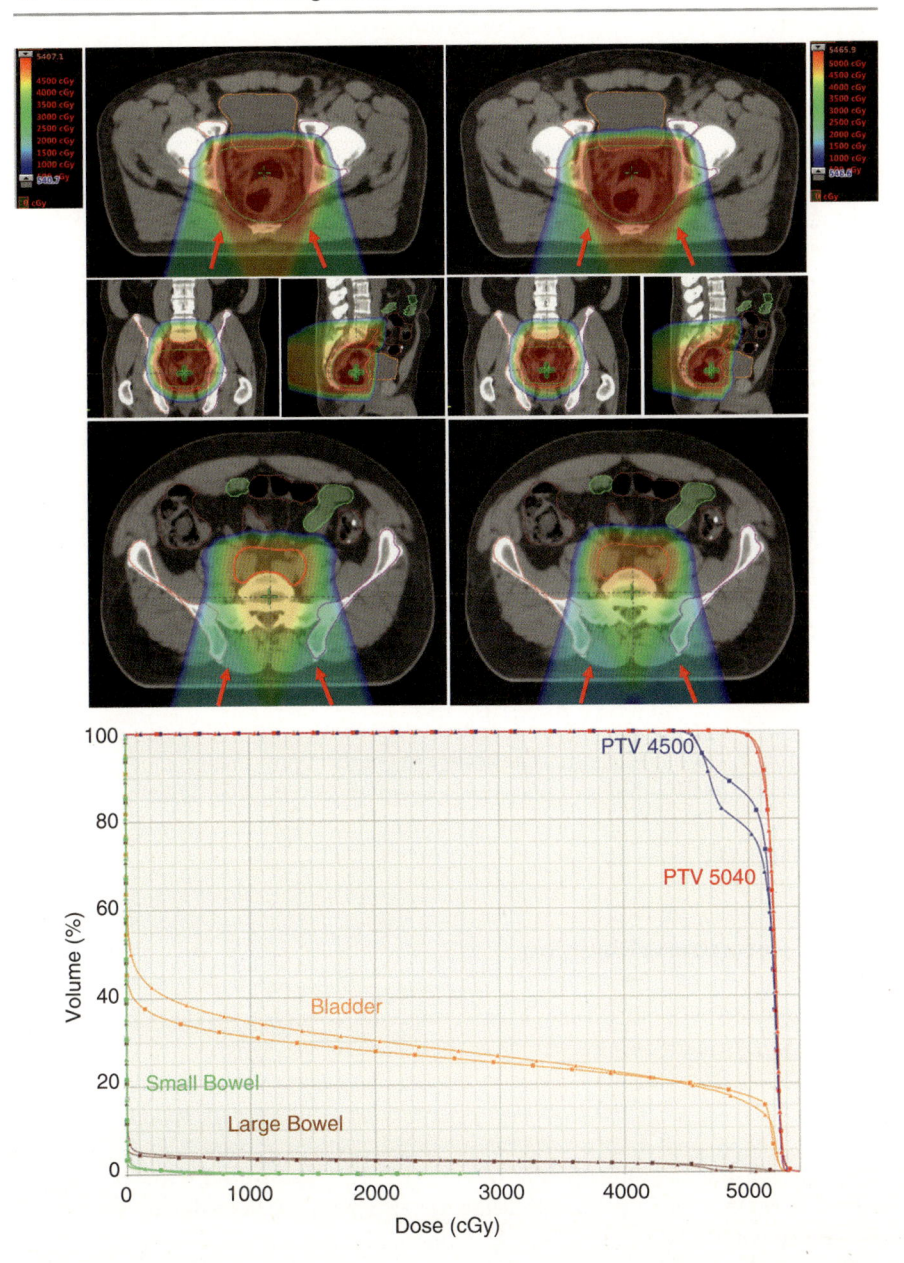

Fig. 16.1 Comparison of PS and PBS for a "simple" rectal adenocarcinoma target volume. This young man with T3 N1 rectal adenocarcinoma was treated with preoperative chemoradiation using PS PT in the supine position using standard target volumes that did NOT include external iliac or inguinal nodes. Panel A and B show comparative color washes for PS (*left*) and PBS (*right*) using posterior oblique fields (*red arrows*) at different viewing planes. Panel C shows the comparative dose-volume histogram. CTV_4500 (*red*), CTV_5040 (*green*), the bladder (*orange*), small bowel (*light green*), large bowel (*brown*), and bone marrow (*pink*) are contoured, and the bowel and bladder are displayed on the dose-volume histogram, where the PS (*square*) and PBS (*triangle*) plans are compared

16.5 Pencil Beam Scanning

In contrast to PS, the distal and proximal margins are both reduced by 2 mm for PBS planning as no compensator is used (3.5% of CTV depth plus 1 mm). Beam-specific PBS target volumes (PBSTV) are created using those proximal and distal margins of each beam as well as the same CTV to PTV expansions in the directions perpendicular to the beam. PBSTV or PTV, which is larger, is used for plan optimization. Usually, PBSTV is adopted. For cases with serious CT artifacts, increase on distal and proximal margin should be considered to ensure target coverage.

16.5.1 Irregular Targets

Generally speaking, PBS offers a potential advantage over passive scattering when targets are irregular. In the case of rectal adenocarcinomas, the target volumes become more complex when nodal volumes are extended more anteriorly to include external iliac nodes (e.g., T4 tumors involving anterior structures) and/or inguinal nodes (e.g., extensive involvement of the anal sphincter). These types of target volumes are more similar to anal SCC target volumes, discussed in more depth below.

Another strategy using PBS to target simpler rectal adenocarcinoma target volumes is to use opposed laterals. The ability to conform proximally allows for sparing of femoral heads while simultaneously keeping skin dose negligible (Fig. 16.2). We have used this technique to treat some patients who need external iliac nodal volumes included as well.

16.5.2 Robustness Planning

Planning margins do not protect against unpredictable changes that occur during the course of treatment. Proton dose distributions are sensitive to changes of tissue density or position of tissue interfaces. To ensure the target coverage, air cavities in bowel or rectum are often overridden with proper HU, as shown in left panel of Fig. 16.3. If the air cavity in this patient shown in Fig. 16.3 was filled during daily treatment, the target will still be covered. However, there would be significant "overshoot" when the air cavity presents during treatment. Therefore, lateral beams would be less likely to unpredictably deposit dose into more sensitive anterior structures (as opposed to muscle and fat lateral to the target volume).

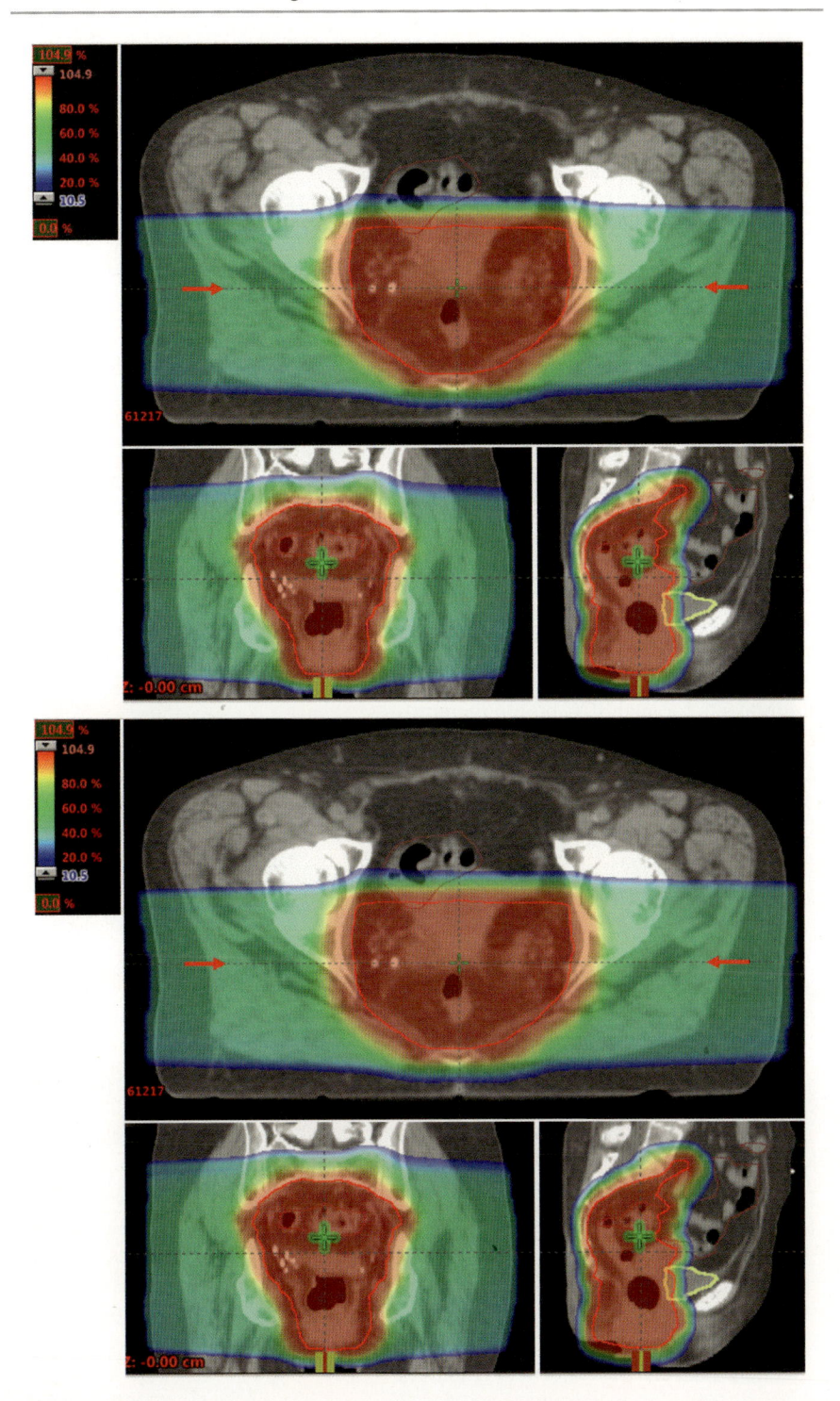

Fig. 16.2 Opposed lateral PBS fields (*red arrows*) for rectal adenocarcinoma. Dose color wash with CTV_4500 (*red*), bladder (*yellow*), and bowel (*brown*) contoured

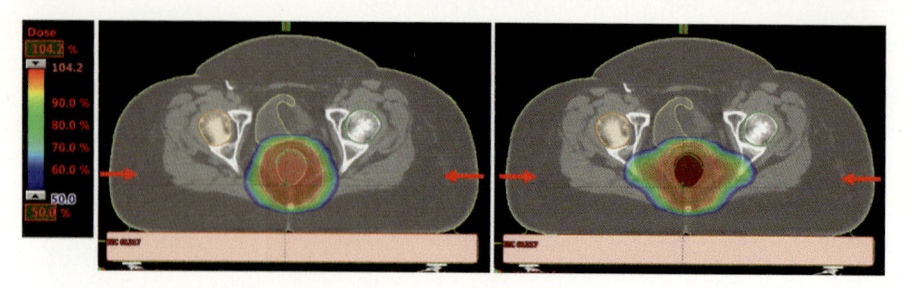

Fig. 16.3 Effect of air in rectum on proton dose distribution. This patient with a rectal lymphoma has significant air in the rectum at the time of simulation treated with opposed lateral PBS beams (*red arrows*). The left panel shows the dose distribution when the air is overridden with tissue equivalent (assuming case of empty rectum). The right panel shows the dose distribution without overriding the air. Both dose color washes are set to 50% of the prescription dose. If posterior beams were used, the "overshoot" would have gone into the bladder instead of the muscle and fat

16.6 Anal Cancer

Special consideration is given to treatment of anal SCC compared to rectal adenocarcinoma. The concurrent chemotherapy is more aggressive, the treatment volumes are larger and more complex, and skin toxicity is a much more significant issue. These clinical considerations are reflected in the more complex technical requirements for anal SCC proton therapy.

16.6.1 Simulation, Target Delineation, Organ at Risk Delineation, and Radiation Dose/Fractionation

- Given the complexity of the treatment volume in anal cancer compared to rectal cancer, CT simulation generally should be performed supine with a comfortably full bladder.
- MRI is helpful for accurate delineation of the extent of anal tumor and involved lymph nodes. PET may also be helpful in identification of involved nodal areas and primary tumor segmentation.
- As in rectal cancer, the GTV and involved nodes should be defined using all imaging modalities, and these should be registered to planning CT for accurate delineation. A further isotropic margin of at least 2 cm should be added to GTV, depending on tumor stage, while respecting anatomical boundaries. Attention must be given, especially for anal verge and perianal lesions, that a 2-cm radial and caudal margin is used to ensure coverage of perianal skin.
- The CTV (elective nodal area) should include inguinal lymph nodes, external and internal iliac lymph nodes, obturator, mesorectal, and presacral space. If appropriate, ischiorectal fossa should be included. The AGITG consensus atlas [20] and the Radiation Therapy Oncology Group (RTOG) elective nodal anorectal atlas [18] are both excellent resources.

- The PTV should be created from CTV as above, but with the larger, more complex target volume, larger expansions may be considered for anal CTV.
- Organs at risk (OAR) is segmented as in rectal cancer with the following additions:

  Due to the myelotoxic concurrent chemotherapy agents used in anal cancer, the total pelvic bone marrow—composed of iliac, lower pelvic, and lumbosacral subdivisions—should be outlined as described by Mell et al. [21].

  In addition, careful attention should be paid to skin dose in anal cancer as radiation dermatitis may be a limiting toxicity for timely completion of therapy. We also use an avoidance structure called "perineal skin" to limit excessive dose to sensitive regions.

  The recommended dosing and fractionation vary depending on the clinical scenario: tumor stage, whether an excisional biopsy has been performed, and the use of a simultaneous integrated boost technique vs sequential boost technique (Table 16.1).

The use of concurrent chemotherapy is standard of care; unless there are medical contraindications to systemic treatment when a higher radiation dose could be considered.

16.6.2 Patient Positioning, Immobilization, and Treatment Verification

Setup accuracy should ideally be ascertained with daily orthogonal X-ray imaging matched to the bony pelvis or volumetric imaging, if available. For advanced stage with bulky disease (primary or lymph nodes), imaging and clinical examination should be considered during the course of treatment (every 1 or 2 weeks) to assess for potential changes in anatomy, as they could have potential impact in dose distribution. Additionally, weight should be monitored as weight loss could lead to overshooting target volumes using proton therapy.

Table 16.1 Recommended radiation doses

Stage	Technique	Elective nodal dose	GTV dose
T1 and non-bulky T2	SIB	42Gy(RBE) in 28F	50.4 Gy(RBE) in 28F
Bulky T2, T3 and T4	SIB	45 Gy(RBE)	54 Gy(RBE) in 30F
Involved nodes	SIB	n/a	50.4–54 Gy(RBE)
Any	Sequential	30–36 Gy(RBE)	Boost to macroscopic 50.4–60 Gy (RBE)

16.7 3D Proton Passive Scattering vs Pencil Beam Scanning Planning

16.7.1 Passive Scattering

There are no reports using PS for anal cancer, therefore principles for treatment of the pelvis (gynecologic, prostate) could be applied. The target volumes for anal cancer are complex compared to rectal cancer since the inguinal nodes are included. Generally, matched fields would be required. Care should be taken to avoid placing match lines on organs at risk (OARs) and any colostomy. Match line feathering can be utilized to reduce excessive hot spots at the match line level.

16.7.2 Pencil Beam Scanning

PBS plans can consist of left- and right-posterior oblique fields to cover volumes encompassing the primary tumor, pelvic nodes, and inguinal nodes [22]. Figure 16.4 shows a plan using right- and left-posterior oblique SFUD (single-field uniform dose or single-field optimization (SFO)) fields in a woman. Of note, a vaginal cylinder was used to maximize sparing of at least the anterior vaginal wall. If a sequential cone down is used for the primary tumor, skin sparing can be

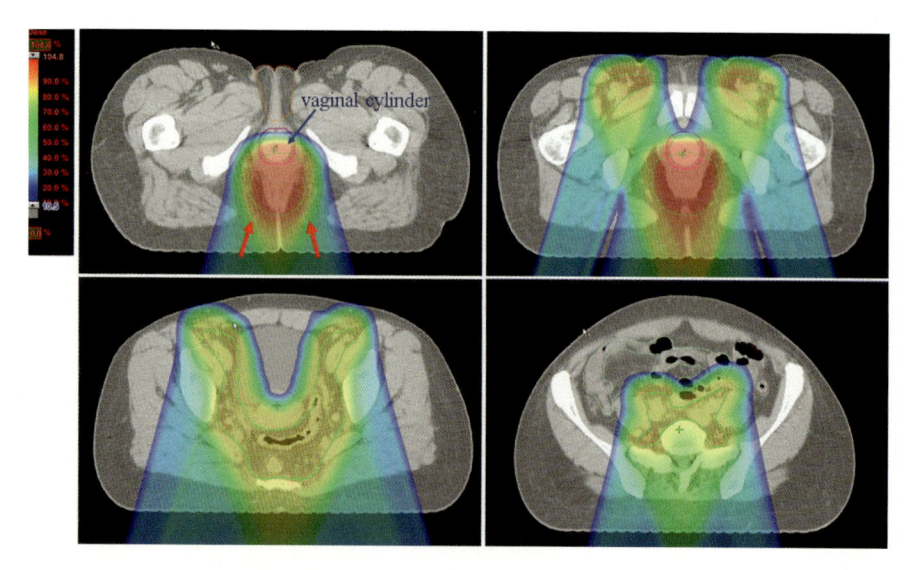

Fig. 16.4 Pencil beam scanning plan using posterior oblique (*red arrows*) SFUD fields for anal cancer. Several axial slices are shown with dose color wash for the initial fields treated to 42 Gy and 50.4 Gy with a simultaneous infield boost. The CTV_4200 (*green contour*) is shown as well as the small bowel (*light green*), large bowel (*brown*), external genitalia (*orange*), and vagina (*pink*). A vaginal cylinder was inserted at the time of simulation and for daily treatments in an effort to spare concentric dose to the entire vagina

achieved using opposed lateral beams. Plans can be optimized using the SFUD technique, allowing each field to uniformly cover the target in order to increase plan robustness.

Alternately, posterior and anterior SFUD fields can be used with an internal "gradient match" where the external iliac volume connects the inguinal nodes and the internal iliac nodes. This fields matching method using volumetric gradient dose optimization (GDO) has been routinely used on craniospinal irradiation for proton PBS technique without match line changes [23]. The GDO involves the use of multiple fields such that in the overlapped junction area, the dose contribution decreases in one field, while this decrease is compensated by increasing dose contribution from the adjacent field. Challenges still exist for opposing beam sets due to the fact of range uncertainties of proton therapy. Cold-dose buffer in the junction has to be deliberately created to prevent potential overlaps between beam sets. To investigate the worst case scenario, often the robustness of the plan is studied by manually introducing setup and range uncertainties. Although this technique may be more sensitive to changes in body weight and position, it can help with challenging volumes, such as a hip replacement as shown in Fig. 16.5.

16.7.3 Dosimetric and Toxicity Comparison

To date there are no data regarding outcomes of patients with anal cancer treated with PT. There are two in silico modeling studies, Ojerholm et al. [22] and Anad et al. [25], reporting that PT offers significant reduction in doses to the small bowel, bladder, and genitalia when compared to seven field IMRT in eight cases [22] and volumetric arc therapy (VMAT) in eight cases [25]. This reduction is more substantial in doses <30 Gy across all organs. Furthermore both studies have shown significant reduction in the pelvic bone marrow dose of clinical relevance.

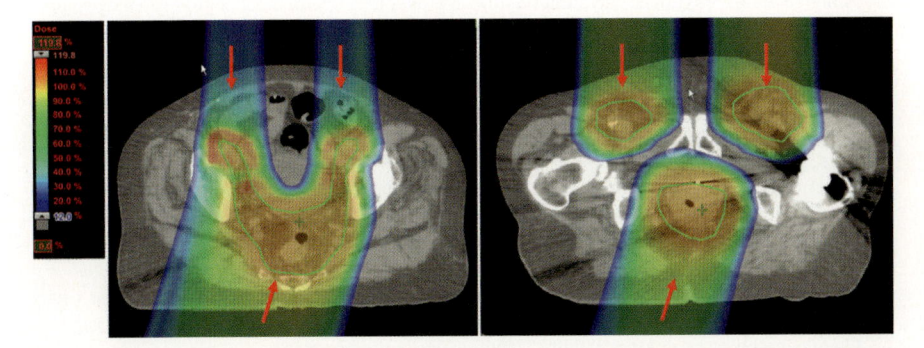

Fig. 16.5 Pencil beam scanning plan for a patient with hip replacement using GDO for anterior and posterior matched fields (*red arrows*). CTV is shown in light green contour

Table 16.2 Recommended dose constraints to organs at risk when using proton beam therapy anal cancer are listed

Organ at risk	Recommended dose constraint
Small bowel	Max dose 54 Gy 120 cc < 15 Gy
Bladder	50% < 35 Gy 35% < 40 Gy 5% < 50 Gy
Femoral heads	Max dose = 50 Gy 50% < 30 Gy 35% < 40 Gy 5% < 44 Gy
Genitalia	50% < 20 Gy 35% < 30 Gy 5% < 40 Gy

These recommendations are adapted from RTOG 0529 protocol [24]. As additional data are accumulated, these constraints will continue to be refined. In clinical practice, the planner should make every effort to achieve the lowest dose possible for all normal tissues while maximizing coverage.

16.7.4 Future Developments

It is crucial that prospective data collection (in a trial or registry) of clinical toxicity and long-term PROMs are undertaken to aid establishing the benefit of protons. MGH currently is running a multi-institutional trial for anal cancer (NCT01858025) to determine the feasibility of PBS with concurrent 5-fluorouracil and mitomycin C. Proton radiotherapy will be considered feasible if grade 3+ skin toxicity seen on this protocol is less than 48% (reported grade 3+ dermatologic toxicity from RTOG 98–11).

References

1. Hong TS, et al. NRG oncology radiation therapy oncology group 0822: a phase 2 study of preoperative Chemoradiation therapy using intensity modulated radiation therapy in combination with Capecitabine and Oxaliplatin for patients with locally advanced rectal cancer. Int J Radiat Oncol Biol Phys. 2015;93(1):29–36.
2. Chopra S, et al. Predictors of grade 3 or higher late bowel toxicity in patients undergoing pelvic radiation for cervical cancer: results from a prospective study. Int J Radiat Oncol Biol Phys. 2014;88(3):630–5.
3. Banerjee R, et al. Small bowel dose parameters predicting grade >/= 3 acute toxicity in rectal cancer patients treated with neoadjuvant chemoradiation: an independent validation study comparing peritoneal space versus small bowel loop contouring techniques. Int J Radiat Oncol Biol Phys. 2013;85(5):1225–31.
4. Robertson JM, et al. The dose-volume relationship of small bowel irradiation and acute grade 3 diarrhea during chemoradiotherapy for rectal cancer. Int J Radiat Oncol Biol Phys. 2008;70(2):413–8.
5. Gunnlaugsson A, et al. Dose-volume relationships between enteritis and irradiated bowel volumes during 5-fluorouracil and oxaliplatin based chemoradiotherapy in locally advanced rectal cancer. Acta Oncol. 2007;46(7):937–44.

6. Tho LM, et al. Acute small bowel toxicity and preoperative chemoradiotherapy for rectal cancer: investigating dose-volume relationships and role for inverse planning. Int J Radiat Oncol Biol Phys. 2006;66(2):505–13.
7. Son CH, et al. Dosimetric predictors of radiation-induced vaginal stenosis after pelvic radiation therapy for rectal and anal cancer. Int J Radiat Oncol Biol Phys. 2015;92(3):548–54.
8. Plastaras JP, Dionisi F, Wo JY. Gastrointestinal cancer: nonliver proton therapy for gastrointestinal cancers. Cancer J. 2014;20(6):378–86.
9. Tatsuzaki H, Urie MM, Willett CG. 3-D comparative study of proton vs. x-ray radiation therapy for rectal cancer. Int J Radiat Oncol Biol Phys. 1992;22(2):369–74.
10. Isacsson U, et al. Comparative treatment planning between proton and X-ray therapy in locally advanced rectal cancer. Radiother Oncol. 1996;41(3):263–72.
11. Colaco RJ, et al. Protons offer reduced bone marrow, small bowel, and urinary bladder exposure for patients receiving neoadjuvant radiotherapy for resectable rectal cancer. J Gastrointest Oncol. 2014;5(1):3–8.
12. Wolff HA, et al. Irradiation with protons for the individualized treatment of patients with locally advanced rectal cancer: a planning study with clinical implications. Radiother Oncol. 2012;102(1):30–7.
13. Dionisi F, B.S., Kirk M, Both S, Vennarini S, McDonough J, Metz JM, Plastaras JP, Pencil Beam Scanning Proton Therapy in the Treatment of Rectal Cancer, in American Society of Radiation Oncology Annual Meeting. 2013: Atlanta, GA.
14. Batra S, et al. Lower rates of acute gastrointestinal toxicity with pencil beam proton therapy relative to IMRT in neoadjuvant chemoradiation for rectal cancer. Int J Clin Oncol. 2015;33(3):696.
15. Berman A, et al. Proton Reirradiation of recurrent rectal cancer: Dosimetric Comparsion, toxicities, and preliminary outcomes. IJPT. 2014.; in press
16. Braendengen M, et al. Delineation of gross tumor volume (GTV) for radiation treatment planning of locally advanced rectal cancer using information from MRI or FDG-PET/CT: a prospective study. Int J Radiat Oncol Biol Phys. 2011;81(4):e439–45.
17. Whaley JT, et al. Clinical utility of integrated positron emission tomography/computed tomography imaging in the clinical management and radiation treatment planning of locally advanced rectal cancer. Pract Radiat Oncol. 2014;4(4):226–32.
18. Myerson RJ, et al. Elective clinical target volumes for conformal therapy in anorectal cancer: a radiation therapy oncology group consensus panel contouring atlas. Int J Radiat Oncol Biol Phys. 2009;74(3):824–30.
19. Moyers MF, et al. Methodologies and tools for proton beam design for lung tumors. Int J Radiat Oncol Biol Phys. 2001;49(5):1429–38.
20. Ng M, et al. Australasian gastrointestinal trials group (AGITG) contouring atlas and planning guidelines for intensity-modulated radiotherapy in anal cancer. Int J Radiat Oncol Biol Phys. 2012;83(5):1455–62.
21. Mell LK, et al. Association between bone marrow dosimetric parameters and acute hematologic toxicity in anal cancer patients treated with concurrent chemotherapy and intensity-modulated radiotherapy. Int J Radiat Oncol Biol Phys. 2008;70(5):1431–7.
22. Ojerholm E, et al. Pencil-beam scanning proton therapy for anal cancer: a dosimetric comparison with intensity-modulated radiotherapy. Acta Oncol. 2015;54(8):1209–17.
23. Lin H, et al. Supine craniospinal irradiation using a proton pencil beam scanning technique without match line changes for field junctions. Int J Radiat Oncol Biol Phys. 2014;90(1):71–8.
24. Kachnic LA, et al. RTOG 0529: a phase 2 evaluation of dose-painted intensity modulated radiation therapy in combination with 5-fluorouracil and mitomycin-C for the reduction of acute morbidity in carcinoma of the anal canal. Int J Radiat Oncol Biol Phys. 2013;86(1):27–33.
25. Anand A, et al. Scanning proton beam therapy reduces normal tissue exposure in pelvic radiotherapy for anal cancer. Radiother Oncol. 2015;117(3):505–8.

Breast Cancer

17

Robert Samstein, David DeBlois, Robert W. Mutter, and Oren Cahlon

Contents

17.1	Introduction	271
17.2	Partial Breast Irradiation	272
17.3	Whole Breast/Chest Wall Plus Regional Nodal Irradiation	274
17.4	Simulation, Target Delineation, and Radiation Dose/Fractionation	278
17.5	Patient Positioning, Immobilization, and Treatment Verification	279
17.6	Three-Dimensional (3D) Proton Treatment Planning	281
	17.6.1 Passive Scattering (PS)/Uniform Scanning (US)	281
17.7	Pencil Beam Scanning (PBS)	282
17.8	Critical Structures	283
17.9	Future Developments	284
References		284

17.1 Introduction

Breast cancer is the most common malignancy of females in the United States with an estimated incidence of >230,000 in 2015 [1]. Radiation therapy plays an important role in prevention of locoregional and distant recurrence which can translate into improvements in overall survival with long-term follow-up [2–4].

R. Samstein • O. Cahlon (✉)
Memorial Sloan Kettering Cancer Center, New York, NY, USA
e-mail: cahlono@mskcc.org

D. DeBlois
ProCure Proton Therapy Center, Somerset, NJ, USA

R.W. Mutter
Mayo Clinic, Rochester, MN, USA

© Springer International Publishing Switzerland 2018
N. Lee et al. (eds.), *Target Volume Delineation and Treatment Planning for Particle Therapy*, Practical Guides in Radiation Oncology, https://doi.org/10.1007/978-3-319-42478-1_17

Adjuvant radiation to the breast is an essential part of breast conservation therapy for most women with early stage breast cancer. For many women with stage 2 and 3 disease, breast/chest wall irradiation in combination with regional nodal irradiation improves outcomes [5, 6].

With continued improvements in cure rates and expected long-term survival in many breast cancer patients, minimizing late toxicities of radiation is essential. Proton therapy may improve the therapeutic ratio by minimizing exposure to the surrounding normal tissue in the thorax, while preserving optimal target coverage. The major potential benefit of protons is thought to be in cardiac avoidance with dose to the heart directly correlated with major cardiac events [7]. In addition, proton therapy can reduce the exposure to nontarget tissues outside of the clinical target volume such as the lungs, soft tissues of the shoulder and back, contralateral breast or chest wall, and dissected axilla, potentially reducing rates of pneumonitis, lymphedema, and secondary cancers and improving other functional outcomes.

Proton therapy has been proposed in breast cancer patients in several settings, including partial breast irradiation (PBI), whole breast radiation (WBRT) with or without regional nodal irradiation (RNI), and postmastectomy radiotherapy (PMRT).

17.2 Partial Breast Irradiation

Early breast conservation trials comparing surgery with or without whole breast radiation therapy demonstrated that most recurrences occur in close proximity to the original tumor bed [2, 8, 9].

Advantages of PBI include a smaller target allowing for accelerated hypofractionation with fewer treatments, which is ultimately more convenient for patients and more cost-effective for the health-care system. A smaller target also decreases normal tissue exposure and may result in decreased toxicity.

PBI can be delivered using IORT, interstitial or intracavitary brachytherapy, and external beam radiation therapy (EBRT) with EBRT being the most common form in the Unites States. Brachytherapy techniques provide better conformality than EBRT but have a more inhomogeneous dose distribution and are more invasive. EBRT is noninvasive and more convenient but less conformal, with more nontarget breast tissue receiving radiation.

Several large phase III clinical trials have randomized early stage breast cancer patients to partial vs. whole breast irradiation. Strnad and colleagues found multicatheter interstitial brachytherapy to be not inferior to adjuvant whole breast irradiation [10]. The 5-year incidence of local recurrence was 1.44% for PBI and 0.92% for WBI, $p = 0.42$. Due to the greater technical complexity and invasiveness of the procedure, interstitial brachytherapy is not widely used in North America for the treatment of breast cancer. Although results from NSABP B-39 and the RAPID trial are still pending, PBI is currently used for select favorable-risk patients with early stage disease, as supported by American Society of Radiation Oncology (ASTRO) consensus guidelines [11].

The TARGIT-A and the ELIOT studies randomized patients to single-dose intraoperative radiation therapy vs. whole breast irradiation (WBI). In TARGIT-A, 5-year local recurrence was significantly higher with IORT compared with WBI (3.3% vs. 1.3%, $p = 0.042$) despite 15.2% of patients with predefined adverse features receiving supplemental WBI in the IORT arm. In the ELIOT trial, the 5-year local recurrence was 4.4% with IORT vs. 0.4% with WBI, $p = 0.0001$. Therefore, at the present time, IORT is only recommended in the setting of a clinical trial [12].

Early toxicity results from the RAPID as well as other reports raised concern of increased adverse cosmesis with PBI [13–16]. Cosmesis has been correlated with the volume of nontarget breast tissue receiving prescription dose [14, 17]. Optimal dose and fractionation for PBI has not been defined, although some data suggest that once daily fractionation may be better tolerated given the relatively large fraction sizes administered with PBI [18, 19].

Proton therapy for PBI has been suggested in order to improve the sparing of tissues outside of the clinical target volume, which could potentially result in improved cosmesis.

An example of PBI beam arrangement and dosimetry can be seen in Fig. 17.1. Dosimetric analyses demonstrated that proton therapy improved sparing of nontarget breast tissue compared with other EBRT techniques. The non-PTV breast volume receiving 50% of the prescription dose was 16.5% with proton therapy, 22.8% with tomotherapy, 33.3% with IMRT, and 40.9% with 3DCRT [20, 21].

One early clinical experience demonstrated increased skin toxicity and telangiectasias with proton therapy delivered via a single beam. In that prospective trial of 98 patients treated at MGH with protons, photons or mixed photons/electrons, a higher rate of telangiectasias (69% vs. 16%), pigmentation changes (54% vs. 22%), and lower rates of good/excellent cosmetic outcomes (62% vs. 94%) were observed

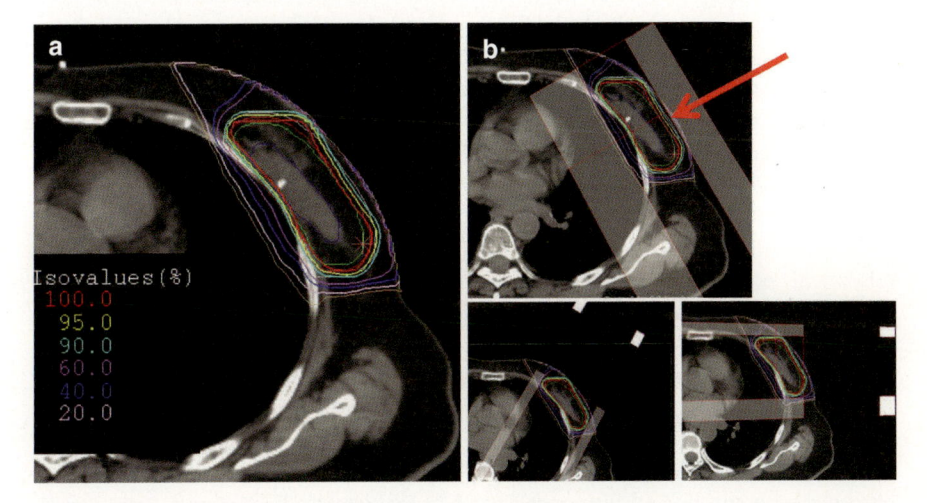

Fig. 17.1 Three field PBI plan with uniform scanning. (**a**) isodose lines for a uniform scanning PBI plan with skin sparing. (**b**) Axial image demonstrating the lightly weighted tangent beam using the aperture edge to spare the skin. Anterior oblique and lateral beams deliver full skin dose

with proton therapy, although there was no difference in patient-reported outcomes [22]. The use of two proton fields was shown to result in a higher proportion of patients with good/excellent cosmesis compared to a single-beam technique [23].

In a larger phase II trial of 90 patients at Loma Linda using 2–4 beams, the 5-year breast tumor recurrence-free survival rate was 97%, and good/excellent cosmetic outcomes were observed in 90% of patients [24, 25]. Therefore, at least two fields per day are recommended by most institutions.

The use of pencil beam scanning proton therapy (PBS) may allow additional skin sparing and improvements in conformality in order to further reduce nontarget breast dose.

17.3 Whole Breast/Chest Wall Plus Regional Nodal Irradiation

Level 1 evidence supports the use of adjuvant radiation to the breast/chest wall and comprehensive regional nodes encompassing the axilla, supraclavicular fossa, and IMN chain, for many patients with stage 2 and 3 breast cancer [4–6, 26–28]. Inclusion of lymph node basins, and in particular the internal mammary nodes (IMN), results in a larger volume of normal tissue and critical organs exposed to radiation with increased treatment morbidity. In addition, most of the debate over whether to incorporate the IMN chain into the target volume is because doing so results in increase heart and lung doses.

A dose-dependent association has been demonstrated between ischemic heart disease and even low radiation doses to the heart [7]. Therefore, the available clinical data suggest that even incremental reductions in dose to the heart will translate to reduced cardiac morbidity in the future. Several photon-based treatment techniques such as heart blocking, breath hold, prone positioning, matched electron/photon fields, and intensity modulated radiotherapy can be used to minimize cardiac dose. However, clinical target volume coverage is often sacrificed in order to achieve the desired cardiac sparing, and there can still be significant exposure to the heart and lung when trying to achieve ideal coverage. A study from MD Anderson showed that only 75–90% of the CTVs received 90% of the prescription dose – well below what is accepted for most disease sites.

Several studies have demonstrated improved target coverage and normal tissue doses with protons compared to 3D conformal photons or IMRT/VMAT [29–35]. These studies are summarized in Table 17.1. In a systematic review of published mean heart doses between 2003 and 2013, the average dose to the heart in tangential photon treatment when the IMN nodes where targeted was 8 Gy compared with 2.6 Gy with protons [36]. More recent proton experience reports have demonstrated even lower mean heart doses in the range of 0.5–1 Gy [32, 37, 38].

Factors that indicate an increased benefit for protons include unfavorable cardiac anatomy with anterior portion of the heart immediately adjacent to the chest wall, lack of breath-hold capability, lack of improvement with breath hold, need for inclusion of the IMNs, and medial tumor and breast reconstruction limiting beam angles.

17 Breast Cancer

Table 17.1 Dosimetric comparisons of OARs for patients treated with proton vs. photon therapy

Study author	Heart mean (Gy RBE) Protons	3DCRT	IMRT	Heart V20 (%) Protons	3DCRT	IMRT	Heart V5 (%) Protons	3DCRT	IMRT	Ipsilateral lung V20 (%) Protons	3DCRT	IMRT	Ispilateral lung V5 (%) Protons	3DCRT	IMRT	Ipsilateral Lung Mean (Gy RBE) Protons	3DCRT	IMRT	Contralateral Breast Mean (Gy RBE) Protons	3DCRT	IMRT
Ares et al. [29][a]	4	18	17	–	–	–	8	43	63	15	39	19	28	82	81	14	42	26	0	2	9
Fagundes et al. [38]	0.9	7.3	10.5	–	–	–	–	–	–	–	–	–	–	–	–	–	–	–	0.2	1.5	3.9
MacDonald et al. [31]	–	–	–	1.6	12.4	–	4.1	35.6	–	–	–	–	–	–	–	–	–	–	–	–	–
Mast et al. [32][b]	0.2	–	2.7	0.1	–	3.5	0.5	–	4.7	2.8	–	12.4	7.7	–	21.9	1.6	–	6.1	–	–	–
Xu et al. [33]	1	3	5	0	4	21	7	24	50	31	36	30	50	70	81	5.5	10	11	0	0	3.5
Bradley et al. [34][a]	0.6	5.9	–	1	6.1	–	2.7	34	–	21.6	35.5	–	35.3	60.5	–	11	17.5	–	–	–	–
Lin et al. [35]	0.01	–	1.6	0.0	–	0.7	0	0	4.3	0	–	12.5	4.7	–	25.2	0.88	–	7.3	–	–	–

– Not reported
[a]Inclusion of internal mammary lymph nodes
[b]Free breathing plans

For most early stage patients receiving whole breast radiation alone with modern treatment planning, there is not likely to be a marked reduction in dose to the normal tissues or improvement in target volume coverage with proton therapy. However, there are some patients with unfavorable anatomy where protons can provide a significant advantage. For example, in patients with a barrel-shaped chest, the lung dose can be high with a tangent approach, and protons can reduce the dose significantly (Fig. 17.2a). In addition, in some patients with left-sided breast cancer, the heart may be fixed to the chest wall, resulting in high doses to the heart and left anterior descending artery with photon tangents. Deep inspiratory breath-hold techniques can often increase the space between the chest wall and heart, reducing cardiac exposure. However, some patients cannot tolerate the procedure and others derive minimal benefit (Fig. 17.2c). Finally, a medial tumor location could necessitate shallow tangents in order to obtain margins on the tumor bed and result in significant contralateral breast dose (Fig. 17.2d).

Early clinical experience using passive scatter techniques have been reported by several institutions including MGH and MSKCC/Princeton Radiation Oncology, with good target coverage, mean heart dose under 1 Gy, and ipsilateral lung V20 12.7–16.5% [31, 37]. Toxicities observed were mild with Grade 2 dermatitis observed in 71.4% and moist desquamation in 28.6% without any Grade 3 skin toxicities [37]. One patient experienced a Grade 3 reconstructive complication. An example of the brisk skin reaction observed can be seen in Fig. 17.3. When skin dose was measured using OSLs, protons dose was similar to that observed in patients treated with bolus with photons. In our experience, the skin reaction with uniform scanning/passive scattered protons is a deep erythema that is more intense than with photons, but the desquamation is typically dry and superficial, and the erythema heals quickly. The skin reaction is more intense in the supraclavicular region than is typically seen with an anterior oblique photon field, and a few patients have had prolonged hyperpigmentation in that area although it does typically ultimately heal completely. Telangiectasias have been identified in a few patients with more than 2 years of follow-up.

Fig. 17.2 Left whole breast RT with DIBH. 43 yo female s/p BCS for T1bN0 IDC of the left breast treated with proton therapy for lung sparing. (**a**) Isodose lines and DVH for photon tangents. (**b**) Isodose lines and DVH for uniform scanning proton plan. Comparison of the DVHs shows that the ipsilateral V20 is reduced from 18% to 8%, V30 from 18% to 2% and V40 from 17% to 0%. (**c**) 53 yo F with pT1cN0, ER/PR+, HER2-, IDC of L breast s/p BCS and AC-T chemo. Accepted for whole breast RT. Did not tolerate DIBH. Tangent fields would have resulted in large portions of the LAD and left ventricle receiving high doses. Patient was therefore simulated for proton therapy and strong target coverage was achieved with near complete cardiac sparing, with a mean heart dose of 0.2 Gy. (**d**) 44 yo F with pT2N0, 4.6 cm, triple negative, poorly differentiated, IDC of upper inner quadrant of left breast s/p BCS/SLNB and AC-T chemo. Simulated for whole breast radiation with DIBH. Although heart was well displaced, because of the location of the tumor bed (green contour) in UIQ, there was still significant spillage into the contralateral breast and a significant portion of the lung receiving full dose. The proton plan gives excellent coverage of the tumor bed and the IMN chain without increasing dose to the lung or contralateral dose

17 Breast Cancer 277

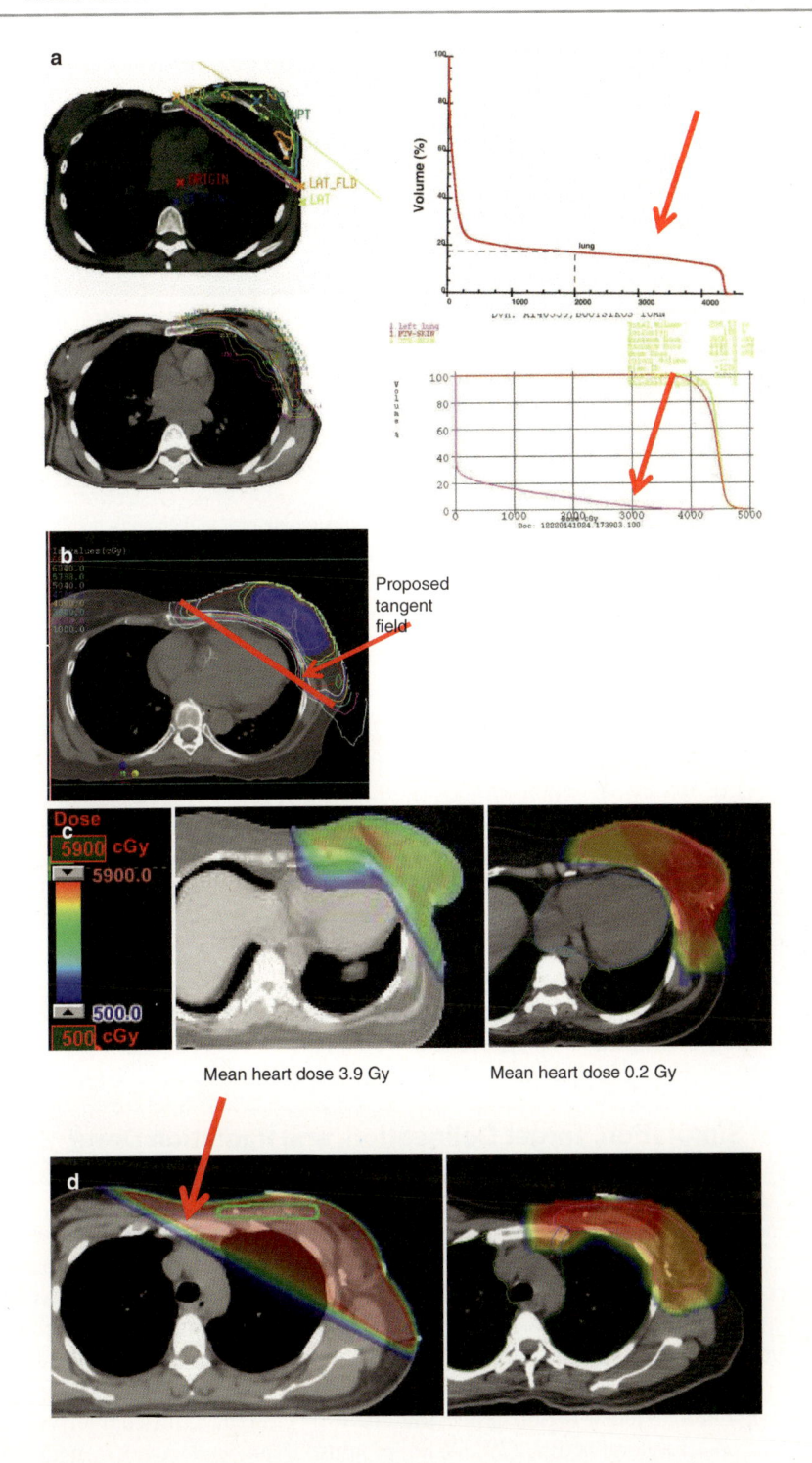

Proposed tangent field

Mean heart dose 3.9 Gy   Mean heart dose 0.2 Gy

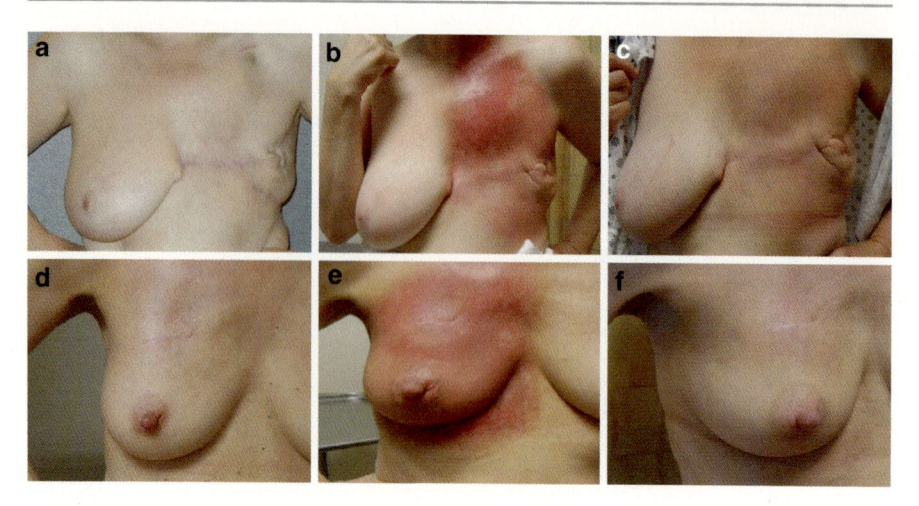

Fig. 17.3 Typical skin reaction observed for patients undergoing proton therapy to the chest wall and regional nodes after mastectomy without reconstruction (**a–c**) and after lumpectomy (**d–f**). *a* and *d*: Baseline. *b* and *e*: end of RT. *c* and *f*: 1 month followup after RT

PBS treatment, as seen in Fig. 17.5, can result in greater skin sparing, if clinically indicated, as well as allow treatment with a single beam, although may be more sensitive to setup uncertainties.

The currently accruing RADCOMP trial randomizes patients to protons vs. photons for breast cancer requiring comprehensive regional nodal irradiation including treatment of the IMNs with a primary endpoint of reduction in cardiac events at 10 years. Other endpoints include health-related quality of life including fatigue and patient-reported body image and function as well as cancer control outcomes. Predictive models to understand the association with radiation dose distribution to the heart with major cardiovascular events and quality of life outcomes will also be developed. The trial is designed to be pragmatic, allowing for treatment at centers across the country with broad eligibility criteria and limited treatment planning requisites. A RADCOMP contouring atlas has also been developed to offer guidance and promote consistency in photon and proton treatment target areas.

17.4 Simulation, Target Delineation, and Radiation Dose/Fractionation

In general, clinical target volume (CTV) should be similar for photon or proton treatment as it defines the area at risk for microscopic disease. However, contouring accuracy is critical with protons given the steep dose gradients. There are areas that the physician may consider including in the proton target volume that historically received significant incidental doses with photons even if not intentionally delineated. The areas where this could make a difference are the posterior supraclavicular fossa, retroclavicular region connecting the IMN contour to the supraclavicular and the posterolateral axilla [39]. With protons, if an area is not specifically contoured, it will receive minimal dose; thus, an atlas for the RADCOMP trial was developed with slight modifications to the RTOG atlas. Guidelines exist as well for contouring of the left anterior descending artery [LAD] [40].

The ribs and intercostals are not included as they are at low risk of microscopic disease, and their exclusion allows the end of range to fall in soft tissue/bone rather than the lungs [41]. In addition, excluding a high-density structure such as the rib reduces the amount of smear necessary and allows for better conformality.

The role of PTV margins for setup uncertainty in breast cancer is unclear. At MSKCC/Princeton Radiation Oncology, a 7 mm margin is added in all directions perpendicular to the beam but not posteriorly (parallel to beam) to avoid expansion into the ribs/lungs and heart. In addition, limited margin is used in the medial supraclavicular fossa to avoid expansion into the esophagus [37]. An expansion is not necessary in the direction of the beam as motion in the beam path has very little dose perturbation. At the Mayo Clinic in Rochester, MN, setup uncertainty analyses of ±5 mm shifts in isocenter along each translation axis and ±3% beam range uncertainty are performed on the CTV and organs at risk as part of routine treatment planning for PBS intensity modulated proton therapy. It should be noted that margins will not compensate for motion or breast tissue deformation.

45–50 Gy (RBE) should be prescribed to the target volumes in 1.8–2.0 Gy fractions. There have been no published reports of hypofractionated schedules for patients being treated to the breast/chest wall and regional lymphatics to date although this is under investigation (NCT02783690).

For proton PBI, contouring should be done similar to photon-based EBRT PBI.

17.5 Patient Positioning, Immobilization, and Treatment Verification

CT simulation should be performed with the arms abducted above the head using a custom mold (alpha cradle, breast board). Due to the en face beams in proton radiotherapy, an "arms down" position can also be considered which can be helpful in patients who have difficulty post axillary surgery or other comorbidities which limit arm mobility. A chin strap and shoulder pulls can be used to assist in reproducibility. IV contrast can assist in defining nodal volumes and OARs, but a non-contrast CT is necessary for dose calculation.

Two matching fields to the chest wall and supraclavicular fossa with uniform scanning or passive scattering are often used. The match line should be feathered, and the fields can be treated daily (4 fields/day) or on alternating days (2 fields/day). A typical beam arrangement is seen in Fig. 17.4.

While most clinical experience to date has been with uniform scanning or passive scattering [31, 34, 37], a pencil beam scanning (PBS) technique has been reported at MGH [42], and as PBS becomes widely available, it will likely become more popular in the future (Fig. 17.5).

Setup accuracy should be confirmed with daily X-ray imaging, or when available, surface imaging such as AlignRT is highly desirable to be employed for interfraction and intrafraction for setup and positioning surveillance.

Fig. 17.4 Typical beam arrangement

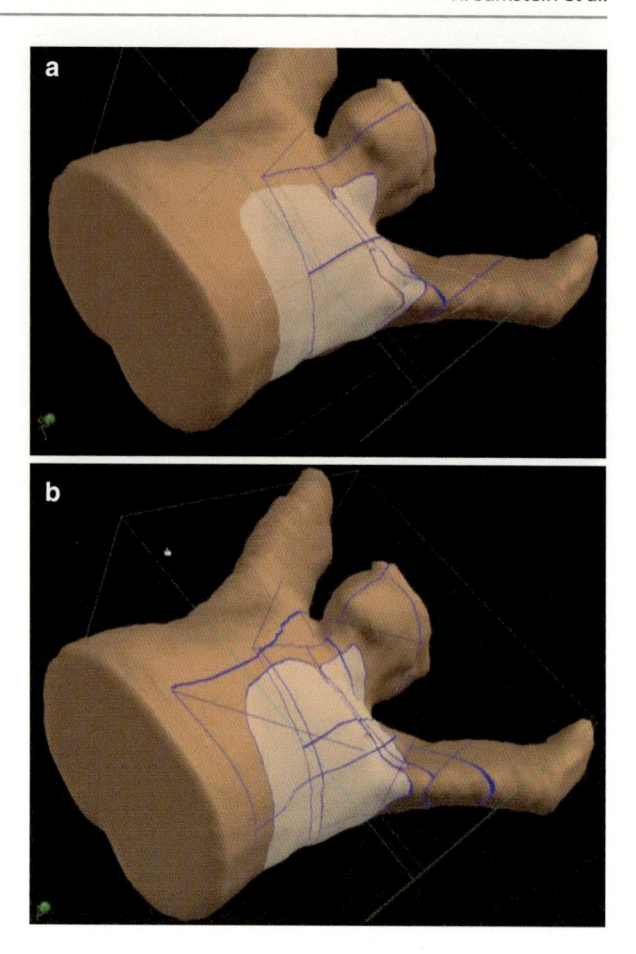

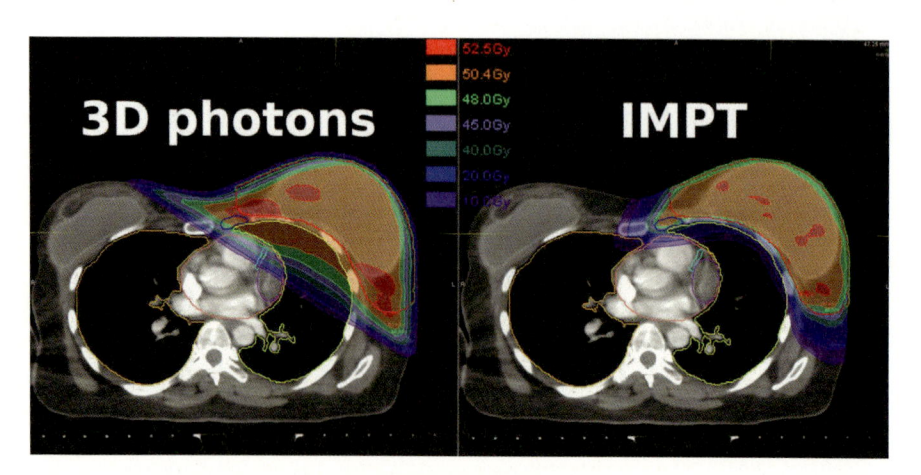

Fig. 17.5 A standard 3D conformal photon plan compared with a proton plan using pencil beam scanning for a patient with locally advanced breast cancer, bilateral implants and inclusion of the internal mammary nodes in the treatment field

End of range uncertainty must be considered in proton therapy related to both setup variability as well as intrafraction motion. Early clinical experience was mostly in the postmastectomy setting, but many centers today are also treating post-lumpectomy patients. Mobile breast tissue in breast conservation patients is a source of setup and range variability, requiring special care when using proton therapy, particularly in patients with pendulous breasts where day-to-day setup uncertainty may be increased. In the postmastectomy setting, with or without reconstruction range uncertainty may be less due to better reproducibility. Low-dose verification CT scans during treatment as well as optical surface tracking technologies such as AlignRT have allowed more robust treatment, including those with intact breasts. In some patients with breast edema, adaptive planning to account for increased range is needed.

Target motion of the chest wall due to respiration has minimal effect, relative to typical setup and beam range uncertainties, due to the relatively low absolute motion in most patients primarily in the direction of the beam [29, 42].

Another potential challenge remains in patients with immediate tissue expander reconstruction due to the metal port perturbing the proton dose distribution. With passive scattering and uniform scanning techniques with anterior beams, a cold spot is created behind the port that can be overcome by increased smearing at the expense of increased heart and lung dose. Thus, tissue expanders have remained a contraindication to proton therapy with those techniques.

The feasibility of treating patients with breast expanders with metallic ports with intensity modulated proton therapy has recently been reported (Mutter, Remmes et al. PTCOG 2016). At the Mayo Clinic, all expanders implanted are made by the same manufacturer. Prior to considering PBS for patients with expanders, a sample expander used in their practice was disassembled, and the water-equivalent thickness of its components was measured. These measurements are used to construct a contouring template in the treatment planning software that is matched to the expander port on the treatment planning images with stopping power override. Two multi-field optimized anterior/oblique beams at ~45° are used in order to provide the best compromise between robust target coverage and ability to limit the dosimetric impact of the expander port and limit hot spots at the skin surface compared with en face single-beam plans. Using this technique in 12 patients, they determined that target coverage and normal tissue dose uncertainties from the expander were clinically acceptable. They cautioned, however, that similarly extensive analyses should be carried out on the physical properties and dosimetric impact of expanders used in each institution's practice prior to considering PBS for these patients [43].

17.6 Three-Dimensional (3D) Proton Treatment Planning

17.6.1 Passive Scattering (PS)/Uniform Scanning (US)

17.6.1.1 Partial Breast Irradiation

Two or three beams are often used for treating partial breast irradiation. In some cases, beams can be manipulated to aid in skin sparing, as seen in Fig. 17.1. However, due to size and location of the disease within the breast, this is not always possible.

17.6.1.2 Whole Breast, Postmastectomy Chest Wall, or Implant Patients with Nodal Basin

Two sets of matching fields to the chest wall and supraclavicular fossa with US or PS are often used. Two isocenters with only a longitudinal shift between them are chosen: a chest wall isocenter and a supraclavicular nodal isocenter. The match lines of the two beam projections must be feathered and not overlap. The fields can be treated daily (4 fields/day) or on alternating days (2 fields/day); alternating days is possible if the individual matched pairs cover the target sufficiently without significant hot spots. A typical beam arrangement is seen in Fig. 17.4. For each pair of matched beams, the minimum air gap that allows the target to fit within the aperture and provides clearance from collisions with the patient or table should be used. The same air gap should be used to allow for a more homogeneous dose distribution at the match lines. However, with larger snout sizes, patients may be able to be treated with a single isocenter and two beam projections that do not require match lines.

Before compensator generation, fiducials in the beam path, such as scar or border wires or BBs, must be contoured and the densities forced to air. This is done as fiducials can disrupt the beam and cause an artificial cold shadow distally.

When planning a breast with an implant, the liquid inside implant may be comprised of varying materials. Some materials may sample as the correct density, while others may not and need to be forced to the correct density.

Range uncertainty in proton therapy must be accounted for, and robustness analysis demonstrates acceptable "worst case scenario" dose profiles [42].

Dose painting and scaling of beams are common to gain coverage and mitigate hot spots.

Lumpectomy boosts are often planned the same as PBI; however, skin sparing is not achievable as the initial portion of treatment cannot spare skin.

Other possible areas to boost include chest wall excluding nodal volumes, chest wall with only internal mammary nodes (IMN) included, or an IMN boost alone.

For chest wall boosts that include the IMN, often fully new fields need not be generated as the boost can be treated with the beams for the initial portion of the plan, with edited apertures if needed to exclude the supraclavicular or axilla nodes.

Chest wall boosts that exclude all nodal volumes may be able to use the beams from the initial portion of treatment as well, provided that the initial did not include IMN. Should this be the case, new fields need to be generated, and the same planning process is followed for the initial treatment.

In some cases, a boost to just the IMN is needed. In these cases, one or two en face beams should be used to cover the target. Care must be taken with the heart as it is distal to the IMN target, and these boosts can increase the heart dose.

17.7 Pencil Beam Scanning (PBS)

PBS planning for breast treatments has a very similar beam geometry to US planning. One to two en face beams should be chosen. Four fields may be necessary if the target is too large, and a two-isocenter technique is required.

Materials in beam path need to be evaluated for forced densities with the same consideration used in US planning.

Beam parameters, such as spot layer distance, spot spacing distance, and spot distance outside of target, should be determined by each institution.

Single field uniform dose (SFUD) should be used to ensure individual beam coverage while maintaining robustness. SFUD should be utilized with robust optimization whenever possible to account for uncertainties, i.e., distal end, setup, and motion uncertainties. If robust optimization is unavailable, Planning Organ at Risk Volume (PRV) and other optimization structures can be used to account for uncertainties.

The use of PBS planning can allow for some skin sparing. In US planning, there is no method to control the proximal end of the beam resulting in potential hot spots on the skin surface. By creating an optimization volume for target and an avoidance structure proximal to the target along the beam path, skin dose can be lowered to less than the prescribed dose.

17.8 Critical Structures

The heart is a critical avoidance structure, especially for left-sided treatments, and should have the mean dose to the organ minimized as much as possible. For treatments with IMN inclusion, the heart and LAD dose must be balanced with coverage to the IMN targets. The esophagus is of concern superiorly in the section of treatments that include the nodal basin targets and should be kept below prescription dose. The lungs should have the V5 and V20 minimized to the ipsilateral lung and all dose to the contralateral lung kept as low as reasonably achievable (ALARA) (Table 17.2).

Table 17.2 Recommended dose constraints to organs at risk when using proton beam therapy. No specific dose constraints have been developed for proton therapy

Organ at risk	Recommended dose constraint
Ipsilateral lung	$V_{20Gy} < 20\%$ $V_{10Gy} < 40\%$ V5 < 50%
Contralateral lung	$V_{20Gy} < 1\%$
Heart	$V_{25Gy} < 5\%$ Max point dose 50 Gy Mean dose <2Gy
Thyroid	Mean dose <20Gy
Esophagus	Max point dose 40 Gy
Contralateral intact breast	Mean dose <5 Gy
Liver	Mean dose <5 Gy
Stomach	Mean dose <2 Gy
Cord	Max point dose <10 Gy

17.9 Future Developments

Mature follow-up of single arm prospective studies as well as the RADCOMP study will better define the clinical benefits of proton therapy.

The use of PBS may allow for better modulation of skin dose and improved conformality in some cases.

References

1. Siegel RL, Miller KD, Jemal A. Cancer statistics, 2015. CA Cancer J Clin. 2015;65:5–29. https://doi.org/10.3322/caac.21254.
2. Fisher B, Anderson S, Bryant J, Margolese RG, Deutsch M, Fisher ER, Jeong J-H, Wolmark N. Twenty-year follow-up of a randomized trial comparing total mastectomy, lumpectomy, and lumpectomy plus irradiation for the treatment of invasive breast cancer. N Engl J Med. 2002;347:1233–41. https://doi.org/10.1056/NEJMoa022152.
3. Clarke M, Collins R, Darby S, Davies C, Elphinstone P, Evans V, Godwin J, Gray R, Hicks C, James S, Mac Kinnon E, Mc Gale P, Mc Hugh T, Peto R, Taylor C, Wang Y, Early Breast Cancer Trialists' Collaborative Group (EBCTCG). Effects of radiotherapy and of differences in the extent of surgery for early breast cancer on local recurrence and 15-year survival: an overview of the randomised trials. Lancet. 2005;366:2087–106. https://doi.org/10.1016/S0140-6736(05)67887-7.
4. EBCTCG (Early Breast Cancer Trialists' Collaborative Group), Mc Gale P, Taylor C, Correa C, Cutter D, Duane F, Ewertz M, Gray R, Mannu G, Peto R, Whelan T, Wang Y, Wang Z, Darby S. Effect of radiotherapy after mastectomy and axillary surgery on 10-year recurrence and 20-year breast cancer mortality: meta-analysis of individual patient data for 8135 women in 22 randomised trials. Lancet. 2014;383:2127–35. https://doi.org/10.1016/S0140-6736(14)60488-8.
5. Whelan TJ, Olivotto IA, Parulekar WR, Ackerman I, Chua BH, Nabid A, Vallis KA, White JR, Rousseau P, Fortin A, Pierce LJ, Manchul L, Chafe S, Nolan MC, Craighead P, Bowen J, Mc Cready DR, Pritchard KI, Gelmon K, Murray Y, Chapman J-AW, Chen BE, Levine MN, MA.20 Study Investigators. Regional nodal irradiation in early-stage breast cancer. N Engl J Med. 2015;373:307–16. https://doi.org/10.1056/NEJMoa1415340.
6. Poortmans PM, Collette S, Kirkove C, Van Limbergen E, Budach V, Struikmans H, Collette L, Fourquet A, Maingon P, Valli M, De Winter K, Marnitz S, Barillot I, Scandolaro L, Vonk E, Rodenhuis C, Marsiglia H, Weidner N, van Tienhoven G, Glanzmann C, Kuten A, Arriagada R, Bartelink H, Van den Bogaert W, EORTC Radiation Oncology and Breast Cancer Groups. Internal mammary and medial supraclavicular irradiation in breast cancer. N Engl J Med. 2015;373:317–27. https://doi.org/10.1056/NEJMoa1415369.
7. Darby SC, Ewertz M, McGale P, Bennet AM, Blom-Goldman U, Brønnum D, Correa C, Cutter D, Gagliardi G, Gigante B, Jensen M-B, Nisbet A, Peto R, Rahimi K, Taylor C, Hall P. Risk of ischemic heart disease in women after radiotherapy for breast cancer. N Engl J Med. 2013;368:987–98. https://doi.org/10.1056/NEJMoa1209825.
8. Liljegren G, Holmberg L, Bergh J, Lindgren A, Tabár L, Nordgren H, Adami HO. 10-year results after sector resection with or without postoperative radiotherapy for stage I breast cancer: a randomized trial. J Clin Oncol. 1999;17:2326–33.
9. Veronesi U, Marubini E, Mariani L, Galimberti V, Luini A, Veronesi P, Salvadori B, Zucali R. Radiotherapy after breast-conserving surgery in small breast carcinoma: long-term results of a randomized trial. Ann Oncol. 2001;12:997–1003.
10. Strnad V, Ott OJ, Hildebrandt G, Kauer-Dorner D, Knauerhase H, Major T, Lyczek J, Guinot JL, Dunst J, Gutierrez Miguelez C, Slampa P, Allgäuer M, Lössl K, Polat B, Kovács G, Fischedick A-R, Wendt TG, Fietkau R, Hindemith M, Resch A, Kulik A, Arribas L, Niehoff

P, Guedea F, Schlamann A, Pötter R, Gall C, Malzer M, Uter W, Polgár C, Groupe Européen de Curiethérapie of European Society for Radiotherapy and Oncology (GEC-ESTRO). 5-year results of accelerated partial breast irradiation using sole interstitial multicatheter brachytherapy versus whole-breast irradiation with boost after breast-conserving surgery for low-risk invasive and in-situ carcinoma of the female breast: a randomised, phase 3, non-inferiority trial. Lancet. 2016;387:229–38. https://doi.org/10.1016/S0140-6736(15)00471-7.
11. Smith BD, Arthur DW, Buchholz TA, Haffty BG, Hahn CA, Hardenbergh PH, Julian TB, Marks LB, Todor DA, Vicini FA, Whelan TJ, White J, Wo JY, Harris JR. Accelerated partial breast irradiation consensus statement from the American Society for Radiation Oncology (ASTRO). Int J Radiat Oncol Biol Phys. 2009;74(4):987–1001.
12. Vaidya JS, Wenz F, Bulsara M, Tobias JS, Joseph DJ, Keshtgar M, Flyger HL, Massarut S, Alvarado M, Saunders C, Eiermann W, Metaxas M, Sperk E, Sütterlin M, Brown D, Esserman L, Roncadin M, Thompson A, Dewar JA, Holtveg HMR, Pigorsch S, Falzon M, Harris E, Matthews A, Brew-Graves C, Potyka I, Corica T, Williams NR, Baum M, TARGIT trialists' group. Risk-adapted targeted intraoperative radiotherapy versus whole-breast radiotherapy for breast cancer: 5-year results for local control and overall survival from the TARGIT-A randomised trial. Lancet. 2014;383:603–13. https://doi.org/10.1016/S0140-6736(13)61950-9.
13. Olivotto IA, Whelan TJ, Parpia S, Kim D-H, Berrang T, Truong PT, Kong I, Cochrane B, Nichol A, Roy I, Germain I, Akra M, Reed M, Fyles A, Trotter T, Perera F, Beckham W, Levine MN, Julian JA. Interim cosmetic and toxicity results from RAPID: a randomized trial of accelerated partial breast irradiation using three-dimensional conformal external beam radiation therapy. J Clin Oncol. 2013;31:4038–45. https://doi.org/10.1200/JCO.2013.50.5511.
14. Liss AL, Ben-David MA, Jagsi R, Hayman JA, Griffith KA, Moran JM, Marsh RB, Pierce LJ. Decline of cosmetic outcomes following accelerated partial breast irradiation using intensity modulated radiation therapy: results of a single-institution prospective clinical trial. Int J Radiat Oncol Biol Phys. 2014;89:96–102. https://doi.org/10.1016/j.ijrobp.2014.01.005.
15. Hepel JT, Tokita M, MacAusland SG, Evans SB, Hiatt JR, Price LL, DiPetrillo T, Wazer DE. Toxicity of three-dimensional conformal radiotherapy for accelerated partial breast irradiation. Int J Radiat Oncol Biol Phys. 2009;75:1290–6. https://doi.org/10.1016/j.ijrobp.2009.01.009.
16. Leonard KL, Hepel JT, Hiatt JR, Dipetrillo TA, Price LL, Wazer DE. The effect of dose-volume parameters and interfraction interval on cosmetic outcome and toxicity after 3-dimensional conformal accelerated partial breast irradiation. Int J Radiat Oncol Biol Phys. 2013;85:623–9. https://doi.org/10.1016/j.ijrobp.2012.06.052.
17. Peterson D, Truong PT, Parpia S, Olivotto IA, Berrang T, Kim D-H, Kong I, Germain I, Nichol A, Akra M, Roy I, Reed M, Fyles A, Trotter T, Perera F, Balkwill S, Lavertu S, Elliott E, Julian JA, Levine MN, Whelan TJ, RAPID trial investigators. Predictors of adverse cosmetic outcome in the RAPID trial: an exploratory analysis. Int J Radiat Oncol Biol Phys. 2015;91:968–76. https://doi.org/10.1016/j.ijrobp.2014.12.040.
18. Livi L, Meattini I, Marrazzo L, Simontacchi G, Pallotta S, Saieva C, Paiar F, Scotti V, De Luca CC, Bastiani P, Orzalesi L, Casella D, Sanchez L, Nori J, Fambrini M, Bianchi S. Accelerated partial breast irradiation using intensity-modulated radiotherapy versus whole breast irradiation: 5-year survival analysis of a phase 3 randomised controlled trial. Eur J Cancer. 2015;51:451–63. https://doi.org/10.1016/j.ejca.2014.12.013.
19. Formenti SC, Hsu H, Fenton-Kerimian M, Roses D, Guth A, Jozsef G, Goldberg JD, Dewyngaert JK. Prone accelerated partial breast irradiation after breast-conserving surgery: five-year results of 100 patients. Int J Radiat Oncol Biol Phys. 2012;84:606–11. https://doi.org/10.1016/j.ijrobp.2012.01.039.
20. Taghian AG, Kozak KR, Katz A, Adams J, Lu H-M, Powell SN, Delaney TF. Accelerated partial breast irradiation using proton beams: initial dosimetric experience. Int J Radiat Oncol Biol Phys. 2006;65:1404–10. https://doi.org/10.1016/j.ijrobp.2006.03.017.
21. Moon SH, Shin KH, Kim TH, Yoon M, Park S, Lee D-H, Kim JW, Kim DW, Park SY, Cho KH. Dosimetric comparison of four different external beam partial breast irradiation techniques: three-dimensional conformal radiotherapy, intensity-modulated radiotherapy,

helical tomotherapy, and proton beam therapy. Radiother Oncol. 2009;90:66–73. https://doi.org/10.1016/j.radonc.2008.09.027.
22. Galland-Girodet S, Pashtan I, MacDonald SM, Ancukiewicz M, Hirsch AE, Kachnic LA, Specht M, Gadd M, Smith BL, Powell SN, Recht A, Taghian AG. Long-term cosmetic outcomes and toxicities of proton beam therapy compared with photon-based 3-dimensional conformal accelerated partial-breast irradiation: a phase 1 trial. Int J Radiat Oncol Biol Phys. 2014;90:493–500. https://doi.org/10.1016/j.ijrobp.2014.04.008.
23. Chang JH, Lee NK, Kim JY, Kim Y-J, Moon SH, Kim TH, Kim J-Y, Kim DY, Cho KH, Shin KH. Phase II trial of proton beam accelerated partial breast irradiation in breast cancer. Radiother Oncol. 2013;108:209–14. https://doi.org/10.1016/j.radonc.2013.06.008.
24. Bush DA, Slater JD, Garberoglio C, Do S, Lum S, Slater JM. Partial breast irradiation delivered with proton beam: results of a phase II trial. Clin Breast Cancer. 2011;11:241–5. https://doi.org/10.1016/j.clbc.2011.03.023.
25. Bush DA, Do S, Lum S, Garberoglio C, Mirshahidi H, Patyal B, Grove R, Slater JD. Partial breast radiation therapy with proton beam: 5-year results with cosmetic outcomes. Int J Radiat Oncol Biol Phys. 2014;90:501–5. https://doi.org/10.1016/j.ijrobp.2014.05.1308.
26. Overgaard M, Jensen MB, Overgaard J, Hansen PS, Rose C, Andersson M, Kamby C, Kjaer M, Gadeberg CC, Rasmussen BB, Blichert-Toft M, Mouridsen HT. Postoperative radiotherapy in high-risk postmenopausal breast-cancer patients given adjuvant tamoxifen: Danish breast cancer cooperative group DBCG 82c randomised trial. Lancet. 1999;353:1641–8. https://doi.org/10.1016/S0140-6736(98)09201-0.
27. Overgaard M, Hansen PS, Overgaard J, Rose C, Andersson M, Bach F, Kjaer M, Gadeberg CC, Mouridsen HT, Jensen MB, Zedeler K. Postoperative radiotherapy in high-risk premenopausal women with breast cancer who receive adjuvant chemotherapy. Danish breast cancer cooperative group 82b trial. N Engl J Med. 1997;337:949–55. https://doi.org/10.1056/NEJM199710023371401.
28. Thorsen LBJ, Offersen BV, Danø H, Berg M, Jensen I, Pedersen AN, Zimmermann SJ, Brodersen H-J, Overgaard M, Overgaard J. DBCG-IMN: a population-based cohort study on the effect of internal mammary node irradiation in early node-positive breast cancer. J Clin Oncol. 2016;34:314–20. https://doi.org/10.1200/JCO.2015.63.6456.
29. Ares C, Khan S, Macartain AM, Heuberger J, Goitein G, Gruber G, Lutters G, Hug EB, Bodis S, Lomax AJ. Postoperative proton radiotherapy for localized and locoregional breast cancer: potential for clinically relevant improvements? Int J Radiat Oncol Biol Phys. 2010;76:685–97. https://doi.org/10.1016/j.ijrobp.2009.02.062.
30. MacDonald SM, Jimenez R, Paetzold P, Adams J, Beatty J, Delaney TF, Kooy H, Taghian AG, Lu H-M. Proton radiotherapy for chest wall and regional lymphatic radiation; dose comparisons and treatment delivery. Radiat Oncol. 2013;8:71. https://doi.org/10.1186/1748-717X-8-71.
31. MacDonald SM, Patel SA, Hickey S, Specht M, Isakoff SJ, Gadd M, Smith BL, Yeap BY, Adams J, Delaney TF, Kooy H, Lu H-M, Taghian AG. Proton therapy for breast cancer after mastectomy: early outcomes of a prospective clinical trial. Int J Radiat Oncol Biol Phys. 2013;86:484–90. https://doi.org/10.1016/j.ijrobp.2013.01.038.
32. Mast ME, Vredeveld EJ, Credoe HM, van Egmond J, Heijenbrok MW, Hug EB, Kalk P, van Kempen-Harteveld LML, Korevaar EW, van der Laan HP, Langendijk JA, Rozema HJE, Petoukhova AL, Schippers JM, Struikmans H, Maduro JH. Whole breast proton irradiation for maximal reduction of heart dose in breast cancer patients. Breast Cancer Res Treat. 2014;148:33–9. https://doi.org/10.1007/s10549-014-3149-6.
33. Xu N, Ho MW, Li Z, Morris CG, Mendenhall NP. Can proton therapy improve the therapeutic ratio in breast cancer patients at risk for nodal disease? Am J Clin Oncol. 2014;37:568–74. https://doi.org/10.1097/COC.0b013e318280d614.
34. Bradley JA, Dagan R, Ho MW, Rutenberg M, Morris CG, Li Z, Mendenhall NP. Initial report of a prospective Dosimetric and clinical feasibility trial demonstrates the potential of protons to increase the therapeutic ratio in breast cancer compared with photons. Int J Radiat Oncol Biol Phys. 2016;95:411–21. https://doi.org/10.1016/j.ijrobp.2015.09.018.

35. Lin LL, Vennarini S, Dimofte A, Ravanelli D, Shillington K, Batra S, Tochner Z, Both S, Freedman G. Proton beam versus photon beam dose to the heart and left anterior descending artery for left-sided breast cancer. Acta Oncol. 2015;54:1032–9. https://doi.org/10.3109/0284186X.2015.1011756.
36. Taylor CW, Wang Z, Macaulay E, Jagsi R, Duane F, Darby SC. Exposure of the heart in breast cancer radiation therapy: a systematic review of heart doses published during 2003 to 2013. Int J Radiat Oncol Biol Phys. 2015;93:845–53. https://doi.org/10.1016/j.ijrobp.2015.07.2292.
37. Cuaron JJ, Chon B, Tsai H, Goenka A, DeBlois D, Ho A, Powell S, Hug E, Cahlon O. Early toxicity in patients treated with postoperative proton therapy for locally advanced breast cancer. Int J Radiat Oncol Biol Phys. 2015;92:284–91. https://doi.org/10.1016/j.ijrobp.2015.01.005.
38. Fagundes MA, Pankuch M, Hartsell W, Ward C, Fang LC, Cahlon O, McNeeley S, Mao L, Lavilla M, Hug E. Cardiac-sparing Postmastectomy proton radiation therapy for women with stage III, loco-regional, breast cancer: a Dosimetric comparison study. Int J Radiat Oncol Biol Phys. 2013;87:S245. https://doi.org/10.1016/j.ijrobp.2013.06.637.
39. Brown LC, Diehn FE, Boughey JC, Childs SK, Park SS, Yan ES, Petersen IA, Mutter RW. Delineation of supraclavicular target volumes in breast cancer radiation therapy. Int J Radiat Oncol Biol Phys. 2015;92:642–9. https://doi.org/10.1016/j.ijrobp.2015.02.022.
40. White BM, Vennarini S, Lin L, Freedman G, Santhanam A, Low DA, Both S. Accuracy of routine treatment planning 4-dimensional and deep-inspiration breath-hold computed tomography delineation of the left anterior descending artery in radiation therapy. Int J Radiat Oncol Biol Phys. 2015;91:825–31. https://doi.org/10.1016/j.ijrobp.2014.11.036.
41. Vargo JA, Beriwal S. RTOG Chest Wall contouring guidelines for post-mastectomy radiation therapy: is it evidence-based? Int J Radiat Oncol Biol Phys. 2015;93:266–7. https://doi.org/10.1016/j.ijrobp.2015.03.001.
42. Depauw N, Batin E, Daartz J, Rosenfeld A, Adams J, Kooy H, MacDonald S, Lu H-M. A novel approach to postmastectomy radiation therapy using scanned proton beams. Int J Radiat Oncol Biol Phys. 2015;91:427–34. https://doi.org/10.1016/j.ijrobp.2014.10.039.
43. Moyers MF, Mah D, Boyer SP, Chang C, Pankuch M. Use of proton beams with breast prostheses and tissue expanders. Med Dosim. 2014;39:98–101. https://doi.org/10.1016/j.meddos.2013.10.006.

Gynecologic malignancies

Jessica E. Scholey, Pamela J. Boimel, Maura Kirk, and Lilie Lin

Contents

18.1　Introduction.. 289
18.2　Simulation, Target Delineation, and Radiation Dose/Fractionation 291
18.3　Proton Treatment Planning 295
　　　18.3.1　Pelvis 296
　　　18.3.2　Local Recurrence or Boost Volumes 296
　　　18.3.3　Re-irradiation... 298
　　　18.3.4　Avoiding Hardware and Sparing OARs 298
18.4　Dosimetric and Toxicity Comparison 298
18.5　Patient Positioning, Immobilization, and Treatment Verification 299
18.6　Future Developments 300
References... 300

18.1　Introduction

- Gynecologic malignancies including endometrial, vulvar, vaginal, and cervical pose a significant challenge for women worldwide with an estimated 83,620 new cases diagnosed in the United States in 2016 [1]. Radiation therapy is routinely

---

L. Lin (✉)
University of Texas-MD Anderson Cancer Center,
1515 Holcombe Blvd Unit 1422, Houston, TX 77030, USA
e-mail: LLLin@mdanderson.org

J.E. Scholey
Department of Radiation Oncology, University of California,
San Francisco, USA

P.J. Boimel • M. Kirk
Department of Radiation Oncology, University of Pennsylvania,
Philadelphia, PA, USA

© Springer International Publishing Switzerland 2018
N. Lee et al. (eds.), *Target Volume Delineation and Treatment Planning for Particle Therapy*, Practical Guides in Radiation Oncology,
https://doi.org/10.1007/978-3-319-42478-1_18

administered to increase local control and overall survival either in the post-hysterectomy or definitive setting. The standard treatment for early-stage cervical and endometrial cancers includes hysterectomy with adjuvant radiation given with or without concurrent chemotherapy depending on the presence of high-risk features [2–7]. The standard treatment for locally advanced cervical cancer is external beam radiation therapy (EBRT) and intracavitary brachytherapy with improved local control and overall survival when given with concurrent chemotherapy [8]. High-risk stage III/IV endometrial cancers are typically treated with hysterectomy and adjuvant radiation, often combined with chemotherapy given either concurrently or sequentially or sandwiched [9].

- The gynecologic target volume includes the pelvis (either post-hysterectomy to treat pelvic lymph nodes or in the definitive treatment of locally advanced cervical cancer to treat the cervix, uterus, parametrium, proximal vaginal, and pelvic lymph nodes), with extended field radiation performed when para-aortic lymph nodes are positive or suspicious for disease. Inguinal lymph node radiation is added for distal vaginal extension or in the treatment of vulvar and vaginal cancers.
- EBRT for gynecologic malignancies has historically been delivered using photons with 2–4 fields to the pelvis, including an extended AP/PA field for treatment of the para-aortic lymph nodes, with the addition of chemotherapy often resulting in significant hematologic and gastrointestinal toxicity. Bone marrow suppression leading to hematologic toxicity with concurrent chemoradiation can necessitate dose reductions in chemotherapy and has been correlated with inferior outcomes [10, 11]. Specifically, the volume of pelvic bone marrow receiving 10–20 Gy has been correlated with increased hematologic toxicity when radiation is given concurrently with cisplatin [12, 13]. In a recent phase II study, bone marrow sparing using intensity-modulated radiation therapy (IMRT) was shown to decrease rates of hematologic toxicity with concurrent cisplatin [14]. IMRT has also been shown to decrease dose to the bowel, rectum, bladder, and bone marrow when treating pelvic and para-aortic lymph nodes versus conventional (3D conformal photon) radiotherapy [15, 16]. However, dose reduction to one OAR with IMRT can often result in increased dose to other OARs and increased integral radiation dose [17]. A recent phase II study of IMRT reported a significant 28% grade ≥ 2 bowel adverse events [18]. The characteristic Bragg peak of protons often translates to a reduction in normal tissue dose when using proton beam radiation therapy (PBRT) with the additional potential to escalate dose and reduce toxicity with combined modality treatment. PBRT may allow for dose escalation to gross disease, fewer chemotherapy dose reductions, and treatment of recurrent disease with little dose to previously irradiated normal tissues.
- Results of early dosimetric studies comparing IMRT alone with mixed IMRT and proton therapy indicate that treatment with proton therapy significantly reduces dose to the small and large bowel as well as kidneys when treating para-aortic lymph nodes [19]. Until recently, the majority of PBRT has been delivered with passive scattering, which can be less conformal and require longer treatment times compared to IMRT. We have recently reported on the clinical feasibility and dosimetric advantages of proton pencil beam scanning (PBS) to reduce normal tissue dose while maintaining target coverage and conformality in the treatment of gynecologic cancers following hysterectomy [20]. PBS was found

to result in a lower volume of bone marrow, bladder, and small bowel treated to low dose (10–30 Gy) compared to IMRT. Initial toxicity estimates have been very encouraging with a low percentage of grade 3 or greater hematologic toxicity. In our experience, PBRT is feasible, allows for combined modality treatment with fewer chemotherapy dose adjustments, and has dosimetric advantages allowing us to meet OAR constraints even when escalating dose to boost gross residual disease or retreating for local recurrence.

18.2 Simulation, Target Delineation, and Radiation Dose/Fractionation

- CT simulation should be performed on a non-contrast CT scan for the purposes of dose calculation. If desired, CT with IV contrast can be subsequently performed and fused to the planning CT for delineation of nodal volumes. Oral contrast may be given to define small and large bowels. Placement of gold seed fiducial markers at the vaginal apex in the postoperative setting or in the cervix in the intact setting may allow for improved target delineation, provided that any artifacts, high-Z materials, or hollow fiducials are overridden appropriately for treatment planning purposes.
- PET-CT-based treatment planning is especially useful for visualization of gross nodal involvement, residual disease, vulvar invasion, sidewall disease, and local recurrence [21–24]. MRI-based brachytherapy treatment planning has been shown to have more accurate delineation of the tumor volume compared to CT-based planning and has been incorporated into consensus guidelines [25–28]. Likewise, MRI can be useful for proton treatment planning prior to brachytherapy to ensure adequate coverage of gross disease. If PET-CT and/or MRI will be used for treatment planning, the scans should optimally be performed at the time of CT simulation using the appropriate immobilization devices and fused with the non-contrast planning CT scan used for dose calculation.
- Robust indexed immobilization is strongly recommended as interfractional vaginal motion can be significant [29–31]. To minimize the impact of bowel gas, patients may be instructed to take anti-gas medication, such as simethicone or Phazyme, with every meal starting approximately 1 week before simulation and throughout the duration of treatment. Patients may be instructed to drink a fixed volume of fluid at some time interval prior to simulation and treatment sessions for a reproducibly full bladder to reduce bladder dose and push bowel away from the fields. For example, at our institution patients are instructed to drink 16 oz of fluid 30 min prior to simulation and each daily fraction. An endorectal balloon inflated with 50–100 cc of water may be employed for target immobilization and to limit anatomical variation.
- To assist in target delineation and to account for internal motion of the target due to variable bladder volume, patients may be scanned initially with a full bladder and rectal balloon and subsequently with an empty bladder and rectal balloon filled to the same volume (Fig. 18.1).
- Patients should be simulated in the supine position using an indexed knee and foot lock to limit hip rotation and encourage fixed flexion at the knees and hips (Fig. 18.2). Positioning of arms should be reproducible and placed so as not to

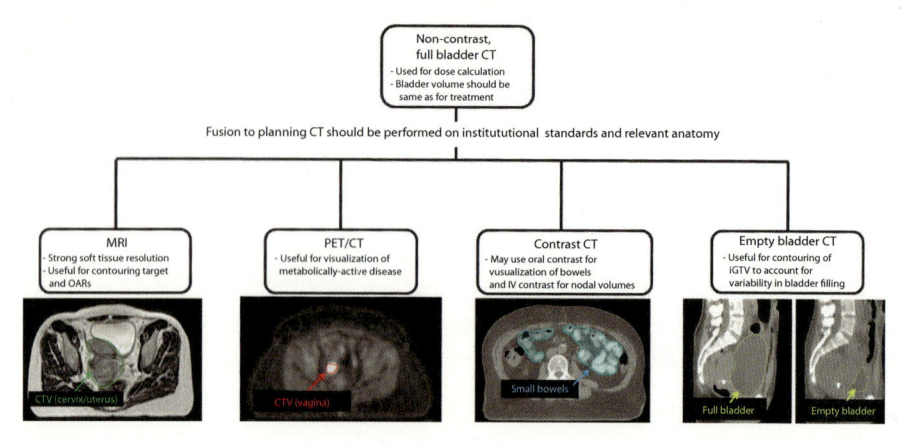

Fig. 18.1 Imaging workflow with clinical examples. It is recommended that images be acquired on the same day and in the same treatment position (see *below*). Image fusions should be performed based on institutional standards and relevant anatomy. For example, image sets at our institution are acquired with the patient in the same treatment position and are fused using rigid registration based on bony anatomy

Fig. 18.2 Recommended setup and immobilization includes indexed knee and foot lock. Hands and arms should rest outside of treatment area, either on the superior chest (shown) or above head if treating para-aortic nodes. *Note: This photo shows options for immobilization, but patient should have minimal clothing on to avoid perturbation of proton beam*

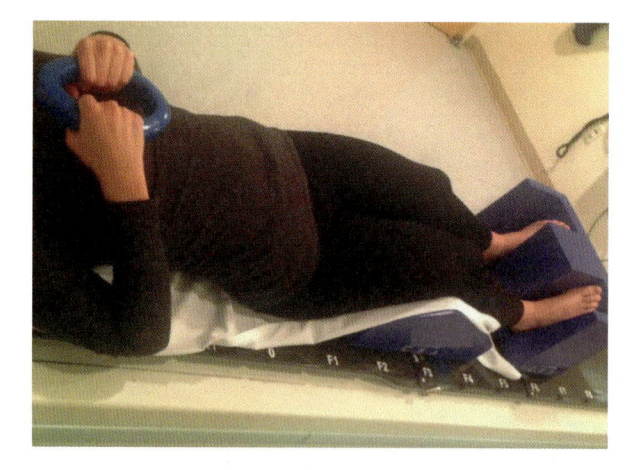

interfere with radiation beams. For example, the patient may hold a ring on the superior chest if treating the pelvis alone but should have arms up using a wing board if including more superior fields to target para-aortic volumes.
- Target and OAR contouring of the post-hysterectomy pelvis should follow RTOG guidelines [32]. The CTV should include the pelvic lymph nodes (common iliac, internal and external iliac, obturator, and presacral when treating cervical cancer and endometrial when there is cervical/parametrial involvement) and the proximal vaginal cuff (3 cm). When treating patients with an intact cervix, the CTV should include the proximal vagina, cervix, uterus, parametrium, ovaries, and pelvic lymph nodes as previously described [33]. The entire mesorectum should be included if there is pelvic sidewall involvement. A nodal CTV should be con-

toured which includes a 7 mm expansion around the vasculature [34]. When contouring para-aortic lymph nodes, use generous margins in the left para-aortic region (including the entire space between the aorta and left psoas muscle), which is the most common location for para-aortic lymph node metastasis [35].
- Internal motion of the vagina caused by changes in bladder volume can be accounted for by fusing the full and empty bladder CT scans and expanding the vagina CTV to include the proximal vagina and paravaginal tissue in both scenarios (iCTV) (Fig. 18.3).
- OARs include small and large bowels, rectum, pelvic bone marrow (including bone marrow in the lower pelvis, ilium, and lumbosacral spine), kidneys, femoral heads, and bladder. Individual loops of small and large bowel are contoured within the field and 2 cm above the PBS target [15]The rectum is contoured from the anus to the rectosigmoid junction.
- To account for variations in patient positioning and setup, a PTV is created such that nodal CTVs are expanded by 7–8 mm and vaginal CTVs are expanded by 10–13 mm. In proton therapy, the PTV accounts for lateral uncertainties and is used for recording and reporting purposes.
- Proton beam range uncertainty can be of concern in proton radiotherapy. To mitigate this uncertainty, either robust optimization can be used or a PBS-specific optimization structure can be created for planning purposes when a single-field optimization planning technique is employed. At our institution, an optimization structure is created by adding a margin of 3.5% of the beam range to the CTV in the beam direction to account for uncertainty in the conversion from Hounsfield unit (HU) values to proton stopping power, and an additional 1 mm margin can be added to correct for beam calibration uncertainty (Fig. 18.4). Specific uncertainty values employed should be evaluated on an institutional basis.
- Artifacts caused by high-density materials should be contoured and assigned a predetermined density or HU value. Gas in the rectum and small and large bowels should be contoured to the density or HU value of the surrounding soft tissue to account for interfractional variation in gas. Any contrast existing in the simulation CT that will not be present for treatment should also be contoured and assigned HU value appropriately (Fig. 18.5).

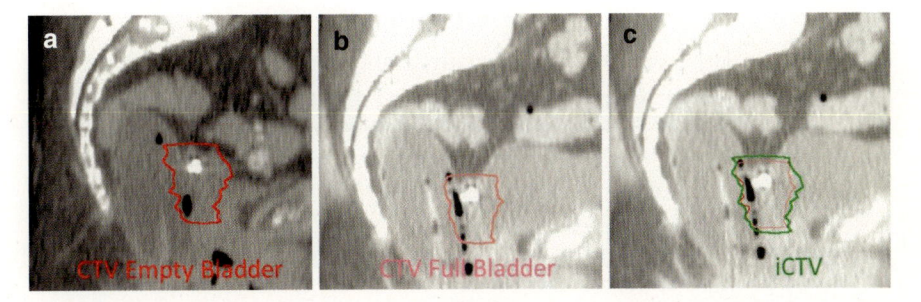

Fig. 18.3 To account for internal motion caused by variable bladder volume, a vaginal CTV should include the CTV contoured on the empty bladder scan (**a**) and full bladder scan (**b**). The iCTV volume should encompass both CTV volumes (**c**)

Fig. 18.4 Pencil beam scanning target volume (PBSTV) optimization structure is created by adding a margin of 3.5% of the beam range plus 1 mm to CTV structure in the direction of the beam

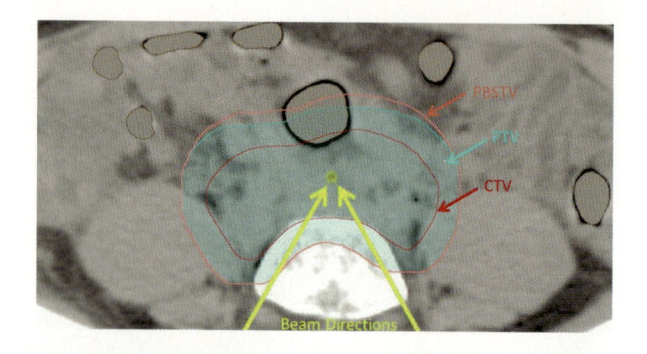

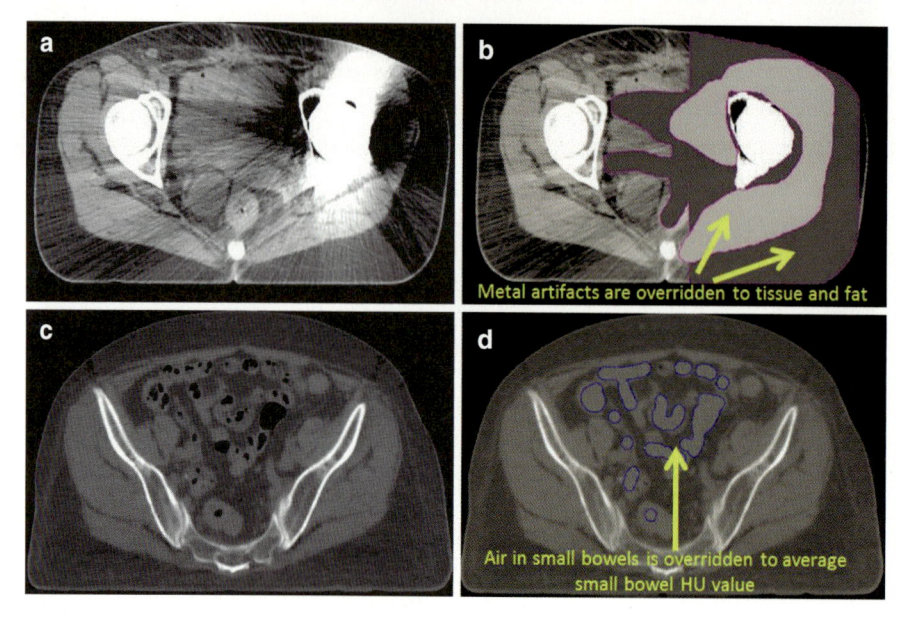

Fig. 18.5 (**a**) Artifacts caused by hip replacement. (**b**) Artifacts should be manually contoured and HU values assigned to nearby fat or tissue. (**c**) Air in bowels. (**d**) Air in bowels should be overridden and assigned to appropriate HU value in planning CT

- All proton doses are provided in relative biologic effectiveness (*RBE* = 1.1). Planned dose is typically 45–50.4 Gy delivered in 1.8 Gy daily fractions but can vary depending on the clinical scenario. At our institution, dose and fractionation for proton therapy follows the same regimen as employed for photon therapy. A dose of 45 Gy is administered when a brachytherapy boost will be added both for definitive treatment of locally advanced cervical cancer and for post-hysterectomy endometrial cancer patients who receive vaginal brachytherapy following whole-pelvis radiation. A dose of 50.4 Gy is administered when treating with EBRT alone for post-hysterectomy high-risk cervical cancer and endometrial cancer. For high-risk endometrial cancer with pelvic disease (i.e., stage II–III endometrial cancer), a dose of 50.4 Gy may be administered followed by

18 Gynecologic malignancies

Table 18.1 Recommended target volumes and radiation doses (in Gy RBE) for common clinical scenarios

Clinical scenario	Target	Dose (Gy RBE)
Pelvic and para-aortic lymph nodes	*Cervix*: Common iliac, internal and external iliacs, obturator, presacral nodes *Endometrial*: Only add presacral lymph nodes if there is cervical or parametrial involvement *Distal vaginal/vulvar invasion*: Add inguinal lymph nodes *Para-aortic nodes*: Extend contour up to the level of the renal hilum (T12)	50.4 Gy in 1.8 Gy fractions to the pelvic lymph nodes 45 Gy in 1.8 Gy fractions to para-aortic lymph nodes Gross nodal boost to 60–66 Gy in 2 Gy fractions
Post-hysterectomy pelvis	Pelvic lymph nodes as above, 3 cm proximal vaginal cuff *Cervix*: Include presacral space, clips, and/or mesorectum if there is pelvic sidewall extension	50.4 Gy in 1.8 Gy fractions 45 Gy in 1.8 Gy fractions with vaginal brachytherapy (VB HDR 3–4 Gy/fx, 3fx)
Intact cervix	Cervix, uterus, parametria, ovaries, proximal vagina + pelvic lymph nodes	45 Gy in 1.8 Gy fractions Boost to 60–66 Gy in 2 Gyfx to positive lymph nodes or parametrial/adnexal/sidewall disease depending on location and accounting for brachytherapy dose T&O brachytherapy boost (HDR-5.5–6 Gy/fx, 5 fx)
Isolated local recurrence	Gross disease alone	60–66 Gy in 2 Gy fractions

vaginal brachytherapy. A dose of 45 Gy is administered to para-aortic lymph nodes if treating. A higher dose per fraction (e.g., 2 Gy/fx) may be given for total dose of 60–66 Gy for conedowns to smaller targets, for example, when boosting gross residual disease, positive lymph nodes, or isolated local recurrences. Guidelines are suggested below but should be tailored for each individual patient and clinical scenario while also accounting for dose to organs at risk (Table 18.1).

18.3 Proton Treatment Planning

Due to the complicated geometry of target volumes, PBS is generally preferred over passive scattering when treating gynecologic cancers with protons. Because of the high potential of interfraction variability in pelvis anatomy, our institution currently treats with single-field uniform dose (SFUD) PBS plans as opposed to intensity-modulated proton therapy (IMPT).

18.3.1 Pelvis

- Careful consideration of beam angles is imperative in proton planning, particularly when treating pelvic regions as there can be significant variations in weight and volume of the bladder and bowel. For this reason, anterior beams are generally avoided. To minimize the impacts of changes in patient anatomy, a posterior beam arrangement is recommended. Two posterior oblique beams angled 10–30 degrees from the posterior have been used at our institution (Figs. 18.6, 18.7 and 18.8). In some cases two lateral beams have been used (Fig. 18.9). Clinical trials are currently ongoing which investigate alternative planning approaches, for example, a single posterior beam planning technique for SFUD proton PBS [36]. Choice of beam arrangement may vary depending on proton beam spot size, potential skin sparing, and institutional and clinical judgment.
- During planning, avoid using beam angles that result in fluence entering through immobilization devices or sharp edges of the couch, as these may not be reproducible during patient setup.
- For patients with mobile anterior tissue (Fig. 18.7), a posterior beam arrangement (consisting of 1–2 beams depending on the spot size) provides a more stable beam path than lateral or anterior beams do, as this technique avoids daily anatomical modifications to the beam pathway.

18.3.2 Local Recurrence or Boost Volumes

- When treating small volumes of gross disease to higher doses (i.e., boost to positive lymph nodes or recurrent disease), beams should be selected which have the shortest and most homogeneous and reproducible path length.

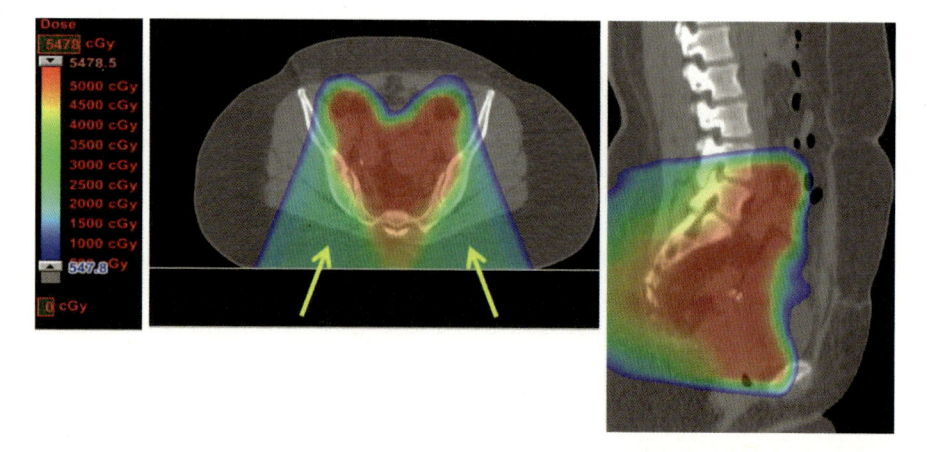

Fig. 18.6 Standard beam orientation for treating the pelvis using SFUD at the University of Pennsylvania. Two posterior oblique beams of angle 30° from posterior are used in this example

18 Gynecologic malignancies

Fig. 18.7 For patients with mobile anterior tissue, posterior beam arrangements are recommended over lateral or anterior beam arrangements, which may be affected by daily anatomical variations due to tissue positioning (delineated by *arrows* in above figure)

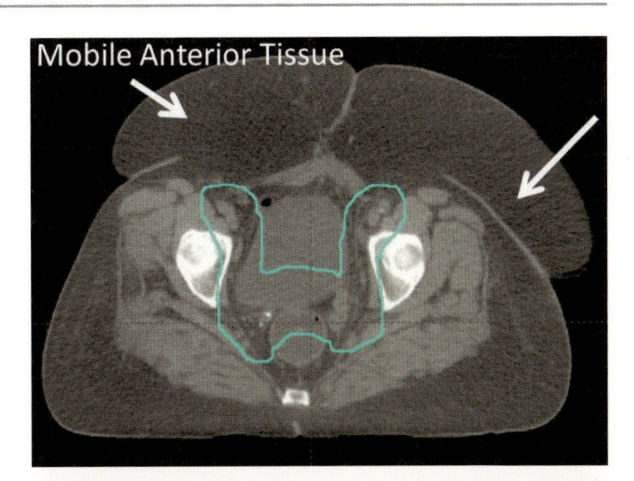

Fig. 18.8 A patient with localized nodal recurrence was treated with two left posterior oblique beams using PBS

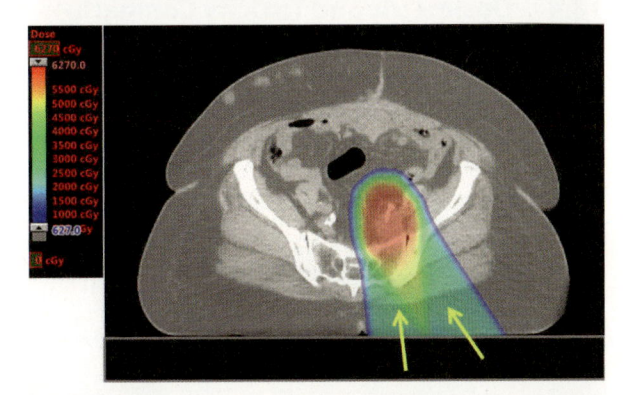

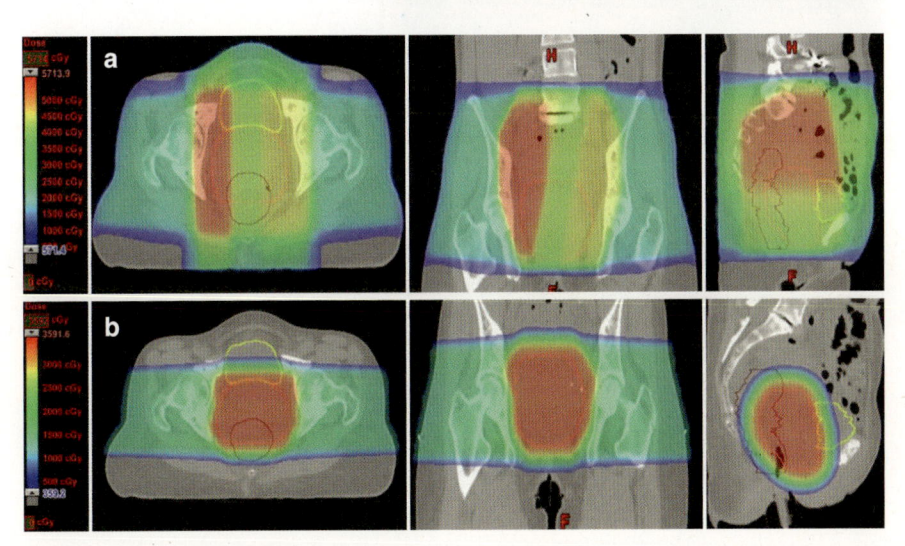

Fig. 18.9 (a) Dose distribution from previous four-field box photon irradiation to a dose of 39.6 Gy with a boost to 55.6 Gy and (b) dose distribution for re-irradiation using protons. In this case, lateral beams were selected for re-irradiation to minimize additional dose to bowel and bladder as no imminent anatomical deformation of the patient external contour was identified

18.3.3 Re-irradiation

- PBRT can be used in patients who have had previous radiation to help limit dose to tissues that have already been irradiated.

18.3.4 Avoiding Hardware and Sparing OARs

- Avoid using beams that traverse through hardware or organs with volume variability due to physiological changes, for example, bladder or bowel. Beams may also be selected to avoid specific organs that may be of clinical concern (e.g., the kidneys) (Fig. 18.10).

18.4 Dosimetric and Toxicity Comparison

- Dose to normal tissues should be low as reasonably achievable without compromising target coverage. The recommendations in Table 18.2 are adapted from IMRT dose constraints outlined in RTOG 0418 and RTOG 1203, along with institutional photon treatment planning objectives. In practice, dose limits should be carefully considered for each patient by the clinical team (Table 18.3).

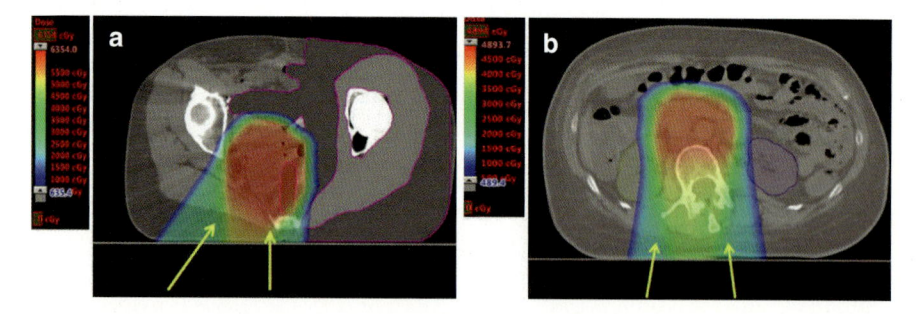

Fig. 18.10 (a) Patient with unilateral hip replacement was treated using a posterior and right posterior oblique beam arrangement to avoid beams traversing through hardware or artifacts. (b) Partial kidney sparing was achieved using posterior oblique beams angled 10° from the posterior for a patient receiving radiation to the para-aortic nodes adjacent to the kidneys

Table 18.2 Recommended dose constraints (in RBE) to organs at risk when using PBRT for treatment of gynecologic malignancies

Organ at risk	Recommended dose constraint
Pelvic bone marrow	V10 Gy < 95%, V20 Gy < 76%
Large bowel	V40 Gy < 30% and V40 Gy < 300 cc
Small bowel	V40 Gy < 30% and V40 Gy < 300 cc
Kidney	V18 Gy < 66%
Bladder	V45 Gy < 35% or ALARA
Rectum	V40 Gy <60 or ALARA
Femoral heads	V30 Gy < 15%

18 Gynecologic malignancies

Table 18.3 OAR dosimetric comparison of IMRT versus PBS with posterior oblique beams for treatment of gynecologic malignancies [20]

Characteristic	Dosimetric comparison of IMRT vs. PBS*
Bladder	Volume receiving 0–35 Gy was significantly lower with PBS than with IMRT. No significant difference between IMRT and PBS for doses >35 Gy
Small bowel	Volume receiving 0–32 Gy was significantly lower with PBS than with IMRT. No significant difference between IMRT and PBS for doses >32 Gy
Large bowel	Volume receiving 0–31 Gy was significantly lower with PBS than with IMRT. Volume receiving 48–58 Gy was significantly lower with IMRT than with PBS
Pelvic bone marrow	Volume receiving 0–29 Gy (specifically V10 Gy and V20 Gy) was significantly lower with PBS than with IMRT. Volume receiving >35 Gy was significantly lower with IMRT
Rectum	V20 Gy and V45 Gy were significantly lower with IMRT than with PBS

*All doses listed in Gy RBE)

18.5 Patient Positioning, Immobilization, and Treatment Verification

- Treatment positioning should be performed using the same immobilization techniques as used in simulation, including consistent bladder filling as previously described.
- Localization should be performed daily by matching bony anatomy in orthogonal kV x-ray imaging. If available, volumetric imaging (CBCT) can be used to verify soft tissue positioning including bladder volume and rectal balloon placement. If volumetric imaging is not available on the proton treatment machine, contrast can be added to the water used to fill the indexed endorectal balloon to assist in kV x-ray alignment and to verify rectal balloon placement. Daily SSD or air gap measurements can assist in identifying changes in weight.
- If proton rooms are not equipped with volumetric imaging, weekly verification CT scans can be used to monitor anatomical variations (e.g., weight loss, tumor changes, and variability in bladder and bowel volume). These factors are important to evaluate as they can cause significant dosimetric changes to the radiation plan. Providing feedback to patients on bladder filling and gas management can result in more consistent preparation for treatment. Continuous communication between the treatment delivery team, physician, physicists, and planner is recommended to timely identify and correct for any patient-related changes which may impact the dose distribution (Fig. 18.11).

Fig. 18.11 A patient who experienced considerable change in weight over the course of 6 weeks. Proton beam path length is adversely affected by weight variation; therefore, adequate monitoring of weight is essential

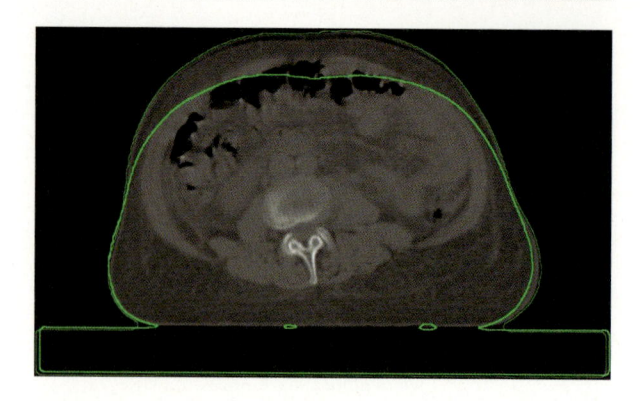

18.6 Future Developments

- The utilization of proton beam radiotherapy is increasing; however, proton beam range uncertainty remains a concern, particularly in the treatment of pelvic malignancies which contain a high level of anatomical variability. Many groups are investigating methods to mitigate this uncertainty, for example, in the use of dual energy CT [37, 38], proton computed tomography [39, 40], and in vivo measurements which may be used to detect the Bragg peak [41, 42].
- The University of Pennsylvania has reported on the use of SFUD in treating gynecologic malignancies using PBS. To our knowledge, no results have been reported on the use of IMPT in treating gynecologic cancers. IMPT may give superior dose distributions and higher OAR sparing; however, IMPT plans are more sensitive to uncertainties. The clinical implementation of robust optimization in treatment planning systems may provide a realization for IMPT in treating gynecologic malignancies in the future.

References

1. Siegel RL, et al. Cancer Statistics, 2016. CA Cancer J Clin. 2016;66:7–30.
2. Sedlis A, et al. A randomized trial of pelvic radiation therapy versus no further therapy in selected patients with stage IB carcinoma of the cervix after radical hysterectomy and pelvic lymphadenectomy: a Gynecologic Oncology Group Study. Gynecol Oncol. 1999;73(2):177–83.
3. Rotman M, et al. A phase III randomized trial of postoperative pelvic irradiation in stage IB cervical carcinoma with poor prognostic features: follow-up of a gynecologic oncology group study. Int J Radiat Oncol Biol Phys. 2006;65(1):169–76.
4. Peters WA III, et al. Concurrent chemotherapy and pelvic radiation therapy compared with pelvic radiation therapy alone as adjuvant therapy after radical surgery in high-risk early-stage cancer of the cervix. J Clin Oncol. 2000;18(8):1606–13.
5. Keys HM, et al. A phase III trial of surgery with or without adjunctive external pelvic radiation therapy in intermediate risk endometrial adenocarcinoma: a Gynecologic Oncology Group study. Gynecol Oncol. 2004;92(3):744–51.

6. Scholten AN, et al. Postoperative radiotherapy for stage 1 endometrial carcinoma: long-term outcome of the randomized PORTEC trial with central pathology review. Int J Radiat Oncol Biol Phys. 2005;63(3):834–8.
7. Sorbe B, et al. External pelvic and vaginal irradiation versus vaginal irradiation alone as postoperative therapy in medium-risk endometrial carcinoma–a prospective randomized study. Int J Radiat Oncol Biol Phys. 2012;82(3):1249–55.
8. Rose PG, et al. Concurrent cisplatin-based radiotherapy and chemotherapy for locally advanced cervical cancer. N Engl J Med. 1999;340:1144–53.
9. Greven K, et al. Final analysis of RTOG 9708: adjuvant postoperative irradiation combined with cisplatin/paclitaxel chemotherapy following surgery for patients with high-risk endometrial cancer. Gynecol Oncol. 2006;103(1):155–9.
10. Mauch P, et al. Hematopoietic stem cell compartment: acute and late effects of radiation therapy and chemotherapy. Int J Radiat Oncol Biol Phys. 1995;31(5):1319–39.
11. Parker K, et al. Five years' experience treating locally advanced cervical cancer with concurrent chemoradiotherapy and high-dose-rate brachytherapy: results from a single institution. Int J Radiat Oncol Biol Phys. 2009;74(1):140–6.
12. Mell LK, et al. Dosimetric predictors of acute hematologic toxicity in cervical cancer patients treated with concurrent cisplatin and intensity-modulated pelvic radiotherapy. Int J Radiat Oncol Biol Phys. 2006;66(5):1356–65.
13. Albuquerque K, et al. Radiation-related predictors of hematologic toxicity after concurrent chemoradiation for cervical cancer and implications for bone marrow-sparing pelvic IMRT. Int J Radiat Oncol Biol Phys. 2011;79(4):1043–7.
14. Klopp AH, et al. Hematologic toxicity in RTOG 0418: a phase 2 study of postoperative IMRT for gynecologic cancer. Int J Radiat Oncol Biol Phys. 2013;86(1):83–90.
15. Portelance L, et al. Intensity-modulated radiation therapy (IMRT) reduces small bowel, rectum, and bladder doses in patients with cervical cancer receiving pelvic and para-aortic irradiation. Int J Radiat Oncol Biol Phys. 2001;51(1):261–6.
16. Song WY, et al. Dosimetric comparison study between intensity modulated radiation therapy and three-dimensional conformal proton therapy for pelvic bone marrow sparing in the treatment of cervical cancer. J Appl Clin Med Phys. 2010;11(4):3255.
17. Lin A, et al. Intensity-modulated radiation therapy for the treatment of anal cancer. Clin Colorectal Cancer. 2007;6(10):716–9.
18. Jhingran A, et al. A phase II study of intensity modulated radiation therapy to the pelvis for postoperative patients with endometrial carcinoma: Radiation Therapy Oncology Group trial 0418. Int J Radiat Oncol Biol Phys. 2012;84(1):e23–8.
19. Milby AB, et al. Dosimetric comparison of combined intensity-modulated radiotherapy (IMRT) and proton therapy versus IMRT alone for pelvic and para-aortic radiotherapy in gynecologic malignancies. Int J Radiat Oncol Biol Phys. 2012;82(3):e477–84.
20. Lin L, et al. Initial report of pencil beam scanning proton therapy for posthysterectomy patients with gynecologic cancer. Int J Radiat Oncol Biol Phys. 2016;95(1):181–9.
21. Tsai C, et al. A prospective randomized trial to study the impact of pretreatment FDG-PET for cervical cancer patients with MRI-detected positive pelvic but negative para-aortic lymphadenopathy. Int J Radiat Oncol Biol Phys. 2010;76(2):477–84.
22. Kidd EA, et al. Clinical outcomes of definitive intensity-modulated radiation therapy with fluorodeoxyglucose-positron emission tomography simulation in patients with locally advanced cervical cancer. Int J Radiat Oncol Biol Phys. 2010;77(4):1085–91.
23. Kidd EA, et al. Lymph node staging by positron emission tomography in cervical cancer: relationship to prognosis. J Clin Oncol. 2010;28(12):2108–13.
24. Simcock B, et al. The role of positron emission tomography/computed tomography in planning radiotherapy in endometrial cancer. Int J Gynecol Cancer. 2015;25(4):645–9.
25. Viswanathan AN, et al. Computed tomography versus magnetic resonance imaging-based contouring in cervical cancer brachytherapy: results of a prospective trial and preliminary guidelines for standardized contours. Int J Gynecol Cancer. 2007;68(2):491–8.

26. Haie-Meder C, et al. Recommendations from gynaecological (GYN) GEC-ESTRO working group (I): concepts and terms in 3D image based 3D treatment planning in cervix cancer brachytherapy with emphasis on MRI assessment of GTV and CTV. Radiother Oncol. 2005;74(3):235–45.
27. Dimopoulos JCA, et al. Recommendations from gynaecological (GYN) GEC-ESTRO working group (IV): basic principles and parameters for MR imaging within the frame of image based adaptive cervix cancer brachytherapy. Radiother Oncol. 2012;103(1):113–22.
28. Viswanathan AN, et al. Comparison and consensus guidelines for delineation of clinical target volume for CT- and MR-based brachytherapy in locally advanced cervical cancer. Int J Radiat Oncol Biol Phys. 2014;90(2):320–8.
29. Harris EE, et al. Assessment of organ motion in postoperative endometrial and cervical cancer patients treated with intensity-modulated radiation therapy. Int J Radiat Oncol Biol Phys. 2011;81(4):e645–50.
30. Jhingran A, et al. Vaginal motion and bladder and rectal volumes during pelvic intensity-modulated radiation therapy after hysterectomy. Int J Radiat Oncol Biol Phys. 2012;82(1):256–62.
31. Ma DJ, et al. Magnitude of interfractional vaginal cuff movement, implications for external irradiation. Int J Radiat Oncol Biol Phys. 2012;82(4):1439–44.
32. Small W Jr, et al. Consensus guidelines for delineation of clinical target volume for intensity-modulated pelvic radiotherapy in postoperative treatment of endometrial and cervical cancer. Int J Radiat Oncol Biol Phys. 2008;71(2):428–34.
33. Lim K, et al. Consensus guidelines for delineation of clinical target volume for intensity-modulated pelvic radiotherapy for the definitive treatment of cervical cancer. Int J Radiat Oncol Biol Phys. 2011;79(2):348–55.
34. Taylor A, et al. Mapping pelvic lymph nodes: guidelines for delineation in intensity-modulated radiotherapy. Int J Radiat Oncol Biol Phys. 2005;63(5):1604–12.
35. Kabolizadeh P, et al. Are radiation therapy oncology group para-aortic contouring guidelines for pancreatic neoplasm applicable to other malignancies - assessment of nodal distribution in gynecological malignancies. Int J Radiat Oncol Biol Phys. 2013;87(1):106–10.
36. NCT01600040, Proton Beam Teletherapy for Post-Hysterectomy Cancers of the Uterus and Cervix; 2012 May 14. Available from: https://clinicaltrials.gov/ct2/show/record/NCT01600040.
37. Yang M, et al. Theoretical variance analysis of single- and dual-energy computed tomography methods for calculating proton stopping power ratios of biological tissues. Phys Med Biol. 2010;55(5):1343–62.
38. Hunemohr N, et al. Experimental verification of ion stopping power prediction from dual energy CT data in tissue surrogates. Phys Med Biol. 2013;59(1):83–96.
39. Hansen DC, et al. A simulation study on proton computed tomography (CT) stopping power accuracy using dual energy CT scans as benchmark. Acta Oncol. 2015;54(9):1–5.
40. Hansen DC, et al. Fast reconstruction of low dose proton CT by sinogram interpolation. Phys Med Biol. 2016;61(15):5868–82.
41. Kurosawa S, et al. Prompt gamma detection for range verification in proton therapy. Curr Appl Phys. 2012;12(2):364–8.
42. Polf JC, et al. Detecting prompt gamma emission during proton therapy: the effects of detector size and distance from the patient. Phys Med Biol. 2014;59(9):2325–40.

Prostate Cancer

19

Neil K. Taunk, Chin-Cheng Chen, Zhiqiang Han, Jerry Davis, Neha Vapiwala, and Henry Tsai

Contents

19.1	Introduction	303
19.2	Simulation	304
19.3	Target Delineation and Prescription	306
19.4	Patient Positioning, Immobilization, and Treatment Verification	310
19.5	Treatment Planning	311
19.6	Planning Constraints	314
References		314

19.1 Introduction

1. In the USA, other than skin cancer, prostate cancer is the leading cancer diagnosis in men, estimated to represent 21% of new cancer diagnoses in men in 2016. Due to improvements in early detection and treatment, prostate cancer mortality has been decreasing since the 1990s [1]. Most patients are diagnosed with non-metastatic disease, and those who opt for intervention are typically managed with radiation therapy (RT) with or without androgen deprivation therapy (ADT) or surgery.
2. The NCCN classification system stratifies patients into pretreatment risk groups based on risk of disease progression and to assist decision-making. This includes very low-, low-, intermediate-, and high-risk groups.

N.K. Taunk (✉) • N. Vapiwala
University of Pennsylvania, Philadelphia, PA, USA
e-mail: Neil.Taunk@uphs.upenn.edu

C.-C. Chen • Z. Han • J. Davis • H. Tsai
Procure Proton Therapy Center, Somerset, NJ, USA

3. RT may be delivered by external beam (intensity-modulated radiation therapy or particle therapy), brachytherapy, or a combination of the two. High-risk and unfavorable intermediate-risk disease is typically managed with RT and ADT [2]. Some patients who opt for surgery may go on to have adjuvant RT and/or ADT.
4. Control rates after RT for prostate cancer are excellent. Significant improvements in local control and/or toxicity have been made with dose-escalated RT, intensity-modulated RT (IMRT), image-guided RT (IGRT), hypofractionated RT, and addition of ADT to patients with intermediate- or high-risk disease [3–5]. Five-year biochemical relapse-free survival after dose-escalated RT is 98%, 85%, and 70% for low-, intermediate-, and high-risk groups, respectively [6].
5. The most common acute and late genitourinary (GU) toxicity during and after prostate RT is irritative urinary symptomatology including urgency, frequency, and hesitancy, all of which may be exacerbated by pretreatment lower urinary tract symptoms or benign prostatic hyperplasia. Erectile dysfunction may occur in approximately one third of men [7]. The Common Terminology Criteria for Adverse Events (CTCAE) Grade 2 gastrointestinal toxicity (rectal bleeding) is encountered in approximately 5% of patients 10 years after treatment [8]. Severe late toxicity including urinary stricture, rectal fistula, and secondary malignancy is relatively uncommon.
6. The benefit of proton therapy in the definitive treatment of prostate cancer may be best realized with potential reduction in acute and late GU and GI toxicities [9]. Rates of Grade 2+ late GU and GI toxicities with IMRT may approach 10–15% and 5–10%, respectively [6, 10]. IMRT/IGRT have allowed for the safe delivery of high-dose RT. Proton therapy may improve the therapeutic ratio by reducing GI toxicity including rectal bleeding, potentially reducing the risk of secondary, radiation-induced malignancy due to the markedly reduced integral dose from lack of exit dose.

19.2 Simulation

1. To aid in daily prostate image guidance, three fiducial markers are implanted in the prostate under transrectal ultrasound guidance (Figs. 19.1 and 19.2). Markers should be radiographically visible and cause minimal streak artifact on CT scan [11]. In our practice, we generally recommend markers that have <10% dose perturbation [12]. These markers should ideally be placed approximately 3–5 days prior to simulation to allow time for resolution of prostate hemorrhage/edema and any fiducial migration.
2. At the time of fiducial placement, a hydrogel spacer (e.g., Augmenix SpaceOAR™) can be inserted to provide temporary physical separation of the anterior wall of the rectum from the prostate (Fig. 19.3). This allows for improved sparing of the anterior rectal wall from the high-dose region of treatment.
3. CT simulation is required in all patients. For dose calculation, a non-contrast CT should be obtained. Intravenous contrast is not required but may assist with target delineation of pelvic nodal volumes.

19 Prostate Cancer

Fig. 19.1 The fiducial marker and an expansion structure expanded from the marker by 1 mm for daily fiducial registration

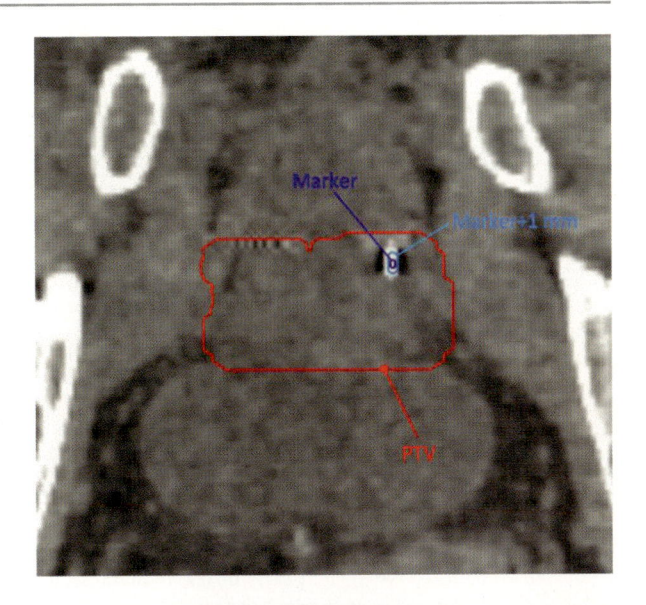

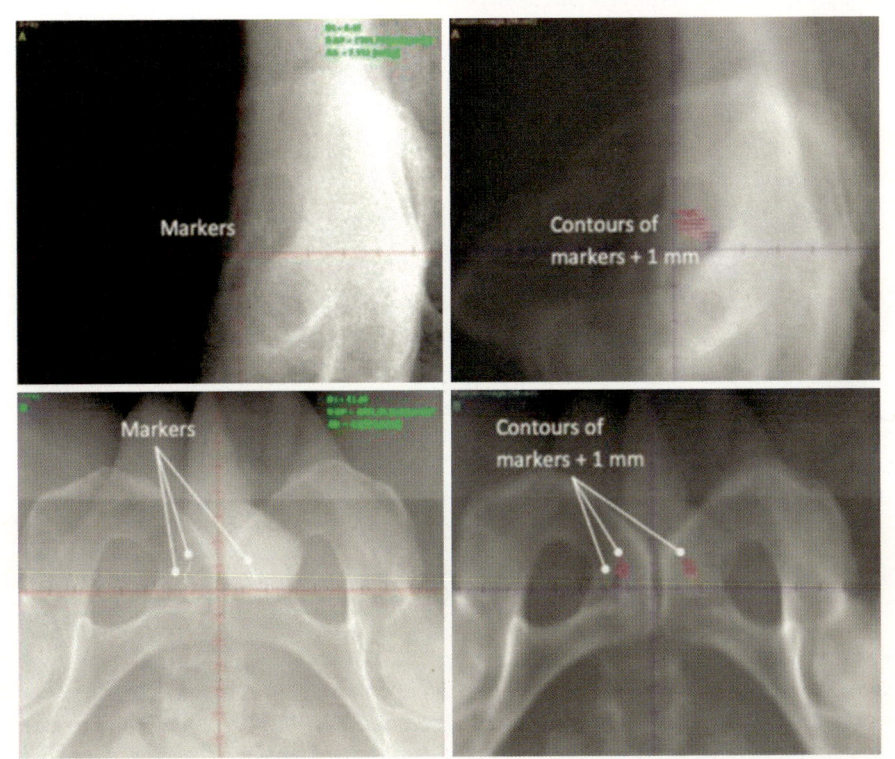

Fig. 19.2 Orthogonal X-ray images for a prostate patient with three fiducial markers. The markers can be aligned with the expanded contour with a 1-mm margin to account for a 2-mm setup uncertainty

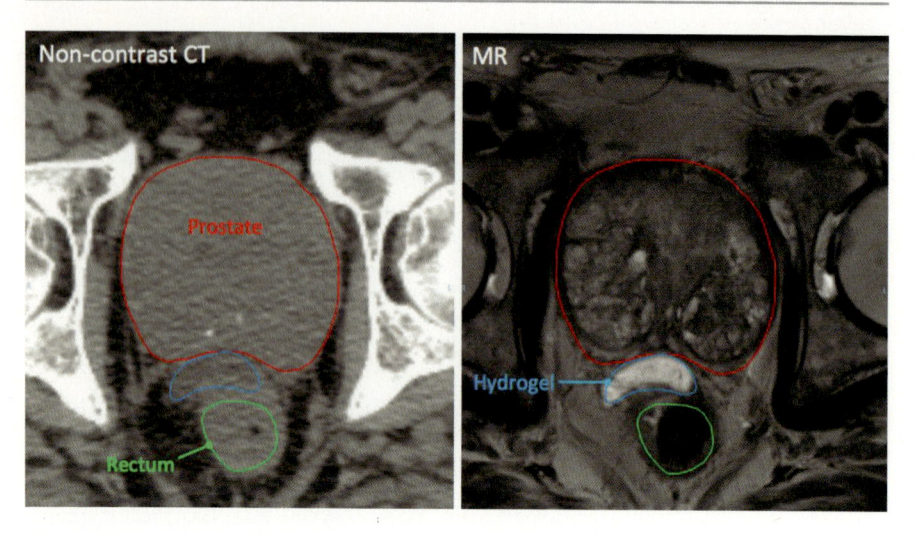

Fig. 19.3 Prostate contoured using the ancillary magnetic resonance (MR) image registered to the non-contrast computed tomography (CT) image. In this case, a hydrogel spacer had been placed between the prostate and rectum, which can be clearly discriminated on the MR images

4. Axial CT images at 1.25-mm intervals are captured from approximately the top of L4 to 5 cm below the ischial tuberosities. The patient is supine on the table immobilized in an indexed customized vacuum-lock cushion or alpha-cradle. Orthopedic metal artifact reduction (OMAR) technology may be helpful in reducing CT streak artifact in patients with prosthetic hips; however, the accuracy of the Hounsfield unit (HU) numbers will still have to be validated.
5. Multiparametric magnetic resonance imaging (MRI) is highly recommended to assist in prostate contouring in all patients. MRI may be particularly helpful in patients with orthopedic hip prostheses as metal streak artifact may make it difficult to contour the prostate accurately.
6. High-resolution, T2 axial MR images through the pelvis/prostate should be registered to the non-contrast planning CT for accurate target delineation paying special attention to soft-tissue alignment.

19.3 Target Delineation and Prescription

1. For low-risk prostate cancer patients, the clinical target volume (CTV) includes the entire prostate. For intermediate-risk patients, we typically include the proximal seminal vesicles (SV) as part of the initial CTV54 and boost the prostate alone in CTV79.2 (Fig. 19.4). If OAR constraints are not exceeded, the entire initial volume may be treated to the full prescription dose. Dose-escalated radiation is certainly recommended, but dose used may vary with institution from 74 to 82 Gy(RBE) [13, 14].

Fig. 19.4 Target volumes and organs at risk for the initial phase (54 Gy(RBE) in 30 fractions) of an intermediate-risk prostate cancer

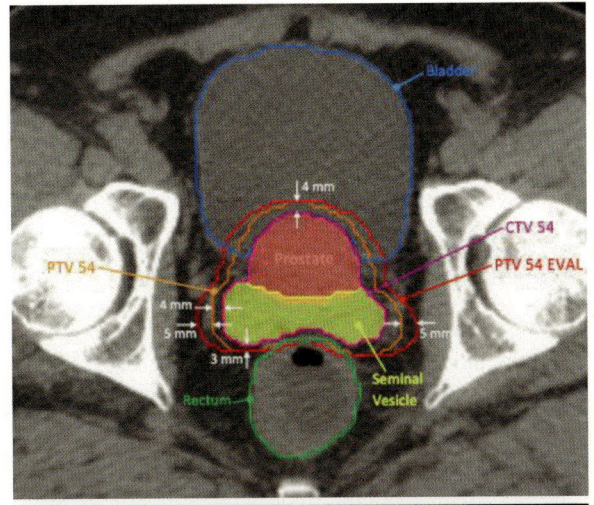

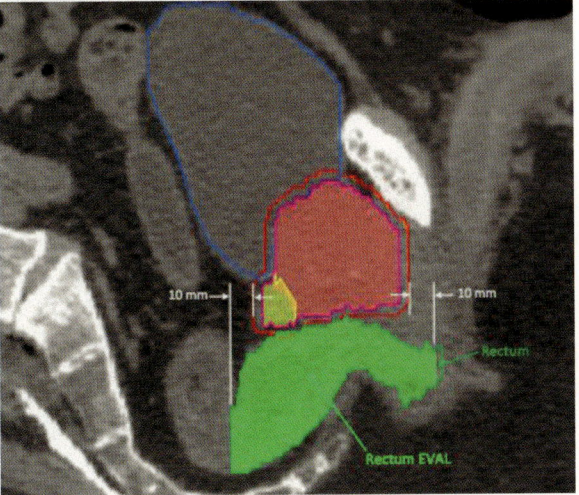

2. For high-risk prostate cancers, the initial CTV45 includes the entire prostate and SVs. The CTV45 may also include the pelvic nodes for physicians who treat the pelvis. The pelvic volume includes the external and internal iliac nodes and obturator nodes contoured as per the Radiation Therapy Oncology Group (RTOG) Pelvic Lymph Node Atlas.
3. When contouring the CTV, every effort should be made to include suspicious lesions and areas of extracapsular penetration (ECE) or seminal vesical invasion (SVI). ECE and SVI are best visualized on the fusion MRI. Review of contours with a diagnostic radiologist can be helpful in distinguishing areas of tumor from normal structures. The prostate apex can be difficult to see clearly on CT, so correlation with MRI is typically helpful in ensuring adequate coverage of the prostate apex. MR imaging is also helpful in the identification of and contouring of

spacer hydrogels. Uncertainties related to image fusion should be considered in the treatment planning process.
4. To aid in image guidance registration, fiducial markers should be contoured with the use of the appropriate window and level setting to allow for proper visualization. Fiducial marker contours should correlate reasonably with the physical dimension specifications provided by vendors. An extra 1-mm margin is then added to the fiducial contour for the low- and intermediate-risk patients, and a 2-mm margin is added for high-risk patients to create registration structures in the IGRT software. On the DRRs, these "grape" or "cloud" structures will represent the region to which fiducial markers should be registered for correct prostate alignment.
5. Setup uncertainty is estimated to be up to 2–3 mm with the use of two to three implanted fiducial markers. The planning target volume (PTV) considering the setup uncertainty would be expanded from the CTV depending on the stage. For low-risk patients, the PTV margin expansion should be 2 mm posteriorly and 3 mm in other directions. For intermediate- and high-risk prostate patients, the PTV margin expansion around prostate is 3 mm posteriorly and 4 mm elsewhere. However, this may vary with institutional practice and difference in patient setup. For example, an alternative approach is to use a 5-mm uniform expansion for optimization and an additional institution-specific 1 mm for range uncertainty [10, 13].
6. Additional margin for range uncertainty is added to the PTV in the lateral directions when an opposed lateral beam arrangement is utilized, creating a PTV-EVAL structure. Adequate dose coverage of the PTV-EVAL is used to assess plan robustness and adequacy of coverage. In our clinical practice, an additional margin of 5 mm is added to the PTV along the beamline axis to create to the PTV-EVAL. Figure 19.5 shows a composite margin 9 mm expanded from the CTV to the PTV-EVAL to account for range uncertainty. Alternatively the margins can be calculated as indicated in Chap. 3.
7. Required normal structures to be contoured include the rectum, bladder, left and right femoral heads, large intestine, small bowel, and penile bulb. A RECTUM-EVAL structure is also created as a plan evaluation structure that is defined as the circumferential rectal wall extending 1 cm superior and inferior to the PTV.

19 Prostate Cancer 309

Fig. 19.5 The delineations of tumor/treatment volumes and organ at risks for a high-risk prostate cancer. The nodes will receive a dose of 45 Gy(RBE), and there is no PTV NODE EVAL since the range uncertainty is considered with the 7-mm margin expanded from CTV NODE

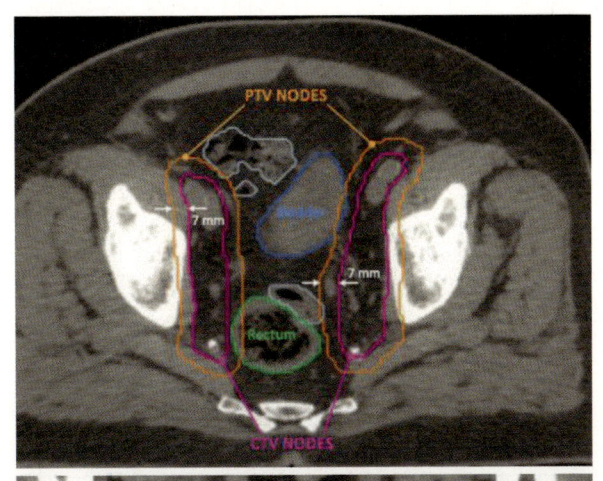

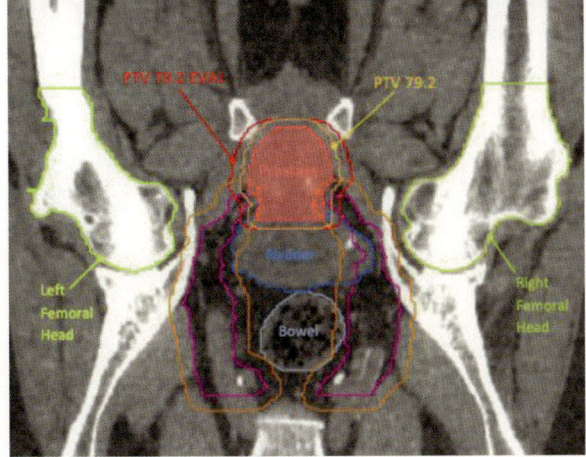

19.4 Patient Positioning, Immobilization, and Treatment Verification

1. Bladder filling is practiced at most institutions to help keep as much of the bladder wall away from the high-dose region and also to help move the small bowel superiorly, away from the target region. Patients are instructed to drink 20 ounces of water 30–60 min prior to simulation and daily treatment. The volume and timing may need to be adjusted at the time of simulation based on the adequacy of bladder filling seen on the simulation CT.
2. Simulation and treatment with an endorectal balloon or rectal saline instillation is recommended as a method of maintaining a consistent rectal shape and for prostate immobilization (Fig. 19.6) [9]. The rectal balloon is typically filled with 50–60 cm^3 of saline. However, other institutions may use 100 cm^3 of saline in a rectal balloon [10]. With saline instillation, up to 100 cm^3 of saline is inserted into the rectum via a lubricated, flexible rubber catheter. If necessary, bowel gas can be removed via the catheter, as well. Daily setup accuracy should be assessed with a daily pair of orthogonal X-ray images using the implanted fiducial markers or cone beam

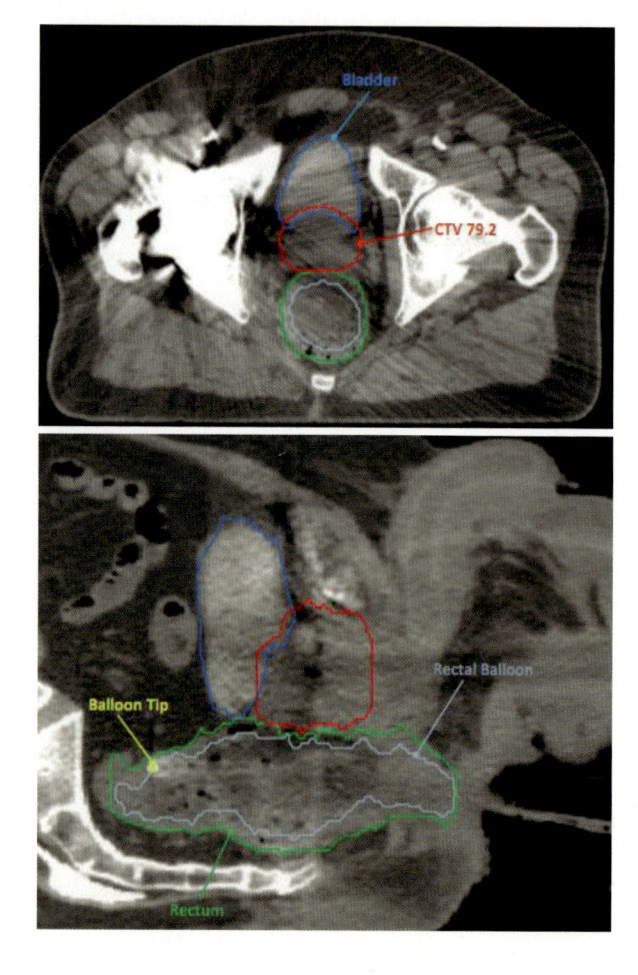

Fig. 19.6 Use of a rectal balloon for an intermediate-risk prostate cancer with right-sided hip prosthesis

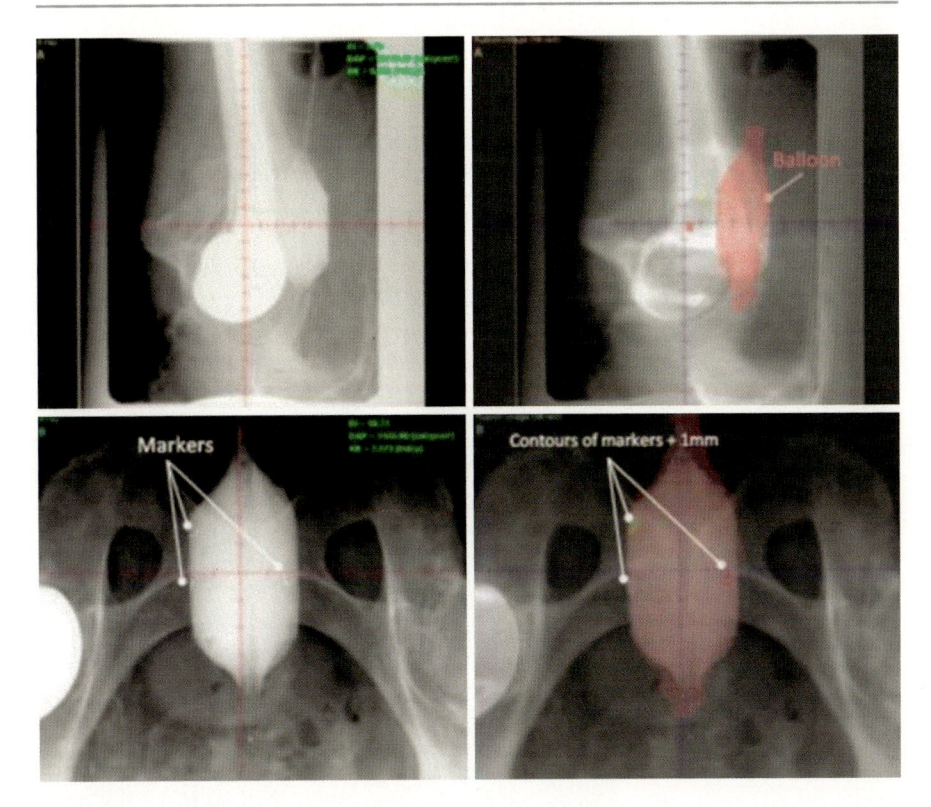

Fig. 19.7 A rectal balloon filled with diluted contrast is used to aid in daily setup for a prostate patient with a hip prosthesis. The fiducial markers are clearly visible on the PA film, and the contrast-filled balloon assists in the lateral view

  CT. Cone beam CT can also verify bladder volume and endorectal balloon placement. In patients with prosthetic hips, fiducial markers may be difficult to visualize through the metallic hip, and a contrast-filled rectal balloon may be helpful in identifying the prostate/anterior rectal wall interface on a daily basis (Fig. 19.7).
3. Large discrepancies between fiducial registration and approximate bony registration may indicate an issue with setup. An effort to reduce bony anatomy discrepancy should be attempted to limit this discrepancy to <5–7 mm. Quality assurance or "QA" CTs may be helpful in understanding the nature of setup inconsistency whether it be related to bladder/rectal filling, patient positioning, or bowel gas.

19.5 Treatment Planning

1. The prostate ± seminal vesicles are typically treated with coplanar, opposed left and right lateral fields with a single isocenter. Two fields or a single alternating lateral field can be treated on a daily basis [15]. Patients who require treatment to the pelvic nodes are treated also with opposed lateral fields. The superior portions of the nodal volumes require treatment with two fields daily, with each

lateral field treating the ipsilateral nodal volumes. These fields are then matched inferiorly with beams that treat the central prostate volume (Fig. 19.8).
2. An alternative approach for patients with a metallic hip prosthesis is to use anterior oblique-oriented beams [16]. A typical beam arrangement for a patient with a right hip prosthesis may be a left lateral, right anterior oblique, and left anterior oblique beams. Anteriorly oriented beams may be sensitive to changes in rectal or bladder filling (Fig. 19.9). Alternatively a posterior oblique can be used in combination with a lateral beam. Thus, QA CTs may be relatively more important in these cases to ensure that the rectal and bladder anatomy remains consistent.
3. Whichever approach is used, daily coverage of the CTV considering the setup and range uncertainty is critical to minimize risk of local failure. In addition,

Fig. 19.8 The dose distributions of a high-risk prostate treatment plan using two matched opposed lateral pencil beam scanning (PBS) fields

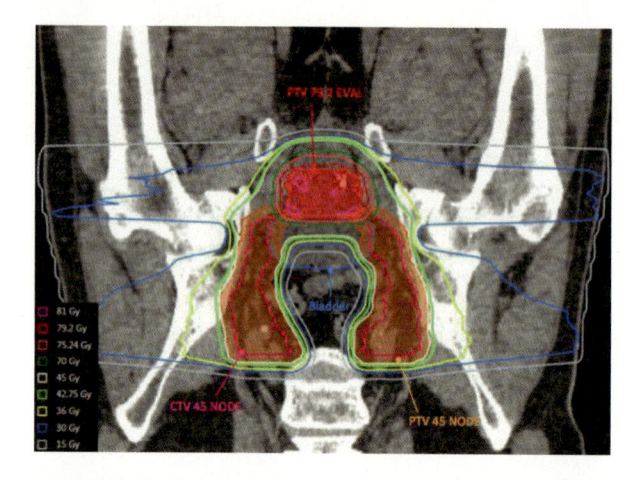

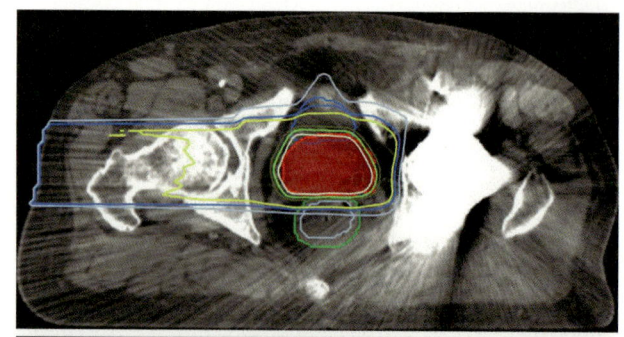

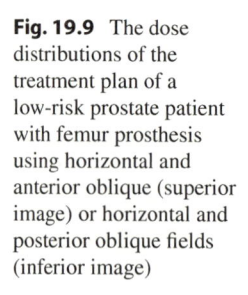

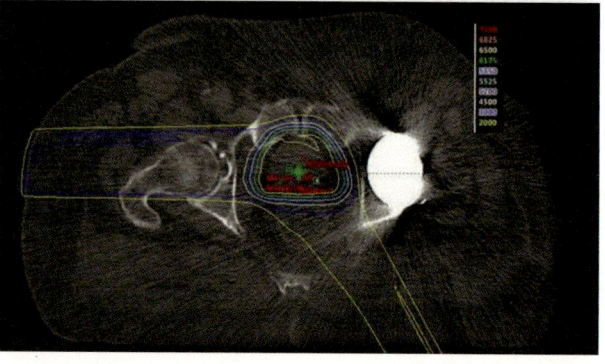

Fig. 19.9 The dose distributions of the treatment plan of a low-risk prostate patient with femur prosthesis using horizontal and anterior oblique (superior image) or horizontal and posterior oblique fields (inferior image)

19 Prostate Cancer

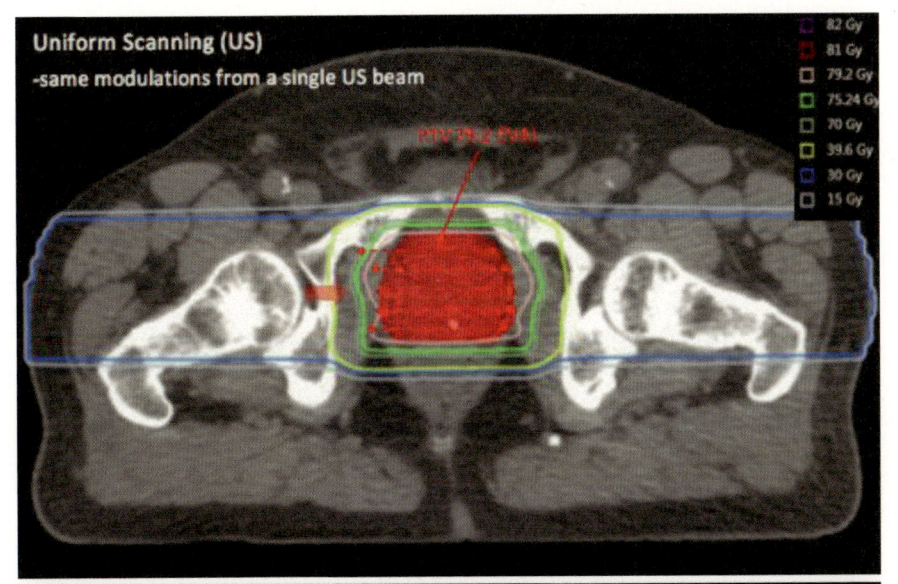

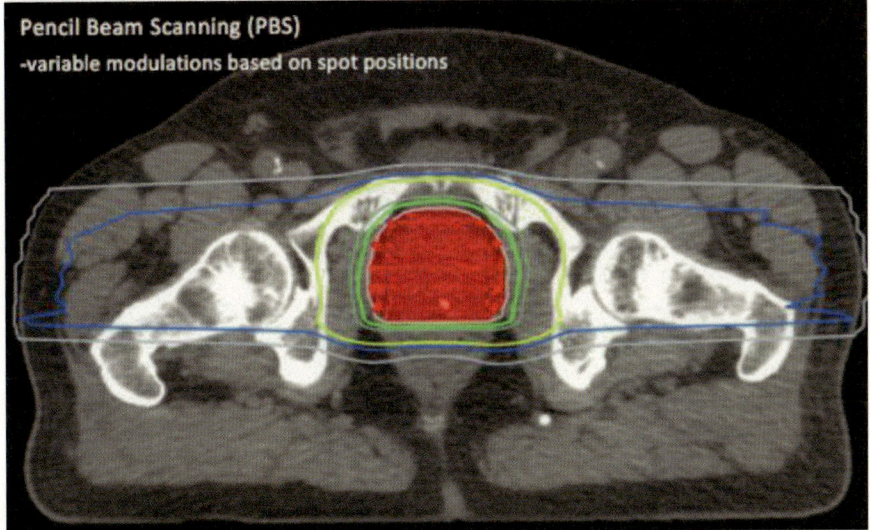

Fig. 19.10 The comparison of dose distributions of prostate treatment plans using uniform scanning (US) and pencil beam scanning (PBS) techniques. The *red dash lines* represent the spread-out Bragg peak (modulation) in the US plan and spot positioning in the PBS plan, respectively

every attempt should be made to reduce the volume of bladder and rectal wall that receives high-dose radiation [17].

4. Pencil beam scanning (PBS) allows treatment of the target volume spot by spot along a 3D grid without the use of tissue compensators or custom apertures. PBS in general provides highly conformal dose distributions as compared to uniform scanning techniques. PBS allows for variable modulation distances as compared to uniform scanning in which range modulation is the same for all spots, resulting in reduced proximal conformality of the beam (Fig. 19.10) [18–20].

Table 19.1 Target volume coverage goals and normal tissue dose constraints in proton treatment planning for prostate cancer

Target		Recommended coverage		
PTV-EVAL V98		≥99.5%		
PTV-EVAL V100		≥95%		
OAR	Normal organ tolerances	Prescription		
		All Rx's Gy(RBE)	≤ 60 Gy(RBE)	> 60 Gy(RBE) Hard constraints
Bladder	Bladder $V_{81Gy(RBE)}$	<1 cm^3		
	Bladder $V_{70Gy(RBE)}$	<25%		
Bladder (post prostatectomy)	Bladder $V_{65Gy(RBE)}$	<40%		
	Bladder $V_{40Gy(RBE)}$	<60%		
Rectum	Rectum-EVAL $V_{70Gy(RBE)}$	<13%		<70Gy(RBE)
	Rectum $V_{70Gy(RBE)}$	<10%		
	Rectum $V_{65Gy(RBE)}$	<17%		
	Rectum $V_{81Gy(RBE)}$	<1 cm^3		
	Rectum $V_{50Gy(RBE)}$	<55%		
Rectum (post prostatectomy)	Rectum $V_{65Gy(RBE)}$	<25%		
	Rectum $V_{40Gy(RBE)}$	<45%		
Penile bulb	Mean dose	<52.5Gy(RBE)		
Femoral heads	Femoral heads $V_{50Gy(RBE)}$	<1.0 cm^3		
Bowel	Bowel 1.0 cm^3		≤55Gy(RBE)	≤ 60Gy(RBE)
	Bowel 0.03 cm^3			≤ 64Gy(RBE)

19.6 Planning Constraints

1. Target volume coverage goals and normal tissue dose constraints for prostate proton therapy are summarized in Table 19.1. Trade-offs between target coverage and normal tissue dose should be determined by the treating physician and take into account the unique clinical factors of the individual case.

References

1. Siegel RL, Miller KD, Jemal A. Cancer statistics, 2016. CA Cancer J Clin. 2016;66(1):7–30.
2. Zumsteg ZS, Zelefsky MJ. Short-term androgen deprivation therapy for patients with intermediate-risk prostate cancer undergoing dose-escalated radiotherapy: the standard of care? Lancet Oncol. 2012;13(6):e259–69.
3. Zelefsky MJ, et al. High dose radiation delivered by intensity modulated conformal radiotherapy improves the outcome of localized prostate cancer. J Urol. 2001;166(3):876–81.
4. Sharifi N, Gulley JL, Dahut WL. Androgen deprivation therapy for prostate cancer. JAMA. 2005;294(2):238–44.

5. Arcangeli G, et al. A prospective Phase III randomized trial of hypofractionation versus conventional fractionation in patients with high-risk prostate cancer. Int J Radiat Oncol Biol Phys. 2010;78(1):11–8.
6. Cahlon O, et al. Ultra-high dose (86.4 Gy) IMRT for localized prostate cancer: toxicity and biochemical outcomes. Int J Radiat Oncol Biol Phys. 2008;71(2):330–7.
7. Robinson JW, Moritz S, Fung T. Meta-analysis of rates of erectile function after treatment of localized prostate carcinoma. Int J Radiat Oncol Biol Phys. 2002;54(4):1063–8.
8. Zelefsky MJ, et al. Incidence of late rectal and urinary toxicities after three-dimensional conformal radiotherapy and intensity-modulated radiotherapy for localized prostate cancer. Int J Radiat Oncol Biol Phys. 2008;70(4):1124–9.
9. Mouw KW, et al. Clinical controversies: proton therapy for prostate cancer. Semin Radiat Oncol. 2013;23(2):109–14.
10. Fang P, et al. A case-matched study of toxicity outcomes after proton therapy and intensity-modulated radiation therapy for prostate cancer. Cancer. 2015;121(7):1118–27.
11. Habermehl D, et al. Evaluation of different fiducial markers for image-guided radiotherapy and particle therapy. J Radiat Res. 2013;54(suppl 1):i61–8.
12. Giebeler A, et al. Dose perturbations from implanted helical gold markers in proton therapy of prostate cancer. J Appl Clin Med Phys. 2009;10(1):2875.
13. Coen JJ, et al. Acute and late toxicity after dose escalation to 82 GyE using conformal proton radiation for localized prostate cancer: initial report of American College of Radiology Phase II study 03-12. Int J Radiat Oncol Biol Phys. 2011;81(4):1005–9.
14. Moon DH, Efstathiou JA, Chen RC. What is the best way to radiate the prostate in 2016? Urol Oncol. 2017;35(2):59–68.
15. Tang S, et al. Impact of intrafraction and residual interfraction effect on prostate proton pencil beam scanning. Int J Radiat Oncol Biol Phys. 2014;90(5):1186–94.
16. Cuaron JJ, et al. Anterior-oriented proton beams for prostate cancer: a multi-institutional experience. Acta Oncol. 2015;54(6):868–74.
17. Michalski JM, et al. Radiation dose–volume effects in radiation-induced rectal injury. Int J Radiat Oncol Biol Phys. 2010;76(3, Supplement):S123–9.
18. Christodouleas JP, et al. The effect of anterior proton beams in the setting of a prostate-rectum spacer. Med Dosim. 2013;38(3):315–9.
19. Tang S, et al. Improvement of prostate treatment by anterior proton fields. Int J Radiat Oncol Biol Phys. 2012;83(1):408–18.
20. Underwood T, et al. Can we advance proton therapy for prostate? Considering alternative beam angles and relative biological effectiveness variations when comparing against intensity modulated radiation therapy. Int J Radiat Oncol Biol Phys. 2016;95(1):454–64.

Adult Intracranial Tumors

20

Natalie A. Lockney, Zhiqiang Han, Kevin Sine, Dominic Maes, and Yoshiya Yamada

Contents

20.1	Introduction	317
20.2	Simulation, Target Delineation, and Radiation Dose/Fractionation	318
20.3	Patient Positioning, Immobilization, and Treatment Verification	320
20.4	Three-Dimensional (3D) Proton Treatment Planning	320
20.4.1	Uniform Scanning (US)	320
20.4.2	Pencil Beam Scanning (PBS)	322
20.5	Uniform Scanning vs. Pencil Beam Scanning Comparisons	325
20.5.1	Proton Stereotactic Radiosurgery (SRS)	325
20.5.2	Dosimetric and Toxicity Comparison	325
20.6	Future Developments	325
References		326

20.1 Introduction

1. Approximately 0.6% of the population will be diagnosed with cancer of the central nervous system (CNS), representing 1.4% of all new cancer cases in the United States [1]. In adults, the most common histology for primary brain tumors is meningioma (24%), followed by glioblastoma (23%), and astrocytoma (14%) [2]. While meningiomas are the most common benign intracranial tumors, glioblastoma is the most common malignant primary brain tumor. Over the past 10 years, 5-year survival rates for CNS tumors have remained relatively stable

---

N.A. Lockney • Y. Yamada (✉)
Memorial Sloan Kettering Cancer Center, New York, NY, USA
e-mail: yamadaj@mskcc.org

Z. Han • K. Sine • D. Maes
ProCure Proton Therapy Center, Somerset, NJ, USA

© Springer International Publishing Switzerland 2018
N. Lee et al. (eds.), *Target Volume Delineation and Treatment Planning for Particle Therapy*, Practical Guides in Radiation Oncology,
https://doi.org/10.1007/978-3-319-42478-1_20

ranging between 23 and 36% [1]. Radiotherapy is utilized for a variety of intracranial tumor types in the definitive, postoperative, and salvage settings depending on the tumor histology and clinical scenario.
2. Proton therapy has been used for both benign and malignant intracranial neoplasms including glioma [3–7], meningioma [8–12], acoustic neuroma [13, 14], and pituitary adenoma [15–18]. The majority of studies evaluating clinical outcomes and toxicities of intracranial proton radiotherapy are retrospective in nature and include some prospective studies as well. There are currently no results of randomized control trials comparing photon versus proton radiotherapy.
3. Due to the dose tolerance of many critical intracranial structures such as the brainstem and optic nerves, the optimal doses necessary to achieve adequate tumor local control may not be reached. Therefore, proton therapy has emerged as an attractive modality to spare toxicity to dose-limiting structures in the brain while allowing potential increased dose to tumor targets. As local control has been shown to be superior for meningiomas treated with higher relative biological effectiveness (RBE) [19] and studies have demonstrated central in-field recurrence as the most common pattern of recurrence in glioblastoma [20], dose escalation is attractive for these malignant tumors in particular. Dose escalation studies using proton therapy have been performed for meningioma [21], low-grade glioma [3], and high-grade glioma [4, 5], though dose escalation in low-grade glioma showed increased toxicity with no meaningful therapeutic benefit.

20.2 Simulation, Target Delineation, and Radiation Dose/Fractionation

1. CT simulation should be performed with intravenous iodinated contrast, when not contraindicated. For the purposes of dose calculation, a non-contrast CT needs to be acquired first and employed in planning proton therapy (see Chap. 3).
2. Magnetic resonance imaging (MRI) with intravenous contrast, when not contraindicated, should also be performed for accurate delineation of extent of gross tumor in soft tissue and also for extent of edema. For patients who have undergone resection of their brain tumors, both preoperative and postoperative MRIs should be used. MRI can also be helpful for delineation of critical normal structures such as the optic chiasm.
3. MRI images should be registered to the non-contrast planning CT for accurate target delineation, including both T1 contrast-enhanced and T2 FLAIR images. Uncertainties related to image fusions should be considered in the treatment planning process (Chap. 3).
4. Refer to Table 20.1 for the recommended dosing and fractionation, which may vary depending on the clinical scenario.
5. Clinical target volumes (CTV) should be expanded according to institutional standard, typically by 3–5 mm, to create a planning target volume (PTV), employed for recording and reporting purposes [22].
6. Concurrent chemotherapy with temozolomide is used for high-grade gliomas [23].

20 Adult Intracranial Tumors

Table 20.1 Recommended target volumes and radiation doses

Clinical scenario	Target volume	Target definition[a]	Dose and fractionation
Glioma, high grade, postoperative vs. definitive if unresectable or inoperable	GTV1	T1-enhancing disease, abutting surgical bed if applicable + FLAIR	46 Gy (RBE) at 2 Gy (RBE) per fraction to GTV/CTV1 with 14 Gy (RBE) to GTV/CTV2 = 60 Gy (RBE) total[b]
	CTV1	GTV1 + 2 cm	
	GTV2	T1-enhancing disease	
	CTV2	GTV2 + 2 cm	
Glioma, low grade, with STR or high-risk features	GTV	T1-enhancing disease or FLAIR for non-enhancing tumors	50.4 vs. 54 Gy (RBE) at 1.8 Gy (RBE) per fraction
	CTV	GTV + 1 cm margin	
Meningioma, low grade, if unresectable, inoperable, or recurrent	GTV	T1-enhancing disease including dural tail and abutting surgical bed if applicable	50.4 vs. 54 Gy (RBE) at 1.8 Gy (RBE) per fraction
	CTV	GTV + 0.5 cm margin	
Meningioma, high grade, postoperative vs. definitive if unresectable or inoperable	GTV	T1-enhancing disease including dural tail and abutting surgical bed if applicable	60 Gy (RBE) at 2 Gy (RBE) per fraction
	CTV	GTV + 0.5 cm margin	
Acoustic neuroma	GTV	T1-enhancing disease	54 Gy (RBE) at 1.8 Gy (RBE) per fraction
	CTV	GTV	
Craniopharyngioma, with STR	GTV	Residual tumor + tumor bed	54 Gy (RBE) at 1.8 Gy (RBE) per fraction
	CTV	GTV + 1.0 cm margin	
Pituitary tumors, nonfunctioning	GTV	T1-enhancing disease	45–50 Gy (RBE) at 1.8 Gy (RBE) per fraction
	CTV	GTV + 0.5 cm margin	
Pituitary tumors, functioning	GTV	T1-enhancing disease	50.4–54 Gy (RBE) at 1.8 Gy (RBE) per fraction
	CTV	GTV + 0.5 cm margin	

Abbreviations: *STR* subtotal resection, *GTV* gross tumor volume, *CTV* clinical target volume, *RBE* relative biological effectiveness
[a]Based on magnetic resonance imaging (MRI) fusion
[b]Alternatively, GTV = T1-enhancing disease and abutting surgical bed if applicable and CTV = GTV + 1.5 cm margin + inclusion of all FLAIR, all to 60 Gy (RBE) with no cone down

20.3 Patient Positioning, Immobilization, and Treatment Verification

1. Simulation and treatment is recommended to be performed in the supine position with a three-point mask.
2. Setup accuracy should be confirmed with daily orthogonal X-ray imaging or volumetric imaging.
3. In-room CT imaging (i.e., cone beam CT) is ideally used for treatment verification, and, if unavailable, verification CT scans performed in the treatment position are recommended to assess for potential changes in patient anatomy (i.e., seroma shrinkage) which can result in a change in the patient dose distribution (Fig. 20.1). If available, in-room CT imaging is recommended weekly. Verification CT scans in the treatment position are recommended as needed based on individual patient cases, such as the presence of seroma cavity and any apparent changes in surface anatomy.
4. Weekly to monthly MRIs are recommended for monitoring cyst growth, particularly for craniopharyngioma. For changes in anatomy, replanning may be required to ensure cyst changes have not extended beyond the treatment field or altered dose distributions to normal tissues (Fig. 20.2).

20.4 Three-Dimensional (3D) Proton Treatment Planning

20.4.1 Uniform Scanning (US)

1. Three-field plans are typically utilized (2–4 beams, Fig. 20.3), preferably with the shortest and most homogeneous radiologic depths.

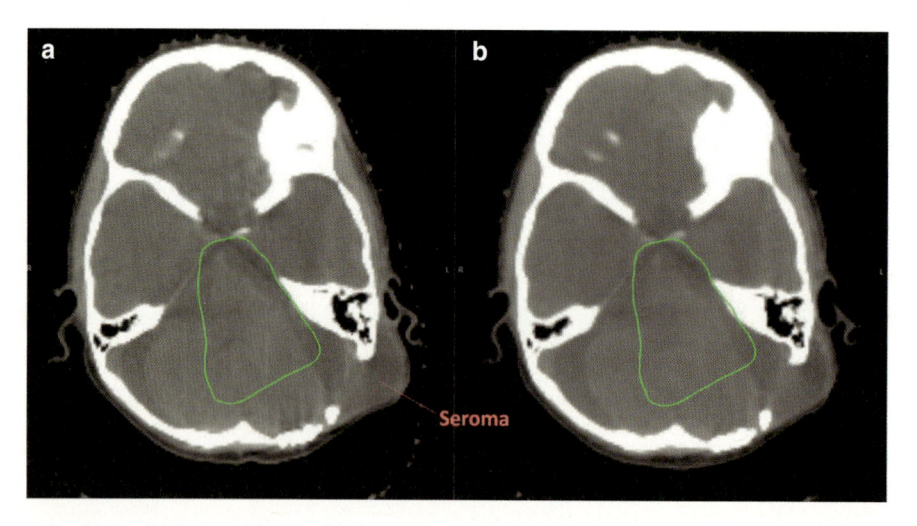

Fig. 20.1 Anatomical changes during proton treatment. (**a**) Planning simulation scan of a posterior fossa target. (**b**) Verification CT 1 week into treatment demonstrating significant seroma shrinkage. This required replanning for accurate delivery of the intended plan

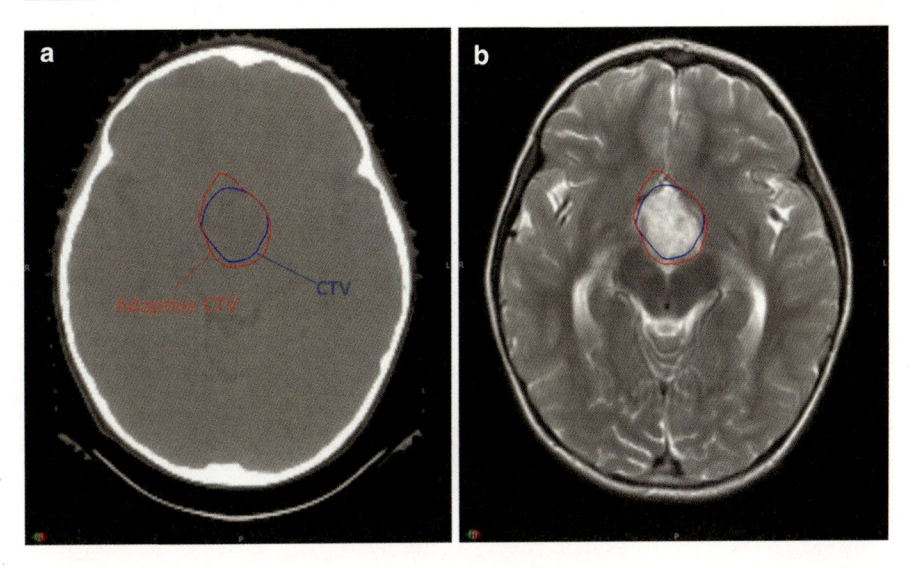

Fig. 20.2 Anatomical changes during proton treatment. (**a**) Planning simulation scan of a suprasellar target. (**b**) Verification MRI 4 weeks after initial scan demonstrating significant cyst growth. This required replanning for accurate delivery of the intended plan

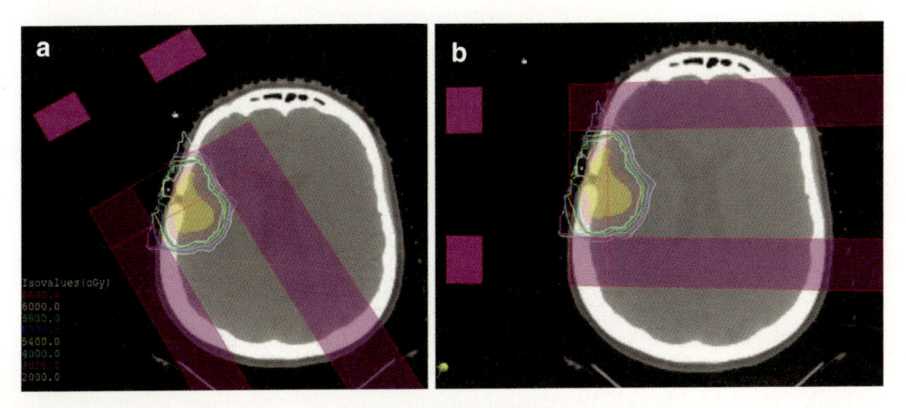

Fig. 20.3 Uniform scanning plan for treatment of a right frontal lobe atypical meningioma with typical two-beam arrangement including (**a**) anterior oblique and (**b**) lateral beams

2. In the planning process, care should be taken not to overlap the distal ends of more than two beams, and no more than one beam should range into the same location of an organ at risk (OAR), especially at levels of serial structures. To visualize the distal end of a beam, the modulation of each beam can be changed to 0.5 cm and the 90% isodose line location for each individual beam can be examined. If excessive distal end overlap between beams is present, alternate beam angles and/or range feathering techniques should be considered. Figure 20.4 demonstrates a three-field beam arrangement mitigating distal end overlap by utilizing various beam angles.

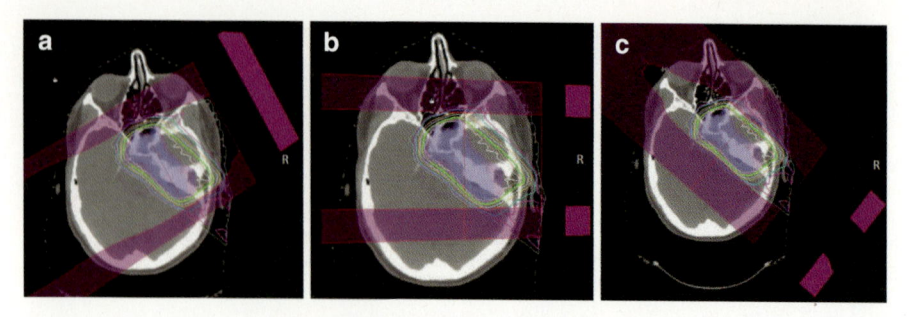

Fig. 20.4 Uniform scanning plan for the treatment of a right skull base meningioma with typical three-beam arrangement including (**a**) posterior oblique, (**b**) anterior oblique, and (**c**) lateral beams

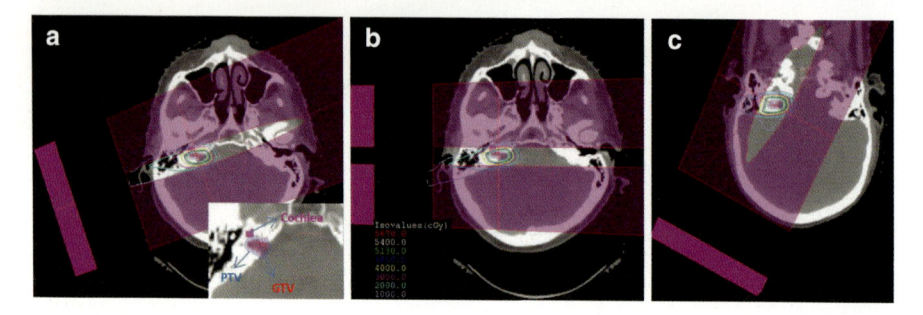

Fig. 20.5 Uniform scanning plan for treatment of an acoustic neuroma tumor with typical three-beam arrangement including (**a**) posterior oblique, (**b**) lateral beams, and (**c**) superior oblique beams

3. Plan robustness is evaluated by analyzing the over and under ranged plans based on the relevant range uncertainties as determined by each center. In analyzing plan robustness, all critical organs at risk should be within their respective dose tolerances and target dose coverage to the CTV should be achieved in both the over and under ranged treatment plans.
4. For acoustic neuroma cases, the ipsilateral cochlea is a critical avoidance structure, and care should be taken to minimize the mean dose as low as reasonably achievable (ALARA) while ensuring 100% GTV V95 coverage. In this case an aperture can be used to minimize the lateral penumbra dose to the cochlea as can be seen in Fig. 20.5.

20.4.2 Pencil Beam Scanning (PBS)

1. The same two- to four-beam arrangement shown in Fig. 20.4 may also be used with PBS; however, in many cases, using a two-field beam arrangement provides sufficient target coverage. As in the case of uniform scanning, it is also important to ensure that there is minimal overlap of beam distal ends.

2. PBS plan optimization is similar to IMRT planning in that it is planned inversely to target and OAR optimization volume(s). The optimization volumes are created by the planner by taking into account proton beam-specific uncertainties. Some treatment planning systems (TPS) are equipped with robust planning optimization. This takes into account these beam-specific/setup uncertainties in the optimization process. When robust optimization is not available in the TPS, planning organ at risk volumes (PRV) and target optimization volumes can be utilized in the treatment planning process to achieve similar results.
3. PBS provides conformal plans with superior skin sparing compared to uniform scanning, particularly when the target volume does not extend to the surface. In most cases, PBS can provide superior proximal conformality. Avoidance structures can also be created with dose-limiting objectives to decrease the skin dose. However, in many instances, the volume will extend to the patient surface, and the advantage of skin sparing even with PBS may be limited (Fig. 20.6).
4. In CNS cases, it is often preferable to use single-field uniform dose (SFUD) as it results in the most robust treatment plan (Figs. 20.7 and 20.8). Each beam should be evaluated individually to ensure adequate coverage and then compositely to evaluate OAR constraints and hot spots. As robust optimization matures in the clinical environment, IMPT may be used more extensively further enhancing the dosimetric gains.
5. IMPT is the method of choice for optimal normal tissue sparing for tumors that wrap around critical OARs (e.g., brainstem, optic chiasm). For the majority of these cases, SFUD is possible; however, some cases might require IMPT or a mix of the two techniques in order to meet currently recommended dose constraints while maintaining plan robustness. (Table 20.2).

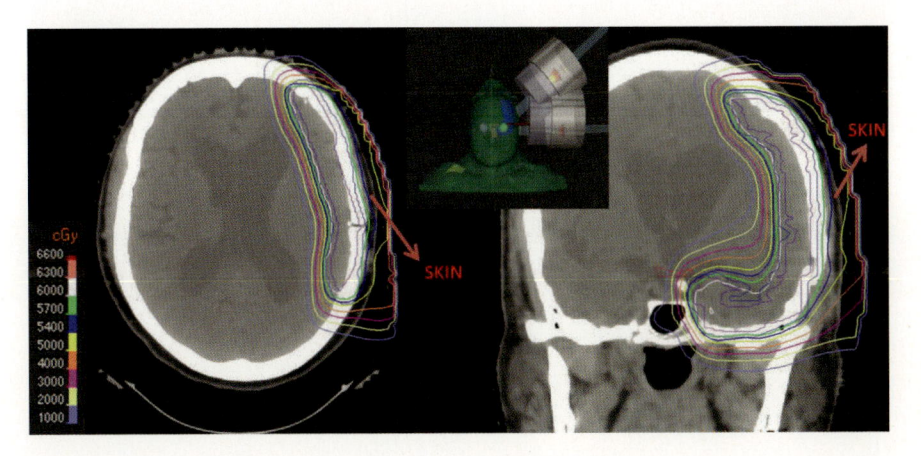

Fig. 20.6 PBS plan with SFUD for treatment of an atypical meningioma of the left frontotemporal brain with sparing of proximal skin

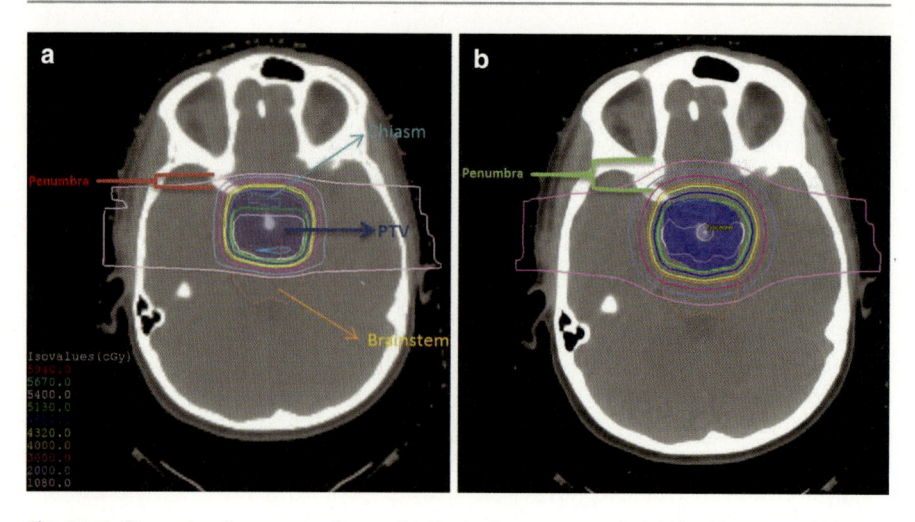

Fig. 20.7 Example of coverage of a craniopharyngioma target using (**a**) uniform scanning with field-in-field technique versus (**b**) pencil beam scanning with SFUD. In such cases, pencil beam scanning often offers an advantage in sparing OAR under prescription dose while ensuring PTV V95 coverage. However, due to lack of aperture, PBS plan has larger penumbra compared with the uniform scanning plan which could be mitigated using a small spot size or apertures

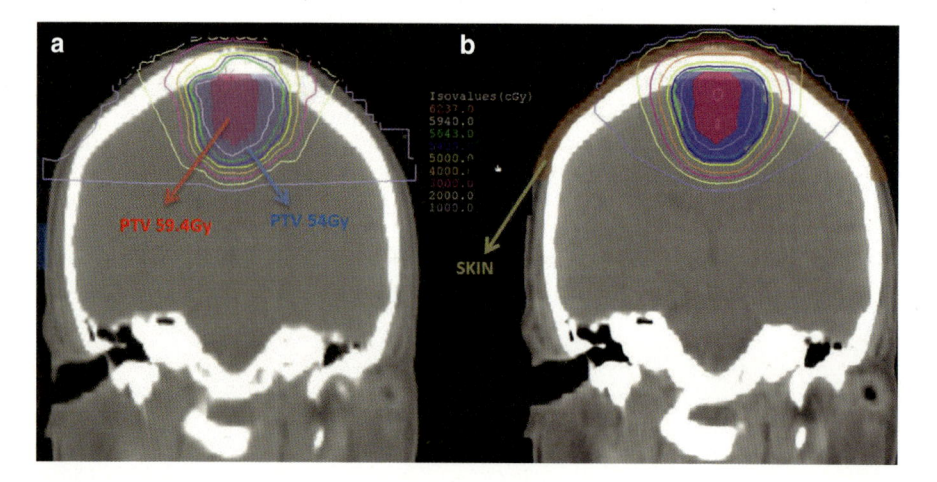

Fig. 20.8 Example of coverage of centralized meningioma target using (**a**) uniform scanning versus (**b**) pencil beam scanning with SFUD using the same beam arrangement. In such cases, pencil beam scanning often offers superior conformity allowing for enhanced brain and skin sparing

20 Adult Intracranial Tumors

Table 20.2 Recommended dose constraints to organs at risk for the treatment of intracranial tumors with proton radiotherapy

Organ at risk	Recommended dose constraint
Brainstem	0.05 cc ≤ 60 Gy/max dose 64 Gy
Cochlea	Max dose ≤50 Gy
Optic nerves and optic chiasm	0.05 cc ≤ 60 Gy
Spinal cord	0.1 cc ≤ 50 Gy/surface max ≤64 Gy
Retina	Dose to 0.1 cc ≤ 45 Gy/max dose ≤60 Gy
Lens	Max dose ≤10 Gy or ALARA

These recommendations are adapted from institutional photon/IMRT treatment planning. Doses are reported in Gy (RBE) for proton therapy (RBE = 1.1)

20.5 Uniform Scanning vs. Pencil Beam Scanning Comparisons

20.5.1 Proton Stereotactic Radiosurgery (SRS)

1. Stereotactic proton radiation can be used to deliver conformal, high-dose radiation to the target. Protons as opposed to photons may offer superior conformality, particularly for larger lesions not amenable to photon stereotactic radiation.

20.5.2 Dosimetric and Toxicity Comparison

1. The organs at risk (OARs) for intracranial tumors include optic structures, the brainstem, cochlea, and eloquent cortex. Unsurprisingly, vision, hearing, and neurocognitive function are critical for patient quality of life.
2. Proton radiotherapy for intracranial tumors has demonstrated superior avoidance of critical structures compared to photon therapy, particularly for targets nearby critical structures [24, 25]. In comparison of 3D conformal radiotherapy (3DCRT), stereotactic radiation (SRS), intensity-modulated photon radiotherapy (IMRT), and radiotherapy with protons with spot scanning (PBS) or passive scattering (PS) for intracranial tumors, PBS and SS were shown to have decreased mean doses to the brainstem, contralateral optic nerve, and eyes [26].
3. While studies have demonstrated superior sparing of critical structures with proton therapy compared to photon therapy, whether this has tangible reduction in patient-reported toxicity and brain function needs to be further studied.

20.6 Future Developments

1. Future studies may help further elucidate the optimal dosing for intracranial tumor as well as the potential benefits of proton therapy on brain function, especially when IMPT matures and is routinely employed in the clinic.

References

1. Howlader N, Noone AM, Krapcho M, et al., editors. SEER Cancer Statistics Review, 1975–2013. Bethesda, MD: National Cancer Institute. http://seer.cancer.gov/csr/1975_2013/, based on November 2015 SEER data submission, posted to the SEER web site, April 2016
2. Surawicz TS, McCarthy BJ, Kupelian V, et al. Descriptive epidemiology of primary brain and CNS tumors: results from the Central Brain Tumor Registry of the United States, 1999–1994. Neuro-Oncology. 1999;1:14–25.
3. Fitzek MM, Thornton AF, Harsh G, et al. Dose-escalation with proton/photon irradiation for Daumas-Duport lower-grade glioma: results of an institutional phase I/II trial. Int J Radiat Oncol Biol Phys. 2001;51:131–7.
4. Fitzek MM, Thornton AF, Rabinov JD, et al. Accelerated fractionated proton/photon irradiation to 90 cobalt gray equivalent for glioblastoma multiforme: results of a phase II prospective trial. J Neurosurg. 1999;91:251–60.
5. Mizumoto M, Tsuboi K, Igaki H, et al. Phase I/II trial of hypofractionated concomitant boost proton radiotherapy for supratentorial glioblastoma multiforme. Int J Radiat Oncol Biol Phys. 2010;77:98–105.
6. Tatsuzaki H, Urie MM, Linggood R. Comparative treatment planning: proton vs. X-ray beams against glioblastoma multiforme. Int J Radiat Oncol Biol Phys. 1992;22:265–73.
7. Shih HA, Sherman JC, Nachtigall LB, et al. Proton therapy for low-grade gliomas: results from a prospective trial. Cancer. 2015;121:1712–9.
8. Slater JD, Loredo LN, Chung A, et al. Fractionated proton radiotherapy for benign cavernous sinus meningiomas. Int J Radiat Oncol Biol Phys. 2012;83:633–7.
9. Boskos C, Feuvret L, Noel G, et al. Combined proton and photon conformal radiotherapy for intracranial atypical and malignant meningioma. Int J Radiat Oncol Biol Phys. 2009;75:399–406.
10. Wenkel E, Thornton AF, Finkelstein D, et al. Benign meningioma: partially resected, biopsied, and recurrent intracranial tumors treated with combined proton and photon radiotherapy. Int J Radiat Oncol Biol Phys. 2000;48:1363–70.
11. Combs SE, Welzel T, Habermehl D, et al. Prospective evaluation of early treatment outcome in patients with meningiomas treated with particle therapy based on target volume definition with MRI and ^{68}Ga-DOTATOC-PET. Acta Oncol. 2013;52:514–20.
12. Weber DC, Schneider R, Goitein G, et al. Spot scanning-based proton therapy for intracranial meningioma: long-term results from the Paul Scherrer Institute. Int J Radiat Oncol Biol Phys. 2012;83:865–71.
13. Harsh GR, Thornton AF, Chapman PH, et al. Proton beam stereotactic radiosurgery of vestibular schwannomas. Int J Radiat Oncol Biol Phys. 2002;54:35–44.
14. Bush DA, McAllister CJ, Loredo LN, et al. Fractionated proton beam radiotherapy for acoustic neuroma. Neurosurgery. 2002;50:273–5.
15. Kjellberg RN, Shintani A, Frantz AG, et al. Proton-beam therapy in acromegaly. N Engl J Med. 1968;278:689–95.
16. Petit JH, Biller BM, Yock TI, et al. Proton stereotactic radiotherapy for persistent adrenocorticotropin-producing adenomas. J Clin Endocrinol Metab. 2008;93:393–9.
17. Petit JH, Biller BM, et al. Proton stereotactic radiosurgery in management of persistent acromegaly. Endocr Pract. 2007;13:726–34.
18. Ronson BB, Schulte RW, Han KP, et al. Fractionated proton beam irradiation of pituitary adenomas. Int J Radiat Oncol Biol Phys. 2006;64:425–34.
19. McDonald MW, Plankenhorn DA, McMullen KP, et al. Proton therapy for atypical meningiomas. J Neuro-Oncol. 2015;123:123–8.
20. Milano MT, Okunieff P, Donatello RS, et al. Patterns and timing of recurrence after temozolomide-based chemoradiation for glioblastoma. Int J Radiat Oncol Biol Phys. 2010;78:1147–55.

21. Chan AW, Bernstein KD, Adams JA, et al. Dose escalation with proton radiation therapy for high-grade meningiomas. Technol Cancer Res Treatment. 2012;11:607–14.
22. ICRU. Prescribing, recording, and reporting proton-beam therapy (ICRU Report 78). J ICRU. 2007;7:1–210. https://doi.org/10.1093/jicru/ndm021.
23. Stupp R, Mason WP, van den Bent MJ, et al. Radiotherapy plus concomitant and adjuvant temozolomide for glioblastoma. N Engl J Med. 2005;352:987–96.
24. Baumert BG, Lomax AJ, Miltchev V, et al. A comparison of dose distributions of proton and photon beams in stereotactic conformal radiotherapy of brain lesions. Int J Radiat Oncol Biol Phys. 2001;49:1439–49.
25. Miralbell R, Cella L, Weber D, et al. Optimizing radiotherapy for orbital and paraorbital tumors: intensity-modulated X-ray beams vs. intensity-modulated proton beams. Int J Radiat Oncol Biol Phys. 2000;47:1111–9.
26. Bolsi A, Fogliata A, Cozzi L. Radiotherapy of small intracranial tumours with different advanced techniques using photon and proton beams: a treatment planning study. Radiother Oncol. 2003;68:1–14.

Primary Spine Tumors

21

Anuradha Thiagarajan and Yoshiya Yamada

Contents

21.1	Introduction	329
21.2	Simulation/Treatment Planning Considerations	331
21.3	Proton Beam Experience for Primary Spine Tumors	333
21.3.1	Giant Cell Tumors	333
21.3.2	Meningiomas	334
21.3.3	Schwannomas	335
21.3.4	Chordomas	336
21.3.5	Osteosarcomas	339
21.3.6	Chondrosarcomas	340
21.3.7	Hemangiopericytomas/Solitary Fibrous Tumors	341
21.3.8	Ewing Sarcomas	343
References		344

21.1 Introduction

1. Radiation therapy is an extremely important modality in the management of primary spine tumors. However, the relative radioresistance of many of these tumors requires high doses for durable local tumor control. In general, radiation doses in excess of 70 Gy are necessary to adequately control macroscopic disease. Likewise, doses greater than 60 Gy in 2 Gy fractions, and preferably over

A. Thiagarajan (✉)
Department of Radiation Oncology, National Cancer Centre Singapore,
11 Hospital Drive, Singapore 169610, Singapore
e-mail: anu_thiagarajan@hotmail.com

Y. Yamada
Department of Radiation Oncology, Memorial Sloan-Kettering Cancer Center,
1275 York Ave, New York, NY 10021, USA

© Springer International Publishing Switzerland 2018
N. Lee et al. (eds.), *Target Volume Delineation and Treatment Planning for Particle Therapy*, Practical Guides in Radiation Oncology,
https://doi.org/10.1007/978-3-319-42478-1_21

66 Gy, are required to treat positive microscopic margins. Traditional concepts of spinal cord tolerance establish the TD5/5 (the dose at which there is a 5% probability of a complication within 5 years) at 45–54 Gy in 2 Gy fractions, beyond which there appears to be a significantly increased risk of developing radiation myelitis [1]. In addition to the spinal cord, toxicities to paraspinal structures, such as small and large bowel, kidneys, and esophagus, must also be considered during spinal irradiation. Unfortunately, the radiation tolerances of these organs range from 23 to 65 Gy. The requirement to adhere to these normal tissue constraints severely limits the dose that can be delivered to spine tumors using conventional radiotherapy techniques and hence curbs the probability for achieving durable local tumor control and, potentially, cure. The need to deliver dose-escalated radiation therapy while minimizing treatment-related morbidity has led to the development of novel radiotherapy techniques such as image-guided intensity-modulated radiation therapy. In addition, there has been a renewed focus on charged particle therapy, in particular, proton beam therapy, the subject of the current chapter.
2. The principal advantage of proton beam therapy in treating spine tumors lies in its dose distribution. In contrast to conventional photon-based radiotherapy where, after a short buildup region, energy deposition decreases exponentially with increasing depth in tissue, the physical characteristics of the proton beam result in increasing energy deposition with penetration distance with the majority of the energy being deposited at the end of a linear track, in what is termed the Bragg peak [2] (Fig. 21.1). Beyond the Bragg peak, the position of which is primarily determined by beam energy, there is virtually no exit dose. This region of maximum energy deposition can be positioned within the target for each beam direction, allowing the creation of a highly conformal high-dose region and a reduction in integral dose of approximately 50–60% [3, 4]. The steeper dose gradients and lower integral doses that characterize proton beam therapy make it a highly attractive modality in the management of malignancies arising in the spine.
3. In spite of their well-recognized advantages, proton beam therapy is not without problems and uncertainties. First and foremost, one must consider the biologic unknowns of proton beam therapy [5]. One of the most fundamental challenges of proton beam radiotherapy is RBE uncertainties [6]. In clinical practice, an invariant 1.1 RBE for protons is generally used, but this disregards the growing body of laboratory evidence demonstrating variability in RBE values for protons with depth. Clonogenic cell survival data approximate RBE values for protons (at 2 Gy per fraction) to be 1.1–1.15 from the entrance to the center of the spread-out Bragg peak (SOBP), increasing to 1.35 at the distal edge and 1.7 at the distal falloff [7]. Further, biologic parameters such as tissue type, cell cycle phase, oxygenation level, and alpha/beta ratio have also been shown to influence RBE values in addition to physical parameters such as dose and linear energy transfer (LET) [2, 8, 9]. For instance, RBE values have been found to increase by up to 20% with decreasing alpha/beta ratio [10]. Several strategies to mitigate RBE uncertainties have been proposed in the literature including tapering the SOBP distal edge (by reducing the physical dose within

Fig. 21.1 Depth dose curves for photons, protons, and carbon ions

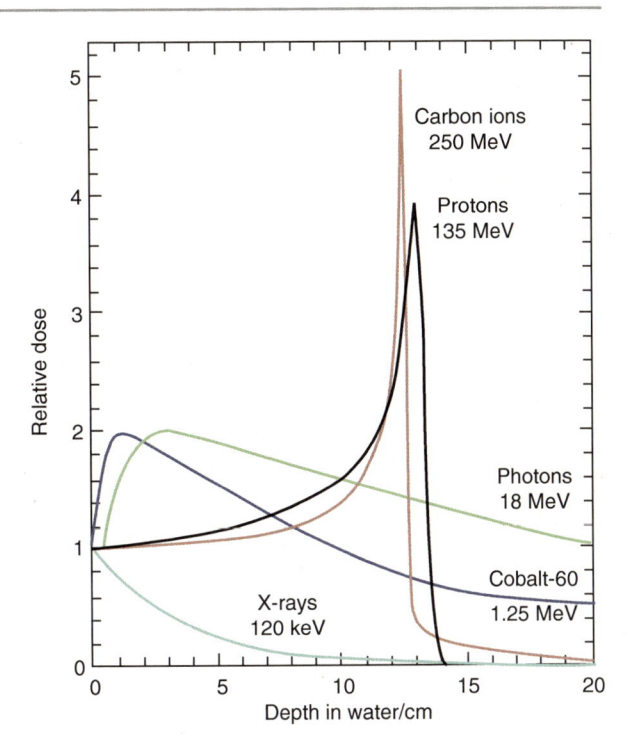

the terminal few millimeters of the proton SOBP), probabilistic and worst-case robust optimization, yielding plans that are less sensitive to range and RBE uncertainties, as well as prioritizing LET optimization within treatment planning attempting to shift LET hotspots into target volumes and away from treatment margins and organs at risk [11].

21.2 Simulation/Treatment Planning Considerations

1. Computed tomography (CT) simulation should be performed with intravenous iodinated contrast, when not contraindicated, to facilitate anatomical delineation. For the purposes of dose calculation, a non-contrast CT needs to be employed in planning proton therapy.
2. Magnetic resonance (MR) imaging is recommended for accurate delineation of the extent of gross disease. Different MR sequences can be useful in delineating normal tissue and target volumes. Contrast enhancement is useful for extraosseous paraspinal and epidural disease. T2 and fat-suppressed T2-weighted images are often very helpful in identifying tumor-bearing areas of many primary tumors of the spine. In the presence of metallic spinal hardware, T2-weighted images can also be useful in assessing the status of the epidural space. Multiplanar imaging is a hallmark of MR imaging and should be utilized in assessing spinal tumors.

3. MR images should be registered to the planning CT for accurate target delineation. Uncertainties related to image fusion should be considered in the treatment planning process.
4. There are unique considerations in treatment planning of spine tumors with proton therapy. The presence of high-density metallic implants in patients with spinal instrumentation, including titanium hardware, introduces considerable uncertainties into the treatment planning process. These uncertainties, primarily pertaining to proton range, may cause significant underdosing of target volumes and/or overdosing of critical structures in the vicinity, and it is critical that the practicing radiation oncologist carefully considers the distribution and magnitude of these effects in plan review. In fact, recent studies of chordoma patients treated with proton beam therapy have shown an inverse association between local tumor control and the presence of titanium-based surgical stabilization [12]. While other factors may have been at play, the dosimetric implications of metallic hardware should be considered.
5. Firstly, CT numbers are used to determine the proton stopping power of tissues in the path of the proton beam. Hence, metallic streak artifacts in the reconstructed CT images can result in errors in the calculated proton range. While proton stopping powers may be manually adjusted in an attempt to mitigate these errors, it is often not straightforward to determine anatomy and tissue density in images that have been degraded by artifacts. Range errors stemming from CT metal artifacts may also be reduced with improved CT image reconstruction methods, which are gradually becoming commercially available. In this regard, it is important to use methods that provide accurate segmentation of metallic implants from surrounding tissue as well as minimize image degradation wrought by metal artifacts.
6. Secondly, pencil beam dose calculation methods are based on water as a reference medium and may not accurately model beam transport through titanium hardware, potentially underestimating dose inhomogeneity and range degradation distal to these implants. Dosimetric analyses have demonstrated that the greater density of metallic implants can affect the range of protons and heavy ions by up to 10 mm and alter the dose by greater than 10% in the high-dose region [12]. Given that the spinal cord is typically only a few millimeters away from the high-dose region, the dosimetric uncertainties associated with metallic implants are unacceptable. One solution to account for these uncertainties is to use a larger number of beams and more conservative range margins. However, a more ideal solution rests in the utilization of dose calculation algorithms that better simulate the physical interactions of protons with high-density metallic implants and, in particular, better model the effect of multiple Coulomb scattering. In this regard, Monte Carlo simulation techniques have been shown to provide more accurate dosimetry in the setting of these spinal fixation devices [13].
7. It is well recognized that patient/tumor motion as well as changes in anatomy during radiation therapy are major causes of geographic misses and unanticipated toxicities. Protons, with their unique beam transmission properties and rapid dose falloff, have been shown to be even more sensitive to these factors

than conventional photon-based techniques [14]. Spinal and paraspinal tumors are relatively static. Hence, tumor motion is not as critical an issue as it is for lung and abdominal tumors which are highly mobile. However, it is imperative that due diligence is paid to rigid immobilization to create a stable and reproducible patient setup on a day-to-day basis. While immobilization in external beam radiation therapy is primarily designed to minimize inter- and intra-fraction patient motion, there are additional aspects that must be considered in proton beam therapy, chief of which is accurately determining and maintaining the target's water equivalent depth along the beam axis. To this end, there are both in-house and commercially available immobilization devices that have been engineered to work with the unique physics of proton beam transmission and designed to keep the range relatively constant for most treatment beam angles. In addition, as proton beam therapy is exquisitely sensitive to changes in patient and tumor anatomy, replanning should be considered if significant tumor shrinkage is anticipated. This may be most relevant for large baseline tumors, located in close proximity to or abutting spinal cord, for which response during the course of treatment may be brisk and without adaptation may result in unanticipated increments in OAR doses. However, precise data on the implementation levels or thresholds for replanning as well as the timing and frequency with which it should be performed is lacking.
8. Normal tissue constraints. Table 21.1 summarizes suggested maximum doses for organs at risk near the spine. In clinical practice, a wide range of doses are considered acceptable.

21.3 Proton Beam Experience for Primary Spine Tumors

21.3.1 Giant Cell Tumors

Giant cell tumors (GCTs) are relatively rare, usually benign skeletal neoplasms occurring primarily in young adults, with a peak incidence in the third and fourth decades. Although the most common location for these tumors is the epiphyses of long bones, they can occur in the axial skeleton, where they may present with local pain and neurologic deficits. In the spine, they are observed most commonly in the

Table 21.1 Dose constraints

Organ at risk	Recommended dose constraint (2 Gy per fraction equivalent dose)
Spinal cord	54 Gy
Cauda equina	60 Gy
Brainstem	60 Gy
Esophagus	65 Gy
Brachial plexus	60 Gy
Bowel	60 Gy
Rectum	70 Gy

sacrum, followed by elsewhere in the mobile spine where they occur in equal incidence in the cervical, thoracic, and lumbar vertebrae. Management of giant cell tumors of the spine is challenging owing to the close proximity to critical neural structures and the frequent vascularity of these tumors. The standard of care for GCTs of the mobile spine and sacrum is en bloc surgical resection where feasible. It is widely recognized that the status of surgical margins is the single best predictor of outcome in GCTs. Following complete resection with wide margins, local control is achieved in 85–90% of cases, but incomplete resection is associated with tumor recurrence in up to 50% of the cases. Therefore, radiotherapy has been advocated by some either as an adjunct to surgery in patients undergoing intralesional or marginal resections or as an alternative treatment in patients with giant cell tumors of the spine that are either unresectable or where resection would result in substantial functional deficits. Although concerns about radiotherapy side effects and in particular the risks of malignant transformation have been raised in the past, the evolution of radiotherapy techniques and the ability to deliver high radiation doses to target volumes with optimal sparing of critical structures have largely allayed these fears. A range of radiotherapy doses have been used in the literature, and when radiotherapy has been used as the primary therapy, local control rates have been satisfactory.

The literature on the use of proton beam therapy for giant cell tumors of the spine is sparse. However, given the concerns that exist about radiation-induced carcinogenesis in a disease that occurs primarily in young adults, proton beam therapy intuitively appears to be a better alternative. There is approximately a 50% reduction in integral dose both with the use of scattered and scanned proton beams compared with photon-based radiotherapy techniques, and mathematical modeling studies in pediatric patients have estimated a twofold or more reduction in risk of radiation-induced malignancies [15]. In a study by Hug et al., eight patients with primary or recurrent giant cell tumors of the axial skeleton were treated with combined high-dose proton and photon radiation therapy at the Massachusetts General Hospital and Harvard Cyclotron Laboratory [16]. The mean target dose was 61.8 CGE. The authors found that 5-year local control rates were excellent (83%) with acceptable rates of morbidity.

21.3.2 Meningiomas

Although spinal meningiomas are far less common than intracranial meningiomas, they account for 25–45% of all spine neoplasms and are the second most common spine tumor in the intradural location after schwannomas. They are most frequently located in the thoracic spine (80%) followed by the cervical spine (15%). They only rarely occur in the lumbar spine (<3%). They primarily affect middle-aged women, and similar to their intracranial counterparts, the vast majority of spinal meningiomas are benign (>90%). Atypical meningiomas and anaplastic/malignant meningiomas account for 5% and 3–5% of all meningiomas, respectively.

The standard of care for spinal meningiomas is surgical resection. Complete resection of the tumor and its dural attachment can often be achieved. Sacrifice of thoracic spinal roots may be required, but where possible, cervical and lumbar nerve roots are preserved. Management of subtotally resected lesions is usually expectant, and symptomatic recurrence is generally managed with further surgery. As with intracranial meningiomas, definitive radiotherapy tends to be reserved for symptomatic primary or recurrent lesions that are considered unresectable owing to technical difficulties or medical comorbidities. In the adjuvant setting, radiotherapy is generally recommended for atypical and anaplastic (grade II and III) meningiomas, regardless of the extent of surgery due to their aggressiveness, their proclivity to recur, and the neurologic morbidity associated with tumor recurrence.

For intracranial meningiomas, radiotherapy doses using conventional photon-based techniques range from 50 to 60 Gy. A dose of 60 Gy is recommended for atypical and anaplastic meningiomas, based on the maximal safe dose deliverable to the surrounding normal brain. Even at this dose, local failures are not uncommon suggesting that strategies that allow safe dose escalation such as proton beam therapy may further optimize outcomes. This may be particularly so in spinal subsites where the tolerability of the spinal cord to radiotherapy is even lower than that of the brain.

The literature on the use of protons in spinal meningioma is limited owing to the rarity of the disease. However, proton beam therapy has been used with success in intracranial and skull base meningiomas (Table 21.1). Hug et al. reported the outcomes of 31 patients with WHO grade II and III meningiomas treated with photon or combined proton–photon irradiation [17]. The total doses ranged from 50 to 68 Gy (RBE) and 40 to 72 Gy (RBE) for grades II and III meningiomas, respectively. Local control was significantly improved with combined proton–photon irradiation compared with photon radiotherapy alone ($P = 0.025$), and survival rates for WHO grade III meningiomas were significantly improved by proton beam therapy and radiation doses >60 Gy (RBE). Similarly, in a study of 24 patients with WHO II and III meningiomas treated by proton and photon beams to a median dose of 65.1 Gy (RBE), Boscos et al. found that survival was significantly associated with total dose [18]. In another recent report on the outcomes of six patients with WHO II and III meningiomas treated at doses of 68.4 Gy (RBE) and 72.0 Gy (RBE), respectively, Chan et al. observed local recurrence in one patient with WHO grade III meningioma. No severe treatment-related toxicity was observed [19].

In addition, in a recent study, Arvold et al. calculated projected second tumor rates in patients with benign meningioma by performing dosimetric comparisons between proton radiotherapy and photon radiotherapy treatment plans and found a 50% reduction in risk of radiation-associated second malignancies with proton beam therapy [20].

21.3.3 Schwannomas

Spinal schwannomas are the most common intradural extramedullary spinal tumors, accounting for approximately 30% of such lesions. They are most frequently seen in the cervical and lumbar spine and only rarely in the thoracic spine.

Although it is virtually impossible to reliably distinguish between schwannomas and neurofibromas radiographically, the former tends to be much more frequently associated with hemorrhage, intrinsic vascular changes (thrombosis, sinusoidal dilatation), cyst formation, and fatty degeneration. As spinal schwannomas generally arise from dorsal nerve roots, patients often present with radiculopathic pain. Sensory changes can also occur in a dermatomal distribution. Weakness is a less common presenting symptom. Myelopathy may occur if the lesion is large. Hence, spinal schwannomas can be debilitating in spite of the fact that they are slow-growing and rarely undergo malignant change. Surgical resection is the management of choice, and gross total resection is usually curative for patients with sporadic tumors. Reported obstacles to complete resection include adhesion of tumor to the spinal cord as a result of hemorrhage, inflammation, or subpial localization as well as attachment of critical structures such as the vertebral artery to extradural components of the tumor.

In general, radiation as a primary treatment modality for benign tumors of the spine such as schwannomas has not been advocated, and descriptions of its role as an adjunct to neurosurgical resection are scarce in the literature. At present, radiotherapy tends to be reserved for patients with technically unresectable disease, patients with medical comorbidities that preclude them from surgery, or those who refuse surgery in favor of noninvasive treatment particularly in the setting of recurrent disease.

In spite of the paucity of published evidence on the utility of radiotherapy as a primary or adjuvant treatment modality in spinal schwannomas, highly conformal photon-based radiotherapy techniques as well as proton therapy have been used with success in patients with vestibular schwannomas. In one report of 88 patients with vestibular schwannoma treated with proton beam stereotactic radiosurgery at the Harvard Cyclotron Laboratory, the 2-year and 5-year local control rates were 95% and 94%, respectively [21]. Excellent facial nerve and trigeminal nerve function preservation rates were achieved. However, only 33% of patients with functional hearing retained serviceable hearing ability, leading the authors to postulate that the use of fractionated proton therapy may have helped diminish this cranial nerve toxicity. Given the similarity in pathology between spinal schwannomas and vestibular acoustic neuromas, this modality may have even greater utility in the management of spinal schwannomas, where the radiation tolerance of the adjacent spinal cord is even more stringent.

21.3.4 Chordomas

Chordomas are rare, slow-growing, locally aggressive bone tumors that arise from the embryonic remnants of the notochord [22]. They exhibit a predominance in men, and the peak incidence occurs between 50 and 60 years of age. In adults, 50% of chordomas occur in the sacrum, 35% at the base of the skull, and the remaining 15% in the cervical, thoracic, and lumbar vertebrae.

Clinically, chordomas of the sacrum and mobile spine can present with localized pain or neurologic deficits corresponding to the spinal level at which they occur.

Unfortunately, the nonspecific nature and insidious onset of these symptoms may lead to delayed diagnosis when disease is already advanced.

Like most complex diseases, care for patients with chordomas is best undertaken in a high-volume quaternary referral center, where the multidisciplinary team members have the necessary expertise in the management of these tumors. Given the rarity of these tumors, there are no randomized clinical trials or large prospective series that define optimal treatment. A landmark study by Fuchs et al. demonstrated that there was a significant difference in recurrence rates between patients who underwent radical en bloc resection of sacral chordomas and those who had subtotal resection [23]. The time to local recurrence was 2.3 years and 8 months, respectively. This finding has since been corroborated by several other case series, supporting aggressive surgical resection in chordomas of the sacrum, mobile spine, and skull base [24, 25]. However, in spite of major advances in surgical interventions, total en bloc resection is achievable in only about half of all sacral chordomas, with much lower rates for chordomas elsewhere. Incomplete or subtotal resection of chordomas, which often arises in the presence of epidural disease, is associated with high rates of recurrence. To combat this, a combined modality approach is recommended, utilizing maximal surgical resection and adjuvant radiation therapy supported by data from small retrospective series.

Historical data evaluating the efficacy of conventional photon-based radiotherapy in the management of skull base chordomas demonstrate poor outcomes with 5-year local control rates less than 25%. However, this must be interpreted with caution as much of this data was accumulated in the era of older surgical and radiotherapy techniques and prior to the advent of MRI. Over the last decade, improvements in surgical techniques and the advent of high-precision radiotherapy in the form of intensity-modulated radiation therapy and image guidance have seen a significant improvement in 5-year local control and survival rates. At Memorial Sloan Kettering Cancer Center, single-fraction SRS via image-guided intensity-modulated radiation therapy has been used in the management of chordomas [26]. Results have been promising with respectable 3- and 5-year local control rates of approximately 71% and 59.1%, respectively, with no serious adverse effects. Likewise, preliminary outcomes of 24 patients with skull base chordoma treated with IG-IMRT at Princess Margaret Cancer Centre, Canada, have demonstrated 5-year overall survival and local control rates of 85.6% and 65.3%, respectively, at a median follow-up of 36 months [27]. The median IG-IMRT dose used was 76 Gy delivered in 2 Gy fractions. The authors conclude by stating that further follow-up was needed to confirm long-term efficacy.

Proton therapy is also an established radiotherapeutic option for the management of sacral chordomas (Table 21.2; Fig. 21.2), and outcomes correlate with dose. In a study by Park et al., 27 patients with sacral chordomas (16 primary and 11 recurrent), most of whom had undergone surgical resection (78%), received photon/proton radiation and followed for a mean time period of 8.8 years [28]. Local control rates for surgery and radiation were 86% for primary and 14% for recurrent chordomas. Among patients receiving definitive radiation, doses of 73 Gy or more resulted in greater local control rates. The authors conclude by recommending 77.4 Gy to unresected chordomas or areas of gross residual disease.

Table 21.2 Published data on proton beam therapy for patients with meningioma

Author	Patients	Radiation modality	Overall survival	Local control	Toxicity
Wenkel et al. [43]	46	Protons and photons, 59.0 GyE	95% and 77% at 5 and 10 years	100% and 88% at 5 and 10 years	20% severe toxicity
Vernimmen et al. [44]	27	Protons 54–61.6 GyE, 16–27 fractions	Not reported	88%	11% late toxicity: ipsilateral partial hearing loss, temporal lobe epilepsy
Noël et al. [45]	51	Protons and photons 60.6 GyE	100% at 4 years	98% at 4 years	4% grade III toxicity. Unilateral hearing loss, complete pituitary deficiency
Boskos et al. [18]	24	34.05 GyE photons and 30.96 GyE protons (total dose 65.01 GyE)	53.2% and 42.6% at 5 and 8 years	46.7% at 5 and 8 years	4% radiation necrosis at 16 months after RT
Pasquier et al. [46]	39	Protons 52.2–66.6 GyE	81.8% at 5 years	84.8% at 5 years	15.5% > grade III

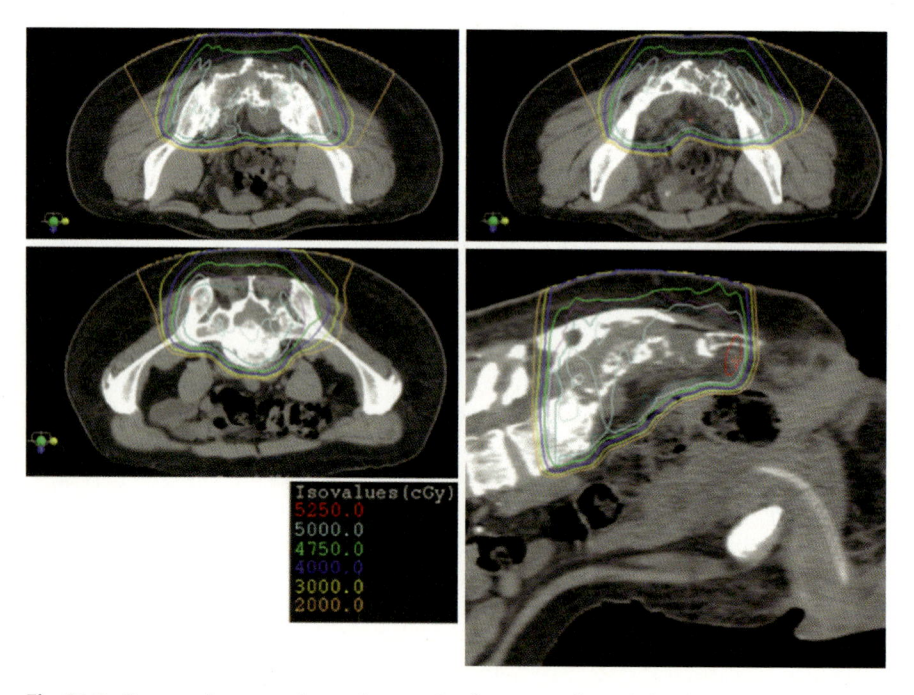

Fig. 21.2 Preoperative proton beam therapy plan for a case of sacral chordoma

A systematic review of the literature on proton beam radiotherapy in patients with skull base chordomas analyzed the outcomes of 416 patients from seven retrospective studies who were treated either exclusively with protons or with a combination of protons plus photons [29]. The majority of these patients had advanced inoperable or incompletely resected tumors. Although there was some heterogeneity of radiation doses and schedules both within and between series, in general, the total radiation dose was 70 GyE or greater. The authors reported 5-year local and overall survival rates of 69% and 80%, respectively, with a median follow-up of 46 months.

In conclusion, the clinical data for modern proton and photon-based radiotherapy show similar results, and choice is generally dictated by both geographic and financial accessibility to proton facilities. High-level evidence of benefit does not exist for unequivocal recommendation of proton-based treatment [30, 31].

21.3.5 Osteosarcomas

Osteosarcomas are primary malignant bone tumors characterized by the production of osteoid or immature bone from neoplastic cells. Although they are the second most common primary malignant tumor occurring in the bone, spinal involvement is rare, accounting for less than 5% of all cases.

Spine osteosarcomas are most commonly located in the sacrum, followed by the thoracic and lumbar spine segments, and, then, the cervical spine. Clinically, spine osteosarcomas present almost universally with gradually progressive pain, and two-thirds of patients exhibit some degree of neurologic impairment.

As with osteosarcomas of the extremities, optimal management for spine osteosarcomas is multimodal, comprising of neoadjuvant chemotherapy followed by wide en bloc excision if feasible and, subsequently, further systemic therapy. Obtaining adequate surgical margins is particularly challenging in the spine. In one study evaluating the relationship between surgical margin status and local recurrence in spine sarcomas, the resection was classified as wide, marginal, or intralesional in 23%, 10%, and 67% of patients, respectively [32]. Resection margins were histologically positive in 60% of cases and associated with a fivefold increased risk of local recurrence. In addition, if the tumor abuts or invades dura, although en bloc resection (vertebrectomy), followed by stabilization and fusion may be possible, surgery is fraught with the risk of tumor seeding into the CSF space. Patients with osteosarcomas of the sacrum fare particularly poorly. In one study that included 12 patients with primary high-grade osteosarcoma of the sacrum, only two patients who underwent surgery had wide excision to negative margins [33]. Although total sacrectomy may improve local control, it comes at the cost of significant morbidity to the patient with neurologic and sexual dysfunction being almost inevitable [34].

Radiation therapy for local control may be considered as the primary modality in patients who decline surgery or in whom there is no effective function-preserving surgical option. It may also have a role in the adjuvant setting following incomplete resections.

Historically, the prognosis for spine osteosarcomas has been inferior to stage-matched extremity osteosarcomas, with reported rates of 5-year survival ranging between 30 and 40%. This may at least in part be attributable to the usage of suboptimal radiotherapy doses prior to the advent of three-dimensional or volumetric image guidance and more conformal radiotherapy techniques. Newer radiation techniques and modalities such as IG-IMRT, proton beam irradiation, and carbon ion radiotherapy now permit safe dose escalation to target volumes while limiting doses to the spinal cord, and preliminary outcomes have been promising.

In a study by Ciernik et al., 55 patients with unresected and incompletely resected osteosarcomas in various anatomic subsites including the spine were offered proton-based radiotherapy. The mean dose was 68.4 Gy, and 58.2% (11–100%) of the total dose was delivered with protons. Local tumor control after 3 and 5 years was 82% and 72%, respectively. Five-year disease-free survival was 65% and 5-year overall survival was 67% [35].

21.3.6 Chondrosarcomas

Chondrosarcomas are malignant cartilage-forming tumors, comprising approximately 10% of all primary bone tumors. If hematologic malignancies of bone are excluded, they are the third most common primary malignant bone tumor after osteosarcoma and Ewing sarcoma. However, spinal chondrosarcomas are relatively infrequent, accounting for less than 10% of all chondrosarcomas and 5% of all spinal tumors. These tumors have a predilection for the thoracic spine and typically originate in the vertebral body and extend into the spinal canal and paraspinal soft tissue. The most common presenting symptom in chondrosarcoma is pain. Other symptoms include a palpable mass and neurologic deficits in approximately 50% of patients.

These malignancies are relatively resistant to radiotherapy and chemotherapy, and wide en bloc surgical resection is the management of choice [36]. Intralesional resections almost always result in tumor recurrence. Both IG-IMRT and proton beam therapy have been used in the adjuvant setting following incomplete resections with promising results. In a recent report looking at preliminary outcomes following high-dose IG-IMRT, 18 patients with skull base chondrosarcomas treated with a median dose of 70 Gy were followed for a median time period of 67 months [27]. Favorable 5-year overall survival and local control rates were found (87.8% and 88.1%, respectively) with acceptable adverse event rates.

The most extensive radiotherapy data for chondrosarcoma, however, comes from proton beam therapy (Table 21.3). The largest series that analyzed the outcomes of 200 patients with skull base chondrosarcomas treated with proton beam therapy showed excellent 10-year local control and survival rates of 98% and 99%, respectively [37]. The median radiotherapy dose was 72 GyE. A subsequent review of the literature demonstrated similar results [38].

In a treatment planning comparison study of intensity-modulated photon and proton therapy for paraspinal sarcomas, the authors found that both IMRT and

Table 21.3 Published data on proton beam therapy for patients with chordomas

Author	Patients	Radiation modality	Local control	Toxicity
Santoni et al. [47]	96	Protons 66.6 GyE or 72 GyE	–	Temporal lobe necrosis 7.6 and 13.2% at 2 and 5 years
Terahara et al. [48]	115	Protons 66.6–79.2 GyE	5-year LC 59%, 10-year LC 44%	–
Hug et al. [49]	33	Protons, 50.4 GyE bis 78.6 GyE	5-year LC 59%	7% of grades III and IV
Colli and Al-Mefty [50]	53	Protons vs. conventional RT	4-year LC 90.0% vs. 19.4%	–
Igaki et al. [51]	13	Protons or protons + photons, 72 GyE	5-year LC 50%	–
Weber et al. [52]	18	Protons, 74 GyE	3-year LC 87.5%	3-year complication-free survival 82.2%
Noel et al. [53]	100	Photons vs. protons, 67 GyE	2- and 4-year LC 86.3% and 53.8%	8 patients visual deficits, one patient symptomatic temporal lobe necrosis; 22 patients hearing deterioration; hormonal deficits in 16 patients
Ares et al. [54]	42	Protons, 73.5 GyE	5-year LC 81%	6% high-grade toxicity

IMPT produced similar levels of tumor conformality [39]. However, a reduction in nontarget integral dose was demonstrated in IMPT plans. The significance of this is twofold. The first is the potential for improved toxicity outcomes, in particular, radiation carcinogenesis. In addition, OAR integral doses could be critically important in the following settings: reirradiation, preoperative radiation therapy, as well as concurrent and sequential chemoradiotherapy. The second is the potential for dose escalation, and this study demonstrated that dose escalation to 93 CGE was possible in all patients within OAR dose constraints irrespective of tumor size, location, and geometry. Whether this translates to improved oncologic outcomes remains to be seen. In short, there are no randomized trials comparing these different contemporary radiotherapy techniques, and the advantages of proton beam therapy are primarily theoretical.

21.3.7 Hemangiopericytomas/Solitary Fibrous Tumors

Hemangiopericytomas are uncommon tumors of the central nervous system (CNS), constituting approximately 1% of all CNS tumors. Originally thought to arise from capillary pericytes, they have been categorized as fibroblastic with no evidence of pericytic differentiation in the updated WHO classification and are thought to lie on the same spectrum as solitary fibrous tumors. The distribution of hemangiopericytomas within the CNS is similar to that of meningiomas. They primarily arise within the brain, and spinal hemangiopericytomas are exceedingly rare, with less than 100 cases reported worldwide. The majority of these tumors are located in the intradural extramedullary compartment. They have been observed to occur throughout the spine but demonstrate some prevalence for the cervical and thoracic spine. If feasible, en bloc resection of the tumor along with the dura is the mainstay of management. Preoperative embolization is recommended to reduce intraoperative blood loss as these tumors are typically highly vascular. Given the rarity of this disease entity, there is a paucity of literature on the role of adjuvant radiotherapy, and much of the available evidence derives from retrospective studies with inherent biases. Available studies have not shown a consistent advantage with postoperative radiotherapy in improving disease-free survival and/or overall survival. Hence, the utility of radiotherapy is best decided on a case-by-case basis in the context of a multidisciplinary discussion and is generally reserved for subtotal resections, when high-risk features, e.g., high grade, are observed or when the morbidity of surgery is considered unacceptably high particularly in the case of recurrent tumors (Table 21.4).

Combs et al. analyzed the use of high-precision photon-based radiotherapy in patients with hemangiopericytoma, including two patients who had primary hemangiopericytoma of the spine [40]. The median RT dose was 54 Gy. The authors demonstrated an overall survival rate of 100% at 5 years and 64% at 10 years for patients treated with a combination of surgical and RT approaches. Progression-free survival after RT was 80% and 61% at 3 and 5 years, respectively.

The role of proton irradiation in the management of hemangiopericytomas of the spine has yet to be defined. However, the physical benefits of protons, namely, the potential to dose escalate as well as the ability to reduce OAR volumes receiving low to intermediate doses, provide future opportunities for dose–response studies to assess if higher doses translate into better local tumor control and survival as well as studies evaluating late side effects such as second malignancies.

Table 21.4 Published data on proton beam therapy for patients with chondrosarcomas

Author	Patients	Radiation modality	Local control	Toxicity
Hug et al. [49]	25	Protons, 70.7 GyE	5-year LC 75%	7% of grades III and IV
Noel et al. [53]	18	Protons + photons, 67 GyE	3-year LC 85%	–
Weber et al. [52]	11	Protons, 68 GyE	3-year LC 100%	3-year complication-free survival 82.2%
Ares et al. [54]	22	Protons, 68.4 GyE	5-year LC 94%	6% high-grade toxicity
Rosenberg et al. [37]	200	Protons + photons, 72.1 GyE	5-year LC 98%	–

21.3.8 Ewing Sarcomas

Ewing sarcomas are malignant, poorly differentiated, small round blue cell tumors that arise in bone and soft tissues. They most commonly present in the second decade of life, and there is a slight male predilection with a male-to-female ratio of 1.5:1. They primarily affect Caucasians and are rare in Blacks and Asians. They commonly arise in the long bones of the extremities and pelvis. Although the vertebrae are the most common bony site of metastatic involvement in Ewing sarcomas, primary Ewing sarcoma of the spine is relatively rare with a reported incidence of 5–8% of all cases. The sacrum and lumbar spine are most commonly affected followed by thoracic and then cervical spine. In the mobile spine, the bulk of lesions have their epicenter in the posterior elements with extension into the vertebral body. In the sacrum, the ala tends to be the most frequently affected site. In addition, spinal canal invasion is evident in the vast majority of cases. Approximately three-quarters of all patients present with clinically localized disease. However, Ewing sarcoma is considered a systemic disease, and subclinical metastatic disease is present in the bulk of patients. In 20–25% of patients who present with overt metastatic disease, common sites of metastases include the lungs and bone/bone marrow.

Typical presentations include localized pain and neurologic impairment. Occasionally, a palpable mass or swelling may be noted. Constitutional symptoms such as fever, malaise/fatigue, weight loss, or anemia are present in 10–20% of patients at the time of presentation and are generally indicative of advanced disease.

As Ewing sarcoma is considered a systemic disease, most modern treatment plans utilize initial induction chemotherapy followed by local treatment followed subsequently by further chemotherapy. These general principles of management applied to Ewing sarcoma occurring elsewhere in the body hold true for spinal locations as well. In a neurologically stable patient with Ewing sarcoma of the spine, initial chemotherapy after biopsy is recommended prior to any definitive local therapy either in the form of radical en bloc resection or radiation therapy. Neoadjuvant chemotherapy typically comprises of vincristine, dactinomycin, and cyclophosphamide (VAC). Following completion of chemotherapy, if tumor restaging studies demonstrate no evidence of metastases, then radical en bloc spondylectomy should be considered because the risk of local recurrence is lower and long-term survival may be improved compared with intralesional excision or radiation therapy alone. However, in cases which are clearly unresectable following induction chemotherapy or where a function-preserving surgical option is lacking as a result of tumor location or extent, definitive radiation therapy alone is recommended. In general, all patients are selected for local therapy in such a way that they are treated with surgery or radiotherapy but not both since combined use exposes them to the morbidities of both modalities. However, postoperative radiotherapy is indicated in the presence of microscopic or gross residual disease following surgery. Following local therapy, adjuvant chemotherapy is resumed, typically for several months.

In patients with progressive neurologic deficits and impending paralysis secondary to spinal cord compression, or in patients with primary mechanical instability or impending instability, prompt decompressive surgery and/or stabilization procedures must be undertaken prior to commencement of systemic therapy. These patients subsequently also require radiation therapy.

The use of proton beam therapy as part of the treatment of Ewing sarcoma of the spine has not been extensively examined in the literature. However, this approach may be particularly beneficial for Ewing sarcomas arising in the spine, and the reasons for this are twofold. Firstly, radiotherapy doses to primary tumors involving the vertebral body using conventional photon irradiation are often limited to ~45 Gy because of proximity of the spinal cord. Doses of at least 55.8 Gy are necessary for adequate local tumor control in unresectable tumors. For patients undergoing postoperative radiotherapy, doses of 45–50.4 Gy are recommended for microscopic disease. The utilization of proton beam therapy enables safe dose escalation. Secondly, patients treated for Ewing sarcoma have been observed to be at high risk for the development of second malignancies with genetic factors, chemotherapy and radiotherapy likely all playing a contributory role. Proton beam therapy has been shown to reduce integral dose to nontarget tissues by approximately 50%, hence reducing the risk of radiation carcinogenesis [41]. In fact, proton beam irradiation has been approved for use in Children's Oncology Group protocols.

Rombi et al. analyzed the initial clinical outcomes in 30 pediatric patients with Ewing sarcoma treated with proton therapy at the Francis H. Burr Proton Therapy Center at Massachusetts General Hospital [42]. The median dose was 54 Gy with a median follow-up of 38.4 months. The 3-year actuarial rates of event-free survival, local control, and overall survival were 60%, 86%, and 89%, respectively. The authors found that proton therapy was well-tolerated, with mostly mild to moderate skin reactions. At the time of publication, the only serious late effects were four hematologic malignancies, which are known risks of topoisomerase and anthracycline exposure. The pediatric patients in this study were treated with passive beam technology. Increasingly, patients can be treated with spot-scanned protons which offer better dose conformality and has the capability to further reduce skin dose, nontarget integral dose, and, hence, radiation-induced second malignancies.

References

1. Emami B, et al. Tolerance of normal tissue to therapeutic irradiation. Int J Radiat Oncol Biol Phys. 1991;21:109–22.
2. Newhauser WD, Zhang R. The physics of proton therapy. Phys Med Biol. 2015;60:R155–209.
3. Mitin T, Zietman AL. Promise and pitfalls of heavy-particle therapy. J Clin Oncol Off J Am Soc Clin Oncol. 2014;32:2855–63.
4. DeLaney TF. Proton therapy in the clinic. Front Radiat Ther Oncol. 2011;43:465–85.
5. McGowan SE, Burnet NG, Lomax AJ. Treatment planning optimisation in proton therapy. Br J Radiol. 2013;86:20120288.
6. Paganetti H, van Luijk P. Biological considerations when comparing proton therapy with photon therapy. Semin Radiat Oncol. 2013;23:77–87.
7. Paganetti H. Relative biological effectiveness (RBE) values for proton beam therapy. Variations as a function of biological endpoint, dose, and linear energy transfer. Phys Med Biol. 2014;59:R419–72.

8. Tommasino F, Durante M. Proton radiobiology. Cancers. 2015;7:353–81.
9. Engelsman M, Schwarz M, Dong L. Physics controversies in proton therapy. Semin Radiat Oncol. 2013;23:88–96.
10. Paganetti H. Significance and implementation of RBE variations in proton beam therapy. Technol Cancer Res Treat. 2003;2:413–26.
11. Underwood T, Paganetti H. Variable proton relative biological effectiveness: how do we move forward? Int J Radiat Oncol Biol Phys. 2016;95:56–8.
12. Verburg JM, Seco J. Dosimetric accuracy of proton therapy for chordoma patients with titanium implants. Med Phys. 2013;40:071727.
13. Paganetti H. Range uncertainties in proton therapy and the role of Monte Carlo simulations. Phys Med Biol. 2012;57:R99–117.
14. De Ruysscher D, Sterpin E, Haustermans K, Depuydt T. Tumour movement in proton therapy: solutions and remaining questions: a review. Cancers. 2015;7:1143–53.
15. Miralbell R, Lomax A, Cella L, Schneider U. Potential reduction of the incidence of radiation-induced second cancers by using proton beams in the treatment of pediatric tumors. Int J Radiat Oncol Biol Phys. 2002;54:824–9.
16. Hug EB, Fitzek MM, Liebsch NJ, Munzenrider JE. Locally challenging osteo- and chondrogenic tumors of the axial skeleton: results of combined proton and photon radiation therapy using three-dimensional treatment planning. Int J Radiat Oncol Biol Phys. 1995;31:467–76.
17. Hug EB, et al. Management of atypical and malignant meningiomas: role of high-dose, 3D-conformal radiation therapy. J Neuro-Oncol. 2000;48:151–60.
18. Boskos C, et al. Combined proton and photon conformal radiotherapy for intracranial atypical and malignant meningioma. Int J Radiat Oncol Biol Phys. 2009;75:399–406.
19. Chan AW, Bernstein KD, Adams JA, Parambi RJ, Loeffler JS. Dose escalation with proton radiation therapy for high-grade meningiomas. Technol Cancer Res Treat. 2012;11:607–14.
20. Arvold ND, et al. Projected second tumor risk and dose to neurocognitive structures after proton versus photon radiotherapy for benign meningioma. Int J Radiat Oncol Biol Phys. 2012;83:e495–500.
21. Weber DC, et al. Proton beam radiosurgery for vestibular schwannoma: tumor control and cranial nerve toxicity. Neurosurgery. 2003;53:577–86. discussion 586–8
22. George B, Bresson D, Herman P, Froelich S. Chordomas: a review. Neurosurg Clin N Am. 2015;26:437–52.
23. Fuchs B, Dickey ID, Yaszemski MJ, Inwards CY, Sim FH. Operative management of sacral chordoma. J Bone Joint Surg Am. 2005;87:2211–6.
24. Osaka S, Osaka E, Kojima T, Yoshida Y, Tokuhashi Y. Long-term outcome following surgical treatment of sacral chordoma. J Surg Oncol. 2014;109:184–8.
25. Ruggieri P, Angelini A, Ussia G, Montalti M, Mercuri M. Surgical margins and local control in resection of sacral chordomas. Clin Orthop Relat Res. 2010;468:2939–47.
26. Yamada Y, et al. Preliminary results of high-dose single-fraction radiotherapy for the management of chordomas of the spine and sacrum. Neurosurgery. 2013;73:673–80. discussion 680
27. Sahgal A, et al. Image-guided, intensity-modulated radiation therapy (IG-IMRT) for skull base chordoma and chondrosarcoma: preliminary outcomes. Neuro-Oncology. 2015;17:889–94.
28. Park L, et al. Sacral chordomas: impact of high-dose proton/photon-beam radiation therapy combined with or without surgery for primary versus recurrent tumor. Int J Radiat Oncol Biol Phys. 2006;65:1514–21.
29. Amichetti M, Cianchetti M, Amelio D, Enrici RM, Minniti G. Proton therapy in chordoma of the base of the skull: a systematic review. Neurosurg Rev. 2009;32:403–16.
30. Jahangiri A, et al. Factors predicting recurrence after resection of clival chordoma using variable surgical approaches and radiation modalities. Neurosurgery. 2015;76:179–85. discussion 185–176
31. Combs SE, Laperriere N, Brada M. Clinical controversies: proton radiation therapy for brain and skull base tumors. Semin Radiat Oncol. 2013;23:120–6.
32. Talac R, et al. Relationship between surgical margins and local recurrence in sarcomas of the spine. Clin Orthop Relat Res. 2002;397:127–32.

33. Ozaki T, et al. Osteosarcoma of the spine: experience of the Cooperative Osteosarcoma Study Group. Cancer. 2002;94:1069–77.
34. Wuisman P, Lieshout O, Sugihara S, van Dijk M. Total sacrectomy and reconstruction: oncologic and functional outcome. Clin Orthop Relat Res. 2000;381:192–203.
35. Ciernik IF, et al. Proton-based radiotherapy for unresectable or incompletely resected osteosarcoma. Cancer. 2011;117:4522–30.
36. Bloch O, Parsa AT. Skull base chondrosarcoma: evidence-based treatment paradigms. Neurosurg Clin N Am. 2013;24:89–96.
37. Rosenberg AE, et al. Chondrosarcoma of the base of the skull: a clinicopathologic study of 200 cases with emphasis on its distinction from chordoma. Am J Surg Pathol. 1999;23:1370–8.
38. Amichetti M, Amelio D, Cianchetti M, Enrici RM, Minniti G. A systematic review of proton therapy in the treatment of chondrosarcoma of the skull base. Neurosurg Rev. 2010;33:155–65.
39. Weber DC, Trofimov AV, Delaney TF, Bortfeld T. A treatment planning comparison of intensity modulated photon and proton therapy for paraspinal sarcomas. Int J Radiat Oncol Biol Phys. 2004;58:1596–606.
40. Combs SE, Thilmann C, Debus J, Schulz-Ertner D. Precision radiotherapy for hemangiopericytomas of the central nervous system. Cancer. 2005;104:2457–65.
41. Schneider U, et al. The impact of IMRT and proton radiotherapy on secondary cancer incidence. Strahlenther Onkol. 2006;182:647–52.
42. Rombi B, et al. Proton radiotherapy for pediatric Ewing's sarcoma: initial clinical outcomes. Int J Radiat Oncol Biol Phys. 2012;82:1142–8.
43. Wenkel E, et al. Benign meningioma: partially resected, biopsied, and recurrent intracranial tumors treated with combined proton and photon radiotherapy. Int J Radiat Oncol Biol Phys. 2000;48:1363–70.
44. Vernimmen FJ, et al. Stereotactic proton beam therapy of skull base meningiomas. Int J Radiat Oncol Biol Phys. 2001;49:99–105.
45. Noel G, et al. Functional outcome of patients with benign meningioma treated by 3D conformal irradiation with a combination of photons and protons. Int J Radiat Oncol Biol Phys. 2005;62:1412–22.
46. Pasquier D, et al. Atypical and malignant meningioma: outcome and prognostic factors in 119 irradiated patients. A multicenter, retrospective study of the Rare Cancer Network. Int J Radiat Oncol Biol Phys. 2008;71:1388–93.
47. Santoni R, et al. Temporal lobe (TL) damage following surgery and high-dose photon and proton irradiation in 96 patients affected by chordomas and chondrosarcomas of the base of the skull. Int J Radiat Oncol Biol Phys. 1998;41:59–68.
48. Terahara A, et al. Analysis of the relationship between tumor dose inhomogeneity and local control in patients with skull base chordoma. Int J Radiat Oncol Biol Phys. 1999;45:351–8.
49. Hug EB, et al. Proton radiation therapy for chordomas and chondrosarcomas of the skull base. J Neurosurg. 1999;91:432–9.
50. Colli BO, Al-Mefty O. Chordomas of the skull base: follow-up review and prognostic factors. Neurosurg Focus. 2001;10:E1.
51. Igaki H, et al. Clinical results of proton beam therapy for skull base chordoma. Int J Radiat Oncol Biol Phys. 2004;60:1120–6.
52. Weber DC, et al. Results of spot-scanning proton radiation therapy for chordoma and chondrosarcoma of the skull base: the Paul Scherrer Institut experience. Int J Radiat Oncol Biol Phys. 2005;63:401–9.
53. Noel G, et al. Radiation therapy for chordoma and chondrosarcoma of the skull base and the cervical spine. Prognostic factors and patterns of failure. Strahlenther Onkol. 2003;179:241–8.
54. Ares C, et al. Effectiveness and safety of spot scanning proton radiation therapy for chordomas and chondrosarcomas of the skull base: first long-term report. Int J Radiat Oncol Biol Phys. 2009;75:1111–8.

Sarcoma

22

Curtiland Deville, Matthew Ladra, Huifang Zhai, Moe Siddiqui, Stefan Both, and Haibo Lin

Contents

22.1	Introduction/Background	348
22.2	Simulation, Target Delineation, and Radiation Dose/Fractionation	349
22.3	OAR Dose Constraints	352
22.4	Patient Positioning, Immobilization, and Treatment Verification	353
22.5	3D Proton Treatment Planning	353
	22.5.1 Passive Scattering (PS)	353
22.6	Pencil-Beam Scanning (PBS)	360
22.7	Future Developments	364
	22.7.1 IMPT	364
References		365

C. Deville (✉) • M. Ladra
Department of Radiation Oncology and Molecular Radiation Sciences,
Johns Hopkins University School of Medicine,
401 N Broadway, Weinberg Suite 1440, Baltimore, MD 21231, USA
e-mail: cdeville@jhmi.edu

H. Zhai • H. Lin
Department of Radiation Oncology, University of Pennsylvania, Philadelphia, PA, USA

M. Siddiqui
Provision Health, Knoxville, TN, USA

S. Both
Department of Radiation Oncology, University Medical Center Groningen,
Groningen, The Netherlands
e-mail: s.both@umcg.nl

© Springer International Publishing Switzerland 2018
N. Lee et al. (eds.), *Target Volume Delineation and Treatment Planning for Particle Therapy*, Practical Guides in Radiation Oncology,
https://doi.org/10.1007/978-3-319-42478-1_22

22.1 Introduction/Background

Sarcomas represent a relatively rare and heterogeneous malignancy of mesenchymal origin occurring in the soft and connective tissues and bone throughout the body with an expected 12,310 new cases and 4990 deaths for soft tissue sarcoma (STS) and 3300 new cases and 1490 deaths for bone and joints in the United States in 2016 [1]. The most common sites of involvement are the extremity (59%: lower 46%, upper 13%), trunk (18%), retroperitoneum (13%), and head and neck (9%) [2].

There are over 100 histologic subtypes as classified by the World Health Organization (WHO) with the most common subtypes being undifferentiated/unclassified STS (previously malignant fibrous histiocytoma), liposarcoma, leiomyosarcoma, synovial sarcoma, and malignant peripheral nerve sheath tumor (MPNST), which is technically of ectodermal origin; molecular genetics are continuously refining these classifications [3]. Tumor size and grade are most highly associated with risk for distant metastasis [4]. While isolated nodal involvement (N1 M0) is uncommon at presentation (0.9%), the subtypes most commonly involved are epitheloid, clear cell, rhabdomyosarcoma, synovial, and angiosarcoma [5].

Limb salvage surgery and radiation have become the mainstay of extremity STS management with amputation generally reserved for salvage, based on randomized evidence demonstrating comparable outcomes to upfront amputation [6, 7]. Local control rates approach 85–90% for high-grade and 90–100% for low-grade extremity STS, respectively [8]. Extrapolating from such data, this combined modality approach of surgery and radiation has also become the mainstay for non-extremity STS.

For retroperitoneal STS, an ongoing randomized trial by the EORTC [9] is currently exploring adjuvant radiation, while dose painting to the high-risk margin during preoperative IMRT reported 80% actuarial, two-year local control rate [10], and is similarly being explored in a nonrandomized, multi-institutional study along with IMPT [11].

Preoperative radiotherapy may be pursued at the risk of increased wound healing complication depending on tumor location for the benefit of reduced, often irreversible radiation fibrosis, lymphedema joint stiffness, bone fracture, and other late radiation sequelae compared to postoperative radiation [12]. Given the complexity of STS management, referral to multidisciplinary subspecialists is associated with reduced local recurrence [13].

Neoadjuvant and adjuvant chemotherapy (largely ifosfamide and doxorubicin-based regimens) may be considered for large (≥ 8 cm), high-grade tumors due to up to 50% incidence of metastatic failure, albeit with limited evidence of benefit [14].

Select small, low-grade tumors may be managed with surgery alone [15].

Unresectable, recurrent, and/or medically inoperable patients may undergo definitive radiation (with or without chemotherapy) with reported 5-year local control, disease-free survival, and overall survival rates of 60%, 36%, and 52%, respectively, for patients receiving 63 Gy or more, including some receiving proton therapy [16], and there is additional history of using particle therapy for primary and recurrent soft tissue and bone sarcomas based on the favorable dose deposition and potential to dose escalate in this setting [17, 18].

While skull base chordomas have higher local failure rates than chondrosarcomas, patients with unresected chordomas may have their disease locally controlled with high-dose proton therapy, making it desirable to neurologically intact patients with upper sacral chordomas or those declining surgery [19–21].

For patients with axial osteosarcomas, local control can be enhanced with high-dose, proton-based RT [22]. Target volume doses and OAR constraints in osteosarcoma are often less than those used with chordoma/chondrosarcoma due to the concern for nerve and bowel toxicity when given alongside MAP (methotrexate, doxorubicin, cisplatin) chemotherapy [19].

Carbon ion radiotherapy offers the additional advantage of high LET and thus increased BED and has been utilized in the management of various sarcoma types largely in Asia with compelling results [23, 24]; however, it is not currently available in the United States and will not be further reviewed in this chapter.

22.2 Simulation, Target Delineation, and Radiation Dose/Fractionation

CT simulation may be performed with or without intravenous iodinated contrast, when not contraindicated, to facilitate anatomical delineation. For the purposes of dose calculation, a non-contrast CT needs to be employed in planning proton therapy (see Chap. 3). 4D motion assessment is advised for upper abdominal tumors.

Magnetic resonance imaging (MR) is recommended for accurate delineation of the extent of gross tumor (T1 post-contrast) as well as radiographic assessment of tumor-related edema (T2 or FLAIR) and generally obviates the need for IV contrast on the co-registered CT.

Positron emission tomography (PET) may be helpful for identification of metabolically active gross disease and identification of involved or suspicious lymph nodes.

PET and MR images should be registered to the planning CT for accurate target delineation. Uncertainties related to image fusion should be considered in the treatment planning process (Chap. 3).

The recommended dosing and fractionation vary depending on the clinical scenario as delineated in Table 22.1.

A relative biological effectiveness (RBE) factor of 1.1 (relative to 60 Co) is employed, and proton doses below are reported in Gy (RBE).

Target volumes should be expanded according to institutional standard accounting for immobilization and image guidance as delineated in Table 22.1 to create a planning target volume (PTV) for recording and reporting purposes [25].

Avoid circumferential irradiation of the limb to reduce the risk of lymphedema and functional deficit.

Full prescription dose to skin over areas commonly traumatized (e.g., the elbow, knee, shin) should be avoided. This is particularly relevant with proton therapy when passive scattering is employed since no skin-sparing effect is obtained.

Treat biopsy scar if it is not subsequently resected after radiotherapy.

Table 22.1 Recommended target volumes and radiation doses

Indication	Target	Definition	Dose
Extremity and trunk (adapted from [7])			
Pre-op	GTV	Gross tumor on T1-weighted, gadolinium-enhanced MR	
	CTV	4 cm craniocaudal and 1.5 cm radial expansion cropped from beyond fascia and uninvolved bone and including any "suspicious" tumor-associated edema on T2-weighted MR	45–50.4 Gy in 1.8 or 2 Gy (consider post-op boost for positive margin 16–18 Gy)
	PTV	5–10 mm depending on daily IGRT and institutional standard	
Post-op	CTV1	Tumor bed with similar 4 cm craniocaudal and 1.5 cm radial expansion cropped from bone and including surgically violated tissues, scar, and drain site (if feasible) and any "suspicious" tumor-associated edema on T2-weighted MR	45–50.4 Gy in 1.8 or 2 Gy
	CTV2	Tumor bed with 1.5 cm margin	60–61.2 Gy (R0 resection)
			66–66.6 Gy (R1)
			74–74.8 Gy (R2; definitive or postoperative gross disease)
	PTVs	5–10 mm depending on daily IGRT and institutional standard	
Retroperitoneum (adapted from [35])			
Pre-op	iGTV	Contour GTV incorporating 4D motion to account for internal margin	45–50.4 Gy in 1.8 or 2 Gy

	ITV	iGTV +1.5 cm (CTV expansion):
		• If tumor extends to inguinal canal, expand iGTV by 3 cm inferiorly
		• Crop ITV at interfaces:
		  – 0 mm: retroperitoneal compartment, bone, kidney, liver
		  – 3 mm: under skin surface
		  – 5 mm: bowel and air cavity	

	HRITV	Retroperitoneal high-risk margin [36]: • Area considered to be at high risk for positive margins following resection • Contour on every axial CT slice with a thickness of about 1.5 cm • Generally includes areas of tumor located along posterior retroperitoneal musculature, posterolateral abdominal wall, ipsilateral para- and prevertebral space, major vessels, or organs that the surgeon would leave in situ	simultaneous in-field boost is being explored: 2.3 Gy × 25 = 57.5 Gy (ref. [10]) Dose escalation protocol under study (ref. [11]) 2.15 Gy × 28 = 60.2 Gy 2.2 Gy × 28 = 61.6 Gy 2.25 Gy × 28 = 63 Gy
	PTVs	5 mm (if frequent 3D IGRT)	
		9–12 mm (if no 3D IGRT)	

Post-op	ITV	Tumor bed +1.5 cm (CTV expansion cropped as detailed above)	45–50.4 Gy in 1.8 Gy or 2 Gy
	HRITV	Tumor bed, retroperitoneal high-risk and positive margins	60–66.6 Gy (as feasible via planning)
	PTVs	5 mm (if frequent 3D IGRT) 9–12 mm (if no 3D IGRT)	
Pelvic and spine chordoma and osteosarcoma proton guidelines (adapted from ref. [19, 20])			
Definitive	GTV	Gross tumor on T1-weighted, gadolinium-enhanced MR	
	CTV1	1–2 cm expansion cropped from beyond fascia and uninvolved bone and including any "suspicious" tumor-associated edema on T2-weighted MR. For spinal lesions the volume includes the vertebral bodies immediately above and below the involved level	45–50.4 Gy RBE in 1.8 Gy RBE
	CTV2	0.5–1 cm expansion cropped to exclude uninvolved bone or organs	64.8 Gy RBE (osteo)–72 Gy RBE (chordoma) in 1.8 Gy RBE
	CTV3	GTV only	72 Gy RBE (osteo)–77.4 Gy RBE (chordoma) in 1.8 Gy RBE
	PTV	Per institutional standard	
Post-op	CTV1	Tumor bed with a 1.5–2 cm expansion, tailored to include all surgically manipulated tissues including scars, drain sites, and stabilization hardware	45–50.4 Gy RBE in 1.8 Gy RBE
	CTV2	Tumor bed with 5 mm margin	70.2–72 Gy RBE in 1.8 Gy RBE
	CTV3	Any residual gross disease	72–77.4 Gy RBE in 1.8 Gy RBE
	PTV	Per institutional standard	

Consultation with the orthopedic or surgical oncologist in the pre-op setting to define the high-risk margin areas of concern [36] or preferred normal tissues to spare [26] and in the post-op setting to review the surgical bed and any areas of concern for positive margin and microscopic residual is recommended.

22.3 OAR Dose Constraints

1. Extremity and trunk (adapted from RTOG 0630 [27])
2. Beam orientation should try to avoid treating the:
   (a) Full circumference of an extremity
   (b) Anus, vulva and scrotum, lung
   (c) Skin to full dose over commonly traumatized areas (e.g., the elbow, knee, shin) and femoral head/neck
3. If the tumor is close to the following structures:
   (a) Anus volume receiving 30 Gy (RBE) (V30) < 50%
   (b) Vulva V30 < 50%
   (c) Testis V3 < 50%, if the patient prefers to reserve fertility
   (d) Total lungs V20 < 20%
   (e) Femoral head/neck V60 < 5% or D_{max} 59 Gy when feasible
   (f) Any joint (including shoulder, elbow, and knee) V50 < 50%
   (g) Kidney V14 < 50%
   (h) Longitudinal strip (1–2 cm) of skin and subcutaneous tissue of an extremity V20 < 50%
   (i) Weight-bearing bone infield V50 < 50% Gy, except when:
      • Tumor invades the bone.
      • There is circumferential involvement of the tumor more than a quarter of the bone.
      • The bone will be resected in a subsequent surgical resection.
4. Retroperitoneal Sarcoma (from ref. [35]):
   (a) Liver mean dose <26 Gy (to planned residual liver)
   (b) Stomach and duodenum V45 < 100%; V50 < 50%, D_{max} 56 Gy
   (c) Kidney if 1 is resected V18 < 15% (remaining kidney)
   (d) Kidney if both will remain mean dose <15 Gy, V18 < 50%
   (e) Spinal cord maximum dose 50 Gy
   (f) Peritoneal cavity (small and large bowel bag) V15 < 830 cm^3, V45 < 195 cm^3
   (g) Small bowel if contoured as individual loops V15 < 120 cm^3, V55 < 20 cm^3
   (h) Large bowel if contoured as individual loops V60 < 20 cm^3
   (i) Rectum V50 < 50%
   (j) Testicles ALARA, V3 < 50% for fertility, D_{max} <18 Gy; consider cryopreservation in young men
   (k) Ovaries D_{max} <3Gy for fertility; consider cryopreservation in young women
   (l) Bladder V50 < 100% (if necessary)
   (m) Perineum (including anus and vulva) V30 < 50% if possible
   (n) Femoral head D_{max} <50Gy if possible, V40 < 64%, mean dose <37%

5. Sacral/spine chordoma and osteosarcoma proton constraints (adapted from ref. [19, 20]):
   (a) Skin ≤66 Gy (RBE)
   (b) Spinal cord ≤54 Gy RBE to center and cord surface ≤63 Gy RBE over a length of 5 cm or less
   (c) Cauda equina ≤70.2 Gy RBE except areas in direct contact with tumor (≤77.4 Gy RBE)
   (d) Sacral Nerves ≤77.4 Gy RBE
   (e) Small bowel ≤50.4 Gy RBE (entire) and ≤57.6 Gy RBE for <50% circumference of single loop
   (f) Large bowel <66 Gy RBE to <1/3 of circumference over length of 5 cm
   (g) Rectum posterior 1/3 < 77.4 Gy RBE and <70.2 Gy RBE over 5 cm

22.4 Patient Positioning, Immobilization, and Treatment Verification

Simulation and treatment should be conducted in the appropriate supine or prone, head- or feet-first position with customized indexed immobilization depending on the anatomic site as demonstrated in the representative case examples that follow.

Setup accuracy should be ascertained with daily orthogonal X-ray imaging or ideally with volumetric imaging when available.

In-room CT imaging (i.e., cone-beam CT) is ideally used for treatment verification. When in-room 3D imaging is not available, off-line verification CT scans with the patient in treatment position are recommended periodically during the course of treatment to assess for potential changes in anatomy (i.e., due to weight loss, tumor swelling, etc.) and potential changes in the accuracy of the dose distribution (see Case 4 below). Consider rescanning every other week for preoperative and definitive cases and at least once midcourse during treatment for postoperative cases, though there are exceptions to this depending on the clinical scenario.

22.5 3D Proton Treatment Planning

22.5.1 Passive Scattering (PS)

1. As the historically most commonly used proton technique, PS can still play a useful role with its advantages of faster delivery and being more robust and forgiving of organ and tumor motion compared to scanning-beam techniques later discussed. These make it useful for treating targets with considerable intra- and inter-fraction motion.
2. There are no absolute rules on selecting field orientation; however, the following guidelines are often used to decide the optimal beam angle:
   (a) Avoidance of critical OARs, ranging into critical OARs, beam path heterogeneities, and anatomy or organs that may vary in positioning or filling
   (b) Minimization of path length and motion effects

3. In practice, two or more fields are employed to improve the robustness of the treatment plan against the delivery uncertainties.
4. Considering the range uncertainties from multiple sources such as energy fluctuation of the delivery machine (~1 mm), compensator manufacturing (~2 mm), and conversion of the CT Hounsfield number into proton's stopping power (~3.5% of distal depth of CTV), distal and proximal margins are applied to the CTV to ensure sufficient target coverage. The distal margin is calculated by 3.5% of distal CTV depth plus 3 mm, while proximal margin is 3 mm plus 3.5% of proximal CTV depth [28]. The 3.5% may vary institutionally based on the technology and methodology employed.
5. Compensator smearing factor globally modifies the compensator design so that variations in tissue densities along the beam path (i.e., bone, air cavity) related to motion and setup uncertainties are taken into consideration. Brass aperture or multi-leaf collimator is employed to modify the lateral field shape.
6. Treatment plans are optimized with requirement that at least 95% of the CTV received the prescribed dose according to ICRU [29] (Varian Eclipse version 11.0.30 was the treatment planning system (TPS) used for all STS cases below, and dose calculations were performed on a 2.5 × 2.5 × 2.5 mm^3 grid).

Case 1 Preoperative lower extremity case: 10 cm gluteal STS in a young female of child bearing potential treated in 25 fractions at 2 Gy (RBE) = 50 Gy (RBE).

1. *Simulation*: CT imaging from L1 to the knee with 1.5 mm slice thickness in the prone position with arms above her head and legs straight in a vac-lock bag for appropriate, customized immobilization (Fig. 22.1). The secondary imaging was MR imaging with IV contrast.
2. *Planning*: A three-field plan utilizing an RPO (right posterior oblique field), LAO (left anterior oblique field), and LIPO (left inferior posterior oblique field) were selected with maximal sparing of OARs and the shortest, simplest beam paths (Fig. 22.2); typically 2–3 fields with the shortest and most homogeneous radiologic depths should be utilized.
3. Distal margins of 7–10 mm and proximal margins of 3–4 mm were used for proton planning. The optimized plan utilized two 4 inch compensator and one 3 inch compensator. Smearing factor of 10 mm and boarder smoothing factor of 15 mm were adopted during compensator design. Three mm motion and setup errors were considered to be a good estimation for the case and were used for smearing calculation.
4. Care was taken not to overlap the distal ends of more than two beams, and no more than 50% of the dose ranged out into an OAR, especially at levels of serial structures (Chap. 3).

22 Sarcoma

Fig. 22.1 Gluteal STS prone setup and immobilization

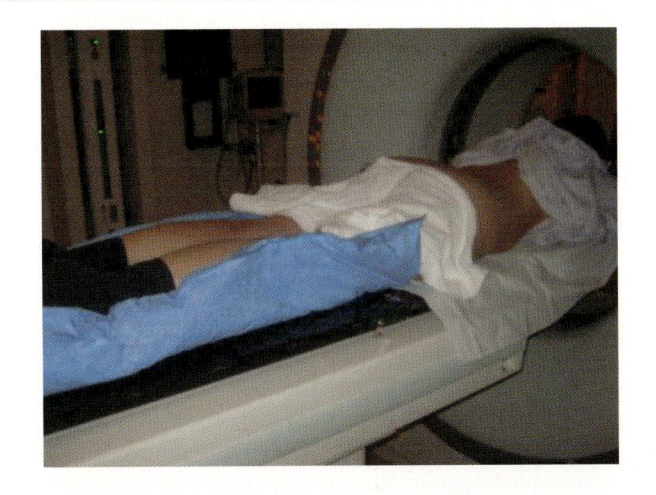

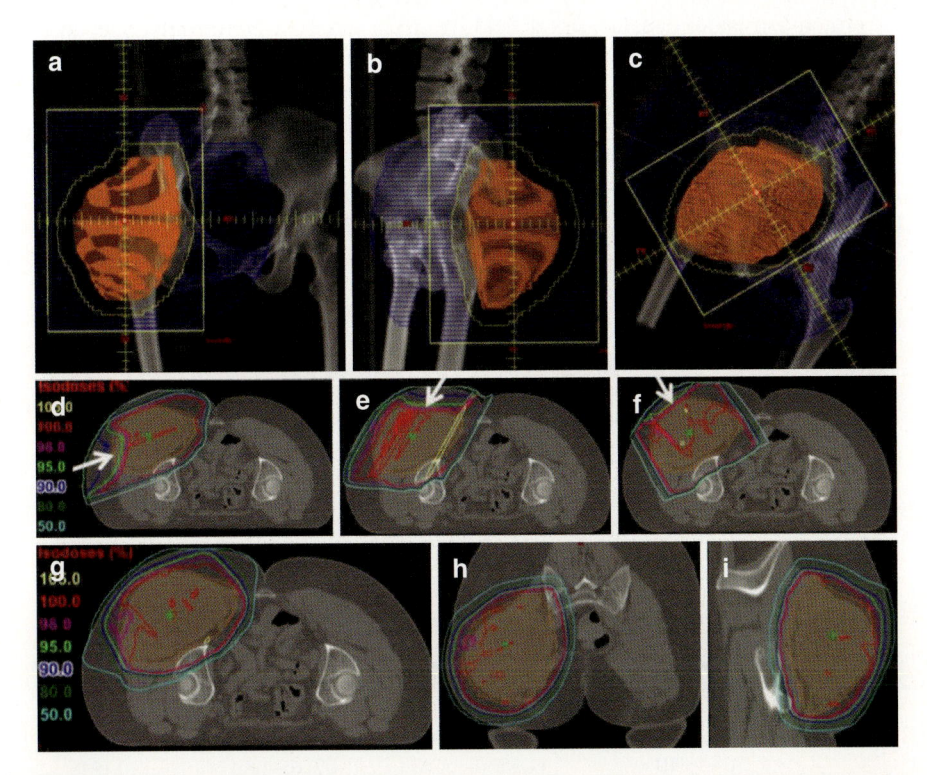

Fig. 22.2 Passive-scattering plan for Case 1, treatment of a gluteal sarcoma with three-beam arrangement including an RPO (right posterior oblique field), LAO (left anterior oblique field), and LIPO (left inferior posterior oblique field). Beam's eye view ((**a**), (**b**), (**c**)), dose contribution from individual field ((**d**), (**e**), (**f**)), and composite dose from axial, sagittal, and coronal view ((**g**), (**h**), (**i**)) are shown. The orange structure represents the CTV

5. For most extremity cases, PS or uniform scanning (US) can be used with excellent results. The target volume for most cases may extend superficially, often just below the skin, resulting in little opportunity for skin sparing. The skin dose with US/PS is similar to the prescription dose, likely slightly higher than with intensity-modulated photon radiation therapy (IMRT) and similar to IMRT with bolus.
6. For extremity cases, the goal is to spare the uninvolved bone, joint, normal soft tissues, including those potentially being used for flaps, and other adjacent OARs depending on the tumor location. As these are generally distal to the target, comparable normal tissue sparing may be achieved with passive or scanned beams.
7. A dosimetric comparison of PS and IMRT is shown in Fig. 22.4. Reduction of nontarget integral dose is demonstrated for PS. However, for concave/convex OARs closest to the target volume, for example, the ipsilateral femoral head in this case, the high-dose volume is slightly higher than IMRT despite the benefits in the low- and intermediate-dose region. This is common for PS because fewer treatment fields are typically employed. Given the similar penumbra between proton and photon beams, fewer fields result in less dose conformity. Secondly, due to uncertainties, PS is generally planned on a larger target volume than IMRT as noted in the PS planning section above. PTV is employed for recording and reporting purposes [25] (Fig. 22.3).
8. Other PS and IMRT dosimetric comparisons: for retroperitoneal and intraabdominal sarcomas, a dosimetric study of eight cases comparing 3DCRT, IMRT, and 3DPT using passive-scattering technique found that 3DPT was able to significantly reduce the integral dose and dose to adjacent OARs while maintaining comparable coverage as noted in Table 22.2 adapted from [30].

Table 22.2 In-silico Comparison of IMRT and 3DPT for retroperitoneal and intraabdominal sarcomas adapted from [30]

		IMRT	3DPT	T-test (P value)
Conformity index		0.751 (0.675–0.820)	0.691 (0.555–0.759)	0.0519
Small bowel	Median V15	52.15% (15.8–71.4)	16.4% (8.1–36.9)	*0.0005*
	Median V45	4.65% (0.8–28.4)	6.3% (2–13.2)	0.9999
Kidney (ipsilateral)	Mean dose	34.1 (4.7–52.7)	22.5 (0–53.3)	0.2160
	V5	98.5% (15.9–100)	58.7% (0.2–100)	0.3119
	V10	85.2% (11.6–100)	57.6% (0–100)	0.3270
	V20	75.3% (7.9–100)	55.5% (0–100)	0.4443
Kidney (contralateral)	Mean dose	6.4 (0–17.0)	0 (0–1.4)	*0.0320*
	V5	49.9% (0–100)	0% (0–8.2)	*0.0493*
	V10	11.5% (0–66.8)	0% (0–4.8)	0.1916
	V20	0% (0–28.6)	0% (0–1.6)	0.9800
Liver	Mean dose	15.7 (2.3–26.8)	2.4 (0–23.8)	*0.0161*
Integral dose	Mean (J)	400 (205–587)	126 (40–209)	*0.0161*

Dose reported in Gy (IMRT) and cobalt gray equivalent (proton)
V5 volume receiving 5 Gy, J joules

22 Sarcoma

Fig. 22.3 Cumulative dose-volume histogram for target volumes and OARs for Case 1, a three-field passive-scattering plan for treatment of a gluteal sarcoma

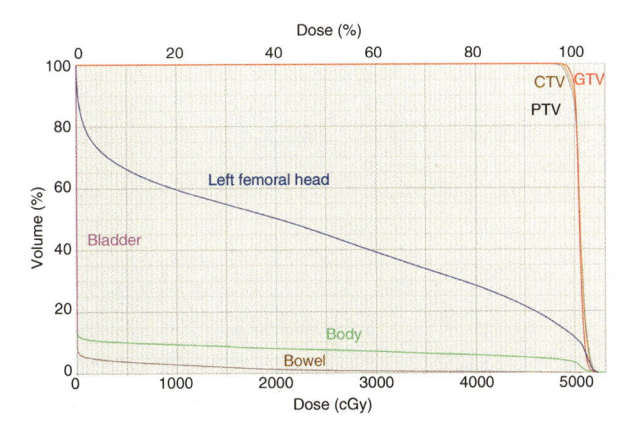

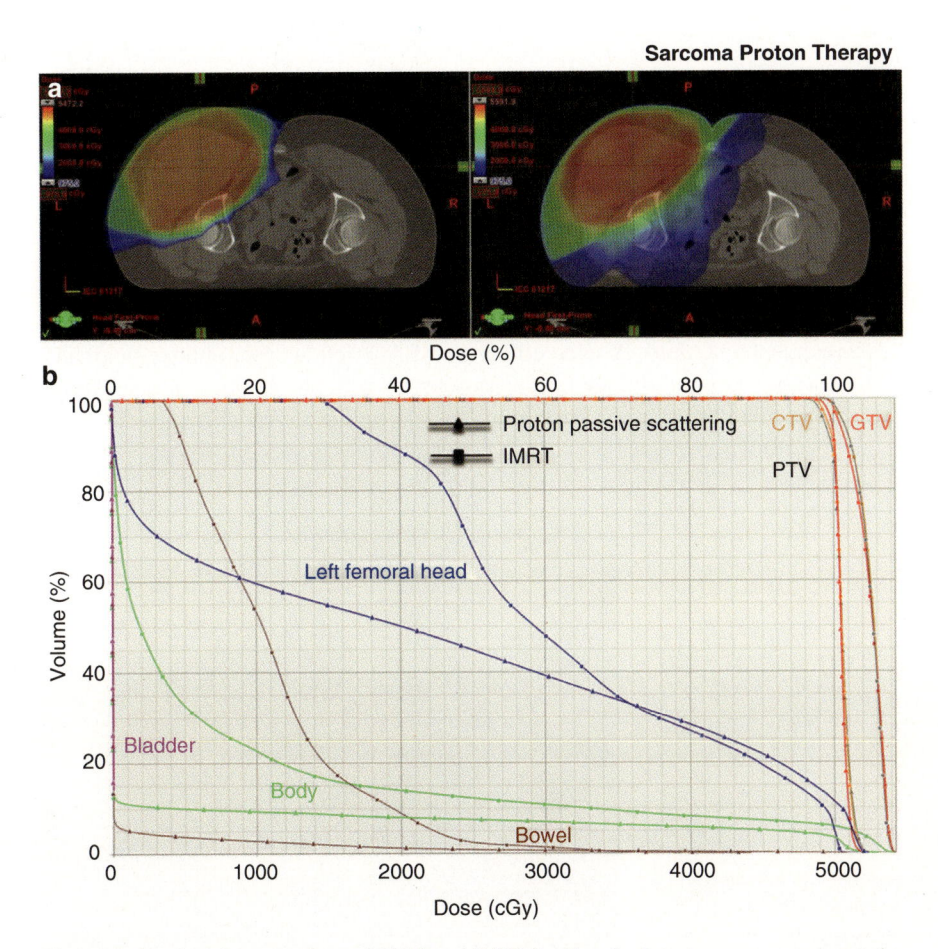

Sarcoma Proton Therapy

Fig. 22.4 Dosimetric comparison of 3DPT and IMRT for Case 1, gluteal sarcoma: representative dose distribution (**a**) and DVH comparison (**b**)

Case 2 Preoperative upper extremity/thoracic case: 63-year-old male with high-grade pleomorphic sarcoma of right pectoralis major insertion just inferior to the shoulder, cT2bN0M0G3, s/p 6 cycles of neoadjuvant chemotherapy, treated in 25 fractions at 2 Gy (RBE) = 50 Gy (RBE).

1. *Simulation*: CT imaging from vertex through diaphragm with 1.5 mm slice thickness in the supine position with bolster under the knees, the head turned to the left with left arm straight by side and right arm akimbo in a vac-lock bag for appropriate, customized immobilization (Fig. 22.5). The patient was offset to the left on the table. The secondary imaging was MR imaging with IV contrast.
2. *Planning*: A two-field PS plan utilizing an LAO (left anterior oblique field) and RSAO (right superior anterior oblique field) was selected with the shortest, simplest beam paths maximal sparing the shoulder, lower neck, and central thoracic OARs (Fig. 22.6). Similar PS planning considerations as detailed in the case above.

Case 3 Preoperative lower extremity case: 18-year-old female with myxoid liposarcoma of the medial knee/distal thigh, treated in 25 fractions at 2 Gy (RBE) = 50 Gy (RBE).

1. *Simulation*: CT imaging from pelvis through knee with 1.5 mm slice thickness in the feet-first, supine position with involved knee built up and slightly elevated in a vac-lock bag for appropriate, customized immobilization (Fig. 22.7). The secondary imaging was MR imaging with IV contrast.
2. *Planning*: A two-field, PS plan utilizing an LAO (left anterior oblique field) and RAO (right anterior oblique field) was selected with the shortest, simplest beam paths maximal sparing the knee joint, vessels, and posterior normal soft tissues (Fig. 22.8) with similar PS planning considerations as detailed above.

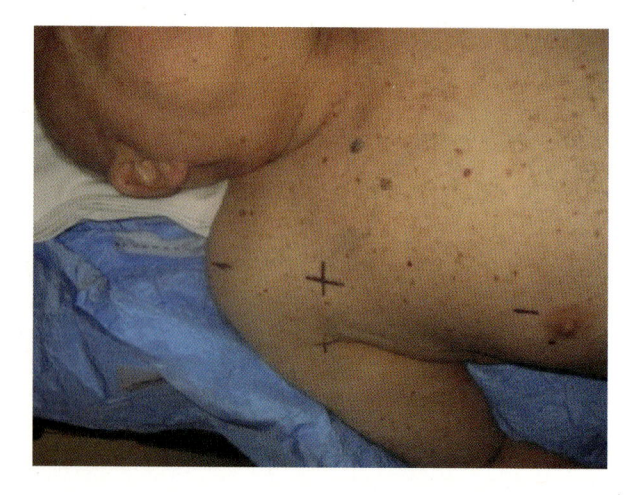

Fig. 22.5 Preoperative upper-extremity/thoracic case setup and immobilization

22 Sarcoma

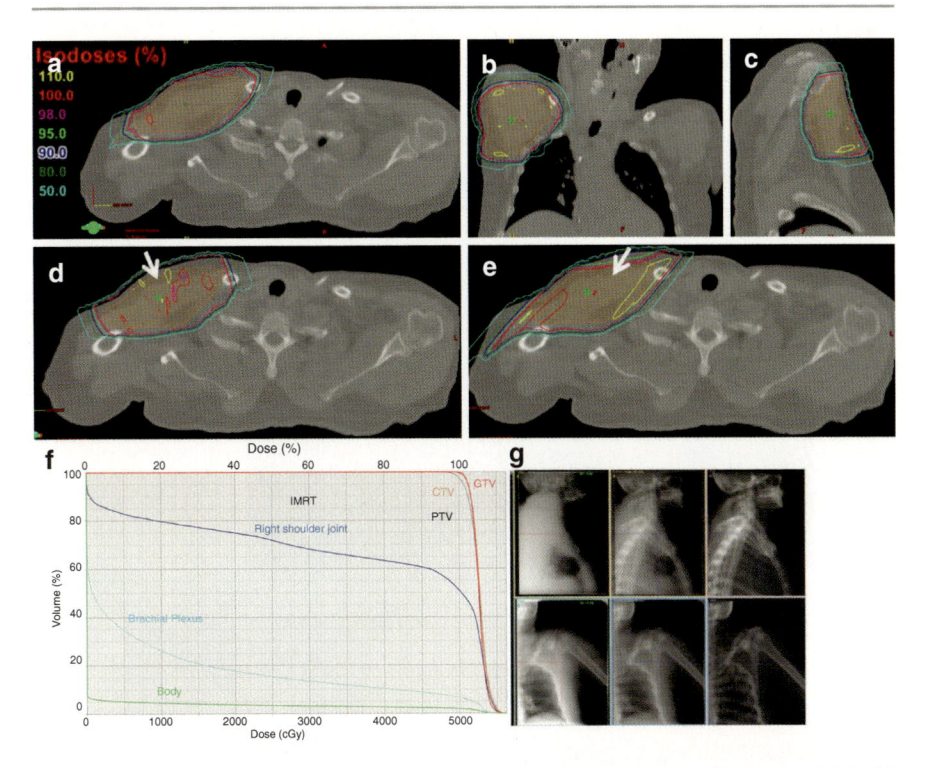

Fig. 22.6 Passive-scattering plan for treatment of an upper-extremity/thoracic sarcoma field with two-field beam arrangement including an LAO (left anterior oblique field) and RSAO (right superior anterior oblique field). Composite dose from axial, sagittal, and coronal view ((**a**), (**b**), (**c**)), dose contribution from individual field ((**d**) and (**e**)), DVH (**f**), and representative daily kV IG technique (**g**)

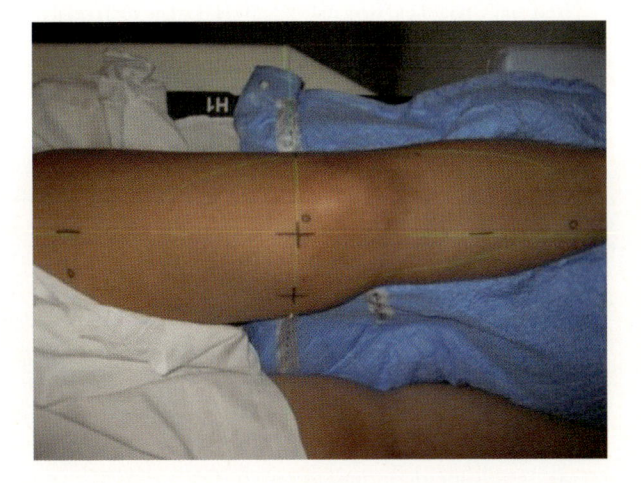

Fig. 22.7 Preoperative extremity (medial knee/distal thigh) supine setup and immobilization

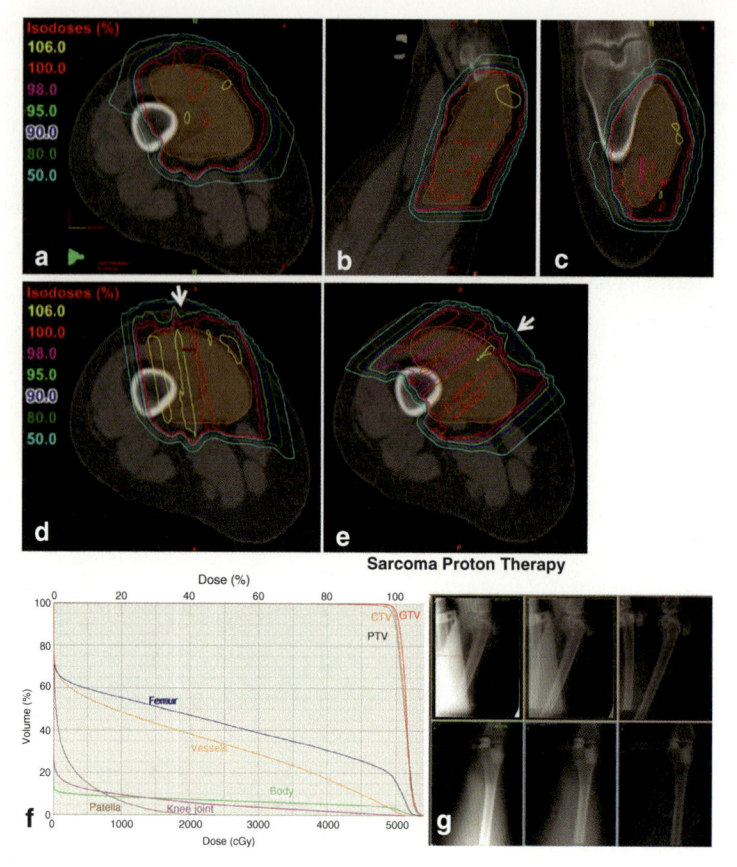

Fig. 22.8 Passive-scattering plan for treatment of a lower extremity/knee sarcoma field with two-field beam arrangement including an LAO (left anterior oblique field) and RAO (right anterior oblique field). Composite dose from axial, sagittal, and coronal view ((**a**), (**b**), (**c**)), dose contribution from individual field ((**d**) and (**e**)), DVH (**f**), and representative daily kV IG technique (**g**)

22.6 Pencil-Beam Scanning (PBS)

1. PBS provides proton therapy the ability to conform the dose in a 3-dimensional fashion using one beam.
2. Compared to PS, PBS provides the advantages of more conformal target dose, especially proximally, larger treatment field size, less neutron dose, and elimination of the time and resources required for the use of aperture and compensators. As no compensator is used, distal and proximal margins are both 2 mm shorter for PBS compared to PS.
3. PBS plans are separated into two categories depending on their treatment planning optimization method:
   (a) Single-field optimization (SFO) or SFUD (single field uniform dose)—based on field-specific optimization. The goal of the optimization is that

each individual field uniformly covers the whole-target volume (though, in practice, the dose homogeneity requirement may be relaxed due to dose constraints of adjacent/overlapping OARs). It has limited OAR sparing when the OAR is located proximal to the beam (Chap. 3).
 (b) Multi-field optimization (MFO or IMPT)—this category, on the other hand, has no requirements for individual fields. Instead, the optimization is performed for all fields together to achieve the target coverage as well as additional dose constrains of OARs, i.e., each field may only cover part of the target with modulated intensity, while the composition of all fields provides full coverage of the target (Chap. 3).
4. Given the same treatment fields and geometry, SFO is generally considered to be more robust than IMPT against delivery uncertainties, while IMPT may offer more OAR sparing in certain clinical circumstances (Fig. 22.9j). Until PBS becomes more mature, SFO plans are generally recommended whenever feasible, with IMPT reserved only for cases where it is deemed clinically necessary. IMPT is often used in combination with SFO or IMRT as part of multimodality therapy [31].
5. A simple and well-accepted approach to improve SFO robustness is using multiple fields. Multiple fields with larger angular separation reduce the concerns of range uncertainties and effect of potential uncertainties in RBE. Additionally, the dose heterogeneities resulting from interplay effects can be smoothed out simply as the cold and hot spots are generally located in different positions for different fields.
6. A simultaneous integrated boost approach is available for both SFO and IMPT, which can provide the potential for dose escalation.
7. When the target size is greater than the maximum PBS field size, abutting fields using gradient dose matching method can be easily and safely employed to cover the whole target without match line changes [32].

Case 4 Retroperitoneal sarcoma, postoperative case: 61-year-old female with left-sided retroperitoneal sarcoma s/p resection with multiple positive margins and sparing of ipsilateral kidney, treated in 35 fractions at 1.8 Gy (RBE) = 63 Gy (RBE).

1. *Simulation*: 4DCT imaging from diaphragm through pelvis with 1.5 mm slice thickness in the supine position in a vac-lock bag for appropriate, customized immobilization. The secondary imaging was MR imaging with IV contrast.
2. *Planning*: For both the initial ITV and sequential conedown to the HRITV, a two-field PBS plan utilizing a posterior field (PO) and left posterior oblique field (LPO) was selected using SFO to spare the adjacent bowel, kidney, and other OARs (Fig. 22.9).
3. Verification scan at fraction 7 shows that CTV coverage is within 1% of planned coverage, and all OAR doses are the same or lower than were planned; PTV coverage reduced by apparent postoperative weight gain (Fig. 22.10).

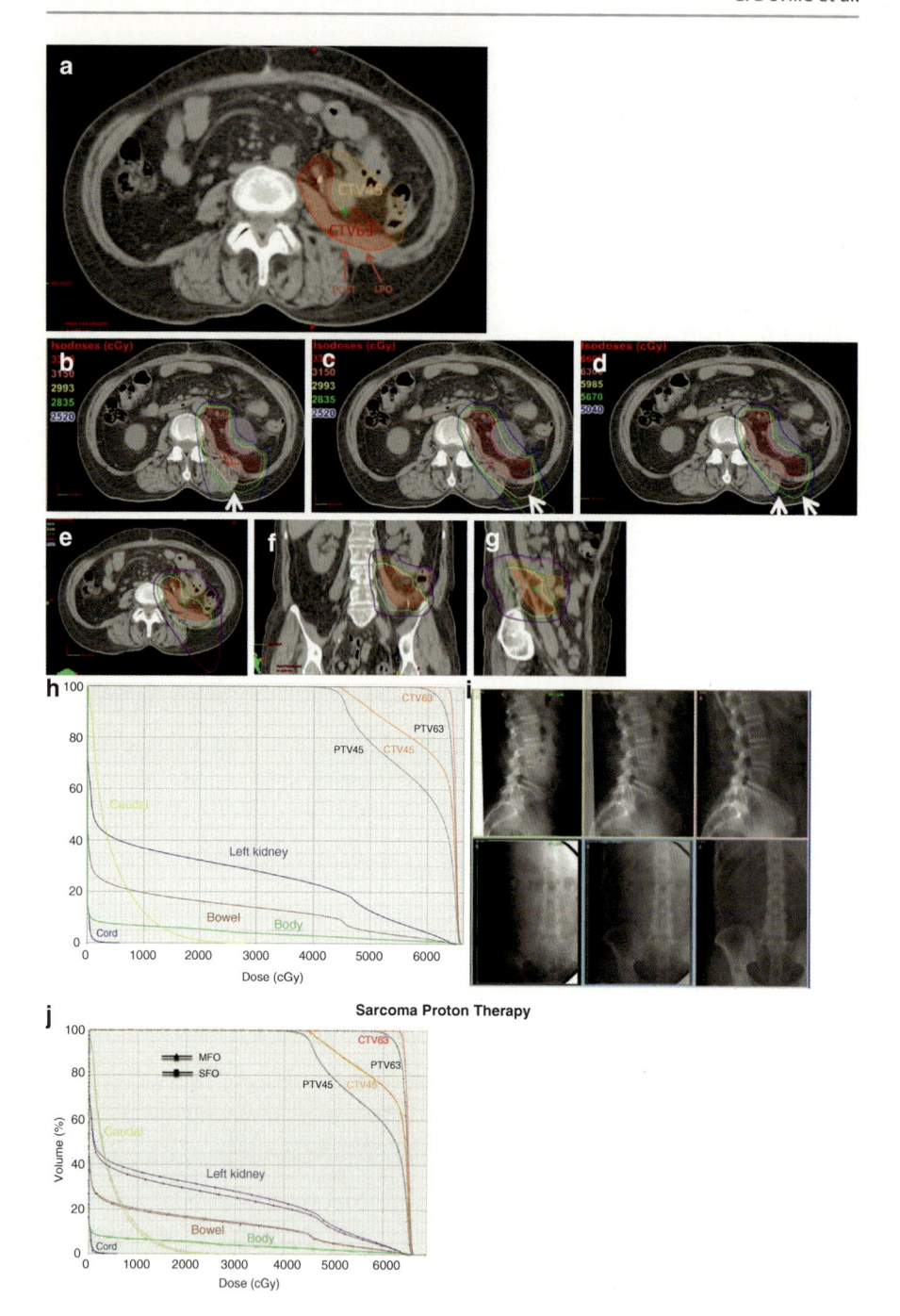

Fig. 22.9 PBS SFO plan for postoperative treatment of a retroperitoneal sarcoma with two-field arrangement including posterior field (PO) and left posterior oblique field (LPO). Initial ITV (CTV45) and HRITV (CTV63) (**a**), dose contribution from individual initial fields ((**b**), (**c**)), composite initial fields (**d**), composite dose from axial, sagittal and coronal view ((**e**), (**f**), (**g**)), DVH (**h**), representative daily kV IG technique (**i**), and DVH comparison of SFO and MFO (**j**)

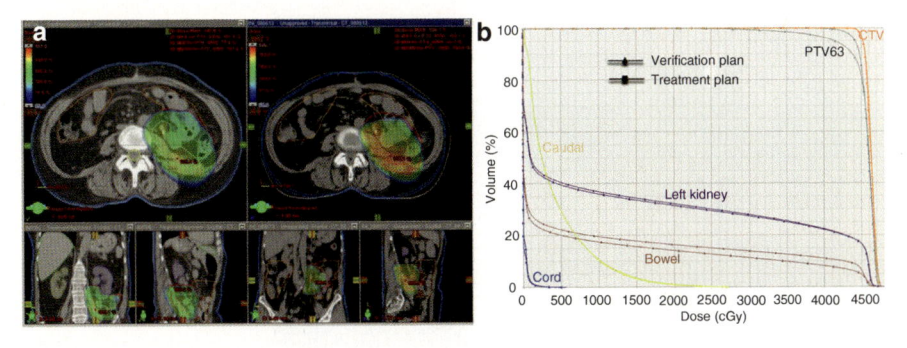

Fig. 22.10 Dosimetric comparison of initial and verification plans for a postoperative retroperitoneal sarcoma case: representative dose distribution (**a**) and DVH comparison (**b**)

Case 5 Pelvic chordoma, definitive RT: 46-year-old female with a sacral chordoma. After multidisciplinary discussions, patient declined surgery due to desire for bowel and bladder preservation. She was treated in 43 fractions at 1.8 Gy RBE = 77.4 Gy RBE. A three-phase plan was used including CTV 50.4 (GTV + 2 cm), CTV 70.4 (GTV + 0.5 cm), and CTV 77.4 (GTV only). All volumes were tailored to omit appropriate OARs. Prior to CT simulation, a spacer was surgically implanted to displace small bowel away from the tumor (Fig. 22.11).

1. *Simulation*: 3DCT imaging of the pelvis with 1.5 mm slice thickness in the supine position in a vac-lock bag for customized immobilization. The secondary imaging was MR imaging with IV contrast.
2. *Planning*: For both the initial CTV 50.4 and CTV 70.4, a three-field (PA, LPO, RPO) SFO PBS plan was used (Fig. 22.11). For the CTV 77.4 a single PA field was used for optimal bowel sparing (Fig. 22.11). A proton-specific PTV margin was used for setup uncertainty:
   (a) In the case where a single beam is used, care must be taken to ensure adequate compensation for range uncertainty and to account for possible increased RBE at the end of the range.
   (b) The range uncertainty depends on the depth of penetration and the anatomical stability of the tissues proximal to the target, e.g., tumor shrinkage and setup uncertainties.
   (c) Robust optimization will allow building a certain degree of range and setup uncertainties into the calculation, which can be evaluated using a robust analysis of the beam. However, anatomical changes cannot be estimated and have to be evaluated using volumetric imaging during the course of treatment. For shallow targets, the range uncertainty is typically small.
   (d) In this case, robustness settings of 0.5 cm uniform patient-position uncertainty and a 3.5% range uncertainty were used during the three-field phases. For the single PA field, 0.6 cm uniform patient-position uncertainty and a 3% range uncertainty were used. End-of-range RBE effects can now be simulated with Monte Carlo techniques.

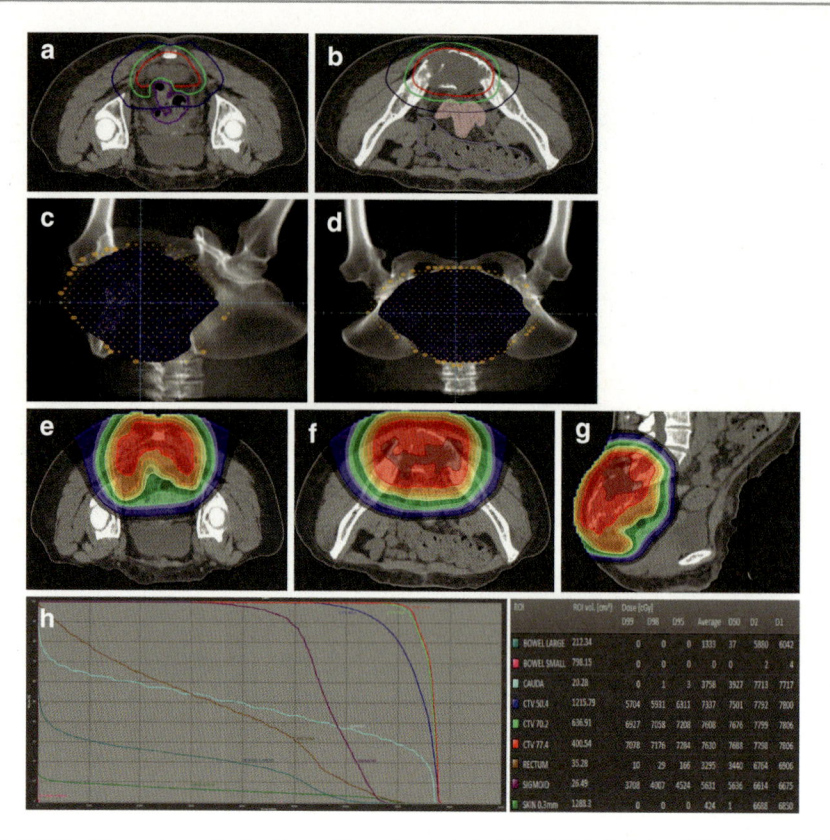

Fig. 22.11 The contours for the three-phase plan included CTV 50.4 (*blue*) = GTV + 2 cm, CTV 70.4 (*green*) = GTV + 0.5 cm, and CTV 77.4 (*red*) = GTV only (A and B). The surgically placed spacer is shown in pink (**b**). Beam's eye view of the LPO field (**c**) and PA field (**d**) with the CTV 50.4 volume shown in blue and the PBS spot placement overlaid in orange. Dose distributions for the composite SFO PBS plan are shown ((**e**), (**f**), (**g**)) alongside the DVH (**h**). Notably, the CTV 77.4 coverage was intentionally reduced to respect rectal and bowel constraints. The placement of a spacer significantly limited the dose to the small bowel

22.7 Future Developments

22.7.1 IMPT

1. IMPT, in particular, as dose painting to the high-risk margin is in the early stages of utilization and exploration.
2. Like photon IMRT, IMPT allows for more flexibility and dose modulation in planning than SFO. By employing multiple fields from differing incident angles, IMPT provides more potential for OARs sparing especially for those overlapping the target volume.
3. The main concern in employing IMPT exclusively is reduced treatment robustness. By incorporating robustness directly into the optimization stage or through

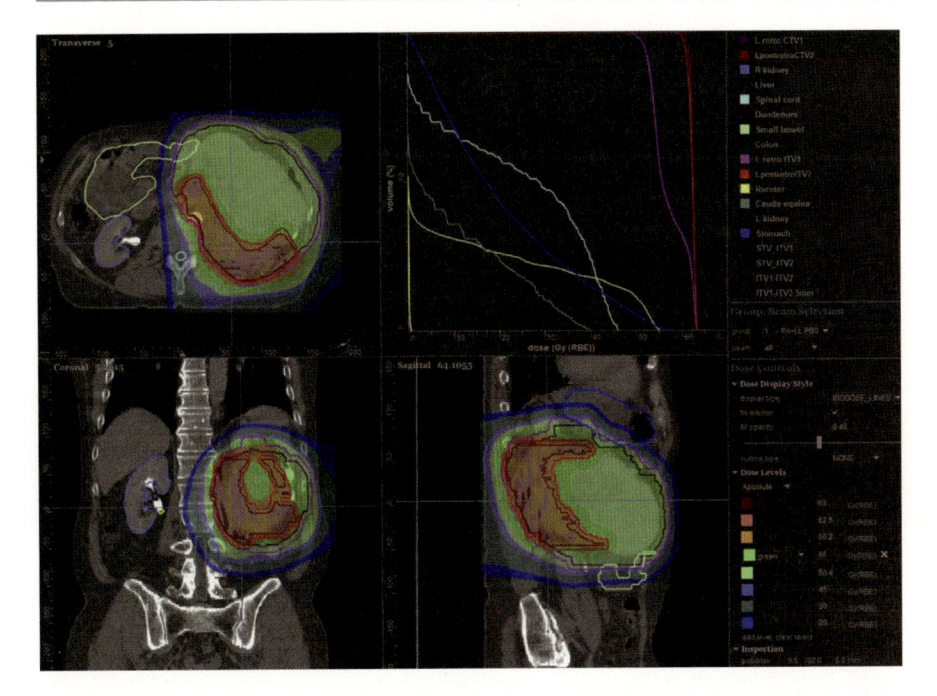

Fig. 22.12 IMPT intensity-modulated proton therapy plan for patient with a retroperitoneal leiomyosarcoma being treated on a study of preoperative radiation dose escalation to the high-risk posterior margin. The average-risk clinical target volume received 50.4 Gy (RBE) and the high-risk posterior margin received 60.2 Gy (RBE) (from [34])

the manipulation of starting conditions of the IMPT optimization (robust optimization and multi-criteria optimization [33]), the flexibility of IMPT is exploited to make the plan more robust against range uncertainties, setup error, and organ motion [34] (Fig. 22.12).

References

1. Siegel RL, Miller KD, Jemal A. Cancer statistics, 2016. CA Cancer J Clin. 2016;66(1):7–30.
2. Lawrence W Jr, Donegan WL, Natarajan N, Mettlin C, Beart R, Winchester D. Adult soft tissue sarcomas. A pattern of care survey of the American College of Surgeons. Ann Surg. 1987;205(4):349–59.
3. Doyle LA. Sarcoma classification: an update based on the 2013 World Health Organization Classification of Tumors of Soft Tissue and Bone. Cancer. 2014;120(12):1763–74.
4. Christie-Large M, James SL, Tiessen L, Davies AM, Grimer RJ. Imaging strategy for detecting lung metastases at presentation in patients with soft tissue sarcomas. Eur J Cancer. 2008;44(13):1841–5.
5. Johannesmeyer D, Smith V, Cole DJ, Esnaola NF, Camp ER. The impact of lymph node disease in extremity soft-tissue sarcomas: a population-based analysis. Am J Surg. 2013;206(3):289–95. https://doi.org/10.1016/j.amjsurg.2012.10.043. Epub 2013 Jun 24 PubMed

6. Rosenberg SA, Tepper J, Glatstein E, Costa J, Baker A, Brennan M, DeMoss EV, Seipp C, Sindelar WF, Sugarbaker P, Wesley R. The treatment of soft-tissue sarcomas of the extremities: prospective randomized evaluations of (1) limb-sparing surgery plus radiation therapy compared with amputation and (2) the role of adjuvant chemotherapy. Ann Surg. 1982;196(3):305–15.
7. Haas RL, Delaney TF, O'Sullivan B, Keus RB, Le Pechoux C, Olmi P, Poulsen JP, Seddon B, Wang D. Radiotherapy for management of extremity soft tissue sarcomas: why, when, and where? Int J Radiat Oncol Biol Phys. 2012;84(3):572–80.
8. McGee L, Indelicato DJ, Dagan R, Morris CG, Knapik JA, Reith JD, Scarborough MT, Gibbs CP, Marcus RB Jr, Zlotecki RA. Long-term results following postoperative radiotherapy for soft tissue sarcomas of the extremity. Int J Radiat Oncol Biol Phys. 2012;84(4):1003–9.
9. https://clinicaltrials.gov/ct2/show/NCT01344018?term=NCT01344018&rank=1. Accessed 24 June 2016.
10. Tzeng CW, Fiveash JB, Popple RA, Arnoletti JP, Russo SM, Urist MM, Bland KI, Heslin MJ. Preoperative radiation therapy with selective dose escalation to the margin at risk for retroperitoneal sarcoma. Cancer. 2006;107(2):371–9.
11. https://clinicaltrials.gov/ct2/show/NCT01659203?term=NCT01659203&rank=1. Accessed 24 June 2016.
12. Davis AM, O'Sullivan B, Turcotte R, Bell R, Catton C, Chabot P, Wunder J, Hammond A, Benk V, Kandel R, Goddard K, Freeman C, Sadura A, Zee B, Day A, Tu D, Pater J, Canadian Sarcoma Group; NCI Canada Clinical Trial Group Randomized Trial. Late radiation morbidity following randomization to preoperative versus postoperative radiotherapy in extremity soft tissue sarcoma. Radiother Oncol. 2005;75(1):48–53.
13. Gustafson P, Dreinhöfer KE, Rydholm A. Soft tissue sarcoma should be treated at a tumor center. A comparison of quality of surgery in 375 patients. Acta Orthop Scand. 1994;65(1):47–50.
14. Pervaiz N, Colterjohn N, Farrokhyar F, Tozer R, Figueredo A, Ghert M. A systematic meta-analysis of randomized controlled trials of adjuvant chemotherapy for localized resectable soft-tissue sarcoma. Cancer. 2008;113(3):573–81.
15. Pisters PW, Pollock RE, Lewis VO, Yasko AW, Cormier JN, Respondek PM, Feig BW, Hunt KK, Lin PP, Zagars G, Wei C, Ballo MT. Long-term results of prospective trial of surgery alone with selective use of radiation for patients with T1 extremity and trunk soft tissue sarcomas. Ann Surg. 2007;246(4):675–81. discussion 681-2
16. Kepka L, DeLaney TF, Suit HD, Goldberg SI. Results of radiation therapy for unresected soft-tissue sarcomas. Int J Radiat Oncol Biol Phys. 2005;63(3):852–9.
17. Weber DC, Rutz HP, Bolsi A, Pedroni E, Coray A, Jermann M, Lomax AJ, Hug EB, Goitein G. Spot scanning proton therapy in the curative treatment of adult patients with sarcoma: the Paul Scherrer institute experience. Int J Radiat Oncol Biol Phys. 2007;69(3):865–71.
18. Guttmann DM, Frick MA, Carmona R, Deville Jr C, Levin WP, Berman AT, Chinniah C, Hahn SM, Plastaras JP, Simone II CB. A prospective study of proton reirradiation for recurrent and secondary soft tissue sarcoma. Radiother Oncol. 2017 Aug;124(2):271–276.
19. DeLaney TF, Liebsch NJ, Pedlow FX, et al. Phase II study of high-dose photon/proton radiotherapy in the management of spine sarcomas. Int J Radiat Oncol Biol Phys. 2009;74:732–9.
20. Rotondo RL, Folkert W, Liebsch NJ, et al. High-dose proton-based radiation therapy in the management of spine chordomas: outcomes and clinicopathological prognostic factors. J Neurosurg Spine. 2015;23:788–97.
21. Noël G, Habrand JL, Jauffret E, de Crevoisier R, Dederke S, Mammar H, Haie-Méder C, Pontvert D, Hasboun D, Ferrand R, Boisserie G, Beaudré A, Gaboriaud G, Guedea F, Petriz L, Mazeron JJ. Radiation therapy for chordoma and chondrosarcoma of the skull base and the cervical spine. Prognostic factors and patterns of failure. Strahlenther Onkol. 2003;179(4):241–8.
22. Ciernik IF, Niemierko A, Harmon DC, Kobayashi W, Chen YL, Yock TI, Ebb DH, Choy E, Raskin KA, Liebsch N, Hornicek FJ, Delaney TF. Proton-based radiotherapy for unresectable or incompletely resected osteosarcoma. Cancer. 2011;117(19):4522–30.
23. Kamada T, Tsujii H, Blakely EA, Debus J, De Neve W, Durante M, Jäkel O, Mayer R, Orecchia R, Pötter R, Vatnitsky S, Chu WT. Carbon ion radiotherapy in Japan: an assessment of 20 years of clinical experience. Lancet Oncol. 2015;16(2):e93–e100.

24. Sugahara S, Kamada T, Imai R, Tsuji H, Kameda N, Okada T, Tsujii H, Tatezaki S, Working Group for the Bone and Soft Tissue Sarcomas. Carbon ion radiotherapy for localized primary sarcoma of the extremities: results of a phase I/II trial. Radiother Oncol. 2012;105(2):226–31.
25. ICRU. ICRU Report 78. Prescribing, recording, and reporting proton-beam therapy. J ICRU. 2007;7(2). doi:https://doi.org/10.1093/jicru/ndm021.
26. O'Sullivan B, Griffin AM, Dickie CI, Sharpe MB, Chung PW, Catton CN, Ferguson PC, Wunder JS, Deheshi BM, White LM, Kandel RA, Jaffray DA, Bell RS. Phase 2 study of preoperative image-guided intensity-modulated radiation therapy to reduce wound and combined modality morbidities in lower extremity soft tissue sarcoma. Cancer. 2013;119(10):1878–84.
27. Wang D, Zhang Q, Eisenberg BL, Kane JM, Li XA, Lucas D, Petersen IA, DeLaney TF, Freeman CR, Finkelstein SE, Hitchcock YJ, Bedi M, Singh AK, Dundas G, Kirsch DG. Significant reduction of late toxicities in patients with extremity sarcoma treated with image-guided radiation therapy to a reduced target volume: results of radiation therapy oncology Group RTOG-0630 Trial. J Clin Oncol. 2015;33(20):2231–8.
28. Moyers MF, Miller DW, Bush DA, et al. Methodologies and tools for proton beam design for lung tumors. Int J Radiat Oncol Biol Phys. 2001;49(5):1429–38.
29. ICRU. Prescribing and reporting photon beam therapy. Report 62. Washington, D.C.: International Commission on Radiation Units and Measurements; 1999.
30. Swanson EL, Indelicato DJ, Louis D, Flampouri S, Li Z, Morris CG, Paryani N, Slopsema R. Comparison of three-dimensional (3D) conformal proton radiotherapy (RT), 3D conformal photon RT, and intensity-modulated RT for retroperitoneal and intra-abdominal sarcomas. Int J Radiat Oncol Biol Phys. 2012;83(5):1549–57.
31. Lomax AJ. Intensity modulated proton therapy and its sensitivity to treatment uncertainties 2: the potential effects of inter-fraction and inter-field motions. Phys Med Biol. 2008;53(4):1043–56.
32. Lin H, Ding X, Kirk M, Liu H, Zhai H, Hill-Kayser CE, Lustig RA, Tochner Z, Both S, McDonough J. Supine craniospinal irradiation using a proton pencil beam scanning technique without match line changes for field junctions. Int J Radiat Oncol Biol Phys. 2014;90(1):71–8.
33. Albertini F, Hug EB, Lomax AJ. The influence of the optimization starting conditions on the robustness of intensity-modulated proton therapy plans. Phys Med Biol. 2010;55(10):2863–78.
34. DeLaney TF, Haas RL. Innovative radiotherapy of sarcoma: proton beam radiation. Eur J Cancer. 2016;62:112–23.
35. Baldini EH, Wang D, Haas RL, Catton CN, Indelicato DJ, Kirsch DG, Roberge D, Salerno K, Deville C, Guadagnolo BA, O'Sullivan B, Petersen IA, Le Pechoux C, Abrams RA, DeLaney TF. Treatment guidelines for preoperative radiation therapy for retroperitoneal sarcoma: preliminary consensus of an International Expert Panel. Int J Radiat Oncol Biol Phys. 2015;92(3):602–12.
36. Baldini EH, Bosch W, Kane JM III, Abrams RA, Salerno KE, Deville C, Raut CP, Petersen IA, Chen YL, Mullen JT, Millikan KW, Karakousis G, Kendrick ML, DeLaney TF, Wang D. Retroperitoneal sarcoma (RPS) high risk gross tumor volume boost (HR GTV boost) contour delineation agreement among NRG sarcoma radiation and surgical oncologists. Ann Surg Oncol. 2015;22(9):2846–52.

Mediastinal Lymphoma

23

Bradford S. Hoppe, Stella Flampouri, Christine Hill-Kayser, and John P. Plastaras

Contents

23.1	Introduction	369
23.2	Simulation, Target Delineation, Radiation Dose, and Fractionation	371
23.3	Passive-Scattering Treatment Planning	373
23.4	Pencil-Beam Scanning	376
	23.4.1 Irregular and Noncontiguous Targets	376
	23.4.2 Long/Wide Targets	378
	23.4.3 Motion Management	378
	23.4.4 Beam-Angle Selection	378
23.5	Future Developments	379
References		379

23.1 Introduction

Hodgkin lymphoma (HL) is a rare diagnosis, with only 9000 cases diagnosed in the USA annually [1]; however, it is the most common malignancy diagnosed in adolescents and young adults 15–19 years of age [2]. Radiation is currently used as primary treatment for early-stage nodular lymphocyte-predominant HL and as consolidation after chemotherapy in early-stage classic HL and bulky mediastinal stage III/IV as well as for slowly responding sites of disease. Approximately 60–70% of

B.S. Hoppe (✉) • S. Flampouri
Department of Radiation Oncology, University of Florida College of Medicine, 2000 SW Archer Road, Gainesville,, FL 33710, USA
e-mail: bhoppe@floridaproton.org

C. Hill-Kayser • J.P. Plastaras
Department of Radiation Oncology, University of Pennsylvania Perelman School of Medicine, Philadelphia, PA, USA

© Springer International Publishing Switzerland 2018
N. Lee et al. (eds.), *Target Volume Delineation and Treatment Planning for Particle Therapy*, Practical Guides in Radiation Oncology, https://doi.org/10.1007/978-3-319-42478-1_23

HL patients will have mediastinal involvement, and 30% of all HL patients will receive radiation [3].

Non-Hodgkin lymphoma (NHL) is comprised of over 100 subtypes with approximately 66,000 cases diagnosed in the USA annually [1]. Primary mediastinal large B-cell lymphoma (PMLBCL) arises from the thymic B cells and comprises 7% of all diffuse large B-cell lymphomas or 2.4% of all NHL [4]. PMLBCL typically affects younger patients (those in their 30s) with a predominance of females over males (3:2) [5].

Standard treatment for HL incorporates chemotherapy with radiation delivered to all sites of initial involvement for early-stage disease and to bulky mediastinal sites or slowly responding sites for stage III/IV disease. For PMLBCL, dose-adjusted R-EPOCH alone (rituximab, etoposide, prednisone, vincristine sulfate, cyclophosphamide, and doxorubicin hydrochloride) can provide excellent results without radiation, while R-CHOP chemotherapy (rituximab, cyclophosphamide, doxorubicin hydrochloride, vincristine sulfate, and prednisone) requires consolidative radiation.

Based on the favorable outcomes and early age of diagnosis, both PMLBCL and HL survivors are expected to live for several decades. Consequently, late side effects from curative therapy become a significant problem for survivors. Recent trials have focused on reducing late morbidity without compromising cure.

Proton therapy is currently being used for HL and NHL in a variety of clinical settings, most prominently for treatment of the mediastinum. Patients with mediastinal lymphoma are at significant risk of cardiac toxicity from both anthracycline chemotherapy and cardiac radiation, as well as radiation-induced second cancers, including breast cancer, lung cancer, thyroid cancer, and sarcomas, decades after treatment.

Radiation dose to the organs at risk (OARs) has been the best surrogate for predicting the risk of subsequent late toxicity, with increasing dose to the OARs being associated with a higher risk of all reported late effects, except for thyroid cancer (peaking at 15–20 Gy) [6, 7].

Multiple dosimetric studies comparing proton therapy to intensity-modulated radiation therapy (IMRT) and three-dimensional conformal radiation therapy (3DCRT) have been conducted, and all demonstrate that proton therapy can best reduce the radiation dose to the OARs [8–12]. Data from a prospective study conducted at the University of Florida Health Proton Therapy Institute (Jacksonville, FL) are reported in Table 23.1. In this study, all 20 patients enrolled derived a dosimetric benefit from proton therapy over either 3DCRT or IMRT [13].

Early disease-specific results have been favorable for the use of proton therapy in HL and NHL, similar to outcomes for IMRT or 3DCRT, without any grade 3 toxicities [13–15]. Although follow-up is not currently mature for assessment of late effects among lymphoma patients treated with proton therapy, clinical data not specific to lymphoma have demonstrated a reduced risk of secondary cancers when proton therapy is used instead of photon radiation [16].

23 Mediastinal Lymphoma

Table 23.1 Average dose to the organs at risk according to treatment technique for the 20 patients enrolled in the HL01 prospective study at the University of Florida Health Proton Therapy Institute

Characteristic	3D-CRT	IMRT	PT
Heart (mean)	16.5 Gy	12.3 Gy	8.9 Gy
Lung (mean)	11.6 Gy	9.8 Gy	7.1 Gy
Breast (mean)	6.3 Gy	6.0 Gy	4.3 Gy
Thyroid (mean dose)	19.3 Gy	17.7 Gy	15.8 Gy
Esophagus (mean dose)	20.3 Gy	16.4 Gy	13.4 Gy
Total body (integral dose)	123 J	104 J	54 J

23.2 Simulation, Target Delineation, Radiation Dose, and Fractionation

Patient positioning for simulation and treatment requires customization based on patient age, sex, disease distribution, and positioning at the time of the prechemotherapy positron-emission tomography/computed tomography scan. Special care must be taken to determine arm and neck positioning.

Due to the response to chemotherapy, most patients will not have disease present at the time of simulation in all of the regions initially involved at presentation. Modern radiation planning using involved-site radiation therapy (ISRT) requires appropriate image fusion with prechemotherapy imaging to identify the initial sites of involvement [17]. When image fusion is poor, a larger clinical target volume (CTV) expansion is needed to accommodate for the uncertainty, while less expansion is needed when the fusion is more accurate. When disease involves the axilla, supraclavicular, and/or infraclavicular region, arm position (above head, akimbo, or at the side) can greatly impact fusion with the prechemotherapy imaging. This uncertainty and consequently larger CTV may lead to increased dose to the breast and lung. When the axilla is not involved, arm position is less critical.

When treating the thorax, the placement of arms above the head can pull the breasts superiorly and medially and pull the axilla and infraclavicular regions above the lung field, which can help reduce the dose to the lungs depending on the pattern of disease. When considering treatment with lateral fields, the arms above the head can preclude the need for radiation beams to pass through the arms. This position, however, is not comfortable for the patient, may not be easily reproducible, and may require larger margins for setup errors and their effect on proton range. A more comfortable and reproducible position for patients is with their arms at their sides or slightly akimbo. This position may allow the breasts to fall inferiorly and laterally, which, in certain circumstances, can reduce the amount of breast tissue receiving radiation. Angle boards aimed at moving the breasts and heart inferiorly have been used in photon clinics and could theoretically be applied to proton clinics. Aquaplast masks can be used to improve the reproducibility of the neck with respect to the mediastinum when both regions require treatment. Indexed immobilization devices must be routinely employed to maintain the patient's position in the beam.

All patients should undergo a CT simulation with and without intravenous contrast to help identify sites of interest. When the mediastinum or abdomen is involved, breathing motion may affect treatment; therefore, a four-dimensional CT scan is required to determine breathing motion and the appropriate involved tumor volume (ITV) margin. Alternatively, the deep-inspiration breath-hold (DIBH) technique can be used to reduce the breathing motion of the mediastinum with a full breath. DIBH has the added advantage of narrowing the mediastinum while pushing the lung and

Table 23.2 Contouring guidelines for involved-site radiotherapy

	Definitive ISRT	Consolidative ISRT	Consolidative ISRT to bulky disease
GTV (pre-chemo)	Gross disease as seen on PET/CT scan and planning CT sim	Gross disease as seen on prechemotherapy PET/CT scans	Gross bulky and adjacent connected disease as seen on prechemotherapy PET/CT scans
GTV (post-chemo)	Not applicable	Residual disease seen at the time of CT simulation that may be PET-negative (GTVPET-negative) or PET-positive (GTVPET-positive)	Residual disease seen at the time of CT simulation that may be PET-negative (GTVPET-negative) or PET-positive (GTVPET-positive)
CTV	GTV + 2–4 cm margin within nodal stations to encompass sites of subclinical disease	GTVpostchemotherapy + margin that includes sites of involvement of GTVprechemotherapy, while respecting normal tissue and OAR boundaries (i.e., if the lung was not involved, do not extend the CTV into the lung) + margin to account for fusion uncertainties between prechemotherapy imaging and CT simulation + margin to account for subclinical involvement (i.e., connecting uninvolved nodal stations lying between 2 involved sites within 5 cm of each other)	GTVpostchemotherapy + margin that includes sites of involvement of GTVprechemotherapy, while respecting normal tissue and OAR boundaries (i.e., if the lung was not involved, do not extend the CTV into the lung) + margin to account for fusion uncertainties between prechemotherapy imaging and CT simulation + margin to account for subclinical involvement (i.e., connecting uninvolved nodal stations lying between 2 involved sites within 5 cm of each other). Adjacent non-bulky well-responding sites of prior involvement can be excluded if they may lead to excessive irradiation of an OAR if included
ITV	CTV + margin for motion (0–2 cm) or + margin for breath-hold uncertainty with DIBH		
PTV	ITV + margin for set up uncertainties (0.3–1.5 cm)		

CTV clinical target volume, *DIBH* deep-inspiration breath-hold, *GTV* gross tumor volume, *ISRT* involved-site radiation therapy, *OAR* organs at risk, *PET/CT* positron emission tomography/computed tomography

Table 23.3 Recommended dose constraints to organs at risk when using proton beam therapy for mediastinal lymphoma

Organ-at-risk	Recommended dose-constraint
Heart	Mean dose < 15 Gy (RBE); minimize left anterior descending artery, left ventricle, valves
Lungs	Mean dose < 15 Gy(RBE); V20 < 30%
Thyroid	Mean dose <
Breast	Minimize V4

These recommendations are adapted from institutional photon/intensity-modulated radiotherapy treatment planning. As additional data are accumulated, these constraints will continue to be refined. In practice, the treatment planner should make every effort to achieve the lowest dose possible for all normal tissues while maximizing coverage

heart away from the upper mediastinal targets, which can also decrease the dose to OARs for select cases [18, 19].

Target delineation is described in Table 23.2, and OAR dose constraints are considered in Table 23.3.

The radiation dose delivered for mediastinal lymphomas in photon or proton therapy is low (HL, ~20–40 Gy; PMLBCL, 30–45 Gy). Attempts should be made to cover the photon PTV completely. However, in proton therapy geometry does not equal dose, and, therefore, the PTV as a geometrical concept cannot guarantee target coverage even if larger margins are employed. In general, we try to achieve a PTVD95 = 100% and a PTV V95 = 100%; however, due to the concern of OAR dose, we will accept a PTVD95 > 95%. Additionally, ISRT guidelines allow for reducing the CTV volume when adjacent OAR dose constraints are being compromised.

23.3 Passive-Scattering Treatment Planning

The goal of treatment planning for ISRT for lymphoma with passive-scattered proton beams is to irradiate the target with an adequate dose while reducing the integral dose to the patient. Treatment planning is technically challenging because of the size and heterogeneity of the targets, consisting of a number of not always contiguous sub-volumes of varying size, shape, and location. Limitations of the passive-scattering delivery technique of proton beams include the maximum field size and the inability to conform the dose proximally to the target. Advantages to passive-scattering delivery include increased plan robustness to patient and target motion uncertainties relative to pencil-beam scanning (PBS).

Because of the non-isotropic nature of the proton uncertainties lateral and in the direction of each beam, a common planning strategy for passive-scattered proton treatments is to assign the CTV or ITV, if applicable, as the beam target. Depending on the effect of respiratory and cardiac functions on the target position as well as the motion mitigation techniques used, the internal CTV motion margin should be included in the ITV.

Commercial treatment planning systems allow that margins be applied for proton range uncertainties, distally and proximally, directly in the properties of each beam. Various institutions use a formula for inherent range uncertainties similar to that described by Moyers et al. [20]. That margin, applied along the proton beam, accounts for the Hounsfield-number-to-relative-proton-stopping-power conversion, beam-delivery reproducibility, treatment planning-system commissioning accuracy, and compensator design and milling. The effects of setup errors on the proton range are compensated by range compensator smearing (thinning) [21].

To avoid geographical misses lateral to the beam, collimator margins for the lateral penumbra are set to the PTV or to the CTV with an adequate expansion for setup variations. Although visualization of proton beam-specific treatment planning volumes is not currently available, appropriate margins can be set to ensure target coverage along and perpendicular to each beam.

Uncertainties due to potential relative biological effectiveness (RBE) variations along the spread-out Bragg peak can be reduced by using multiple treatment fields. Range feathering can be also employed to reduce potential high end-of-the range RBE effects.

Since mediastinal lymphomas may involve different sites of the mediastinum, such as the anterior mediastinum, superior mediastinum, and/or posterior mediastinum, no single simple principle can be used for treatment planning. General guidelines for beam selection include:

- The use of multiple beams to treat the same part of the target
- Preference for beams with a small path length
- The use of matching beams if the target depth changes significantly
- Match-line changes for sets of matching beams to reduce dose in homogeneities
- No beams crossing the heart

Figure 23.1 shows two potential beam arrangements for a patient with anterior mediastinal disease. In both cases, multiple fields are used; however, in the first plan, these two fields are entering at slightly oblique anterior angles, while in the second plan, they enter with an anterior and posterior field approach. The latter plan not only substantially increases the cardiac dose, as can be seen in the dose-volume histogram comparison and color wash, but also completely traverses the heart to get to the anterior mediastinal disease, which is counter to the goals of avoiding beams that cross the heart and beams that cross volumes of changing density (such as the heart throughout the cardiac cycle). Consequently, patients with anterior mediastinal disease won't benefit from proton therapy if planning is done inappropriately as shown in the dose-volume histogram (DVH).

Patient plans with alternative beam arrangements are shown in Fig. 23.2. In the top case, posterior beams spare both the heart and the breast of the patient. In the next case, both anterior and posterior matching beams were used to reduce the integral dose. In the bottom case, nine beams were used to treat the large target that included the neck, mediastinum, left axilla, spleen, and para-aortics. The ITV is

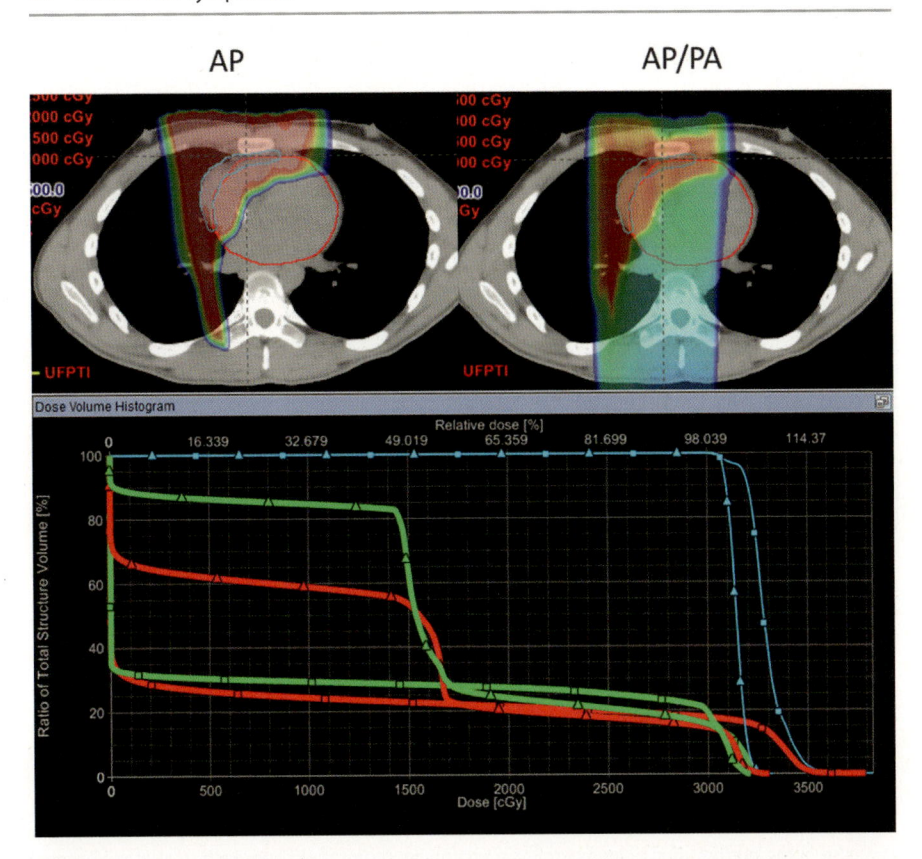

Fig. 23.1 Two potential beam arrangements with the color wash dose distribution for a patient with anterior mediastinal Hodgkin lymphoma. In both cases multiple fields are used; however, in the first plan, these two fields are entering at slightly oblique anterior angles, while in the second plan, they enter with an anterior and posterior field approach. The dose-volume histogram demonstrates the dramatic impact on the heart (*red*) and esophagus (*green*) and PTC (*blue*) with the anterior approach (*squares*) and anterior/posterior approach (*triangles*)

shown in green. The treatment time can vary from 30–90 min depending on the number of isocenters and fields being treated each day.

Plan evaluation is based on target coverage goals, OAR dose constraints, and plan quality indices such as integral dose and dose conformality. Frequently, the plans are normalized to the desired CTV coverage, but PTV coverage requirements are also set to facilitate photon and proton plan comparisons.

The previously discussed margins do not protect against occasional unpredictable changes that occur during the course of treatment, such as lymphoma progression, pleural effusion, pneumonia, or weight loss. Proton dose distributions are sensitive to changes of tissue density or position of tissue interfaces. If image-guided radiation therapy is not based on 3D imaging, repeat verification CT imaging and dose recalculation are recommended to verify the accuracy of the treatment.

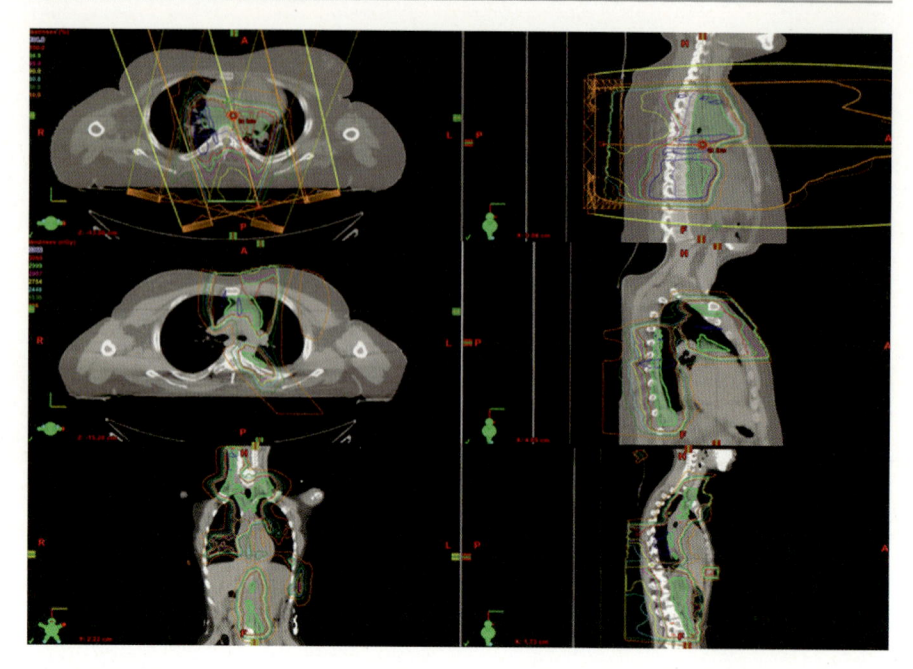

Fig. 23.2 Various beam arrangements for patients with different distributions of mediastinal lymphoma; the involved-site radiotherapy involved tumor volume is contoured in *green*. The case in the top image demonstrates a volume that lies posterior to the heart and consequently benefits from a posterior field approach to protect the heart and breast tissue. The case in the middle image shows a male with posterior mediastinal disease that benefits by treatment with a posterior field, while the superior mediastinal disease and left axillary disease are treated with an anterior field approach. The case in the bottom image demonstrates a complicated nine-field approach to treat a 17-year-old with stage IIIA bulky Hodgkin lymphoma with various matching anterior, posterior, and lateral fields to treat the posterior mediastinum, cervical neck, left axilla, spleen, and para-aortics

23.4 Pencil-Beam Scanning

23.4.1 Irregular and Noncontiguous Targets

Pencil-beam scanning (PBS) offers a potential advantage over double scattering (DS) with regard to conformality around OARs, especially when targets are irregular. PBS is particularly useful when the target volume varies markedly in depth, usually in the superior/inferior direction, or when the target is noncontiguous and extends over a large field size (the PBS maximum field size is 34 cm in the Y axis and 24 cm in the X axis vs. 24 cm for DS). For example, a typical ISRT target volume may encompass the entire depth of the mediastinum above the level of the heart but with a thin shallow extension that drapes in front of the heart (Fig. 23.3). Compared to photons, anterior proton beams can dramatically decrease the mean heart dose, a parameter that has been shown to correlate with the risk of late coronary heart disease [22]. However, due to the margin required for target coverage with proton therapy, the conformality of medium and high doses (range, 25–30 Gy

23 Mediastinal Lymphoma

[RBE]) may be worse than for IMRT. Treating the entire length of the field with DS using a single compensator provides poorly conformal plans for which target "tapering" is exaggerated. Various DS techniques can be used to help improve conformality, including manual compensator editing, splitting fields to use two (or more) compensators, and field matching as described above. Nevertheless, PBS solves many of the treatment planning complications of DS by allowing irregular and noncontiguous targets with homogeneous target coverage and improved sparing of OARs (Fig. 23.4) [12]. PBS allows delivery of 3D conformal treatments with

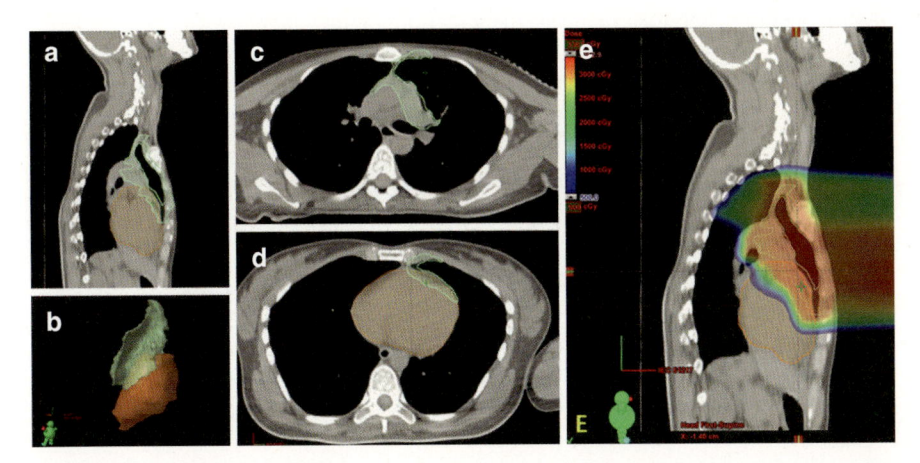

Fig. 23.3 An example of an irregular target volume using the involved-site radiotherapy paradigm in a patient with primary mediastinal large B-cell lymphoma in the anterior mediastinum with chest wall invasion. The involved tumor volume (*light green*) tapers to a thin anterior structure that drapes anterior to the heart (*orange*). Contours shown in (**a**) sagittal, (**b**) 3D rendering, and axial slices at (**c**) the level of left hilum, and (**d**) the most inferior involved tumor volume slice. The pencil-beam scanning proton plan shown in panel E uses a single right anterior oblique field painted twice

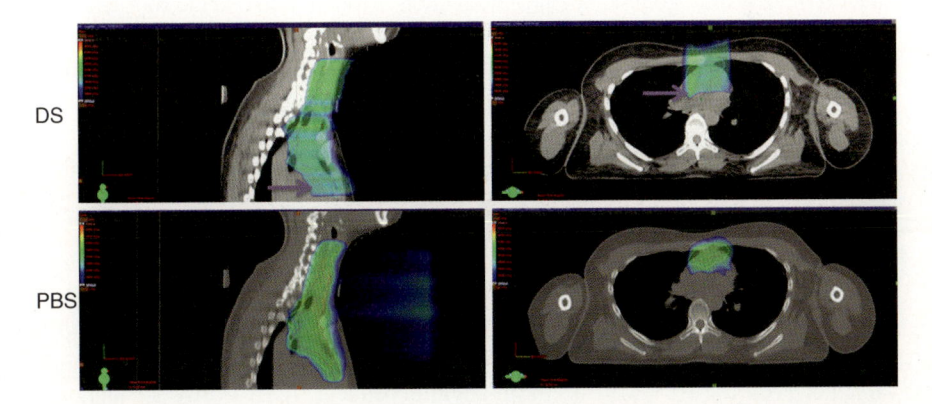

Fig. 23.4 A comparison of double-scatter and pencil-beam scanning proton therapy plans for a patient with Hodgkin lymphoma in the anterior mediastinum and neck. The *arrows* indicate the regions where the double-scatter plan has an increased volume treated to a medium dose (color wash set to 2700 cGy)

one–two fields, with fewer "moving parts," and without the need for multiple custom-built compensators and apertures.

23.4.2 Long/Wide Targets

PBS field sizes tend to be larger than DS field sizes, so longer and wider targets in the beam's eye view can be approached more simply. When treating a large target with DS, field matching may be required. Matched DS fields can be feathered as in photon therapy, but this requires the creation of new apertures for each field. Matched DS fields usually result in hot and/or cold streaks. With the relatively low prescription dose used in lymphoma, these hot spots may not be clinically consequential, but care must be taken to avoid putting a relatively "hot streak" into a critical serial OAR, like a coronary vessel or heart valve. By the same token, a "cold" area within a target volume is suboptimal. Mediastinal lymphoma volumes can be quite long and/or wide, depending on the pattern of disease. Although a classic mantle field is difficult to deliver with proton therapy, regardless of available technology, ISRT fields may be long and narrow, as seen in cases of HL with high neck involvement paired with lower mediastinal disease. In these cases, the larger PBS field sizes allow planning with a single isocenter and without the hot and cold areas that result from feathering. Alternatively, PBS field matching can be easily and safely implemented as described by Lin et al. [23].

23.4.3 Motion Management

Although DIBH can be used with PBS, the beam-on times for single-field treatments are generally longer than with DS, especially if many layers need to be painted. When using PBS with free breathing, target coverage can be degraded due to the interplay effect if motion orthogonal to the beam direction is roughly double the spot size [12, 24]. If the lateral target motion is small compared to the spot size used (approximately half of the spot size), however, repainting and the use of fractionation negate the interplay effect, resulting in adequate coverage. If motion orthogonal on the beam direction is excessive, then techniques to limit motion, such as a compression belt or DIBH, may be employed, or a larger spot size should be used. A larger spot size can be generated by enlarging the air gap between the range shifter and the patient surface.

23.4.4 Beam-Angle Selection

Depending on the location of the target with respect to OARs, optimal beam angles vary; however, the PTV will be beam-angle dependent. A PTV that accounts for uncertainty in the direction of the beam, or an optimization volume including the correction for range uncertainty, is thus created for each beam. For PBS, this is not automatically included in the beam properties in all commercial treatment planning systems. For example, the University of Pennsylvania uses a distal margin of the range × 3.5% + 1 mm and the proximal margin calculated from the difference of the range from the spread-out Bragg peak × 3.5% + 1 mm. The lateral margin is the usual margin for PTV expansion. Generally, beams are selected from one direction or another to maximize the lack of an exit dose. Because there is more skin sparing with PBS compared to DS, overlapping beams on skin is not a major concern. Beams that are angled away from each other slightly allow for improved robustness.

23.5 Future Developments

As PBS technology matures and intensity-modulated proton therapy can be more routinely and robustly deployed, projected dosimetric gains may further increase the benefits of PBS for malignancies requiring radiation treatment to the mediastinum.

References

1. Siegel R, Ma J, Zou Z, Jemal A. Cancer statistics, 2014. CA Cancer J Clin. 2014;64:9–29.
2. Ward E, DeSantis C, Robbins A, Kohler B, Jemal A. Childhood and adolescent cancer statistics, 2014. CA Cancer J Clin. 2014;64:83–103.
3. Goyal G, Silberstein PT, Armitage JO. Trends in use of radiation therapy for Hodgkin lymphoma from 2000 to 2012 on the basis of the National Cancer Data Base. Clin Lymphoma Myeloma Leuk. 2016;16:12–7.
4. Armitage JO, Weisenburger DD. New approach to classifying non-Hodgkin's lymphomas: clinical features of the major histologic subtypes. Non-Hodgkin's Lymphoma Classification Project. J Clin Oncol. 1998;16:2780–95.
5. Jackson MW, Rusthoven CG, Jones BL, Kamdar M, Rabinovitch R. Improved survival with radiation therapy in stage I–II primary mediastinal B cell lymphoma: a surveillance, epidemiology, and end results database analysis. Int J Radiat Oncol Biol Phys. 2016;94:126–32.
6. Inskip PD, Sigurdson AJ, Veiga L, Bhatti P, Ronckers C, Rajaraman P, et al. Radiation-related new primary solid cancers in the childhood cancer survivor study: comparative radiation dose response and modification of treatment effects. Int J Radiat Oncol Biol Phys. 2016;94:800–7.
7. Tseng YD, Cutter DJ, Plastaras JP, Parikh RR, Cahlon O, Chuong MD, et al. Evidence-based Review on the Use of Proton Therapy in Lymphoma From the Particle Therapy Cooperative Group (PTCOG) Lymphoma Subcommittee. Int J Radiat Oncol Biol Phys. 2017; [Epub ahead of print].
8. Chera BS, Rodriguez C, Morris CG, Louis D, Yeung D, Li Z, et al. Dosimetric comparison of three different involved nodal irradiation techniques for stage II Hodgkin's lymphoma patients: conventional radiotherapy, intensity-modulated radiotherapy, and three-dimensional proton radiotherapy. Int J Radiat Oncol Biol Phys. 2009;75:1173–80.
9. Maraldo MV, Brodin NP, Aznar MC, Vogelius IR, Munck af Rosenschold P, Petersen PM, et al. Estimated risk of cardiovascular disease and secondary cancers with modern highly conformal radiotherapy for early-stage mediastinal Hodgkin lymphoma. Ann Oncol. 2013;24(8):2113–8.
10. Hoppe BS, Flampouri S, Su Z, Latif N, Dang NH, Lynch J, et al. Effective dose reduction to cardiac structures using protons compared with 3DCRT and IMRT in mediastinal Hodgkin lymphoma. Int J Radiat Oncol Biol Phys. 2012;84:449–55.
11. Hoppe BS, Flampouri S, Su Z, Morris CG, Latif N, Dang NH, et al. Consolidative involved-node proton therapy for Stage IA-IIIB mediastinal Hodgkin lymphoma: preliminary dosimetric outcomes from a Phase II study. Int J Radiat Oncol Biol Phys. 2012;83:260–7.

12. Zeng C, Plastaras J, James P, Tochner Z, Hill-Kayser C, Hahn S, et al. Proton pencil beam scanning for mediastinal lymphoma: treatment planning and robustness assessment. Acta Oncol. 2016;55:1132–8.
13. Hoppe BS, Flampouri S, Zaiden R, Slayton W, Sandler E, Ozdemir S, et al. Involved-node proton therapy in combined modality therapy for Hodgkin lymphoma: results of a phase 2 study. Int J Radiat Oncol Biol Phys. 2014;89:1053–9.
14. Sachsman S, Flampouri S, Li Z, Lynch J, Mendenhall NP, Hoppe BS. Proton therapy in the management of non-Hodgkin lymphoma. Leuk Lymphoma. 2015;56:2608–12.
15. Hoppe BS, Hill-Kayser CE, Tseng YD, Flampouri S, Elmongy HM, Cahlon O, et al. Consolidative proton therapy after chemotherapy for patients with Hodgkin lymphoma. Ann Oncol. 2017; [Epub ahead of print].
16. Chung CS, Yock TI, Nelson K, Xu Y, Keating NL, Tarbell NJ. Incidence of second malignancies among patients treated with proton versus photon radiation. Int J Radiat Oncol Biol Phys. 2013;87:46–52.
17. Specht L, Yahalom J, Illidge T, Berthelsen AK, Constine LS, Eich HT, et al. Modern radiation therapy for Hodgkin lymphoma: field and dose guidelines from the international lymphoma radiation oncology group (ILROG). Int J Radiat Oncol Biol Phys. 2014;89:854–62.
18. Rechner LA, Maraldo MV, Vogelius IR, Zhu XR, Dabaja BS, Brodin NP, et al. Life years lost attributable to late effects after radiotherapy for early stage Hodgkin lymphoma: The impact of proton therapy and/or deep inspiration breath hold. Radiother Oncol. 2017; [Epub ahead of print].
19. Hoppe BS, Mendenhall NP, Louis D, Li Z, Flampouri S. Comparing Breath Hold and Free Breathing during Intensity-Modulated Radiation Therapy and Proton Therapy in Patients with Mediastinal Hodgkin Lymphoma. Int J Particle Ther. 2017;3:492-6.
20. Moyers MF, Miller DW, Bush DA, Slater JD. Methodologies and tools for proton beam design for lung tumors. Int J Radiat Oncol Biol Phys. 2001;49:1429–38.
21. Urie M, Goitein M, Wagner M. Compensating for heterogeneities in proton radiation therapy. Phys Med Biol. 1984;29:553–66.
22. van Nimwegen FA, Schaapveld M, Cutter DJ, Janus CP, Krol AD, Hauptmann M, et al. Radiation dose-response relationship for risk of coronary heart disease in survivors of Hodgkin lymphoma. J Clin Oncol. 2016;34:235–43.
23. Lin H, Ding X, Kirk M, Liu H, Zhai H, Hill-Kayser CE, et al. Supine craniospinal irradiation using a proton pencil beam scanning technique without match line changes for field junctions. Int J Radiat Oncol Biol Phys. 2014;90:71–8.
24. Zeng C, Plastaras JP, Tochner ZA, White BM, Hill-Kayser CE, Hahn SM, et al. Proton pencil beam scanning for mediastinal lymphoma: the impact of interplay between target motion and beam scanning. Phys Med Biol. 2015;60:3013–29.

Pediatric Tumors

24

Paul B. Romesser, Nelly Ju, Chin-Cheng Chen, Kevin Sine, Oren Cahlon, and Suzanne L. Wolden

Contents

24.1	Introduction	381
24.2	Craniospinal Irradiation	384
	24.2.1 Simulation, Setup, and Planning	384
24.3	Medulloblastoma	387
	24.3.1 Simulation, Setup, and Planning	387
24.4	Retinoblastoma	389
	24.4.1 Simulation, Setup, and Planning	390
24.5	Pediatric Sarcomas	391
24.6	Rhabdomyosarcoma	391
	24.6.1 Simulation, Setup, and Planning	391
24.7	Ewing Sarcoma	393
	24.7.1 Simulation, Setup, and Planning	393
References		395

24.1 Introduction

Pediatric malignancies are uncommon, representing less than 1% of all cancers diagnosed each year. Significant advances in the last 30 years have led to significantly improved survival rates of childhood cancers. Despite these advances, cancer remains the second leading cause of death in children after accidents.

P.B. Romesser • O. Cahlon • S.L. Wolden (✉)
Memorial Sloan Kettering Cancer Center, New York, NY, USA
e-mail: woldens@mskcc.org

N. Ju • C.-C. Chen • K. Sine
Procure Proton Therapy Center, Somerset, NJ, USA

© Springer International Publishing Switzerland 2018
N. Lee et al. (eds.), *Target Volume Delineation and Treatment Planning for Particle Therapy*, Practical Guides in Radiation Oncology,
https://doi.org/10.1007/978-3-319-42478-1_24

Of the approximate 12,000 new cases of pediatric cancer each year in the United States, about 3000 will require radiation therapy in the frontline management [1]. Given the improved outcomes, secondary to well-designed and well-conducted clinical trials, the pediatric community is committed to the design of new trials that not only increase cure rates but that also maximize health-related quality of life in the developing child and adult survivor [2].

A shift from two-dimensional to three-dimensional radiation plans and later to intensity-modulated radiation therapy (IMRT) resulted in increased conformality of treatment plans with a reduction of the treated volume. As organs at risk could be easily identified on computerized tomographic (CT) images, constraints were applied a priori to limit the dose of radiation delivered to the normal tissue while maximizing the dose to the target of interest; this is known as inverse planning. In order to achieve high conformality, the number of beams utilized increased. While inversely planned IMRT increased the conformality of the high-dose regions, it came at the expense of an expansion of the low-dose volume to achieve the optimal constraints.

Proton beam radiotherapy (PBRT) represents yet another stride forward in radiation therapy. The principle advantage of proton therapy over photon or X-ray therapy is the ability to reduce dose to normal tissues given inherent differences in the dose deposition of the proton as compared to the photon, discussed in Chaps. 1–3. Yet questions remain whether the dosimetric advantage of proton therapy actually improves clinical outcomes for patients. In addition, optimal management of uncertainties in proton therapy range, relative biological effectiveness (RBE), and linear energy transfer (LET) is still being studied, and long-term outcomes are needed to verify that the uncertainties do not negatively impact outcomes [3, 4].

Multiple modeling publications have suggested that proton therapy should result in reduced late toxicity by reducing normal tissue exposure. However, long-term clinical outcomes are now just being published, and outcomes are favorable but not conclusive for reduced toxicity, and larger studies with longer follow-up are needed.

Because of the perceived benefit of proton therapy for pediatric tumors, the number of pediatric patients receiving proton therapy annually is rising rapidly. The most commonly treated pediatric tumors with proton therapy are brain tumors and sarcomas.

In the United States, approximately 50% of pediatric proton therapy cases require daily anesthesia due to the young age of patients being treated. Proton patients tend to be younger because it is generally believed that younger patients are more susceptible to the harmful effects of radiation. As many proton centers are freestanding, a strong pediatric anesthesia program is necessary to ensure safe treatment for anesthesia patients.

The majority of pediatric proton patients require concurrent chemotherapy and strong collaboration with a local pediatric oncology program, and hospital is necessary for optimal treatment. A large portion of patients will require hospitalization during the course of RT, and it is important to avoid treatment interruptions.

It is unlikely that a randomized trial comparing protons versus photons for pediatric tumors will ever be conducted. The majority of publications to date have shown that the tumor control outcomes with protons versus photons are comparable and that proton therapy reduces the dose to surrounding organs at risk, but there is little clinical data on reduction in late effects, which is one of the primary cited indications for proton therapy.

To date, most pediatric proton publications have been single institution retrospective series and prospective phase 2 trials. The Children's Oncology Group (COG) now allows the use of proton therapy in most ongoing protocols, and future comparative analyses of photon vs proton patients is anticipated. Furthermore, the Pediatric Proton Consortium Registry is a multi-institutional initiative led by the Massachusetts General Hospital (MGH) to develop robust, prospective outcomes for pediatric proton therapy.

The majority of proton publications to date have been with passively scattered proton therapy. Pencil-beam scanning (PBS) is emerging as the next generation of proton therapy allowing inversely planning with intensity- and energy-modulated proton fields, known as the intensity-modulated proton therapy (IMPT). This technology actively delivers radiation dose on a layer by layer basis, dwelling at specific locations for an amount of time coincident with the planned delivery of dose to provide conformal treatment plans. This represents a significant technological advance over passively scattered or uniform scanning, which are employed in three-dimensional proton planning. As the number of proton centers with PBS in the United States is increasing, it is expected that this will become the most commonly used technique for pediatric proton therapy delivery.

For most pediatric tumors treated with pencil-beam scanning, single-field uniform dose (SFUD) is used mostly for treatment planning to have more robustness. However, IMPT known also as multifield optimization (MFO) is helpful for select spinal tumors for which patch and through fields might have been used in the past, and dose conformality around a critical structure is needed such as the brainstem or spinal cord. MFO does produce improved high-dose conformality around a critical structure but can result in less robust plans; these plans are exquisitely sensitive to motion and set up error and need to be planned and delivered carefully.

PBS also allows for more rapid treatment delivery due to generous setup uncertainties with slow-gradient match. PBS has a larger field size than other proton delivery systems and does not require use of apertures and compensators which slowdown treatment delivery. In addition, omission of compensators and apertures from the beam path reduces neutron contamination, which can be helpful in pediatric patients. For example, at our center a uniform-scanning anesthesia case would typically require 40 min in the treatment room. With PBS, this can be reduced to about 25 min.

The potential disadvantage of PBS is the dependence of spot size. With larger spot sizes, the penumbra of PBS around the field edge could be reduced for shallow tumors compared to the use of apertures in passive scatter (PS) and uniform scanning (US). Today, most treatment planning systems are not capable of using PBS with apertures. It is hoped that most of the commercially available treatment planning systems will be able to accommodate PBS with apertures in the near future.

24.2 Craniospinal Irradiation

Craniospinal irradiation (CSI) is an important radiation technique that is used in the treatment of several pediatric central nervous system malignancies, which require coverage of the entire craniospinal axis given a substantial risk of subarachnoid spread.

Acute side effects of CSI include skin redness/irritation, hair loss, fatigue, nausea, vomiting, decreased appetite, and bone marrow suppression. Late effects include growth retardation, hypothyroidism, hypopituitarism, accelerated heart disease, pulmonary complications, bowel complications, infertility, hearing loss, and radiation-induced secondary malignancies. Efforts to reduce these toxicities have been made by reducing the CSI dose, which is dependent on the primary tumor histology and extent of disease (i.e., microscopic versus gross).

Because of the ability of protons to deposit the majority of their dose within the Bragg peak with little to no exit dose, proton therapy has gained significant interest as a treatment modality for CSI. MD Anderson has compared the dosimetry of proton and photon CSI plans and reported that proton-based CSI provides more homogenous target coverage and improved normal tissue sparing [5]. Many studies have evaluated proton versus photon-based CSI and have a significant reduction in the predictive risk of ototoxicity, pneumonitis, cardiac failure, xerostomia, and hypothyroidism [6].

Both proton and photon CSI will impact axial and cranial growth patterns because the dose to growing bones in the skull and spine is similar. Similarly, differences in neurocognitive effects from the craniospinal portion of treatment would not be expected as by definition the entire brain would receive the same dose with protons and photons, and it is the CSI portion that contributes most to neurocognitive dysfunction.

The major advantages of proton, as compared to photon, CSI plans are seen in the boost fields allowing less normal brain to be treated and lower doses to the cochlea and in the spine fields with decreased dose to the thyroid, esophagus, heart, lungs, and abdominopelvic organs. Given this significant normal tissue-sparing, proton-based CSI has been theorized to decrease the risk of neurocognitive impairment, heart disease, thyroid disease, and secondary malignancies [7–11]. That being said, studies of long-term survivors treated with CSI have demonstrated that the most common secondary malignancies have been brain tumors (high-grade gliomas and meningiomas) as well as spinal sarcomas, none of which are expected to decrease with proton-based CSI as the brain and spine (i.e., the target) are treated to the same dose with both proton and photon-based therapies [2]. Nonetheless based on the ALARA (as low as reasonable achievable) principle, any modality to reduce normal tissue dose may further improve the therapeutic ratio, which is of paramount importance in the developing child [2].

24.2.1 Simulation, Setup, and Planning

CSI requires careful examination of patient setup at simulation and daily treatments. The use of sedation should be considered for patient comfort and to assist with accurate setup depending on patient's age and cognitive development [6].

CSI can be performed in either the supine or prone position, with the supine position preferred as it is more comfortable and reproducible and allows a uniform source-to-skin difference [12].

Immobilization is critical for setup reproducibility. An Aquaplast™ facemask is preferable given the need to carefully immobilize the head and to match the upper spinal and cranial fields. Additional immobilization of the body is preferred, using either Vac-loc™ or Alpha Cradle™ as the majority of patients require an additional matched field in the spine to cover the entire length of the spinal axis.

The CTV_{CSI} should include the entire brain and spinal canal encompassed by the dura matter. Careful attention should be given to the area of the cribriform plate, which commonly extends more caudally and anteriorly in pediatric patients as compared to adults. The inferior border of the CTV_{CSI} should include the cauda equina as defined by spine MR most commonly to the level of the S3 vertebral body.

In growth immature patients, an additional normal tissue target volume (NTTV) should be added to CTV_{CSI} to include the majority of the vertebral bodies as asymmetric irradiation might increase the risk of scoliosis or kyphosis. In growth mature patients, the entire brain and thecal sac alone are treated, allowing for more vertebral body and lung sparing. Figure 24.1 shows the comparison of dose distribution of growth immature and mature CSI patients. Both plans are for a prescription of 36 Gy(RBE).

Clinical target volumes should be expanded according to institutional standard, typically by 3–5 mm, to create a planning target volume (PTV) employed for recording and reporting purposes per ICRU 78.

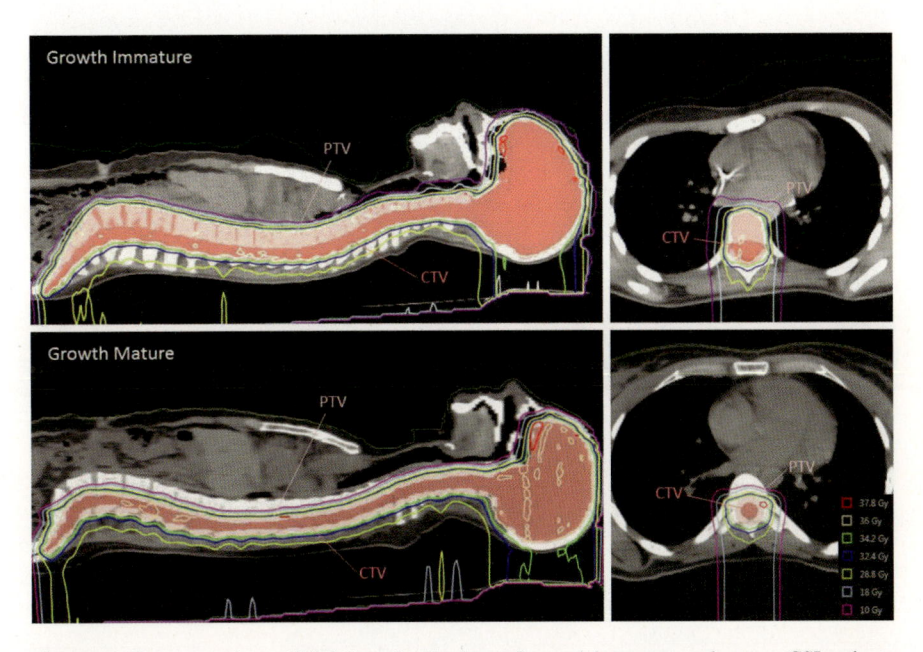

Fig. 24.1 The comparison of PBS dose distributions of growth immature and mature CSI patients

Reproducibility of patient setup should be maximized to minimize dosimetric uncertainties ideally with daily orthogonal X-ray, if available, in order to confirm setup accuracy [6].

With both IMPT and 3D–PBRT, matched fields are required to cover the cranial field and spine field. Often the spine field requires further division secondary to field size limitations. Most commonly two–three matched fields are utilized. Match line feathering should be utilized with both US and PS to reduce hot or cold spots at the match line level; however, with PBS, a dose gradient can be generated to improve homogeneity between matched fields and avoiding the need for match line feathering.

Delivery of CSI with non-PBS techniques requires multiple fields due to a limited field size and feathering of match lines to avoid hot and cold spots. This is labor intensive from both a treatment planning perspective and delivery with multiple plans needed for each respective match line and delivery of multiple fields each day for a lengthy treatment delivery time. With PBS, less fields are needed allowing for a faster delivery, and the slow-gradient matched lines do not require feathering as it is made homogenous within the plan. Figure 24.2 show the comparisons of match lines of spinal fields delivered by non-PBS (uniform scanning) and PBS techniques.

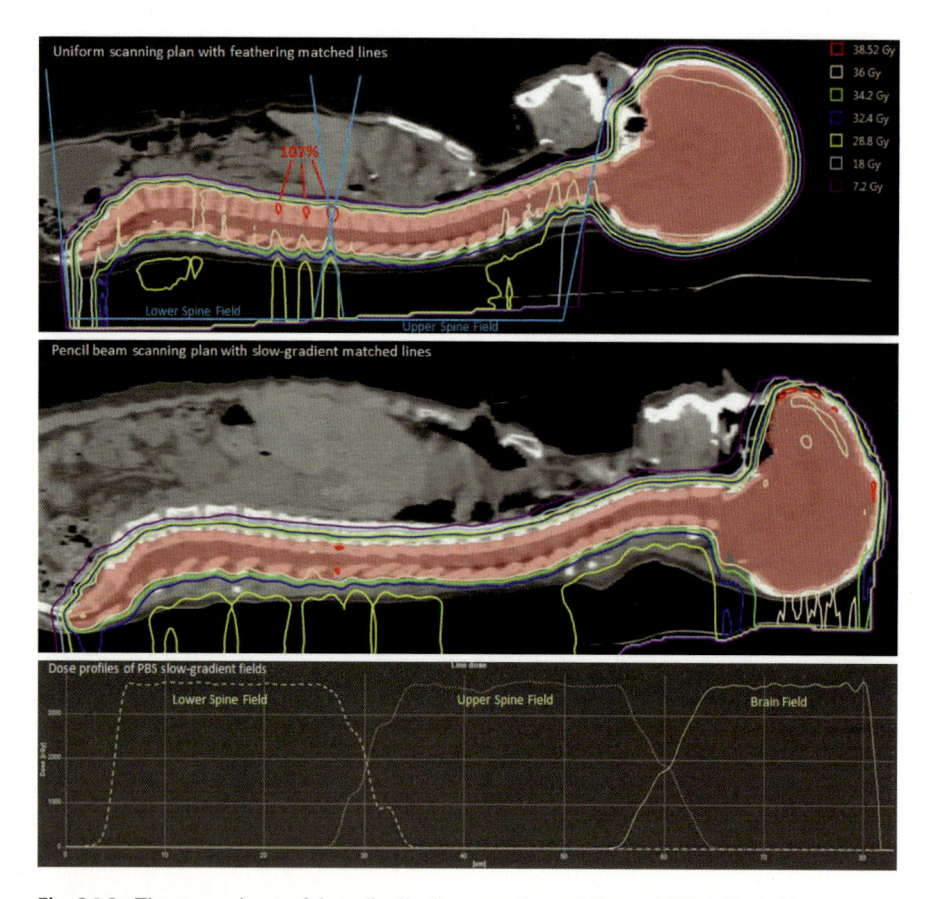

Fig. 24.2 The comparisons of dose distribution around match lines of CSI delivered by non-PBS (uniform scan) and PBS techniques

Both plans are for a prescription of 36 Gy(RBE). Around 107% dose hot spot around the matched lines was found in the uniform-scanning plan.

CSI planning should ensure coverage of the brain and thecal sac by at least the 95% isodose line and good anterior skull-based coverage including the cribriform plate. The spine should be covered with a homogenous dose without excessive hot or cold spots (i.e., >95% but less than 105% of the prescribed dose), and the thyroid, esophagus, heart, and abdominal organs should receive 5% or less of the prescribed dose [13]. Over- and under-range plans should be evaluated with relevant range uncertainties as determined by each center.

24.3 Medulloblastoma

Medulloblastoma is the most common malignant CNS tumor in children. Medulloblastoma arises in the posterior fossa and has a high propensity for leptomeningeal dissemination.

Standard therapy for patients over the age of 3 includes maximal safe surgical resection followed by craniospinal irradiation and chemotherapy.

Treatment regimens are determined by risk category which depends on patient age, extent of surgical resection, presence or absence of CNS dissemination, and histological characteristics [14].

CSI dose depends on risk category with current recommendations of 23.4 Gy(RBE) for standard-risk and 36 Gy(RBE) for high-risk disease.

A boost to a total dose of 54–55.8 Gy(RBE) to the tumor bed is standard of care for both standard- and high- risk groups.

A recent case-matched multi-institutional cohort study compared the clinical outcomes of patients with standard-risk medulloblastoma treated with modern proton and photon therapy and demonstrated no differences in patterns of failure, recurrence-free survival, or overall survival [15].

Additional studies have reported that proton beam radiotherapy results in greater cochlea, pituitary, hypothalamus, parotid, and temporal lobe sparing as compared to photon therapy [16, 17].

Proton beam therapy has been reported to theoretically reduce the risk for secondary malignancies in medulloblastoma patients by a factor of 8–15 when compared to photon-based treatment including intensity-modulated radiation therapy (IMRT) [18].

Unless contraindicated contrast-enhanced MR brain in the pre- and postsurgical setting should be obtained. In addition, given the high propensity for leptomeningeal dissemination, a contrast-enhanced MR spine and lumbar puncture with cerebrospinal fluid cytology should be performed to rule out macroscopic and microscopic tumor dissemination.

24.3.1 Simulation, Setup, and Planning

Simulation parameters and treatment setup are described in the craniospinal section above. In general, treatment planning should start with CSI to sterilize the CSF followed by treatment of the higher-dose boost fields.

Pre- and postoperative contrast-enhanced MR brain scans should be fused, preferably with deformable registration, with the simulation CT scan. If there was radiographic evidence of leptomeningeal dissemination on the MR spine, then fusion is warranted to help aid in contouring. As the patient was likely in different positions on the MR and CT simulation, carefully attention should be paid to verify accuracy on the planning CT scan.

At our institution, we have had excellent success with treating boosting the tumor bed alone [19]. This was confirmed in a recent Children's Oncology Group Study that found that tumor bed boost was as effective as a whole posterior fossa boost. The CTV_{brain_boost} should include the entire GTV, defined as any residual disease in the brain and the postoperative tumor bed, with a 1–1.5 cm margin though respecting anatomic barriers such as bone and tentorium.

Clinical target volumes should be expanded according to institutional standard, typically by 3–5 mm, to create a planning target volume (PTV) employed for recording and reporting purposes per ICRU 78.

While both IMPT and 3D–PBRT can be utilized for the tumor bed boost, published reports to date have been obtained primarily with 3D–PBRT. This technique typically employs three fields (posterior obliques and PA or laterals and PA with the PA usually being the shared beam). IMPT might have a small benefit in terms of added conformality and reduced skin dose, but this depends on the size of the spot used. Publications from MGH have shown that for larger spot sizes, apertures are necessary to produce similar dose distributions as with PS and apertures.

For the boost, with three posteriorly angled portals, special care must be taken to avoid end of range issues within the brainstem. This can be done several different ways: (1) evaluate end of range structures, (2) range feathering, or (3) use of lateral beams (and lateral penumbra) in the brainstem rather than distal edge. Figure 24.3 shows the dose distribution of the posterior fossa tumor bed boost for a prescription of 54 Gy(RBE).

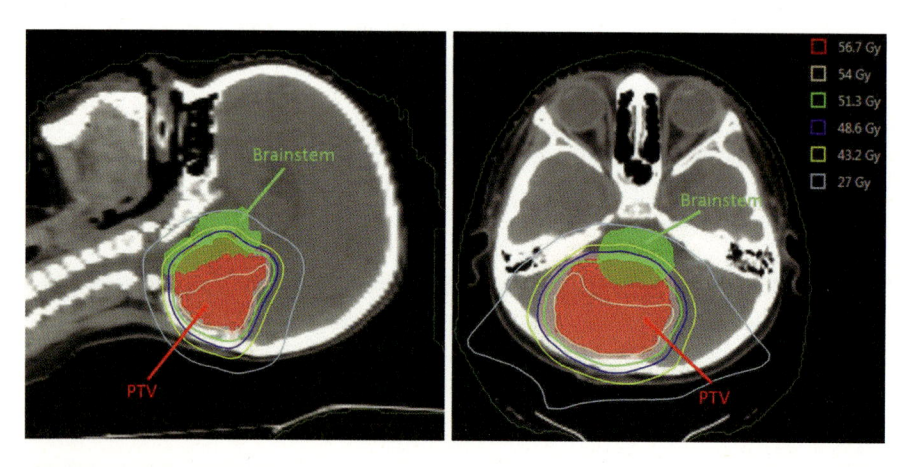

Fig. 24.3 The dose distribution of the posterior fossa tumor bed boost for a prescription of 54 Gy (RBE)

Recent preclinical data suggests that RBE for protons might be higher than 1.1 in some tissues and at some points along the beam path, especially the distal edge of the Bragg peak. The higher RBE of protons at the distal edge might lead to increased brainstem toxicity for patients being treated to the posterior fossa, such as medulloblastoma since beams are often entering posteriorly and ending near the brainstem. Published reports to date have not shown an increase in brainstem toxicity compared to historical controls with photons. However, higher rates of post-RT MRI changes with protons have been reported as compared to photons.

Standard brainstem constraints from adult guidelines have historically been used for pediatric tumors. Recently, pediatric specific brainstem constraints have been identified. Based on the UFPTI data, two additional brainstem constraints are now used routinely in the pediatric proton community: D50 < 52.4 Gy (RBE) and Dmax <60 Gy (RBE) [20].

24.4 Retinoblastoma

Retinoblastoma (RB) is the most common primary ocular malignancy in children.

Retinoblastoma can result from a new or inherited germline mutation of the RB1 tumor suppressor gene, which is an important regulator of the G1-S cell cycle checkpoint. Tumorigenesis requires loss of heterozygosity with a second event leading to inactivation of the second RB1 allele. Patients with a germline mutation in one allele typically present at a very young age (1 year) with multiple tumors in both eyes. Whereas patients without a germline mutation present a little later (3 years) most commonly with a single tumor.

Standard therapy includes multiple curative options including laser therapy, photocoagulation, cryotherapy, ophthalmic artery chemosurgery, intravitreal chemotherapy, plaque brachytherapy, external beam radiation therapy, and enucleation.

While external beam radiotherapy was the preferred treatment option for many years, the use of EBRT has significantly declined because of the morbidity of radiation therapy including a high rate of secondary malignancies, especially in patients with a germline mutation [21].

As treatment outcomes have steadily improved over time, the leading cause of death among patients with hereditary retinoblastoma is second malignancy [22].

In patients with locally advanced radiation, therapy is often still employed in the treatment management, as these tumors are highly responsive to radiotherapy. Given the predisposition for second malignancy development, conformal radiation modalities, such as PBRT, have been favored when radiation therapy is indicated. Proton-based treatment results in a significant reduction in the integral dose and the volume of nontarget tissue receiving low-dose radiation as compared to photon-based radiation modalities [23].

A recent report comparing retinoblastoma patients treated with proton therapy at the Massachusetts General Hospital and those treated with photon therapy at Boston Children's Hospital between 1986 and 2011 reported that PBRT significantly lowered the risk of a radiation induced malignancy in this population [22].

In general we only recommend radiation therapy for patients without a germline mutation or for patients with a germline mutation who have exhausted other treatment options or who have suffered a relapse.

24.4.1 Simulation, Setup, and Planning

Given the average age of these patients, anesthesia is generally recommended for simulation and treatment.

Immobilization with a three-point mask with an oral opening for airway management is recommended.

Reproducibility of patient setup should be maximized ideally with nonionizing radiation image guidance modalities when available, such as optical surface tracking, to help shrink volumetric expansions in order to limit unnecessary irradiation of normal tissues at risk. If non-radiation modalities are unavailable, daily orthogonal X-ray image guidance can suffice. It is preferable to treat patients on a treatment couch with 6-degrees of freedom (vertical, longitudinal, lateral, pitch, roll, and yaw) to help ensure efficient and accurate patient setup.

A pretreatment contrast-enhanced MR orbit should be fused, preferably with deformable registration, with the simulation CT scan to aid in tumor delineation.

At our center, we have treated these in the past with US. PBS can also be used and might lower the skin dose compared to other techniques. For upfront RB cases, a lateral-anterior oblique beam is typically best as shown in Fig. 24.4, but for more advanced/recurrent disease after exenteration, 2–3 beams are usually used (lateral and anterior oblique).

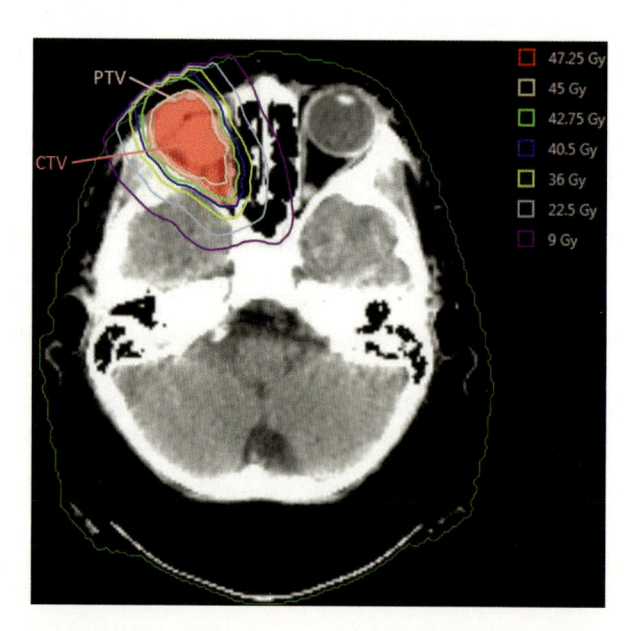

Fig. 24.4 The dose distribution of a single right-anterior oblique PBS field for prescribed 45 Gy (RBE) orbital retinoblastoma relapse following enucleation

24.5 Pediatric Sarcomas

Pediatric sarcomas are an uncommon and diverse group of diagnoses. Ewing sarcoma, rhabdomyosarcoma, and non-rhabdomyosarcoma are the most common sarcomas that require radiation in the frontline management.

Presentation patterns differ since these sarcomas can involve nearly every part of the body. Many rhabdomyosarcomas occur in the head and neck or genitourinary tract, while Ewing sarcomas are common in the extremities and axial skeleton.

24.6 Rhabdomyosarcoma

Rhabdomyosarcoma (RMS) is the most common pediatric soft tissue sarcoma arising from the malignant mesenchyme. RMS has a bimodal incidence with ~2/3 of cases diagnosed in children 6 years of age and younger and ~1/3 diagnosed in adolescents. The more favorable embryonal subtype is more common in younger children, whereas the more aggressive alveolar subtype is more common in adolescents.

Treatment regimens are determined by risk category (low-, intermediate-, and high-risk groups), which depends on site of origin, histology, lymph node involvement, metastatic spread, and extent of surgical resection [14]. Patients with gross residual or unresectable disease (Group III) are treated to 50.4 Gy. Elective nodal irradiation is not commonly practiced unless there is gross or microscopic disease that merits irradiation. All of these patients are treated with intensive chemotherapy regimens.

As treatment outcomes are good in patients with localized disease treated with combined-modality therapy with greater than 70% of patients surviving more than 5 years after diagnosis, there is significant interest in developing effective albeit less toxic treatment options for these patients.

In a recent report on patients treated with PBRT in a prospective phase II protocol, there was no difference in disease control outcomes and a favorable toxicity profile as compared to historical IMRT reports [24].

Dosimetric comparisons of PBRT and IMRT from phase 2 prospective MGH/MDA trial for RMS patients demonstrated that PBRT results in a lower integral dose and improved normal tissue sparing in 26 of 30 organs at risk that were evaluated [25, 26]. Based on this, it would be expected to result in reduced late effects. However, it is important to remember that the facial asymmetry and disfigurement associated with lateralized PM-RMS is not expected to be reduced with protons as the facial bones are usually included in the target volume.

24.6.1 Simulation, Setup, and Planning

The use of sedation should be considered for patient comfort and to assist with accurate setup depending on patient's age and cognitive development.

Immobilization is critical for setup reproducibility. For parameningeal RMS a three-point mask is recommended, except in the setting of nodal irradiation for which a five-point mask is preferred.

Unless contraindicated, contrast-enhanced MRI, CT, and PET scans in the pre-chemotherapy and post-chemotherapy setting should be obtained to help evaluate for intracranial extension, perineural spread, tumor response to chemotherapy, and surgical-resection status. Fusion with the planning CT simulation should be performed, preferably with deformable registration, to help with tumor demarcation.

The GTV_{36Gy} should include all gross and suspected microscopic tumor at the time of diagnosis (pre-chemotherapy) as well as any lymph nodes that may be involved.

The CTV_{36Gy} consists of the GTV_{36Gy} plus a 1 cm margin.

The $GTV_{50.4Gy}$ should include any residual gross disease or suspicious abnormality seen on the post-chemotherapy MRI, CT, and/or PET scans at the primary tumor site and lymph nodes (if initially involved). This will allow for potential field reduction based upon response to induction chemotherapy. In the rare case of a complete radiographic response, then no radiotherapy beyond 36 Gy is warranted.

The $CTV_{50.4Gy}$ consists of a 1 cm expansion from the $GTV_{50.4Gy}$.

Clinical target volumes should be expanded according to institutional standard, typically by 3–5 mm, to create a planning target volume (PTV) employed for recording and reporting purposes per ICRU 78.

For parameningeal-RMS cases, the goal is to spare the oral cavity, lens, retina, brainstem, temporal lobes, pituitary, hypothalamus, lacrimal gland, parotid glands, and spinal cord. In many cases, comparable normal tissue sparing may be achieved with passive- or uniform-scanned proton beams or with PBS. PBS provides more conformal plans with greater control over the proximal end of the beam and an additive advantage of skin sparing. Typically 2–4 field plans have been used to optimize target coverage and OAR sparing. We have typically favored lateral and posterior oblique beams. Anteriorly angled beams often result in unwanted orbital exposure. We have typically tried to avoid superior oblique and vertex beams in young patients to avoid unwanted brain exposure. For patients with tumors near the paranasal sinuses, special consideration should be given to try to avoid anteriorly angled beams traversing through the sinuses when possible. When such beams are needed, verification scans should be done during RT to ensure there has not been filling, which could lead to under dosing of the tumor. Figure 24.5 shows the dose distribution for a parameningeal RMS using uniform-scanning fields with apertures for a prescription of 50.4 Gy (RBE).

Tumor regression can alter dosimetry with proton therapy and must be monitored. While now rarely indicated, for patients undergoing early proton therapy (weeks 0–4), there can be significant regression and verification scans are needed to check for changes accordingly. For these cases, we typically perform a verification scan in week 3 to allow time for a plan modification if needed. For definitive parameningeal-RMS cases treated at week 13 and beyond, the majority of tumor regression has occurred during chemotherapy, and adaptive planning is less likely to be needed.

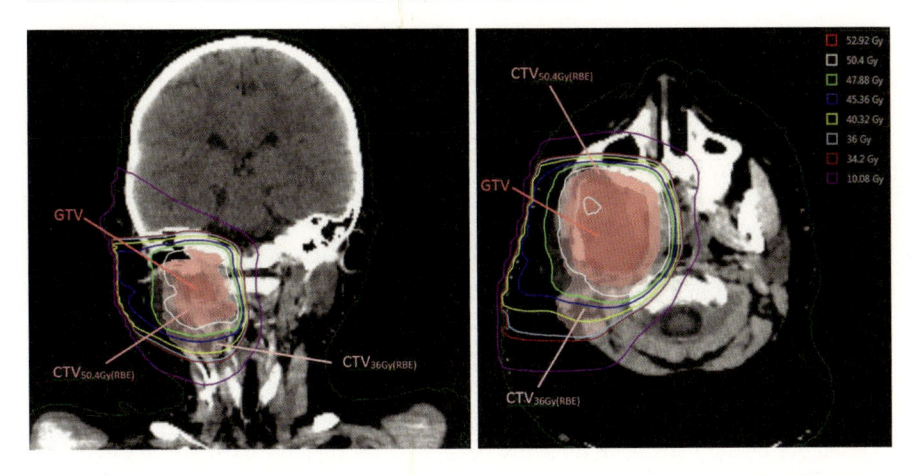

Fig. 24.5 The dose distribution of a parameningeal RMS using uniform-scanning fields with apertures for a prescription of 50.4 Gy (RBE)

24.7 Ewing Sarcoma

Ewing sarcoma is the second most common bone tumor in children but can also arise in soft tissues. It most commonly affects children in the second decade. Ewing sarcoma is highly radiosensitive and may arise from a variety of locations, most commonly from the long bones of the appendicular skeleton or pelvis. Patients with large pelvic/sacral tumors are often managed with definitive radiation. These are excellent cases for proton therapy. Tumors arising in the appendicular skeleton are often managed with surgery and less likely to benefit from proton therapy. Paraspinal tumors can also benefit from proton therapy.

Standard therapy for patients with non-metastatic disease includes induction chemotherapy followed by surgery and/or radiation therapy and adjuvant chemotherapy.

In patients with gross residual or unresectable disease, radiation therapy to 55.8 Gy is recommended, whereas 50.4Gy is recommended for microscopic positive margins postsurgical excision.

Dosimetric studies of various Ewing sarcoma tumor sites have noted that PBRT provides better normal tissue sparing and less integrative dose [1, 27, 28]. Clinical outcomes of Ewing sarcoma patients treated with proton therapy have been excellent and comparable to photon-based treatment plans [29].

24.7.1 Simulation, Setup, and Planning

Given the older age of these patients, sedation is often not indicated.

Unless contraindicated contrast-enhanced MRI of the primary tumor site as well as a PET/CT scan should be obtained to help chemotherapeutic response and extent of surgical-resection status. Fusion with the planning CT simulation should be performed, preferably with deformable registration, to help with tumor demarcation.

The GTV_{45Gy} should include all initial gross disease based on all pre-chemotherapy (and preoperative) scans. The CTV_{45Gy} consists of a 1 cm expansion from the GTV_{45Gy}.

The $GTV_{55.8Gy}$ consists of residual post-chemotherapy soft tissue tumor as well as PRE-chemotherapy abnormalities in bone. The $CTV_{55.8Gy}$ should be a 1 cm expansion from the $GTV_{55.8Gy}$.

If the patient is status postsurgical resection with microscopic margins, the $CTV_{50.4Gy}$ should include the postoperative bed with a 1 cm expansion. If there is any gross residual disease, these should be included in the $GTV_{55.8}$ as noted above.

Clinical target volumes should be expanded according to institutional standard, typically by 3–5 mm, to create a planning target volume (PTV) employed for recording and reporting purposes per ICRU 78.

The 2–4 beam plans have typically been used for patients with pelvic sarcomas. For well-lateralized pelvic tumors, lateral beams are usually heavily weighted with some contribution of anterior and/or posterior beams. Anterior beams traversing through bowel should be used with caution due to day-to-day variations in bowel gas filling. This can lead to under-dosing of the target if not accounted for. We typically generate our compensators with bowel override to ensure coverage. This is a conservative approach that ensures target coverage with slight increase in OAR exposure. For sacral tumors as shown in Fig. 24.6, we usually use primarily

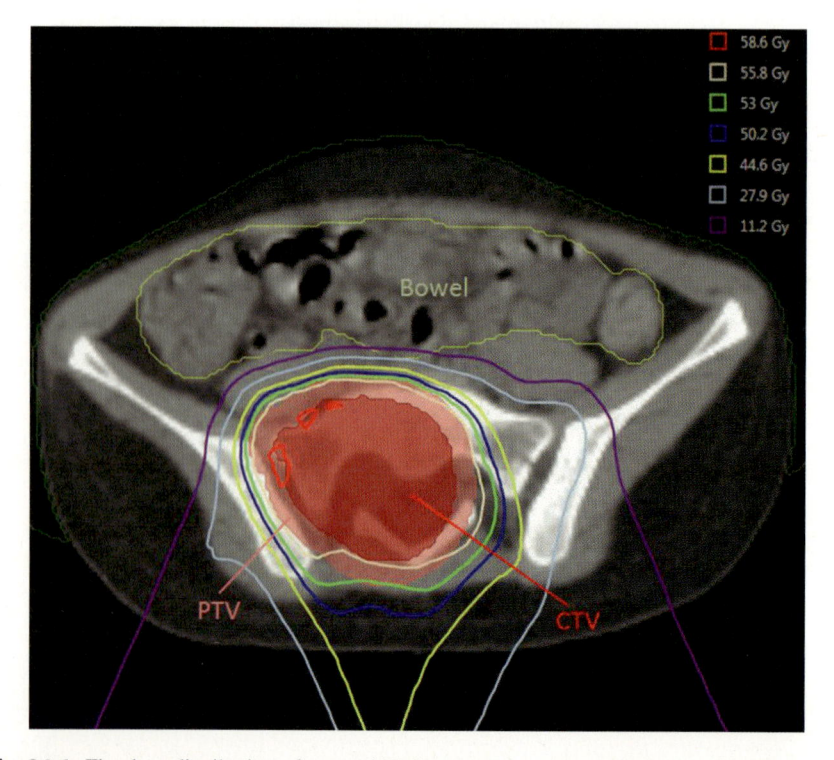

Fig. 24.6 The dose distribution of a sacral Ewing sarcoma using uniform-scanning fields with apertures for a prescription of 55.8 Gy (RBE)

posterior beams to minimize the bowel exposure. However, with US/PS, the skin dose can be high in some areas and can lead to brisk skin reaction. A lateral beam using the aperture edge to block the skin can be used in cases where the PTV does not touch the skin. Alternatively, PBS can be used for skin sparing when available.

References

1. Merchant TE. Clinical controversies: proton therapy for pediatric tumors. Semin Radiat Oncol. 2013;23:97–108.
2. Wolden SL. Protons for craniospinal radiation: are clinical data important? Int J Radiat Oncol Biol Phys. 2013;87:231–2.
3. Merchant TE, Farr JB. Proton beam therapy: a fad or a new standard of care. Curr Opin Pediatr. 2014;26:3–8.
4. Cuaron JJ, Chang C, Lovelock M, et al. Exponential increase in relative biological effectiveness along distal edge of a proton Bragg peak as measured by deoxyribonucleic acid double-strand breaks. Int J Radiat Oncol Biol Phys. 2016;95:62–9.
5. Howell RM, Giebeler A, Koontz-Raisig W, et al. Comparison of therapeutic dosimetric data from passively scattered proton and photon craniospinal irradiations for medulloblastoma. Radiat Oncol. 2012;7:116.
6. Mahajan A. Proton craniospinal radiation therapy: rationale and clinical evidence. Int J Particle Ther. 2014;1:399–407.
7. Zhang R, Howell RM, Giebeler A, Taddei PJ, Mahajan A, Newhauser WD. Comparison of risk of radiogenic second cancer following photon and proton craniospinal irradiation for a pediatric medulloblastoma patient. Phys Med Biol. 2013;58:807–23.
8. Zhang R, Howell RM, Homann K, et al. Predicted risks of radiogenic cardiac toxicity in two pediatric patients undergoing photon or proton radiotherapy. Radiat Oncol. 2013;8:184.
9. Zhang R, Howell RM, Taddei PJ, Giebeler A, Mahajan A, Newhauser WD. A comparative study on the risks of radiogenic second cancers and cardiac mortality in a set of pediatric medulloblastoma patients treated with photon or proton craniospinal irradiation. Radiother Oncol. 2014;113:84–8.
10. Merchant TE, Hua CH, Shukla H, Ying X, Nill S, Oelfke U. Proton versus photon radiotherapy for common pediatric brain tumors: comparison of models of dose characteristics and their relationship to cognitive function. Pediatr Blood Cancer. 2008;51:110–7.
11. Pulsifer MB, Sethi RV, Kuhlthau KA, MacDonald SM, Tarbell NJ, Yock TI. Early cognitive outcomes following proton radiation in pediatric patients with brain and central nervous system tumors. Int J Radiat Oncol Biol Phys. 2015;93:400–7.
12. Singhal M, Vincent A, Simoneaux V, Johnstone PA, Buchsbaum JC. Overcoming the learning curve in supine pediatric proton craniospinal irradiation. J Am Coll Radiol. 2012;9:285–7.
13. Giebeler A, Newhauser WD, Amos RA, Mahajan A, Homann K, Howell RM. Standardized treatment planning methodology for passively scattered proton craniospinal irradiation. Radiat Oncol. 2013;8:32.
14. Cotter SE, McBride SM, Yock TI. Proton radiotherapy for solid tumors of childhood. Technol Cancer Res Treat. 2012;11:267–78.
15. Eaton BR, Esiashvili N, Kim S, et al. Clinical outcomes among children with standard-risk medulloblastoma treated with proton and photon radiation therapy: a comparison of disease control and overall survival. Int J Radiat Oncol Biol Phys. 2016;94:133–8.
16. St Clair WH, Adams JA, Bues M, et al. Advantage of protons compared to conventional X-ray or IMRT in the treatment of a pediatric patient with medulloblastoma. Int J Radiat Oncol Biol Phys. 2004;58:727–34.
17. Lin R, Hug EB, Schaefer RA, Miller DW, Slater JM, Slater JD. Conformal proton radiation therapy of the posterior fossa: a study comparing protons with three-dimensional planned photons in limiting dose to auditory structures. Int J Radiat Oncol Biol Phys. 2000;48:1219–26.

18. Miralbell R, Lomax A, Cella L, Schneider U. Potential reduction of the incidence of radiation-induced second cancers by using proton beams in the treatment of pediatric tumors. Int J Radiat Oncol Biol Phys. 2002;54:824–9.
19. Wolden SL, Dunkel IJ, Souweidane MM, et al. Patterns of failure using a conformal radiation therapy tumor bed boost for medulloblastoma. J Clin Oncol. 2003;21:3079–83.
20. Indelicato DJ, Flampouri S, Rotondo RL, et al. Incidence and dosimetric parameters of pediatric brainstem toxicity following proton therapy. Acta Oncol. 2014;53:1298–304.
21. Mouw KW, Sethi RV, Yeap BY, et al. Proton radiation therapy for the treatment of retinoblastoma. Int J Radiat Oncol Biol Phys. 2014;90:863–9.
22. Sethi RV, Shih HA, Yeap BY, et al. Second nonocular tumors among survivors of retinoblastoma treated with contemporary photon and proton radiotherapy. Cancer. 2014;120:126–33.
23. Krengli M, Hug EB, Adams JA, Smith AR, Tarbell NJ, Munzenrider JE. Proton radiation therapy for retinoblastoma: comparison of various intraocular tumor locations and beam arrangements. Int J Radiat Oncol Biol Phys. 2005;61:583–93.
24. Ladra MM, Szymonifka JD, Mahajan A, et al. Preliminary results of a phase II trial of proton radiotherapy for pediatric rhabdomyosarcoma. J Clin Oncol. 2014;32:3762–70.
25. Ladra MM, Edgington SK, Mahajan A, et al. A dosimetric comparison of proton and intensity modulated radiation therapy in pediatric rhabdomyosarcoma patients enrolled on a prospective phase II proton study. Radiother Oncol. 2014;113:77–83.
26. Kozak KR, Adams J, Krejcarek SJ, Tarbell NJ, Yock TI. A dosimetric comparison of proton and intensity-modulated photon radiotherapy for pediatric parameningeal rhabdomyosarcomas. Int J Radiat Oncol Biol Phys. 2009;74:179–86.
27. Lee CT, Bilton SD, Famiglietti RM, et al. Treatment planning with protons for pediatric retinoblastoma, medulloblastoma, and pelvic sarcoma: how do protons compare with other conformal techniques? Int J Radiat Oncol Biol Phys. 2005;63:362–72.
28. Fogliata A, Yartsev S, Nicolini G, et al. On the performances of intensity modulated protons, RapidArc and helical tomotherapy for selected paediatric cases. Radiat Oncol. 2009;4:2.
29. Rombi B, DeLaney TF, MacDonald SM, et al. Proton radiotherapy for pediatric Ewing's sarcoma: initial clinical outcomes. Int J Radiat Oncol Biol Phys. 2012;82:1142–8.